THE ESSENTIAL LIFE

A SIMPLE GUIDE TO LIVING THE WELLNESS LIFESTYLE

THANK YOU TO THE MANY CONTRIBUTORS FOR THEIR COLLECTIVE GENIUS IN BRINGING THIS WORK TOGETHER AND SHARING A VISION OF HOW PLANTS AND NATURAL REMEDIES BRING NEW LEVELS OF WELLNESS AND POWERFULLY IMPACT OUR LIVES.

2nd EDITION

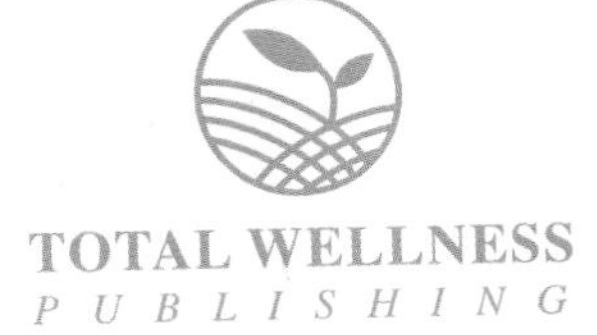

ISBN 9 781495 146442

TABLE OF CONTENTS

SECTION 1
introduction

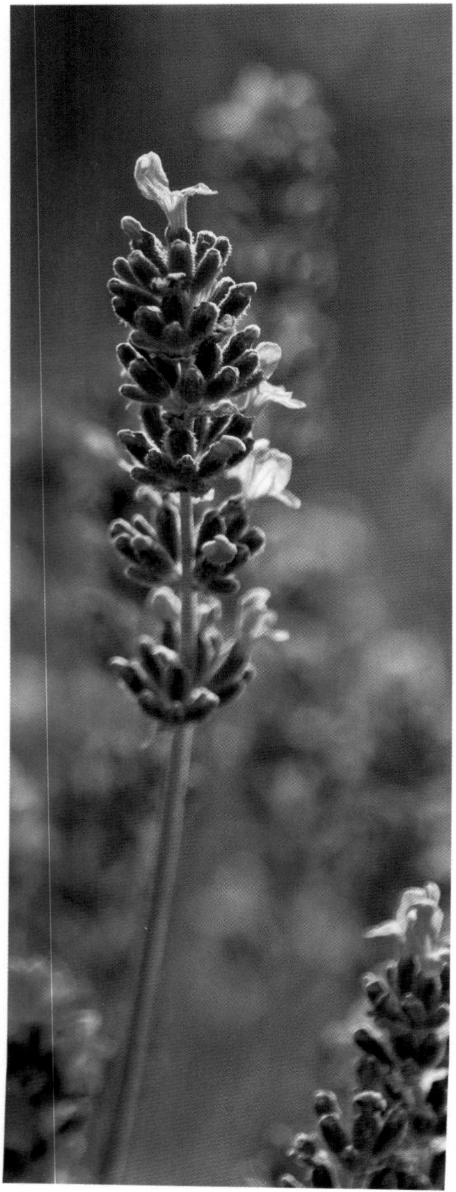

SECTION 2
quick reference

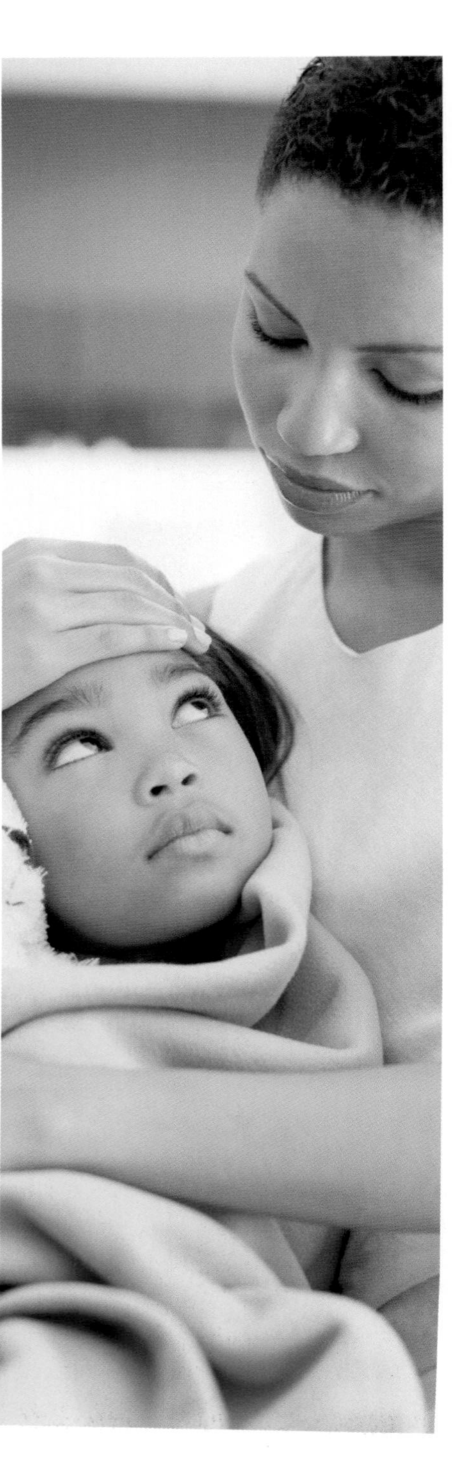

SECTION 3
natural solutions

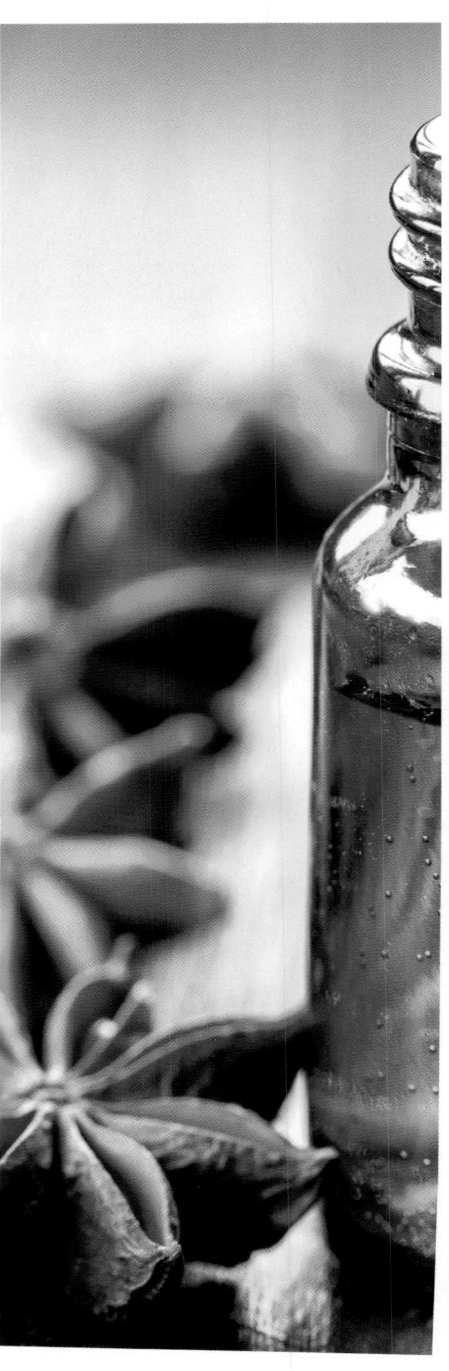

SECTION 4

body systems & focus areas

SECTION 5

natural living recipes

SECTION 6

supplemental

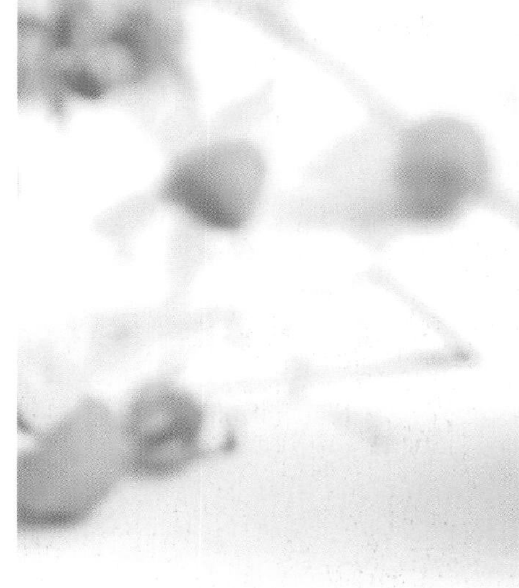

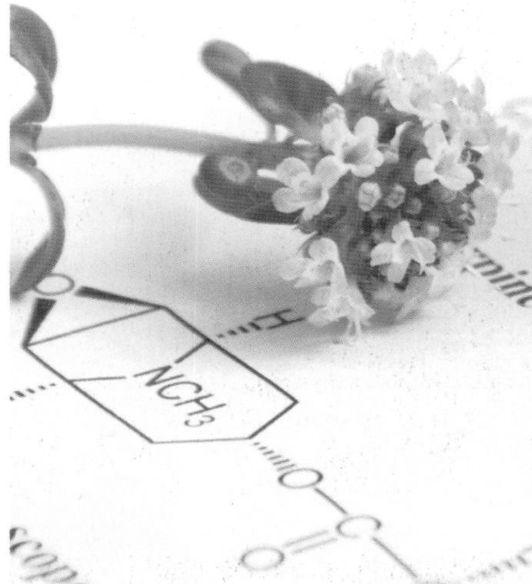

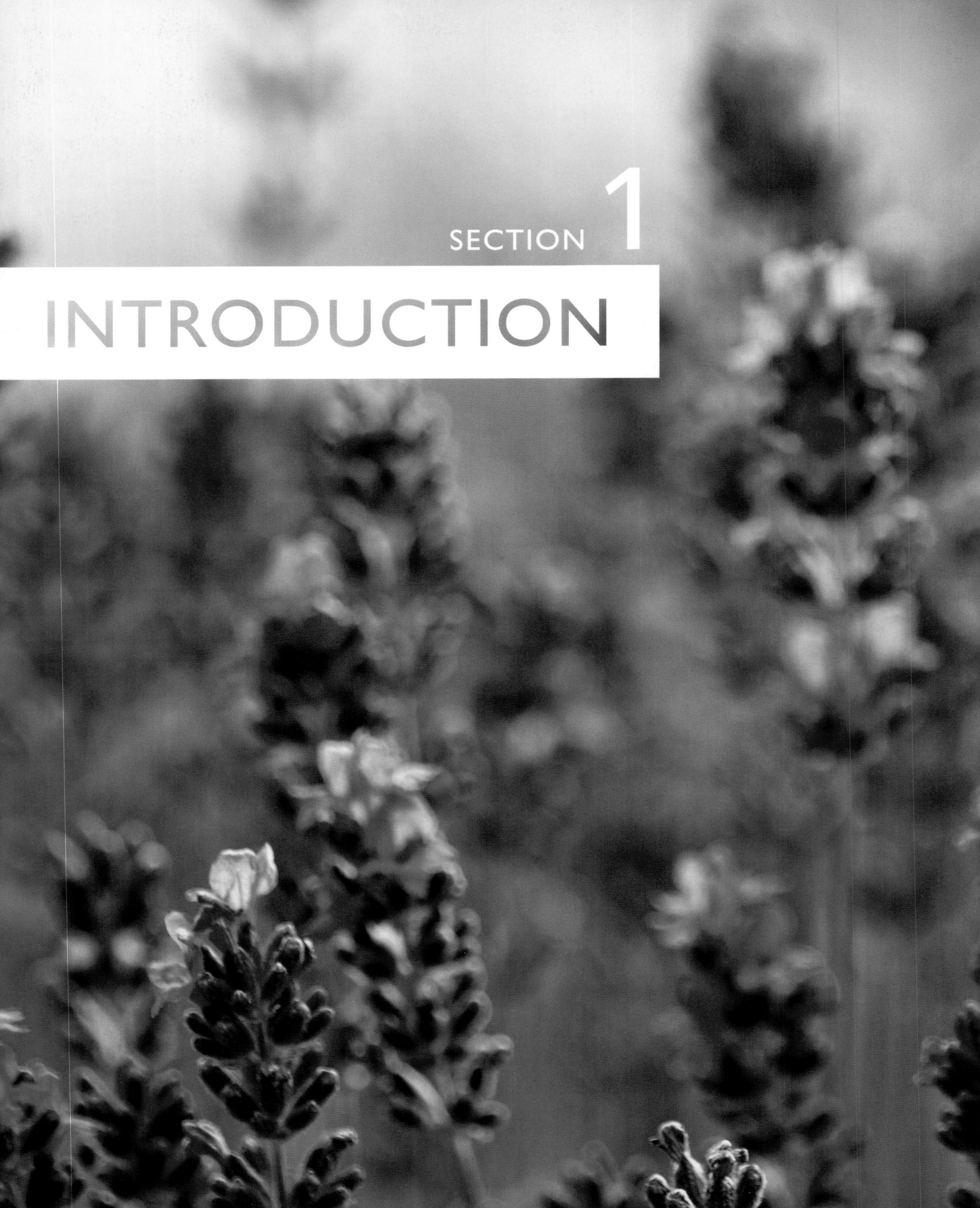

SECTION 1

INTRODUCTION

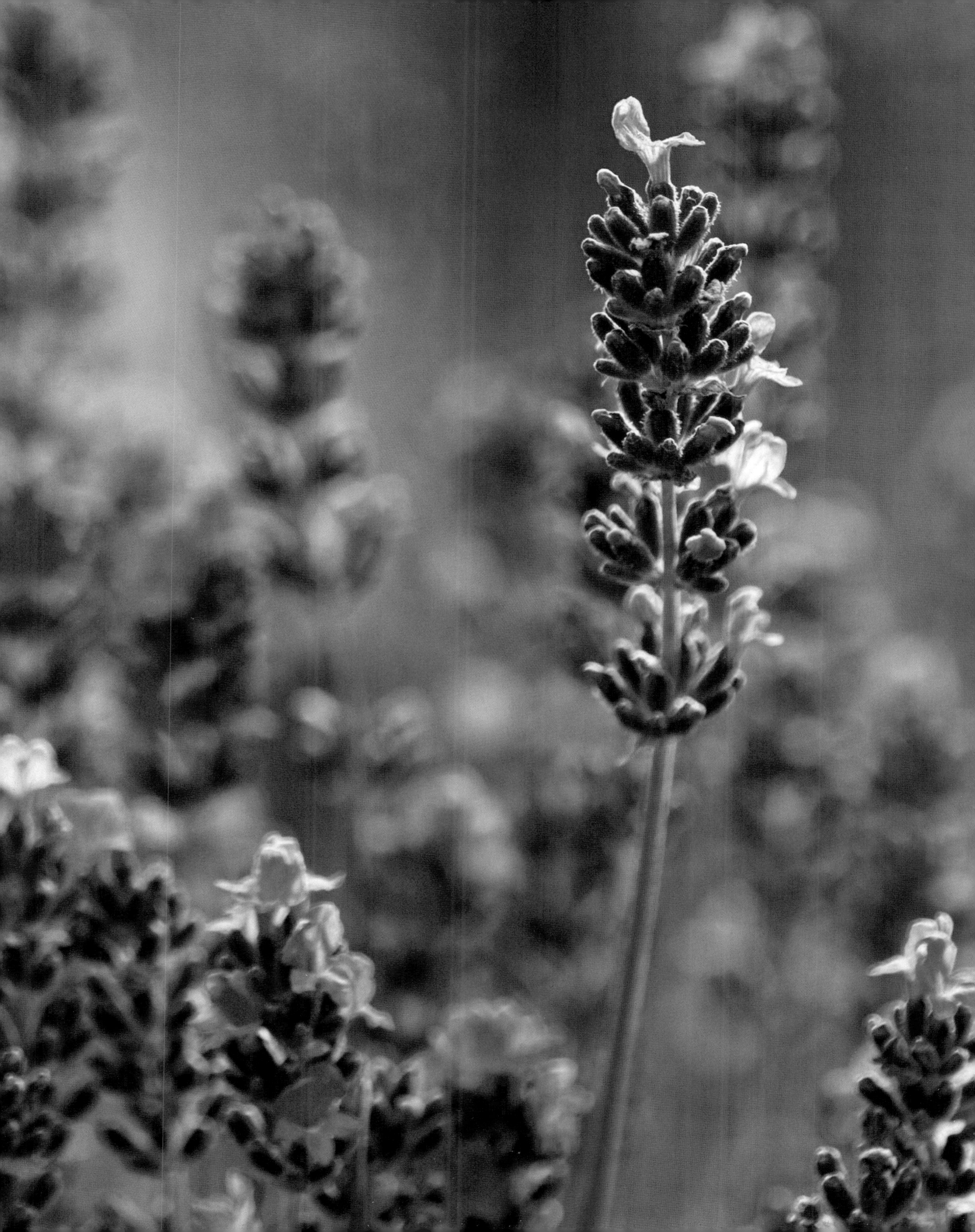

How to Use this Guide

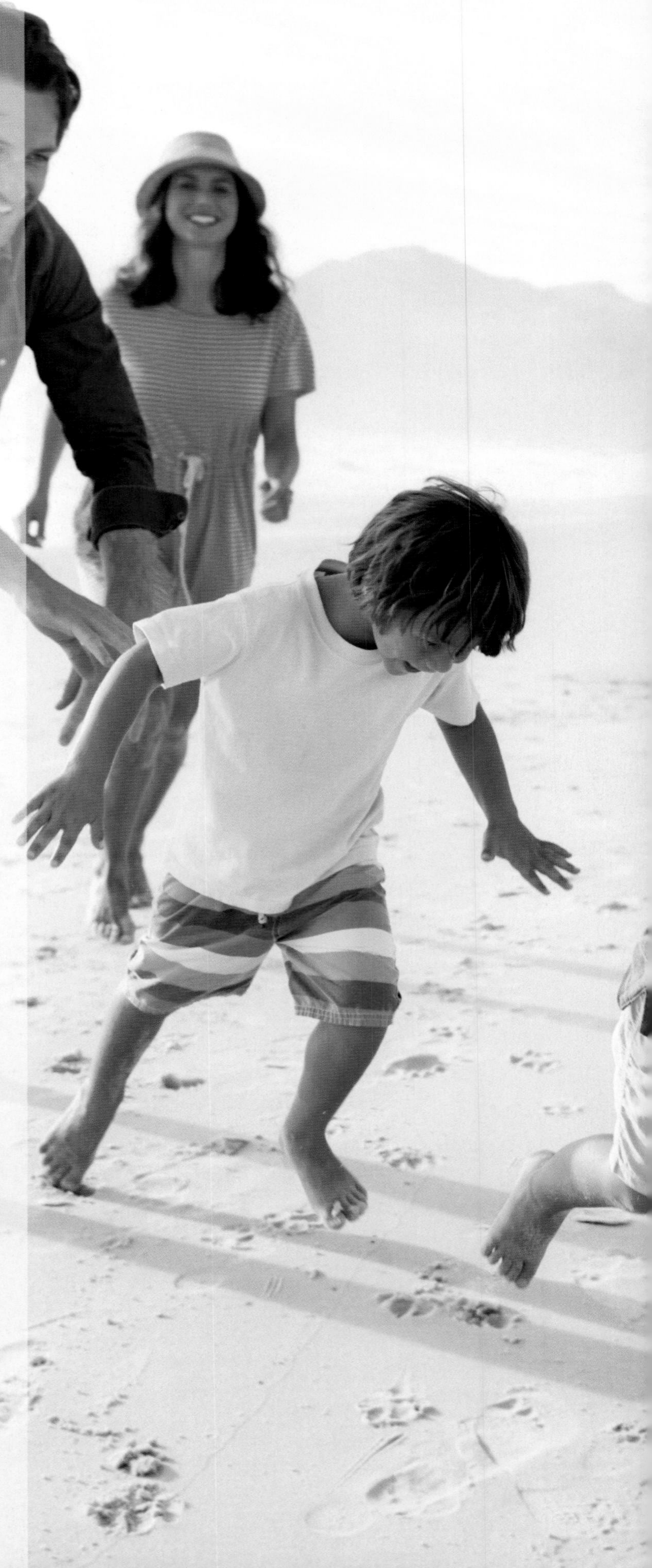

THE ESSENTIAL LIFE is a composition of everything essential for a vibrant life. It's for the new and the experienced essential oil user. It provides both simple, quick-reference information and expert-level knowledge. Its content is intended to enhance your entire lifestyle, and consequently, your life-experience.

Start by learning how to use each section of this book.

SECTION 1: Introduction

Establish a foundation of simple knowledge for using essential oils. Learn what oils are, where they come from, and how to use them effectively and safely.

SECTION 2: Quick Reference

Quickly look up any ailment, and link it to commonly used essential oils with this A-Z index of ailments. Learn basic application methods for recommended remedies.

SECTION 3: Natural Solutions

Become familiar with detailed information about individual essential oils and essential oil blends, as well as supplementary products. Discover how oils are distilled, common uses, basic emotional benefits, and tips for each oil.

SECTION 4: Body Systems

Experience the deepest level of healing knowledge by exploring both disease symptoms and body symptoms in order to support full Body Systems functioning. Learn to address wellness in a holistic way, acknowledging root causes and corresponding healing tools.

SECTION 5: Natural Living

Implement essential oils throughout your lifestyle! Explore and enjoy the benefits of using essential oils for cleaning, cooking, gardening, fitness, intimacy, weight loss, children, pets, on-the-go, and more.

SECTION 6: Supplemental

Explore other in-depth information about essential oils and ailments in the glossary, index, and other resources.

Reach for your oils and refer to this book daily, and enjoy THE ESSENTIAL LIFE!

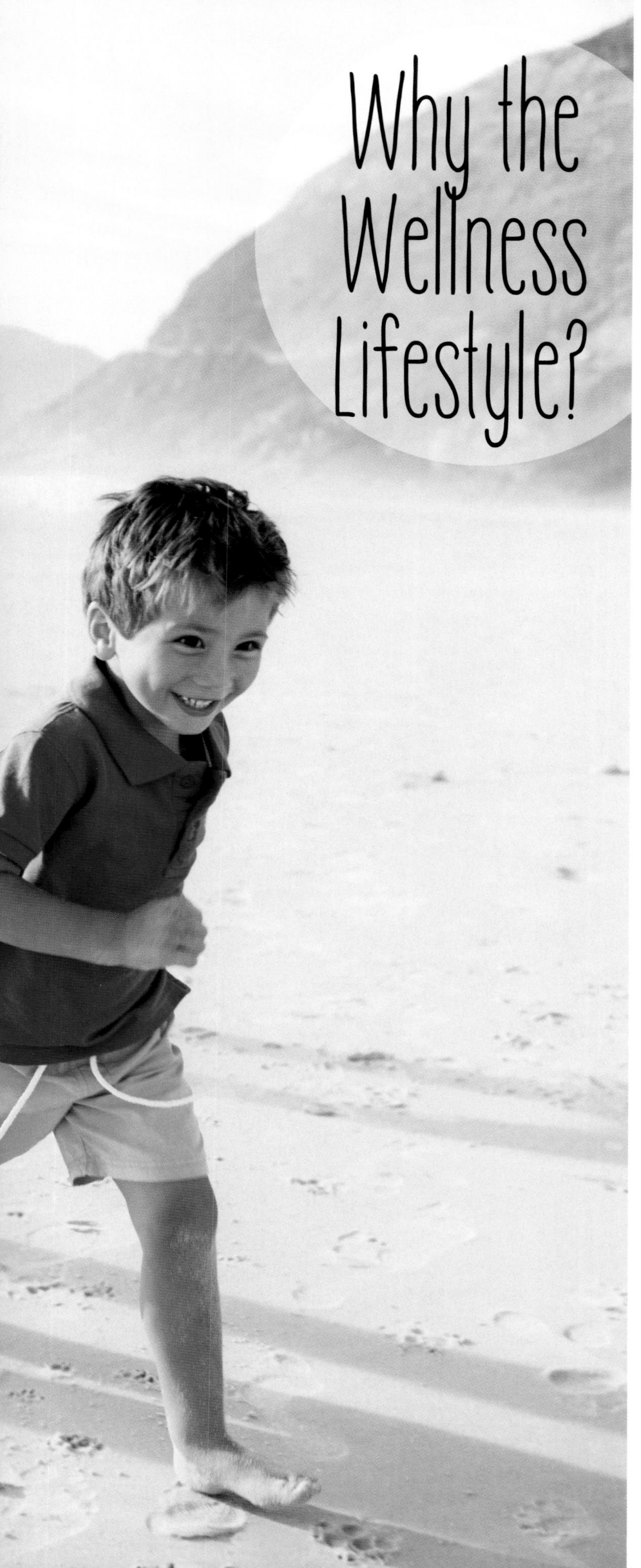

Why the Wellness Lifestyle?

What does it mean to be well? Wellness can be characterized by not merely the absence of disease, but by feeling good and enjoying one's life. How you feel – physically, mentally and emotionally – determines the state of your overall health and well being. It might be said that your health is your greatest asset, since it affects how you think, feel, move, interact, prosper, and achieve. When you don't feel well, every other aspect of your life is impacted.

Poor lifestyle habits put people at high risk for virtually every physical and mental illness. The Centers for Disease Control and Prevention (CDC) report that heart disease is the leading cause of death for men and women, accounting for one in every four deaths in the U.S. According to the National Institute of Mental Health, 75 to 90 percent of all doctor office visits in the U.S. are for stress-related ailments and complaints. Sometimes major life events, such as divorce, loss of a loved one, financial problems, or the birth of a child, can combine with genetic or biologic predispositions to prompt a stress-related health crisis. Our culture often encourages a dependence on doctors, drugs, and health care systems to fix and heal these physical and emotional ailments. Yet it is widely known and accepted within the medical community that learned behaviors and lifestyle choices, such as poor stress management, inadequate nutrition, physical inactivity, insufficient sleep, smoking, and excessive alcohol consumption are major contributors to illness and a diminished quality of life.

Modern medicine tends to fixate on diagnosis and treatment, whereas a wellness lifestyle focuses on education, self-awareness, and prevention. Instead of merely treating disease, the wellness lifestyle addresses its causes - what lies beneath the disease and its symptoms. Our thoughts, feelings, beliefs, habits, and choices are fueling the fires of inflammation, pain, toxicity, and illness in the body. By addressing the root causes of disease rather than merely treating the symptoms we can assist the body in healing itself.

The wave of the future is Integrative Medicine, wherein traditional allopathic treatments work in conjunction with alternative, non-traditional practices to treat the whole person instead of just the disease. In this way, patients and practitioners form a partnership whose goal is to treat the mind, body, and spirit, all at the same time.

Your body is capable of healing itself naturally. Most times, it does not need synthetic medications to take over its job, but simply the right support tools the enable it to do what it was engineered to do. The key to wellness is simply learning what serves the body, then restoring to the to the body what it needs. This will yield lasting healing and continued wellness.

Plant remedies, known as essential oils, have been used throughout the world for millennia and are one of nature's most powerful support tools available to help your body heal itself. Essential oils can be used in many aspects of our daily lives. Typical uses include cleaning, cooking, skin care, animal care, enhancing the air in a room, and supporting the emotional and physical needs of the body.

The overall quality of essential oils is very important when using them therapeutically. The most important factor when selecting essential oils is that they be tested and certified to be pure, potent, genuine, and authentic.

The bottom line to wellness is that each and every day you make choices that affect your health. Ultimately your health rests in your hands. You have the power to live a life of optimal health. We invite you to join us in living the wellness lifestyle, using this book as your guide. Your journey to health and wellness begins here.

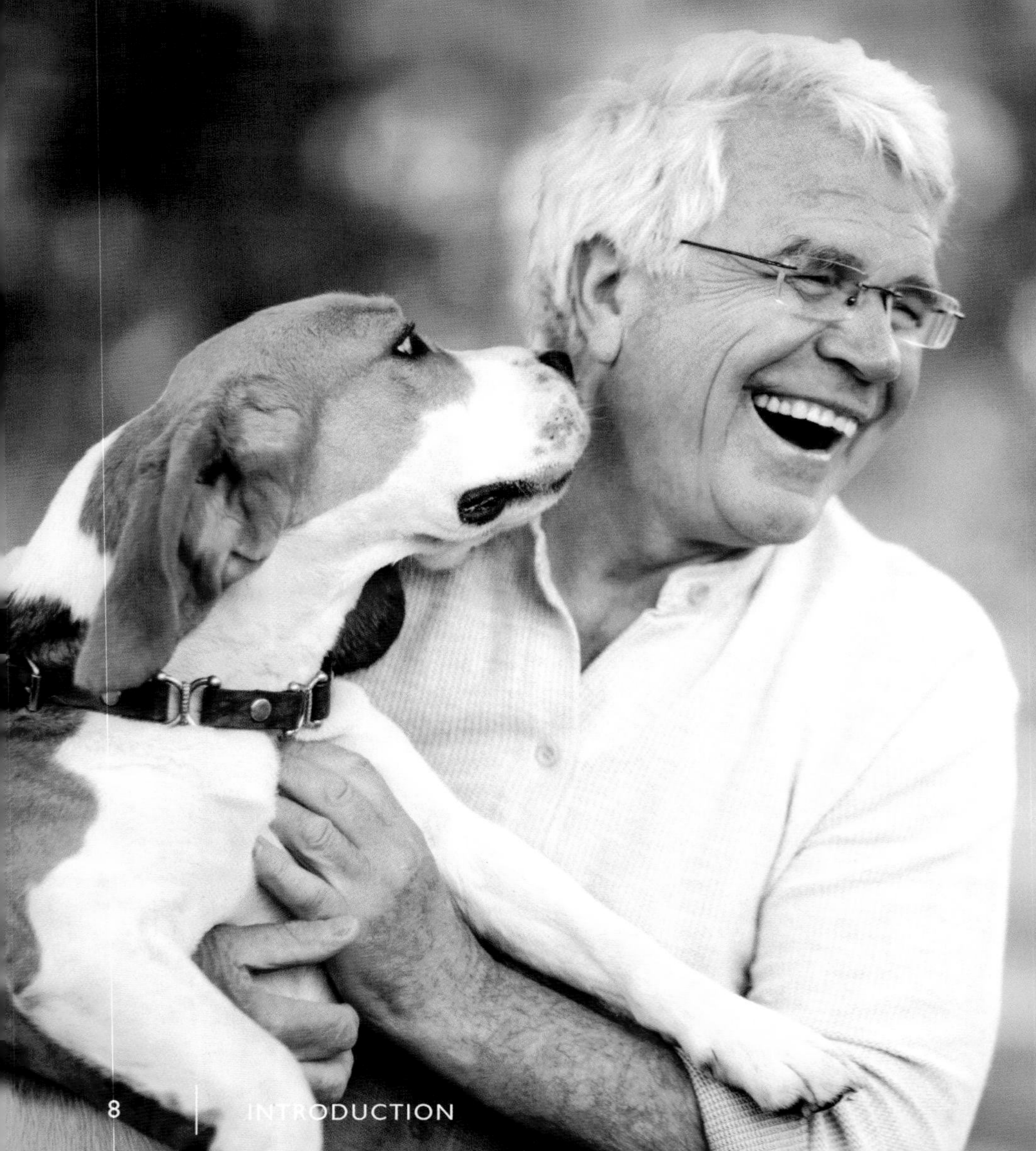

Why Quality Matters

Sourcing

When it comes to sourcing essential oils, the terrain and soil of origin matter. If a field is sprayed with toxic chemicals, or these chemicals are added to the soil, it affects the chemistry of the plants. The distillation process, temperature, and the use of toxic solvents and chemicals for extraction also affect the purity and potency of the essential oil.

Variations in the natural chemistry of oils is permitted, as this is a legitimate expression of nature. As one truly studies the art of growing, harvesting, and distilling essential oils, one discovers the grower's craft and the beauty of this expert human art. Today we experience the best of tradition in growers' expertise and wisdom handed down through the generations, combined with advancements in science, farming, and distillation practices.

Supplier

When it comes to healing, choosing a supplier of essential oils who is well known for quality and efficacy is, well, "essential." Every oil has specific constituents, which provide varying levels of therapeutic effects. Therefore, it is necessary to sort through dozens of species of a single plant source, from a myriad of geographical locations, to find the right combination of therapeutic compounds.

This is one of the supplier's greatest tasks: to responsibly search the world for the highest quality compounds that produce the best possible essential oils nature can provide. One of the best ways this is accomplished is by creating trusted alliances with honest growers and distillers.

Authenticity

Regulation of therapeutic grade essential oils is limited and standards are minimal. This leaves suppliers to self-regulate quality. The term "therapeutic grade" is simply insufficient to identify a level of quality. There exists, therefore, two very distinctly different views. In one, compromised sourcing is permissible and synthetic additives are acceptable components. In the other, true holistic healing requires unprocessed oils that are sourced directly from nature with nothing added. These strict standards allow the oils to remain rich and complex as nature created them. One should expect to pay a higher price for these genuine, authentic, pure, and potent superior-grade essential oils.

Quality

To be truly therapeutic and superior grade, an essential oil needs to be tested and certified as pure, potent, genuine, and authentic. Each of these terms is important and meaningful in reference to measurements of quality. It is vital to note that although chemists have successfully recreated multiple constituents of plants, they have never replicated a complete essential oil. Why? They simply have not discovered or identified every compound nature produces.

Process

To protect and maintain the highest quality essential oils, plants must be patiently harvested by those who are knowledgeable, honest, and committed to gathering only the "one" specie, and who allow the plant proper maturation time.

After harvesting, the plant material is ready for distillation. In order to carefully extract the precious constituents, this process must be conducted gently, slowly, and skillfully. Quality distillation requires reduced pressure and temperature, protecting these essences from being oxidized or destroyed by excessive heat.

Once distillation is complete, the essential oils are moved to distribution companies or to middlemen, known as brokers. As a general rule, the farther down the supply chain you go, the less likely you are to get pure product. Most companies that sell essential oils have no ability (or in many cases no desire) to verify the quality of the oils they receive from their supplier before they pass it on to their customers. Look for companies that work directly with growers, sourced from all over the world.

There is a growing number of products falsely claiming to be an essential oil or to contain essential oils. Too often, these products use fragrant synthetic chemical substitutes o dilute or replace more expensive essential oil extracts. These claims deceive many consumers who believe they are using natural products.

Essential oils are comprised of only three elements: carbon, hydrogen, and oxygen. The molecules in essential oils are

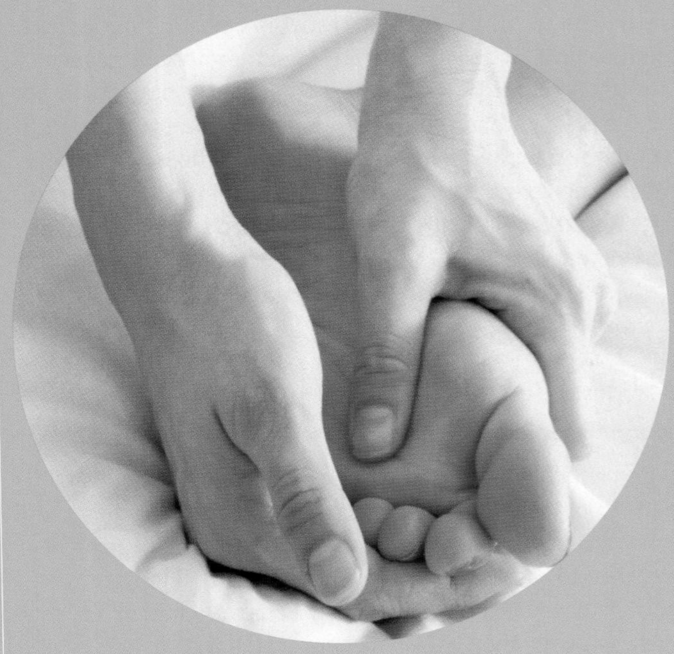

derivatives. Essential oils are volatile organic liquids. There are no vitamins, minerals, essential fatty acids, or hormones in essential oils. Any claim of such ingredients simply reveals the impurity of a product.

Aroma

One of the most telling ways to detect pure, high-quality oils is by the aroma. Superb aroma is earned and is the result of quality plant sourcing, quality distillation processes, and the absence of chemical solvents. Generally, the more pure and "sweet" an aroma, the greater the purity and the better the sourcing.

Supplier Responsibility

It is the distributing company's responsibility to provide the consumer with carefully extracted, pure (no fillers or artificial ingredients) essential oils. Rigorous quality testing, above and beyond the minimum required, helps ensure oils are free of contaminants. Look for companies that verify the quality and purity multiple times prior to making the product available to the consumer. Additionally, the distributor is responsible for labeling products according to FDA GRAS (Generally Regarded As Safe) standards.

Measuring Quality

Measurements of quality fall under specific categories of genuine, authentic, pure, and potent.

Authentic

In the world of essential oils, the term "Authenticity" means:

- The composition of an oil is equal to the plant specified on the label.
- The oil is not a mixture of plant species, rather the plant specified.
- The oil is not the product of a mixture of plants or weeds growing alongside the species.
- The oil is comprised of and distilled from only the plant parts clearly identified.
- In total, the oil is characterized precisely so as to clearly identify its healing qualities through consistently occurring compounds.

Genuine

The term "Genuine" is equivalent to the term "Unadulterated," meaning:

- **The essential oil is 100 percent natural** and contains no addition of any other substances – even other natural substances. It contains NO synthetics, agents, diluents, or additives.
- **The essential oil is 100 percent pure** and contains NO similar essential oil or hybrid, added to extend supply.
- **The essential oil is 100 percent complete** and has been fully distilled. Almost all essential oils are distilled in a single process. Ylang ylang is an exception, as it passes through more than one distillation to be complete. Distillation processes that are disrupted can produce I, II, III, and "extra" essential oil classes.

Pure

Purity alone does not necessarily mean an oil is good quality. A pure oil can be distilled incorrectly or may be obtained from a particular variety of inferior plant species. Additionally, oils may contain contaminants, pesticides, herbicides, solvents, inferior and/or unlabeled plant sources, other unlabeled species, and synthetic compounds. The distillation process may magnify the concentration of these undesirable elements.

Potent

Essential oils are the most potent form of plant material. The chemical constituents found in the plant material will either increase or decrease the potency of the essential oil. The climate and soil composition affect the potency of plant matter. This is why sourcing an oil from its native habitat is essential.

Personal Responsibility

When it comes to obtaining quality essential oils, the consumer must do his own research, use common sense, exercise prudence, and do what is best for himself and his family. Education is key to becoming a skilled user of these potent plant extracts.

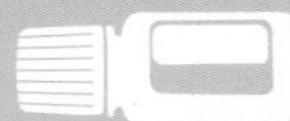

How to Use Essential Oils

Application Methods

Aromatic 

The very term **Aromatherapy** was derived from the fact that essential oils are, by nature, aromatic. Their aromas can elicit powerful physiologic, mental, and emotional responses. Essential oils are also volatile, meaning they evaporate quickly and are rapidly absorbed into the body. The process of conveying aromas to the brain is called olfaction, or simply, smelling. It happens courtesy of the olfactory system.

As a person inhales an essential oil, the molecules of oil go up into the back of each nostril to the postage-sized epithelium patch. There the molecules attach to receptors on the cilia hairs, which convert to nerves on the other side of the mucous patch. These nerves send the odor information to the olfactory bulb in the brain. This means the essential oil itself is not sent to the brain, but instead a neural translation or "message" of the complex chemistry it contains is delivered. The millions of nerves enter the olfactory bulb, which communicates directly with the amygdala, hippocampus, and other brain structures.

The amygdala, a center for emotions in the limbic system, links our sense of smell to our ability to learn emotionally. Here, aromatic information is connected to the emotions of the situation. This capacity to pair the two, information and emotions, is inextricably connected to our survival ability, making essential oils a powerful partner in creating and maintaining emotional health. Inhalation of essential oils is also received through the alveoli of the lungs and, from there, into the bloodstream.

The easiest way to aromatically use essential oils is to open a bottle and simply breathe in the aroma through the nose. This technique is known as **direct inhalation**. To enhance this method, place a drop of an oil or blend in the hands, rub them together, and then cup around the nose and mouth (not necessary to make contact with the face) and breathe in. Additionally, oil drops can be placed on a piece of cloth or tissue, held close to the face, and inhaled.

Diffusing essential oils aromatically is beneficial for affecting mood, killing airborne pathogens, and changing the aroma of a space such as a room, office, or car. Other uses include a targeted approach for relaxing or stimulating the mind. Additionally, one of the most effective ways to impact a respiratory condition is to use a diffuser as an inhalation device, whether being in a room where diffusing is occurring or purposely breathing in the vapor. **Diffusers** are devices that can be used to evaporate an essential oil into a surrounding environment. There are four main types of diffusers: atomizing, vaporizing or humidification, fan, and heat. The best diffusers are atomizing and employ a cold air pump to force the essential oil through an atomizer, separating the oil into tiny particles that create a micro-fine vapor in the air. The essential oil bottle is, in some manner, directly connected to the diffuser, and no water is involved. Atomizing diffusers are normally more expensive and usually create a little bit of noise due to the mechanisms in action. Vaporizing or humidification diffusers employ water with the essential oil and use ultrasonic waves to emit the oil and water particles into the air. Fan and heat diffusers are usually low cost and mainly used for small areas such as cars. The amount of oil used varies with each diffuser type.

Different diffusers provide different capacities for covering the square footage of a room. Other features may include timers, some allowing both constant and intermittent distribution options. Essential oils can be added to water or alcohol (such as vodka) in a **spray bottle** (preferably glass). The mixture can then be sprayed in the air (i.e. air freshener), on surfaces (i.e. countertop), or on the body (i.e. for cooling and soothing benefits).

The best **dosage** for aromatic use of essential oils is smaller doses implemented multiple times throughout the day. It is best to avoid having infants and young children inhale oils at a close distance, as it is harder to determine dosage.

Topical

Because essential oils are fat-soluble, when they are **applied directly** to the skin, their chemical compounds are readily absorbed and enter the bloodstream. This is one reason why quality of oils is important. Many quality oils are safe to use NEAT (defined as: applied topically to the skin with no carrier oil; a carrier oil being a different kind of oil used for dilution such as fractionated coconut oil). One location that is most universally accepted as best for NEAT application is the bottoms of the feet.

The other primary method of distributing essential oils topically is to combine them with a carrier oil, used for both dilution and prevention of evaporation. Using a carrier oil PRIOR to applying an oil slows down the absorption process (does not prohibit), therefore slowing the therapeutic onset. Applying a carrier oil AFTER essential oil application enhances therapeutic onset. Either way, the carrier oil prevents potential rapid evaporation.

By taking the time to massage an essential oil thoroughly into the skin, absorption is enhanced by increasing the blood flow to the area thus allowing the skin to more efficiently absorb valued compounds. Applying essential oils with a carrier oil and then **massaging** the skin or applying warm heat such as a rice bag or **moist cloth compress** helps drive the oil deeper into the tissues. This is especially helpful for muscle pain, body aches, and injured tissue. Carrier oils also protect the skin from irritation. Children, the elderly, and those with sensitive skin or compromised systems are advised to always use a carrier oil.

Some of the more popular **carrier oils** are fractionated coconut oil, virgin coconut oil, jojoba oil, grapeseed oil, almond oil, avocado oil, and extra virgin olive oil. Competing aroma is one consideration when selecting the carrier oil of choice.

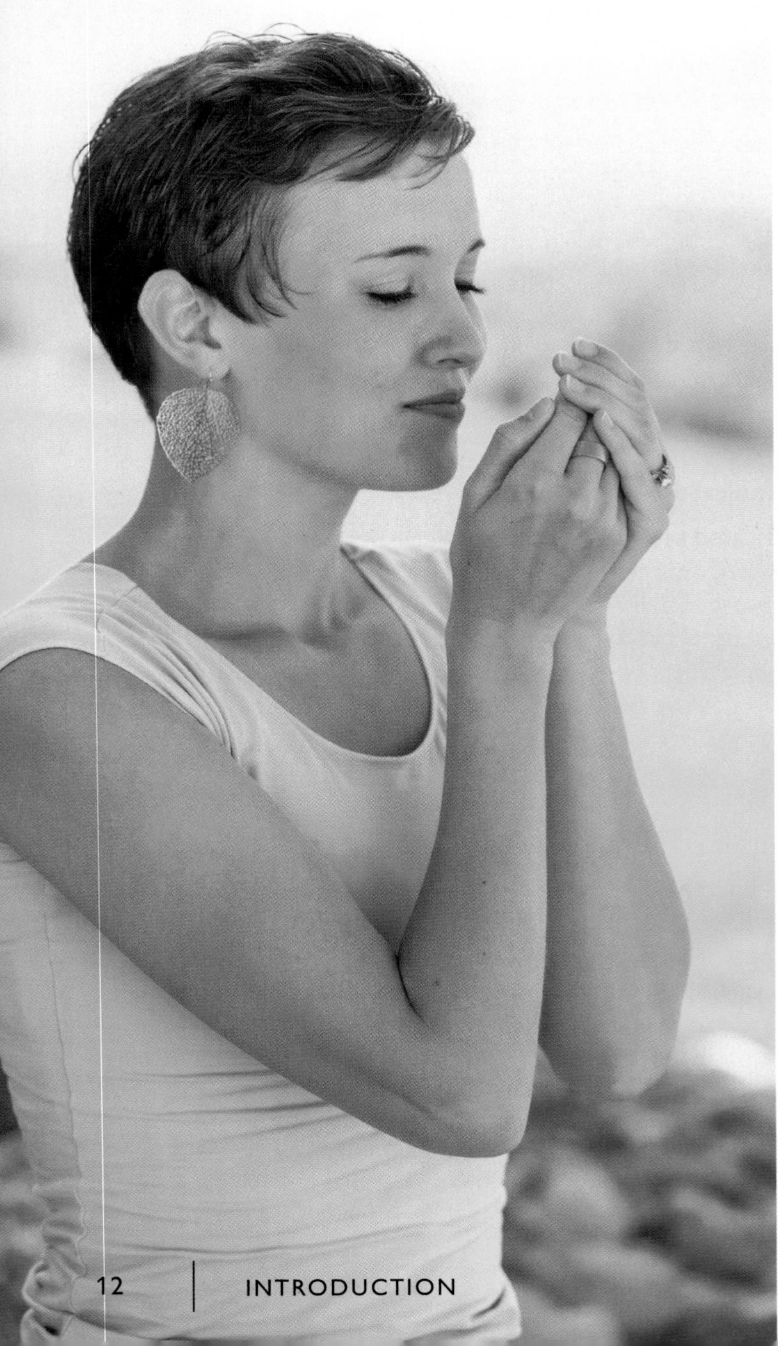

Fractionated coconut oil is a favorite and is created by removing the fatty acids from regular coconut oil, which is solid at 76 degrees. Fractionating, or removing the fatty acids, keeps the oil in a liquid state, making it easier for use in application (i.e. while giving a massage) and to combine with essential oils in containers such as spray and roll-on bottles. The fractionating process also increases shelf life and makes it odorless and colorless. It's great on the skin and doesn't clog the pores.

Topical application methods can vary considerably. Most frequently, oils are simply placed either on the skin of any area of concern or on the bottoms of the feet. Additional methods of distribution can include combining oils in an unscented lotion, or with a carrier oil or water in a spray, balm, or roller bottle. Limiting the number of drops used and diluting is the best way to safely use essential oils topically. It's generally unnecessary to use exaggerated amounts to achieve a therapeutic effect. Every drop of essential oil contains a vast bouquet of potent chemical constituents made by nature to deliver powerful effects in sometimes as little as one or a few drops.

The appropriate **dosage** for topical use of essential oils is different for each individual and should be tailored to their personal circumstances. The age and size of an individual are the biggest considerations as is the individual's overall health status. It is best to use smaller amounts more often rather than greater amounts less often. Start with the lowest amount that makes sense and then increase the dose as needed to achieve the desired outcome. A topical dose of essential oils can be repeated every twenty minutes in an acute situation or every two to six hours as needed otherwise. A recommended ratio for dilution follows:

Babies	0.3 % dilution	(1 drop to 1 tablespoon)
Children	1.0 % dilution	(1 drop to 1 teaspoon)
Adults	2.0-4.0% dilution	(3-6 drops to 1 teaspoon)

When applying essential oils topically, avoid sensitive skin areas such as eyes, inner ears, genitals, and broken, damaged, or injured skin. After applying essential oils the residue can be enjoyed and massaged into the palms for therapeutic benefit. However, if immediate contact with sensitive areas, such as the eyes, is predicted be sure to thoroughly wash hands.

A favorite use for essential oils is in a **bath**, which functions both as a topical and aromatic method. Using an emulsifier such as shampoo, bath gel, milk, or honey with an essential oil before placing in the bath water disperses the oil throughout the water rather than it floating on top. Or add 3 to 10 drops of essential oils to **bath salts** (use amount per product instructions) or 1 cup Epsom salts and then dissolve in bath.

Essential oils can be applied to **reflex points** or nerve endings in the feet or hands. Oils can also be applied to various points on the rim and parts of the ears, referred to as **auricular therapy**, similar to the reflex points on the hands or feet. Refer to "Reflexology" later in this section.

Layering is the process of applying more than one oil to a desired location to intensify the effect of an oil or to address multiple concerns at once. For example, frankincense is often used as the first oil applied to an area on the skin to magnify the effects of subsequent oils layered on top. If an individual is sensitive to or dislikes the smell of an oil(s), they may resist its use. Applying an oil to the bottoms of one's feet (perhaps the least preferred aroma is applied first) and then layering a second and even third oil on top to "deodorize" and create a different aroma can be effective. Putting on socks after application can "contain" the aroma to a degree as an additional option. For example, apply vetiver, layer lavender on top. If satisfactory, then the process is complete. If not, add a third oil such as wild orange or invigorating blend. The last oil applied will be the strongest aroma initially. After time, a more base note oil lingers longer than a top note oil.

Internal

Just as plants are eaten fresh, dried for herbs, used in hot water infusions (tea), taken internally for therapeutic benefits, and used for improved flavor of foods, essential oils can be taken internally for these same uses. We consume essential oils when we eat food. Fresh aromatic plants normally contain 1 to 2 percent by weight of volatile compounds or essential oils. When plants are distilled for the extraction of their essential oils, the properties are concentrated. Essential oils are more potent than whole plant material. Small amounts should be used when taking oils internally.

Essential oils are fat-soluble, so they are readily delivered to all organs of the body, including the brain. They are then metabolized by the liver and other organs. Internal use of essential oils is the most potent method of use, and proper dosing for internal use should be followed according to labeling recommendations and other professional guidelines to avoid unnecessary overuse or toxicity. All ingested food can be toxic if taken in too high of doses. Some traditional essential oil users profess that internal use of essential oils is not safe. However, modern research as well as internal use by hundreds of thousands of users over many years indicates that internal use following appropriate and safe dosing guidelines is perfectly and appropriately safe. Dosage guidelines for internal use vary depending on the age and size of the person as well as an individual's health status.

Essentials oils can be **ingested** internally under the tongue (1 to 2 drops sublingually), in a gelatin cap (often referred to as a "gel cap"), in a vegetable capsule (often referred to as a "veggie cap"), in a tea, in food, or in water. Some essential oils, such as cinnamon and oregano, are best used internally. Heat affects the compounds in an oil. Therefore, it is best to add oils to hot liquids after the heating process has occurred.

Another method of internal essential oil use is **vaginal insertion**. Oils can be diluted in a carrier oil, inserted using a vaginal syringe, and held in place using a tampon. Oils can also be diluted in a carrier oil and then absorbed into a tampon. The tampon is inserted and kept in usually overnight. Essential oils can also be diluted in water and used to irrigate the vaginal area with a vaginal syringe.

Rectal insertion is an appropriate and safe way to apply essential oils, especially for internal conditions. Oils can be deposited into the rectum using a rectal syringe, or oils can be placed in a capsule and the capsule then inserted and retained in the rectum overnight. Consult an aromatherapy professional for using essential oils in **suppositories**.

Keep in mind that a single drop of essential oil is obtained from a large amount of plant material. One drop of essential oil can contain hundreds of compound constituents and is very potent. These two facts should be considered in determining the amount of oil to ingest. For example, it takes one lemon to make about five drops of lemon essential oil. A common internal dose for an adult is 1 to 5 drops of essential oil every one or two to six hours (depending on the oils selected), but preferably no more than 25 drops of essential oils divided into doses in a 24-hour period. This methodology allows the body, especially the liver, time to process each dosage. This dosage should be adjusted for a person's age, size, and health status. For extended internal use a lower daily dose is advised. If a higher dose is desired, consult a healthcare professional.

Some oils are not considered safe to ingest. Those include oils from the needles of trees such as pine essential oil and some bark oils such as cypress and some varieties of eucalyptus. Verifying a "Safe for Supplemental Use" or "Supplement Facts" label on an essential oil bottle serves as guide for oils that are appropriate to be taken internally. Other oils such as wintergreen and birch are required by law to have childproof lids on them, because the benefit of thinning blood could be hazardous to a young child or baby if ingested.

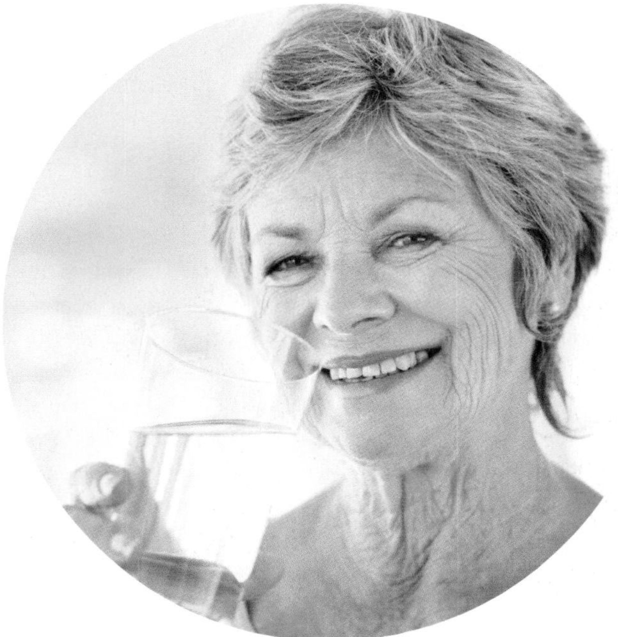

Oil Touch Technique

Essential oils have a powerful effect on well being. These effects are specific and unique to each oil that nature has provided. When we understand these healing properties and how our bodies naturally respond to them, we can use essential oils to promote a superior state of being. The Oil Touch technique provides a way to use these gifts to maximizes emotional and physical healing.

The Oil Touch technique is comprised of four stages. Each stage utilizes two oils or oil blends. Do not substitute other essential oils. Because these essential oils are applied full strength (NEAT) to the skin, it is very important that you use only the highest quality essential oil. Oils need to be both pure and potent. The method of distillation, growing and harvesting standards, plant species, even the region of the world from which it comes, greatly affect the content of the essential oil. Much like the raw materials entering a factory completely determine the end product, an Oil Touch is effective if the essential oil used has consistent and whole chemistry.

What is Oil Touch?

Oil Touch is an interaction between nature's chemistry and neurology (brain and healing communication system). It supports the body to move toward a healing state. Health is created as the body achieves and maintains balance. This balance can be interrupted by heightened stress, environmental toxins, or traumas. Oil Touch promotes balance so healing can continue and is recommended as an integral part of preventive care even for healthy people.

Oil Touch is not a treatment for any specific disease or condition. The body's natural healing abilities are miraculous. Awakening these abilities in others is a simple and precious gift.

How does it Work?

Balance in your body looks something like a series of connected teeter-totters. To illustrate, consider the process of standing up. In order for you to stand and walk, your body is maintaining a delicate balance between falling forward and falling backwards. Just like leaning too much to either side will make you fall over, your body inside is maintaining similar delicate balances. For example, your nervous system is either in a stressed state or a rested state. Like a teeter-totter, both sides can't be high at the same time. Your immune system is the same and will mirror the nervous system's actions. It is either moving infection out of your body or it is pushing it in deeper for you to deal with later. Your body works this way with regard to your senses too. When injured your body sends pain; we call this nocioception. When it is not in pain, it sends good sensations we call proprioception. When all of these are in balance with each other you become more healthy and heal much better. Oil Touch can help restore this balance. It can be compared to re-booting a computer for optimal functioning. This condition is called homeostasis.

The Oil Touch Technique

Oil Touch technique is divided into four stages. Each stage supports a shift in how your body heals and adapts to stress and injury.

Step 1 shifts the nervous system from stress to rest. Step 2 encourages the body to move from the secondary immune system to the primary immune system. Step 3 reduces pain and inflammation. During the entire process, good feeling (proprioception) is stimulated. As the technique progresses, the effects compound, and a dramatic shift occurs in all three factors.

Once your recipient is in this state, they are ready for step 4. In this step, you nudge them back the other direction. The body takes over and finds its balance. This is why it is like re-booting a computer. You turn it off and then back on. The body knows where to stay to get the healing job done right.

In order to do this, you will need to learn a few easy skills and perform them in the right order.

Setting up for an Oil Touch:

You should find a quiet, comfortable place. Using a massage table is best. A headpiece that angles up and down can be helpful for comfort. You may wish to bolster the recipient's ankles with a rolled towel or blanket. Your goal is to make your recipient as comfortable as possible. Your recipient will need a blanket for warmth and modesty as they will need to remove their clothing from the waist up and lie face down on the table. They will have their arms at their sides with their shoes and socks off. They will remain in this position for the duration of the technique. Encourage the recipient to completely relax and receive.

Applying Oil

When applying oil, hold the bottle at a 45-degree angle over the recipient and let a drop fall onto the back. You will typically apply 3 to 4 drops along the spine. It is preferable to start at the low back and move up to the neck. In stage 4 you will apply a couple of drops to each foot.

Distributing the Oil

When distributing along the spine spread the oil from the base of the low back to the top of the head. This is done by gently using the pads of the finger tips. This is a very light touch and is complete when you have spread the oil along the spine with three passes.

Palm Circles through the Heart Area:

Making a triangle with the thumbs and first fingers, place your hands on the center of the back at the level of the heart. Slide the hands in a clockwise fashion over the skin, creating a circle about eight inches wide. Complete three circles and hold for a moment. After pausing, separate the hands, sliding them along the spine. One hand stops on back of the head while the other hand stops and rests just below the waistline. Pause, leaving your hands in this position. Connect with your recipient, and feel their breathing. Focus on being present with them to find a rhythm that is theirs and not yours.

The Alternating Palm Slide:

This movement is a rhythm created by sliding the hands along the surface of the skin. Stand to the side of the recipient, and place your hand on the low back with your fingers pointing away from you at the level just below their waistline. Place your palm against the far side of the spine. Slide your hand away from you with very mild pressure. That is the basic movement. Begin this motion with your fingertips at the spine and lower your palm to their skin as you slide your hand away from you. The slide ends when your hand starts to turn down the recipient's side. Follow your first slide with a second using your other hand and, while alternating hands, move up the body toward the head with each horizontal slide. Keep your touch very light and keep it rhythmic. It is kind of like mowing a lawn, one stroke overlapping the other as it moves up the back toward the head. This movement continues up the back, the shoulders, the neck, and finally up on the head until you reach the level just above the ears.

Repeat this three times, beginning each time at the waistline. Move to the recipient's other side and complete three passes on the opposite side.

5 Zone Activation:

Imagine broad vertical pinstripes running from the waistline to the shoulders, five to the left of the spine and five to the right running parallel with the spine. The two-inch area directly on either side of the spine is Zone 1. The spaces on both sides directly adjacent to Zone 1 are Zone 2 and so forth. Zone 5 is the farthest out, located on both sides at the angle of the ribs where they start to turn down to the recipient's sides. Standing at the head of the table, place both hands on either side of the spine at the waistline as close together as you can. Drag your palms with light pressure up the spine, allowing your fingers to trail behind like the train of a wedding dress. Continue this motion through the neck and head, allowing your hands to gently continue the motion lightly to the crown of the head. That completes Zone 1. Now move to Zone 2. Place your hands at the waistline again, but separate them about two inches (this is Zone 2). Pull your palms up toward the shoulders in a straight line as you did for Zone 1. However, once your hands reach the shoulders, turn the fingertips in, drag your palms out along the shoulder blade, rotate the fingers out, and slide them under the front of the shoulders as you drag your palms lightly back to toward the spine, continue up the neck and head as you did for Zone 1. Repeat for

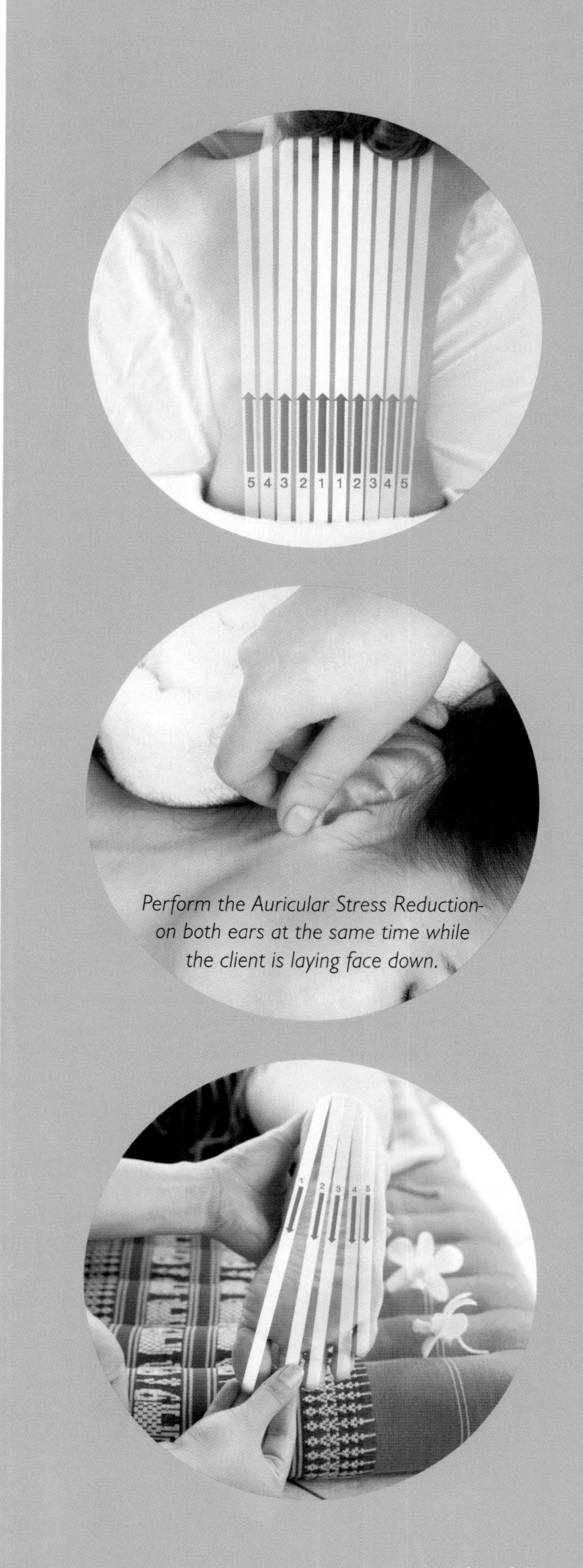

Perform the Auricular Stress Reduction on both ears at the same time while the client is laying face down.

Zones 3, 4, and 5 as you did for zone 2, starting with your hands on the zone just outside the previous one. Complete just one pass per zone.

Auricular Stress Reduction:

Stand at the head of the table. Using your thumbs and forefingers, take hold of both earlobes. Massage them in a circular motion, much like you might rub a penny. Massage along the edge of the ears from the lobe to the top. Drag your fingers back down to the earlobe and repeat three times.

Thumb Walk Tissue Pull:

Stand at your recipient's side near the hips. Place your hands on the back at the waistline with your thumbs on the muscles running directly on either side of the spine. In a circular motion with your thumbs, massage the muscle on either side as you walk up the spine in an alternating fashion until you reach the back of the head. Repeat three times.

Autonomic Balance on the Feet:

There are three steps for the feet. Apply the oils (wild orange and peppermint) together and spread on the bottom of the foot. You may wish to apply some fractionated coconut oil here as well.

Grip the foot with your hands and, using a circular motion with your thumbs similar to the thumb tissue pull, wipe the oil into the skin. Start at the side of the heel and move across it horizontally, then move down one half inch and work your way across the other direction, almost like you are tilling a garden. Repeat this pattern until you reach the end of the forefoot. You will have just pushed the oil quickly into the skin.

Divide the foot into five zones, just like on the back. The strip running from the heal to the big toe is Zone 1, the strip including the second toe is Zone 2, and so forth. To trigger the reflexes in the foot, place one thumb near the other thumb, starting at the heel on the inside (Zone 1), walk down the foot, pushing into the bottom of the foot with the thumbs using medium pressure. Let one thumb trail the other thumb, so each spot is triggered twice. Complete one pass for each of the five zones, continuing to the tips of the toes.

Gripping the foot, swipe down each zone with your thumb as you slightly compress the foot with your hand. Similar to lightly milking a cow, alternating your hands, swipe Zone 1 three times and then continue through all five zones. Make one pass.

Complete these steps again on the second foot.

The Lymphatic Pump:

If your recipient falls asleep let them sleep, or perform the Lymphatic Pump. This will help them get moving again and be less disoriented when they arise. Do this by taking both feet in the hands, saddling your thumbs just in front of the heel at the arch. Push toward the head crisply one time, giving them a forward shake. Their body will rebound back toward you. Repeat the motion, matching the rebound. Create an impulse going back and forth. Do this for about ten seconds and repeat a couple of times.

tips

- If for some reason a particular essential oil cannot be used, do not substitute it with another oil. Just remove it from the technique and use fractionated coconut oil on that stage.
- The Oil Touch technique is designed to be performed on a massage table. If you do not have access to one, adapt, and do the best you can.
- Once you establish contact with your recipient, stay in contact with at least one hand on the body at all times.
- You can use fractionated coconut oil at any time during this process, but if you are using it to lubricate the skin you are pressing too hard. You should be able to perform this on dry skin. Complete the following steps in order, referencing the descriptions above.

STEP 1 Grounding blend
- Apply & distribute oil
- Heart Area Circles

Lavender
- Apply & distribute oil
- Alternating Palm Slide
- 5-Zone Activation
- Auricular Stress Reduction

STEP 2 Melaleuca
- Apply & distribute oil
- Alternating Palm Slides
- 5-Zone Activation

Protective blend
- Apply & distribute oil
- Alternating Palm Slides
- 5-Zone Activation
- Thumb Walk Tissue Pull

STEP 3 Massage blend
- Apply & distribute oil
- Alternating Palm Slides
- 5-Zone Activation

Soothing blend
- Apply & distribute oil
- Alternating Palm Slides
- 5-Zone Activation
- Thumb Walk Tissue Pull

STEP 4 Wild orange & Peppermint
- Apply oil to feet
- Autonomic Balance on feet
- Apply & distribute oil to spine
- Heart Area Circles
- Lymphatic Pump

Safety and Storage

Essential oils are concentrated, potent plant extracts and should be used with reasonable care. Essential oils are very effective and safe when used appropriately. It takes a small amount to induce a powerful therapeutic benefit.

Never apply oils directly to the eyes or ear canals. After applying essential oils, avoid eye contact or the touching of sensitive areas. If essential oils enter the eyes, place a drop of carrier oil, such as fractionated coconut oil or olive oil, in the eye and blink until the oils clear. Never use water, as oils and water don't mix or help with dilution.

Some oils are "warm," creating a heat-like sensation on the skin, and should be diluted with a carrier oil when used topically. These oils can include birch, cassia, cinnamon, clove, eucalyptus, ginger, lemongrass, oregano, peppermint, thyme, and wintergreen. With babies, children, and those with sensitive skin or compromised health, it is particularly important to exercise caution or avoidance with these same oils, as they can be a temporary irritant or overly potent to delicate skin. When using these oils internally, it is best to consume in a gelatin or vegetable capsule.

Some oils contain furocoumarins, a constituent that can cause skin to be photosensitive. Photosensitive oils react to sources of UV rays. The higher the concentration of furanoids, the greater the sensitivity. Oils with concentrated amounts of furanoids include any cold pressed citrus oil such as bergamot, grapefruit, lemon, and lime, with lesser amounts in wild orange. Internal use of these oils is typically not a problem. It is best to wait a minimum of twelve hours after topical application of photosensitive oils before being exposed to UV rays.

Most essential oils applied topically and used reasonably are safe to be used during pregnancy and nursing. Some individuals prefer to avoid internal use during pregnancy and some use essential oils only aromatically during the first trimester. Several oils may be helpful during and after delivery. Internal use of peppermint essential oil should be avoided while nursing as it may reduce milk supply.

Persons with critical health conditions should consult a healthcare professional or qualified aromatherapist before using essential oils and may want to research individual oils prior to using them. In general, those with low seizure thresholds should be cautious in using or avoid altogether fennel, basil, rosemary, birch, and any digestive blend that contains fennel. Those with high blood pressure should be cautious with or avoid thyme and rosemary essential oils.

On occasion a person may experience a cleansing reaction, which takes place when the body is trying to rid itself of toxins faster than it is able. When this happens, increase water intake and decrease application of essential oils, or change the area of application.

safety tips

- Avoid eyes, ears, and nose
- Avoid exposing area of application to sunlight for 12 hours after using citrus oils topically
- Dilute oils for children and sensitive skin with fractionated coconut oil
- Refer to the Natural Solutions section for specific oil safety and usage

The compounds in essential oils are best preserved when stored and kept from light, heat, air, and moisture. Long exposure to oxygen begins to break down and change the chemical makeup of an essential oil. This process is called oxidation, and the oil is said to have "oxidative breakdown." This process is slow but can, over time, promote skin sensitivity with some oils. Citrus oils and blue tinted oils are especially prone to this breakdown. For optimum storage of these types of oils for longer than a year, refrigeration is best. A carrier oil may be added to slow the oxidation process. It's also good practice to keep air space in essential oil bottles to a minimum. The oxidative process for oils that are opened and kept for a long period of time can be slowed by transferring the oils to smaller bottles. Some oils with bigger compounds, such as sesquiterpene compounds (myrrh and sandalwood) actually get better with age. Essential oils can be flammable and should be kept clear of open flame, spark, or fire hazards

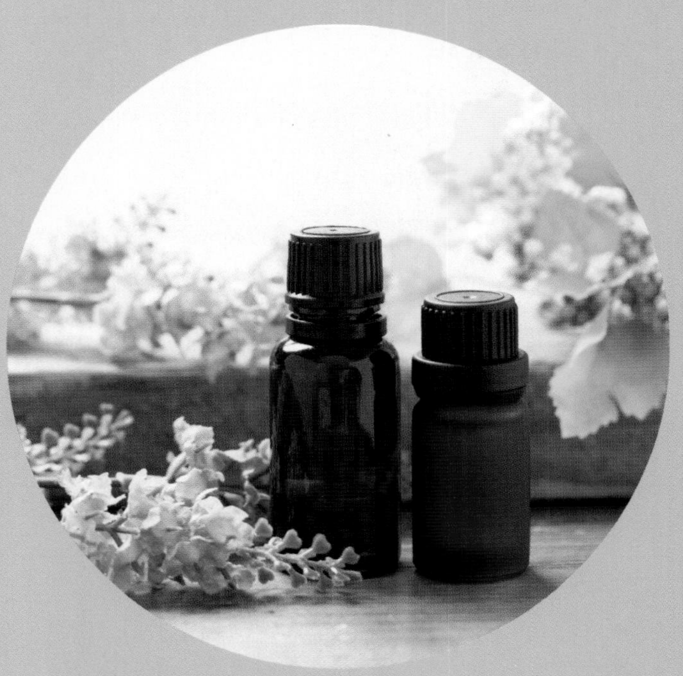

SECTION 2

QUICK REFERENCE

How to Use This Section

Ailments are indexed A-Z. Start by searching for the ailment in question, then note the recommended essential oils for each ailment. Oils are listed in order of most common use. Application methods are also recommended for each oil. Here are key applications for you to choose from:

= Aromatic:

Diffuse with a diffuser.
Inhale from cupped hands (your personal diffuser).
Inhale from oil bottle.
Wear an oil pendant.

= Topical:

Apply to area of pain or concern (dilute as needed).
Apply under nose, back of neck, forehead, or wrists.
To affect entire body, apply to bottoms of feet, spine, or navel.
To affect specific organs or body systems, apply to reflex points on the ears,hands, or feet (See *Reflexology* pg. 426).
*Add warm compress or massage to drive oils deeper into body tissues.

= Internal:

Put a drop or two of oil under tongue, hold a few seconds, and then swallow.
Drink a few drops in a glass of water.
Put a few drops of oil in an empty capsule and swallow.
Put a drop of oil on the back of your hand and lick.

For more specific instruction, see *Application Methods* on page 11. For more in depth information, see *Be a Power User* on page 414.

Frequency:

For acute conditions use every fifteen to twenty minutes until symptoms subside, then apply every two to six hours as needed. For chronic or ongoing conditions repeat one to two times per day, typically a.m. and p.m.

For more information on a particular ailment, see the corresponding *Body Systems* page.

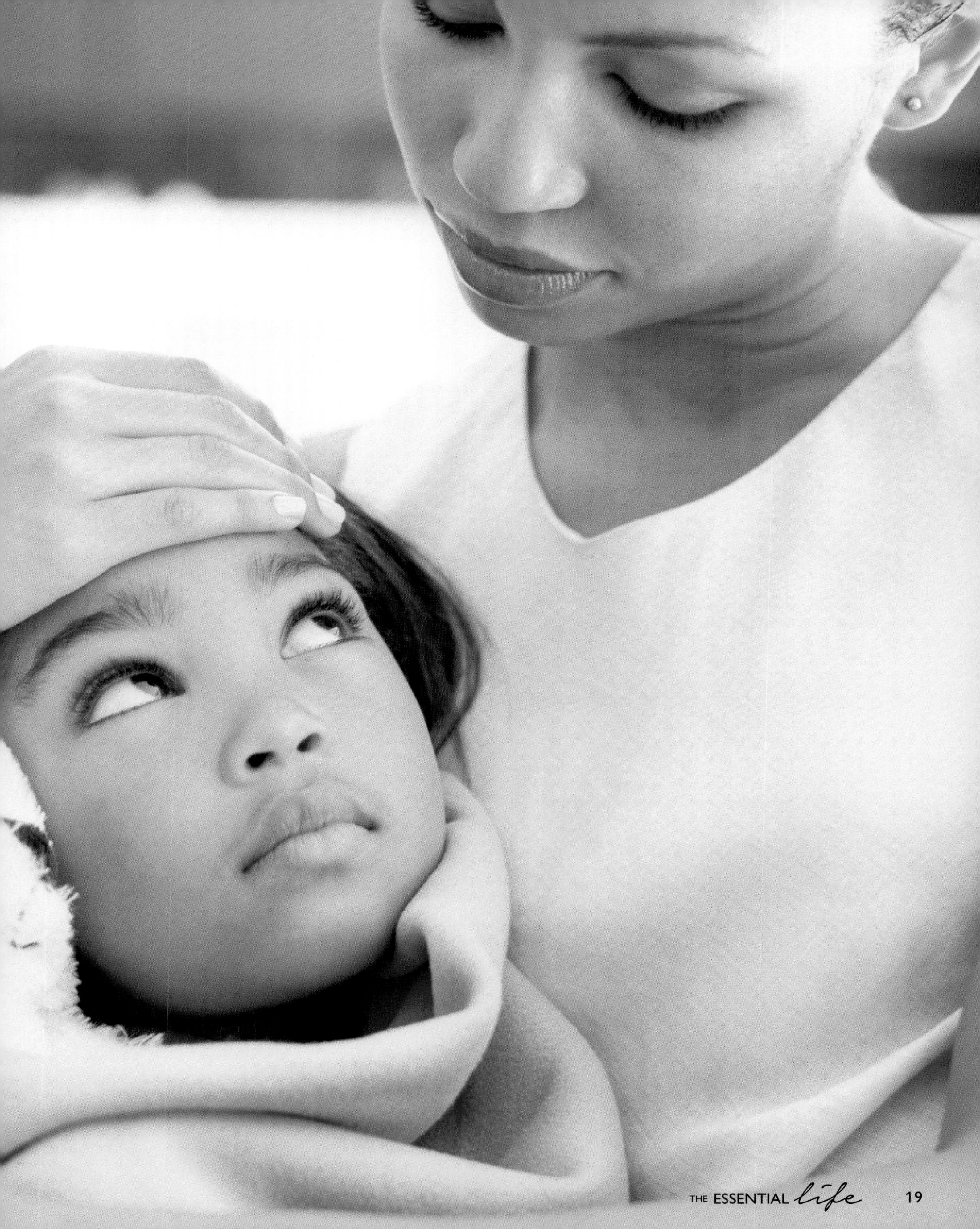

Ailments Index A-Z

STEPS: ❶ Look up ailment. 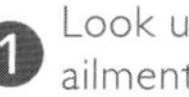 ❷ Choose one or more of the recommended oils. (Order of recommendation is left to right.) 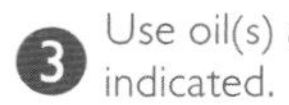 ❸ Use oil(s) as indicated. ❹ Learn more: see the corresponding body system/focus area.

AILMENT	RECOMMENDED OILS AND USAGE	BODY SYSTEM/FOCUS AREA
Abdominal Cramps	Tight, constrictive, commonly intermittent abdominal discomfort; the result of spasm of an internal organ, e.g. bowel spasm related to menstrual cramps or gastroenteritis. digestion blend · peppermint · ginger · clary sage · basil	Pain & Inflammation pg. 294
Abnormal Sperm Morphology	The size and shape of sperm, which means the head should be oval in shape, includes a mid-section and a long, straight tail. If sperm have a double tail, no tail, or a head that is crooked, misshapen, has double heads, or too large, it is considered to be abnormal, and therefore unable to successfully penetrate an egg. detoxification blend · cellular complex blend · rosemary · frankincense · clary sage	Men's Health pg. 276
Abscess (tooth)	A contained collection of liquefied tissue in the body that is known as pus. It is the result of the body's defensive reaction to foreign material. clove · cellular complex blend · cleansing blend · soothing blend · frankincense	Oral Health pg. 291
Absentmindedness	Preoccupation so great that the ordinary insistence on attention is avoided. focus blend · cedarwood · patchouli · vetiver · peppermint	Brain pg. 208
Abuse Trauma	Trauma caused by being intentionally harmed or injured by another person. frankincense · cedarwood · focus blend · joyful blend · comforting blend	Mood & Behavior pg. 279
Aches	A pain identified by persistence, tedium, and, usually, limited intensity. wintergreen · peppermint · soothing blend · cypress · massage blend	Muscular pg. 283; Skeletal pg. 313
Acid reflux	Gastroesophageal reflux disease (GERD) is a chronic digestive disease. GERD happens when stomach acid or, at times, stomach content, flows back into the food pipe (esophagus). The backwash (reflux) irritates the lining of the esophagus and causes GERD. peppermint · digestion blend · lemon · ginger · fennel	Digestive & Intestinal pg. 235
Acidosis	Excess acid in the body due to the accumulation of acid or the depletion of alkaline reserves. Blood pH is abnormally low. fennel · helichrysum · cellular complex blend · lemon · detoxification blend	Detoxification pg. 230
Acne	A common skin disease identified by pimples on the chest, face, and back that occur when pores of the skin become filled with bacteria, oil, and dead skin cells. melaleuca · lemon · skin clearing blend · anti-aging blend · sandalwood	Integumentary pg. 264
Acromegaly	A syndrome that happens when the anterior pituitary gland produces excess growth hormone (GH) after epiphyseal plate closure at puberty. A number of disorders may increase the pituitary's GH output, although most commonly it involves a GH-producing tumor called pituitary adenoma, derived from a distinct type of cell (somatotrophs). grounding blend · frankincense · rosemary · women's blend · detoxification blend	Endocrine pg. 244

Diffuse into the air or inhale from cupped hands.
Apply topically directly to affected areas.
Take internally in a capsule or in a glass of water.
TIP For children use 1-2 drops; for adults use 2-4 drops.

AILMENT	RECOMMENDED OILS AND USAGE	BODY SYSTEM/FOCUS AREA
Actinic Keratosis	A small rough spot on skin that comes from too much sun exposure. It is usually reddish in color, with a rough texture, and often has a white or yellowish scale on top. There may be a prickling pain when touched. anti-aging blend · lavender · frankincense · sandalwood · cedarwood	Autoimmune pg. 200
ADD or ADHD	A disorder characterized by a short attention span, impulsivity, and in some cases hyperactivity. focus blend · cellular complex blend · vetiver · reassuring blend · calming blend	Autoimmune pg. 200
Addison's Disease	Addison's disease is a disorder affecting disrupted functioning of the part of the adrenal gland called the cortex. This results in loss of production of two important chemicals (hormones) normally released by the adrenal cortex: cortisol and aldosterone. clove · basil · cinnamon · protective blend · joyful blend	Endocrine pg. 244
Adenitis	Inflammation of a gland or lymph node. melaleuca · rosemary · lemon · cellular complex blend · invigorating blend	Autoimmune pg. 200
Adrenal Fatigue	Adrenal glands produce a diversity of hormones that are essential to life. The medical term adrenal insufficiency (Addison's disease) refers to deficient production of one or more of these hormones as a result of an underlying disease. rosemary · basil · geranium · detoxification blend · invigorating blend	Endocrine pg. 244 Autoimmune pg. 200
Age Spots	Age spots, or liver spots, are flat tan, brown, or black spots. They vary in size and usually appear on the face, hands, shoulders, and arms. anti-aging blend · frankincense · sandalwood · myrrh · lavender	Integumentary pg. 264
Agitation	Extreme uneasiness, as manifested in depression and other mental disorders. Also referred to as psychomotor agitation. calming blend · soothing blend · frankincense · grounding blend · focus blend	Mood & Behavior pg. 279; Focus & Concentration pg. 255
AIDS or HIV	A severe immunological disorder caused by the retrovirus HIV, resulting in a defect in cell-mediated immune response that is revealed by increased susceptibility to opportunistic infections and to certain rare cancers. cinnamon · protective blend · melissa · clove · helichrysum	Immune & Lymphatic pg. 259
Alcohol Addiction	The frequent intake of large amounts of alcohol, commonly noted by decreased health, social, and physical functioning impairment. cinnamon · detoxification blend · protective blend · metabolic blend · grapefruit	Addictions pg. 190
Alertness	A measure of being mentally keen, active, and rapidly aware of the environment. focus blend · peppermint · frankincense · grounding blend · ginger	Brain pg. 208; Focus & Concentration pg. 255
Alkalosis	Uncommonly high alkalinity of blood and body fluids. rosemary · detoxification blend · protective blend · lemon · wild orange	Detoxification pg. 230
Allergies (insect)	A hypersensitive reaction to an insect allergen; an antigen-antibody reaction is revealed in many forms. lavender · melaleuca · arborvitae	First Aid pg. 251

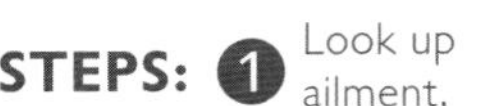
STEPS: ❶ Look up ailment. ❷ Choose one or more of the recommended oils. (Order of recommendation is left to right.) 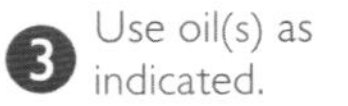 ❸ Use oil(s) as indicated. ❹ Learn more: see the corresponding body system/focus area.

AILMENT	RECOMMENDED OILS AND USAGE	BODY SYSTEM/FOCUS AREA
Allergies (pet dander)	An overreaction of the immune system to ordinarily harmless pet dander, resulting in skin rash, sneezing or wheezing, swelling of mucous membranes, or other unusual conditions. cleansing blend · detoxification blend · women's blend	Allergies pg. 194
Alzheimer's Disease	Alzheimer's disease (AD) is the most typical form of dementia, a neurologic disease defined by loss of mental ability harsh enough to interfere with normal activities of daily living lasting at least six months and not present from birth. cellular complex blend · frankincense · clove · coriander · lemon	Brain pg. 208
Amenorrhea	The nonexistence of menstrual periods. Amenorrhea arises if a woman has missed three or more periods in a row. clary sage · cellular complex blend · frankincense · rosemary · basil	Women's Health pg. 332
Amnesia	Loss of memory. Memory loss may result from two-sided (bilateral) damage to parts of the brain necessary for memory storage, processing, or recall (the limbic system, along with the hippocampus in the medial temporal lobe). frankincense · wild orange · patchouli · peppermint · focus blend	Brain pg. 208
Amyotrophic Lateral Sclerosis	Sometimes called Lou Gehrig's disease, ALS is a rapidly fatal neurological disease that attacks the nerve cells that control voluntary muscles. clove · cellular complex blend · melissa · frankincense · cedarwood	Skeletal pg. 313
Anemia	A condition in which there is an unusually low number of red blood cells in the bloodstream. Major warning signs are shortness of breath, paleness, unusually rapid or strong heart beats, and tiredness. protective blend · basil · cellular complex blend · cinnamon · rosemary	Cardiovascular pg. 216
Aneurysm	A localized, blood-filled dilation of a blood vessel caused by weakening of the vessel wall or disease. cellular complex blend · frankincense · helichrysum · marjoram · cypress	Cardiovascular pg. 216
Anger	A feeling of stress and hostility, usually caused by anxiety sparked by a perceived threat to rights, one's self, values, or possessions. calming blend · grounding blend · focus blend · frankincense · reassuring blend	Mood & Behavior pg. 279
Angina	Pain, discomfort, or strain localized in the chest that is caused by an deficient supply of blood (ischemia) to the heart muscle. It is also at times characterized by a feeling of suffocation, crushing heaviness, or choking. rosemary · cellular complex blend · protective blend · basil · ginger	Cardiovascular pg. 216
Ankylosing Spondylitis	Inflammation of the spine and the sacroiliac joints, which causes pain and stiffness in and around the spine, including the neck and back. soothing blend · wintergreen · birch · massage blend · douglas fir	Skeletal pg. 313
Anorexia	Eating disorder combined with acute fluctuations and loss in body weight. calming blend · frankincense · invigorating blend · joyful blend · uplifting blend	Eating Disorders pg. 240

- (aromatic) Diffuse into the air or inhale from cupped hands.
- (topical) Apply topically directly to affected areas.
- (internal) Take internally in a capsule or in a glass of water.
- TIP For children use 1-2 drops; for adults use 2-4 drops.

AILMENT	RECOMMENDED OILS AND USAGE	BODY SYSTEM/FOCUS AREA
Anosmia	The inability to perceive odor; a lack of functioning olfaction. helichrysum (topical, internal, aromatic); cellular complex blend (topical, aromatic); lemongrass (topical, internal, aromatic); roman chamomile (topical, internal, aromatic); rose (topical, aromatic)	Respiratory pg. 307
Anthrax	An infection caused by the bacterium Bacillus anthracis that essentially affects livestock but can sometimes spread to humans, affecting either the intestines, skin, or lungs. oregano (topical, aromatic); arborvitae (topical, aromatic); thyme (topical, aromatic); detoxification blend (topical, aromatic); clove (topical, aromatic)	Immune & Lymphatic pg. 259
Antiseptic	A substance that hinders the development and growth of microorganisms, without necessarily killing them. arborvitae (topical, aromatic); melaleuca (topical, aromatic); protective blend (topical, aromatic); lemon (topical, aromatic); wild orange (topical, aromatic)	Immune & Lymphatic pg. 259
Anxiety	A mood disorder characterized by emotional, somatic, behavioral, and cognitive components encircling chronic dread, fear, panic attacks, and worry. calming blend (topical, aromatic); grounding blend (topical, aromatic); vetiver (topical, aromatic); frankincense (topical, aromatic); reassuring blend (topical, aromatic)	Mood & Behavior pg. 279
Apathy	A lack of emotion, interest, feeling, and concern, a state of indifference or the suppression of emotions such as concern, excitement, motivation, and/or passion. patchouli (topical, aromatic); rose (topical, aromatic); jasmine (topical, aromatic); grounding blend (topical, aromatic); frankincense (topical, aromatic)	Mood & Behavior pg. 279
Appetite (loss of)	Absence of the desire to eat, induced by psychological drugs or by environmental, social, or other factors. grapefruit (topical, aromatic, internal); metabolic blend (topical, internal); bergamot (topical, internal, aromatic); black pepper (topical, internal); inspiring blend (aromatic)	Weight pg. 327
Appetite Suppressant	A drug that declines feelings of hunger. Most work by increasing levels of serotonin or catecholamine, chemicals in the brain that curb appetite. metabolic blend (internal, topical, aromatic); grapefruit (internal, aromatic); ginger (internal, topical); cinnamon (internal, topical); cassia (internal, topical)	Weight pg. 327
ARDS	Sudden respiratory failure due to the accumulation of fluid in the lungs and an increase in the permeability of the barrier between the capillaries and the air sacs in the lungs. melissa (topical, aromatic); eucalyptus (topical, aromatic); rosemary (topical, aromatic); respiration blend (topical, aromatic); protective blend (topical, aromatic)	Respiratory pg. 307
Arrhythmia	An irregularity in the strength or rhythm of the heartbeat. basil (internal, topical); cellular complex blend (internal, topical); rosemary (internal, topical); ylang ylang (topical, internal); lavender (topical, internal)	Cardiovascular pg. 216
Arteriosclerosis	Any of a group of chronic diseases in which hardening, thickening, and loss of elasticity of the arterial walls result in flawed blood circulation. protective blend (internal, topical); arborvitae (topical); wild orange (internal, topical); juniper berry (internal, topical); cardamom (internal, topical)	Cardiovascular pg. 216
Arthritic Pain	Inflammation of a joint, commonly followed by pain, stiffness, and swelling, resulting from trauma, infection, degenerative changes, metabolic disturbances, or other causes. soothing blend (topical); wintergreen (topical); lemongrass (topical); massage blend (topical); douglas fir (topical)	Skeletal pg. 313; Pain & Inflammation pg. 294
Arthritis (reactive)	Reactive arthritis is a chronic form of arthritis featuring the following three conditions: (1) inflamed joints, (2) inflammation of the eyes (conjunctivitis), and (3) inflammation of the genital, urinary, or gastrointestinal systems. soothing blend (topical); massage blend (topical); white fir (topical); lemongrass (topical); wintergreen (topical)	Autoimmune pg. 200; Pain & Inflammation pg. 294

STEPS: 1 Look up ailment. 2 Choose one or more of the recommended oils. (Order of recommendation is left to right.) 3 Use oil(s) as indicated. 4 Learn more: see the corresponding body system/focus area.

AILMENT	RECOMMENDED OILS AND USAGE	BODY SYSTEM/FOCUS AREA
Asthma	A continual, long-lasting inflammatory disease of the airways. In those susceptible to asthma, this inflammation causes the airways to swell and spasm repeatedly so that the airways narrow. respiration blend, eucalyptus, rosemary, peppermint, cardamom	Respiratory pg. 307
Ataxia	Loss of the capacity to coordinate muscular movement. Also called dyssynergia, incoordination. frankincense, white fir, helichrysum, marjoram, cypress	Brain pg. 208
Atherosclerosis	The increase of a waxy plaque on the inside of blood vessels. marjoram, basil, lavender, melissa, lemon	Cardiovascular pg. 216
Athlete's Foot	A typical fungus infection between the toes in which the skin starts cracking and peeling away, and becomes itchy and sore. melaleuca, massage blend, cardamom, arborvitae	Athletes pg. 197; Candida pg. 212; Integumentary pg. 264
Attachment Disorder (RAD)	A rare but severe condition in which an infant or young child doesn't establish healthy attachments with parents or caregivers. Reactive attachment disorder may develop if the child's basic needs for affection, comfort, and nurturing aren't met and loving, caring, stable attachments with others are not established. frankincense, calming blend, cedarwood, grounding blend, reassuring blend	Mood & Behavior pg. 279
Auditory Processing Disorder	The impaired ability in children to recognize subtle differences between sounds in words even though hearing is normal. frankincense, sandalwood, cellular complex blend, bergamot, vetiver	Brain pg. 208
Autism	A complicated developmental disorder characterized by difficulties with social interaction, verbal and nonverbal communication, and behavioral problems, along with repetitive behaviors and limited focus of interest. frankincense, vetiver, focus blend, geranium, peppermint	Nervous pg. 287; Brain pg. 208
Autoimmune Disorder	An illness that occurs when the body tissues are attacked by its own immune system. cellular complex blend, detoxification blend, lemongrass, digestion blend, ginger	Autoimmune pg. 200
Autointoxication	Self-poisoning caused by endogenous microorganisms, metabolic wastes, or other toxins produced within the body. detoxification blend, cilantro, clove, geranium, thyme	Weight pg. 327
Avoidant Restrictive Food Intake Disorder	An eating disorder that prevents the consumption of certain foods. It is often viewed as a phase of childhood that is generally overcome with age. Also known as selective eating disorder (SED). cinnamon, ginger, invigorating blend, joyful blend, metabolic blend	Eating Disorders pg. 240
Back Muscle Fatigue	A state of fatigue or loss of strength and/or muscle endurance following arduous activity associated with the accumulation of lactic acid in muscles. soothing blend, tension blend, wintergreen, birch, massage blend	Muscular pg. 283

Diffuse into the air or inhale from cupped hands.
Apply topically directly to affected areas.
Take internally in a capsule or in a glass of water.
TIP For children use 1-2 drops; for adults use 2-4 drops.

AILMENT	RECOMMENDED OILS AND USAGE	BODY SYSTEM/FOCUS AREA
Back Pain	A pain in the lumbar, cervical regions or lumbosacral, regions of the back, shifting in sharpness and intensity. Causes may consist of muscle tension or stress on the root of a nerve. soothing blend, massage blend, peppermint, lemongrass, frankincense	Muscular pg. 283
Back Stiffness	Persistent throbbing or stiffness anywhere along the spine, from the base of the neck to the tail bone. massage blend, peppermint, soothing blend, white fir, lemongrass	Muscular pg. 283
Bacteria	One-celled forms of life that are tiny and cause many diseases and infections. thyme, oregano, protective blend, melaleuca, cinnamon	Immune & Lymphatic pg. 259
Bags Under the Eyes	The appearance of swelling in the tissues under the eyes caused by fluid buildup around the eyes. sandalwood, geranium, anti-aging blend, roman chamomile, juniper berry	Integumentary pg. 264
Balance Problems	Balance problems include a wide range of symptoms, from lightheadedness to dizziness. Muscles, joints, and bones (musculoskeletal system), hearing, visual senses, central nervous system, and heart and blood vessels (cardiovascular system) must work normally to have normal balance. ginger, cellular complex blend, cedarwood, grounding blend, vetiver	Brain pg. 208
Baldness	Medically known as alopecia, baldness may be patchy, a condition called alopecia areata. A variant of alopecia areata may involve the entire head: alopecia capitis totalis. cellular complex blend, sandalwood, clary sage, lavender, thyme	Integumentary pg. 264
Basal Cell Carcinoma	A slow-growing, locally invasive but rarely metastasizing neoplasm of the skin derived from basal cells of the hair follicles or epidermis. cellular complex blend, detoxification blend, rosemary, frankincense, clove	Cellular Health pg. 221
Bed Sores	A painful, reddened area of ulcerated skin caused by pressure and lack of movement. They are worsened by exposure to urine or other irritating substances on the skin. Also called a pressure sore, decubitus sore, or decubitus ulcer. massage blend, helichrysum, lavender, myrrh, frankincense	Integumentary pg. 264
Bed-wetting	Involuntary urination while asleep after the age at which bladder control typically happens. cypress, black pepper, massage blend, ylang ylang, reassuring blend	Urinary pg. 324
Bee Sting	An injury caused by the venom of bees, usually followed by swelling and pain. cleansing blend, lavender, melaleuca, roman chamomile, basil	First Aid pg. 251
Bell's Palsy	A weakness or paralysis of the muscles on one side of the face. Damage to the facial nerve that controls muscles on one side of the face causes that side of the face to droop. frankincense, massage blend, grounding blend, peppermint, rosemary	Nervous pg. 287
Benign Prostatic Hyperplasia	A noncancerous case of the prostate that causes overgrowth of the prostate tissue, expanding the prostate and obstructing urination. clary sage, juniper berry, cypress, cedarwood, focus blend	Cellular Health pg. 221

STEPS: **1** Look up ailment. **2** Choose one or more of the recommended oils. (Order of recommendation is left to right.) **3** Use oil(s) as indicated. **4** Learn more: see the corresponding body system/focus area.

AILMENT	RECOMMENDED OILS AND USAGE	BODY SYSTEM/FOCUS AREA
Binge Eating Disorder (BED)	A mental illness marked by recurrent binge eating episodes without the individual's effort to exercise, purge, and/or use of medications like diet pills or laxatives. metabolic blend · renewing blend · cinnamon · cedarwood · joyful blend	Eating Disorders pg. 240
Bipolar Disorder	Commonly called manic depression, a disorder characterized by mood swings and repeated episodes of depression with at least one episode of mania. calming blend · frankincense · reassuring blend · vetiver · bergamot	Brain pg. 208; Limbic pg. 273
Bladder Control	Urinary incontinence is unexpected loss of urine that is sufficient enough in regularity and amount to cause physical and/or emotional concern in the person experiencing it. rosemary · thyme · lemongrass · sandalwood	Urinary pg. 324
Bleeding	The discharge of blood from the vascular system as a result of harm to a blood vessel. myrrh · helichrysum · geranium	Cardiovascular pg. 216
Blisters from Sun	A local swelling of the skin that consists of watery fluid and is caused by infection, burning, or irritation. lavender · myrrh · anti-aging blend · helichrysum · sandalwood	Integumentary pg. 264
Blisters on Feet	A local swelling of the skin that contains watery fluid and is caused by burning or irritation, located one or both feet. myrrh · frankincense · patchouli · lavender · melaleuca	Integumentary pg. 26
Bloating	Any abnormal general swelling of the abdominal area. Symptoms include a feeling of being full or a tight abdomen, which may cause abdominal pain. cilantro · digestion blend · peppermint · ginger · dill	Digestive & Intestinal pg. 235
Blood Clot	A thickened lump in the blood formed by tiny substances called platelets. Clots form to stop bleeding, such as at the site of a cut. helichrysum · myrrh · massage blend · clove · fennel	Cardiovascular pg. 216
Blood Detoxification	A decrease of the toxic properties of poisons. geranium · detoxification blend · clove · cellular complex blend · thyme	Detoxification pg. 230
Blood Pressure (high)	Commonly called hypertension. Blood pressure is the force of blood pushing against the walls of arteries as it flows through them. Arteries are the blood vessels that carry oxygenated blood from the heart to the body's tissues. basil · marjoram · lavender · ylang ylang · cypress	Cardiovascular pg. 216
Blood Pressure (low)	A condition in which a person's blood pressure is not satisfactory for tissue oxygenation or normal perfusion. basil · cellular complex blend · helichrysum · cardamom · rosemary	Cardiovascular pg. 216
Blood Sugar (low)	An uncommonly low concentration of glucose in the circulating blood. metabolic blend · wild orange · cinnamon · coriander · cassia	Blood Sugar pg. 205

Diffuse into the air or inhale from cupped hands.
Apply topically directly to affected areas.
Take internally in a capsule or in a glass of water.
TIP For children use 1-2 drops; for adults use 2-4 drops.

AILMENT	RECOMMENDED OILS AND USAGE	BODY SYSTEM/FOCUS AREA
Blood Sugar Imbalance	A condition in which the body does not handle glucose effectively. Blood glucose levels may fluctuate outside of the body's optimal blood glucose range. cinnamon, cassia, protective blend, metabolic blend, fennel	Blood Sugar pg. 205; Endocrine pg. 244; Candida pg. 212
Blurred Vision	The loss of sharpness of vision and the inability to see fine details. cellular complex blend, lemongrass, helichrysum, frankincense, anti-aging blend	Nervous pg. 287
Body Dysmorphic Disorder	A type of chronic mental illness in which one cannot stop thinking about a minor or imagined flaw in his/her appearance. But to the individual, his/her appearance seems so shameful that he/she does not want to be seen by anyone. clove, frankincense, arborvitae, cellular complex blend, rosemary	Brain pg. 208
Body Myositis	Inflammation of a muscle, especially a voluntary muscle, characterized by pain, tenderness, and sometimes spasm in the affected area. marjoram, lemongrass, massage blend, cypress, wintergreen	Muscular pg. 283
Body Odor	A revolting smell combined with stale perspiration. Freshly secreted perspiration is odorless, but after disclosure to the atmosphere and bacterial movement at the surface of the skin, chemical changes develop to produce the odor. detoxification blend, cilantro, arborvitae, dill, cleansing blend	Detoxification pg. 230
Boils	Boils and carbuncles are bacterial infections of hair follicles and neighboring skin that form pustules (small blister-like swellings which contains pus) around the follicle. myrrh, anti-aging blend, melaleuca, cleansing blend, lavender	Integumentary pg. 264
Bone Pain	Any pain that is associated with an unusual condition within a bone, such as osteomyelitis. soothing blend, white fir, helichrysum, birch, wintergreen	Skeletal pg. 313
Bone Spurs	Osteophytes, frequently referred to as parrot or bone spurs, are bony bumps that form along joint edges. cypress, eucalyptus, wintergreen, massage blend, basil	Skeletal pg. 313
Brain Fog	A condition that affects all ages and which is defined by decreased clarity of thought, confusion, and forgetfulness which may lead to minor depression. peppermint, encouraging blend, frankincense, focus blend, bergamot	Brain pg. 208
Brain Injury	An extremely comprehensive term for any injury occurring in the brain of a living person before, during, or after birth, which is typically understood to be traumatic. frankincense, cellular complex blend, arborvitae, bergamot, peppermint	Brain pg. 208
Breastfeeding (milk supply)	Giving a baby milk from the breast, suckling or nursing. fennel, dill, women's monthly blend, clary sage, basil	Women's Health pg. 332
Breathing Problems	A condition in which respiratory function is insufficient to meet the needs of the body when physical activity increases and places extra claim on it. respiration blend, eucalyptus, douglas fir, peppermint, cardamom	Respiratory pg. 307

QUICK REFERENCE

STEPS: ❶ Look up ailment. ❷ Choose one or more of the recommended oils. (Order of recommendation is left to right.) ❸ Use oil(s) as indicated. ❹ Learn more: see the corresponding body system/focus area.

AILMENT	RECOMMENDED OILS AND USAGE	BODY SYSTEM/FOCUS AREA
Brittle Nails	Brittleness with breakage of finger or toenails. arborvitae · fennel · frankincense · myrrh · lemon	Integumentary pg. 264
Broken Bone	A break in continuity of bone; it may be caused by stress, twisting due to muscle spasm or indirect loss of leverage, or by disease that results in osteopenia. white fir · birch · helichrysum · soothing blend · frankincense	Skeletal pg. 313
Broken Capillaries	Break in the tiniest blood vessels with the smallest diameter. cellular complex blend · metabolic blend · lavender · geranium · cypress	Cardiovascular pg. 216
Broken Heart Syndrome	A temporary heart condition that is often brought on by stressful situations, such as the death of a loved one. Complaints include sudden chest pain or the sensation of a heart attack. basil · clary sage · comforting blend · jasmine · lavender	Cardiovascular pg. 216
Bronchitis	The disease is defined by low-grade chest pains, fever, hoarseness, and vigorous cough. Inflammation of the mucous membrane of the bronchial tubes. respiration blend · eucalyptus · cardamom · thyme · protective blend	Respiratory pg. 307
Bruise	Caused by an injury in which the skin is not broken. white fir · roman chamomile · geranium · helichrysum · soothing blend	Cardiovascular pg. 216; Integumentary pg. 264
Bruised Muscles	Contusions occur when a direct blow or repeated blows from a blunt object strike part of the body, crushing underlying muscle fibers and connective tissue without breaking the skin. birch · helichrysum · soothing blend · white fir · massage blend	Muscular pg. 283
Buerger's Disease	A condition in which the blood vessels swell and can become blocked with blood clots. This eventually damages or destroys skin tissues and may lead to infection. Usually first shows in the hands and feet and may expand to affect larger areas of the arms and legs. arborvitae · black pepper · clary sage · cypress · lemongrass	Cardiovascular pg. 216
Bulimia	A chronic eating disorder involving repeated and secretive episodes of eating, defined by uncontrolled fast ingestion of large quantities of food over a short period of time, followed by self-induced vomiting, purging, and anorexia. Often followed by feelings of guilt, depression, or self-disgust. grapefruit · patchouli · arborvitae · invigorating blend · renewing blend	Eating Disorders pg. 240
Bunions	An unusual enlargement of the joint (the first metatarsophalangeal joint, or MTPJ) at the base of the big toe (hallux). eucalyptus · cypress · ginger · wintergreen · basil	Skeletal pg. 313
Burns	Injuries to tissues caused by electricity, radiation, heat, friction, or chemicals. lavender · frankincense · anti-aging blend · myrrh · helichrysum	Integumentary pg. 264; First Aid pg. 251
Bursitis	Inflammation of the bursae, the fluid-filled sacs that protect against friction between bones and other tissues. It commonly effects the elbows, wrists, ankles, hips, or knees. wintergreen · soothing blend · birch · cypress · douglas fir	Skeletal pg. 313; First Aid pg. 251

Diffuse into the air or inhale from cupped hands.
Apply topically directly to affected areas.
Take internally in a capsule or in a glass of water.
TIP For children use 1-2 drops; for adults use 2-4 drops.

AILMENT	RECOMMENDED OILS AND USAGE	BODY SYSTEM/FOCUS AREA
Calcified Spine	Spine that is hardened by calcium deposits. birch, cellular complex blend, cedarwood, soothing blend, geranium	Skeletal pg. 313
Calluses	Thickened skin due to chronic irritation or rubbing. oregano, skin clearing blend, roman chamomile, cypress	Integumentary pg. 264
Cancer (bone)	A skeletal malignancy occurring as a sarcoma, in an area of accelerated growth or as metastasis from cancer somewhere else in the body. cellular complex blend, frankincense, helichrysum, white fir, lemon	Cellular Health pg. 221
Cancer (brain)	A brain tumor is an intracranial solid neoplasm, a tumor (defined as an uncommon growth of cells) within the brain or the central spinal canal. arborvitae, cellular complex blend, clove, frankincense, myrrh	Cellular Health pg. 221
Cancer (breast)	Breast cancer is caused by the development of malignant cells in the breast. Cancer cells are defined by uncontrolled distribution leading to unusual growth and the ability of these cells to infect normal tissue locally or to spread throughout the body. This process is called metastasis. protective blend, cellular complex blend, rosemary, frankincense, lavender	Cellular Health pg. 221
Cancer (cervical)	A disease in which the cells of the cervix become unusual and start to grow uncontrollably, forming tumors. cellular complex blend, women's blend, frankincense, rosemary, geranium	Cellular Health pg. 221
Cancer (colon)	A disease defined by the development of malignant cells in the lining or epithelium of the first and longest portion of the large intestine. detoxification blend, cellular complex blend, lavender, frankincense, geranium	Cellular Health pg. 221
Cancer (hurthle cell thyroid)	A rare form of cancer that affects the thyroid gland. lemon, rosemary, melissa, clary sage, frankincense	Cellular Health pg. 221
Cancer (liver)	A rather rare form of cancer with a high mortality rate. Liver cancers can be classified into two types. They are either primary, when the cancer starts in the liver itself, or metastatic. geranium, clove, frankincense, thyme, lemongrass	Cellular Health pg. 221
Cancer (lung)	Malignant growths of the lung. Inhaled carcinogens are known to be important predisposing causes, although the exact cause of lung cancer is not known. frankincense, melissa, eucalyptus, thyme, lavender	Cellular Health pg. 221
Cancer (ovarian)	Cancer of the ovaries, the egg-releasing and hormone-producing organs of the female reproductive tract. Malignant or cancerous, cells multiply and divide in an uncommon fashion. cellular complex blend, geranium, clary sage, frankincense, rosemary	Cellular Health pg. 221
Cancer (pancreatic)	The pancreas, located in the abdomen, has endocrine and exocrine functions; cancer cells can develop from both types of functional cells. cellular complex blend, frankincense, coriander, clove, protective blend	Cellular Health pg. 221

QUICK REFERENCE

STEPS: ❶ Look up ailment. ❷ Choose one or more of the recommended oils. (Order of recommendation is left to right.) ❸ Use oil(s) as indicated. ❹ Learn more: see the corresponding body system/focus area.

AILMENT	RECOMMENDED OILS AND USAGE	BODY SYSTEM/FOCUS AREA
Cancer (prostate)	A disease in which cells in the prostate gland become atypical and start to grow uncontrollably, forming tumors. oregano · cellular complex blend · detoxification blend · arborvitae · frankincense	Cellular Health pg. 221
Cancer (skin)	A cutaneous neoplasm created by ionizing radiation; certain genetic defects; chemical carcinogens, including tar products, petroleum, arsenics, and fumes from some molten metals; or overexposure to the sun or other sources of ultraviolet light. geranium · cellular complex blend · anti-aging blend · sandalwood · frankincense	Cellular Health pg. 221
Cancer (throat)	Cancer of the voice the vocal cords, voice box, and other parts of the throat, such as the tonsils and the oropharynx. This type of cancer is rather uncommon. It is often grouped with pharyngeal cancer, which forms in the pharynx and laryngeal cancer, which forms in the larynx. frankincense · cellular complex blend · thyme · lavender · cinnamon	Cellular Health pg. 221
Cancer (tongue)	A form of cancer that begins in the cells of the tongue. geranium · cellular complex blend · detoxification blend · frankincense · cinnamon	Cellular Health pg. 221
Cancer (uterine)	Any cancer that arises in the uterus such as leiomyosarcoma, choriocarcinoma, cervical CA, endometrial CA, and mesodermal mixed tumor. clary sage · cellular complex blend · frankincense · geranium · rosemary	Cellular Health pg. 221
Candida	A variety of yeast like fungi that are generally part of the normal flora of the mouth, skin, intestinal tract, and vagina, but can cause an array of infections. thyme · oregano · arborvitae · melaleuca · protective blend	Digestive & Intestinal pg. 235; Candida pg. 212
Canker Sores	Small yellowish or white sores or ulcers that grow inside the mouth. They are painful, self-healing, and can reappear. birch · metabolic blend · melaleuca · protective blend · oregano	Oral Health pg. 291
Cardiovascular Disease	Cardiovascular diseases include arteriosclerosis, coronary artery disease, heart valve disease, arrhythmia, heart failure, hypertension, orthostatic hypotension, shock, endocarditis, diseases of the aorta and its branches, disorders of the peripheral vascular system, and congenital heart disease. cellular complex blend · basil · coriander · cinnamon · marjoram	Cardiovascular pg. 216
Carpal Tunnel Syndrome	A disorder caused by compression at the wrist of the median nerve supplying the hand, causing tingling and numbness. cypress · lemongrass · massage blend · basil · frankincense	Nervous pg. 287
Cartilage Injury	Injury to fibrous connective tissue found in adults. helichrysum · lemongrass · soothing blend · birch · basil	Skeletal pg. 313
Cataracts	A cloudiness or murkiness in the normally transparent crystalline lens of the eye. This cloudiness can cause a decrease in vision and may lead to blindness. frankincense · cardamom · clary sage · clove · lavender	Nervous pg. 287
Cavities	The carious defect (lesion) produced by destruction of dentin and enamel in a tooth. clove · protective blend · birch · helichrysum · melaleuca	Oral Health pg. 291

Diffuse into the air or inhale from cupped hands.
Apply topically directly to affected areas.
Take internally in a capsule or in a glass of water.
TIP For children use 1-2 drops; for adults use 2-4 drops.

AILMENT	RECOMMENDED OILS AND USAGE	BODY SYSTEM/FOCUS AREA
Celiac Disease	A chronic gastrointestinal disease defined by sensitivity to malabsorption and gluten from the small intestine, resulting in stools with high fat content, diarrhea, and nutritional and vitamin deficiencies. Also called celiac sprue, gluten-sensitive enteropathy, and nontropical sprue. ginger, lemongrass, detoxification blend, digestion blend, metabolic blend	Autoimmune pg. 200; Digestive & Intestinal pg. 235
Cellulite	A fatty deposit causing an uneven or dimpled appearance, commonly found around the thighs. metabolic blend, grapefruit, lemon, wild orange, rosemary	Weight pg. 327
Chapped Skin	Skin that is rough, cracked, or reddened by exposure to cold or excessive moisture evaporation. frankincense, myrrh, roman chamomile, anti-aging blend, topical blend	Integumentary pg. 264
Chemical Imbalance	A disequilibrium of one or more neurotransmitters. Some believe that many, if not all, mental disorders are attributable to a chemical imbalance. cellular complex blend, detoxification blend, cilantro, geranium, frankincense	Brain pg. 208
Chemical Sensitivity Reaction	An allergic condition attributed to extreme sensitivity to various environmental chemicals, such as water, food, air, building materials, or fabrics. detoxification blend, cilantro, wild orange, coriander, arborvitae	Immune & Lymphatic pg. 259
Chest Infection	Infection of the increased visceral cavity of the trunk. detoxification blend, protective blend, cellular complex blend, eucalyptus, melaleuca	Immune & Lymphatic pg. 259
Chest Pain	Chest pain comes in many assortments, ranging from a sharp stab to a dull ache. Some chest pain is described as burning or crushing. In come cases, the pain travels up the neck, into the jaw, and then radiates through to the back or down one or both arms. protective blend, cellular complex blend, rosemary, basil, marjoram	Cardiovascular pg. 216; Pain & Inflammation pg. 294
Chicken Pox	An acute contagious disease, found in children, that is caused by the varicella-zoster virus and classified by skin eruptions, Malaise and minor fever. frankincense, cellular complex blend, thyme, melaleuca, protective blend	Immune & Lymphatic pg. 259
Chiggers	The juvenile form (larvae) of a certain type of mite of the family Trombiculidae. Mites are arachnids (like spiders and ticks). detoxification blend, repellent blend, lemongrass	First Aid pg. 251
Cholera	An intense infectious disease defined by watery diarrhea that is caused by the bacterium Vibrio cholera. detoxification blend, protective blend, cinnamon, respiration blend, rosemary	Immune & Lymphatic pg. 259
Cholesterol (high)	A sterol found in all animal tissues, bile, blood, and animal fats: a precursor of other body steroids. A high level of cholesterol in the blood is suggested in some cases of atherosclerosis, leading to heart disease. metabolic blend, lavender, basil, lemongrass, sage	Cardiovascular pg. 216
Chondromalacia Patella	Abnormal softening or degeneration of cartilage. See also patellofemoral syndrome. birch, soothing blend, cypress, lemongrass, helichrysum	Skeletal pg. 313

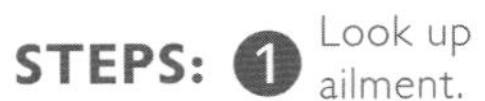

STEPS: 1 Look up ailment. 2 Choose one or more of the recommended oils. (Order of recommendation is left to right.) 3 Use oil(s) as indicated. 4 Learn more: see the corresponding body system/focus area.

AILMENT	RECOMMENDED OILS AND USAGE	BODY SYSTEM/FOCUS AREA
Chronic Fatigue	A debilitating sickness that causes staggering exhaustion and a constellation of immunological and neurological symptoms. massage blend · cellular complex blend · peppermint · basil · protective blend	Energy & Vitality pg. 248
Chronic Pain	Pain that lasts beyond the term of a painful stimulus or injury. Can also refer to cancer pain, pain from a chronic degenerative disease, or pain from an unknown cause. soothing blend · birch · wintergreen · lemongrass · cypress	Pain & Inflammation pg. 294
Circulatory System	An organ system that permits blood to circulate and transport nutrients. Also called the cardiovascular system. melaleuca · massage blend · cypress · basil · rosemary	Cardiovascular pg. 216
Cirrhosis	A continual degenerative disease in which normal liver cells are impaired and are then replaced by scar tissue. detoxification blend · geranium · lemon · frankincense · myrrh	Digestive & Intestinal pg. 235
Clogged Pores	A plug of sebum and keratin within a hair follicle. metabolic blend · cardamom · cilantro · lemon · topical blend	Integumentary pg. 264
Club Foot	A condition in which one or both feet are twisted into an unusual position at birth. The condition is also recognized as talipes or talipes equinovarus. arborvitae · helichrysum · basil · roman chamomile · rosemary	Skeletal pg. 313
Cold Body Temperature	A body temperature below 97.6 degrees Fahrenheit (36.4 degrees Celsius)." Normal" body temperature is 98.6 degrees Fahrenheit (37 degrees Celsius). cinnamon · black pepper · protective blend · eucalyptus · rosemary	Cardiovascular pg. 216
Cold (common)	A viral infection of the upper respiratory system, including the throat, nose, sinuses, Eustachian tubes, larynx, trachea, and bronchial tubes. cardamom · protective blend · melissa · lemon · melaleuca	Immune & Lymphatic pg. 259
Cold Hands/Feet/Nose	Common cardiovascular trigger most common in women, causing vasoconstriction, which triggers the body to conserve heat to maintain the core body temperature. massage blend · cypress · basil · ginger · lemongrass	Cardiovascular pg. 216
Cold Sores	Sensitive, reddish bumps usually located on or around the mouth and lip area, also known as fever blisters. clove · detoxification blend · arborvitae · protective blend · melaleuca	Integumentary pg. 264
Colic	Persistent, unexplained crying in a healthy baby between two weeks and five months of age. dill · cilantro · digestion blend · marjoram · bergamot	Children pg. 225
Colitis	Inflammation of the colon or large bowel which has several causes. The lining of the colon becomes swollen, and ulcers often develop. cardamom · ginger · peppermint · digestion blend · helichrysum	Digestive & Intestinal pg. 235

Diffuse into the air or inhale from cupped hands.
Apply topically directly to affected areas.
Take internally in a capsule or in a glass of water.
TIP For children use 1-2 drops; for adults use 2-4 drops.

AILMENT	RECOMMENDED OILS AND USAGE	BODY SYSTEM/FOCUS AREA
Coma	A state of severe unresponsiveness, in which an individual shows no voluntary movement or behavior. frankincense (topical); cellular complex blend (topical); sandalwood (topical); helichrysum (topical); cedarwood (topical)	Brain pg. 208
Concentration	vetiver (topical, aromatic); reassuring blend (topical, aromatic); focus blend (topical, aromatic); sandalwood (topical, aromatic); cedarwood (topical, aromatic)	Focus & Concentration pg. 255
Concentration (poor)	The inability to focus the mind. focus blend (topical, aromatic); cedarwood (topical, aromatic); reassuring blend (topical, aromatic); vetiver (topical, aromatic); peppermint (topical, aromatic)	Focus & Concentration pg. 255
Concussion	A trauma-induced change in mental status, with amnesia and confusion, and with or without a brief loss of consciousness. frankincense (aromatic, topical); bergamot (aromatic, topical); cypress (aromatic, topical); sandalwood (aromatic, topical); focus blend (aromatic, topical)	Brain pg. 208
Confidence (lack of)	invigorating blend (topical, aromatic); focus blend (topical, aromatic); encouraging blend (topical, aromatic); wild orange (topical, aromatic); jasmine (topical, aromatic)	Limbic pg. 273
Confusion	Impaired orientation in terms of time, place, or person; a disturbed mental state. focus blend (topical, aromatic); frankincense (topical, aromatic); jasmine (topical, aromatic); cedarwood (topical, aromatic); wild orange (topical, aromatic)	Mood & Behavior pg. 279
Congenital Heart Disease	An abnormality in the heart's structure that one is born with. cellular complex blend (internal, topical); marjoram (topical, internal); detoxification blend (topical, internal); protective blend (topical, internal); basil (topical, internal)	Cardiovascular pg. 216
Congestion	The existence of an unusual amount of fluid in a vessel or organ; especially excessive accumulation of blood, due either to increased afflux or to obstruction of return flow. lemon (topical, internal, aromatic); peppermint (aromatic, topical, internal); fennel (topical, internal, aromatic); respiration blend (topical, aromatic); eucalyptus (aromatic, topical, internal)	Respiratory pg. 307
Conjunctivitis	Inflammation or redness of the lining of the white part of the eye and the underside of the eyelid (conjunctiva) that can be caused by infection, allergic reaction, or physical agents like infrared or ultraviolet light. melaleuca (topical, aromatic); rosemary (topical, aromatic); ravensara (topical, aromatic); clary sage (topical, aromatic); melissa (topical, aromatic)	Immune & Lymphatic pg. 259
Connective Tissue Trauma	Injury to tissue that binds and supports other tissue. helichrysum (topical, internal); geranium (topical, internal); lemongrass (topical, internal); ginger (topical, internal); birch (topical)	Muscular pg. 283
Constipation	An intense or chronic condition in which bowel movements occur less often than normal or consist of hard, dry stools that are painful or difficult to pass. digestion blend (internal, topical); detoxification blend (internal, topical); rosemary (internal, topical); lemon (internal, topical); peppermint (internal, topical)	Digestive & Intestinal pg. 235
Convulsions	Also called seizures; a sudden violent contraction of a group of muscles. frankincense (topical); geranium (topical); helichrysum (topical); sandalwood (topical); grounding blend (topical)	Brain pg. 208; Muscular pg. 283; Nervous pg. 287
Corns	A small cone shaped callosity caused by pressure over a bony prominence, usually on a toe. ylang ylang (topical); arborvitae (topical); cellular complex blend (topical); clove (topical)	Integumentary pg. 264

QUICK REFERENCE

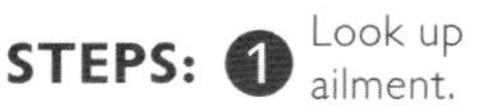

STEPS: 1 Look up ailment. 2 Choose one or more of the recommended oils. (Order of recommendation is left to right.) 3 Use oil(s) as indicated. 4 Learn more: see the corresponding body system/focus area.

AILMENT	RECOMMENDED OILS AND USAGE	BODY SYSTEM/FOCUS AREA
Cortisol Imbalance	An imbalance in the naturally produced hormone generated from the adrenal glands that aids in maintaining homeostasis of the body. Cortisol levels change regularly based on diet, stress, sleep, and exercise. basil, clove, cinnamon, coriander, geranium	Endocrine pg. 244
Cough	A strong release of air from the lungs that can be heard. Coughing protects the respiratory system by clearing it of secretion and irritants. lemon, frankincense, respiration blend, protective blend, cinnamon	Respiratory pg. 307
Cough (whooping)	Also known as pertussis; an extremely contagious disease which causes typical spasms (paroxysms) of uncontrollable coughing. eucalyptus, cypress, clary sage, respiration blend, oregano (dilute heavily)	Respiratory pg. 307
Cramps	A immediate, uncontrolled, spasmodic muscular contraction causing severe pain, often occurring in the leg or shoulder as the result of a strain or chill. soothing blend, arborvitae, cypress, basil, massage blend	Muscular pg. 283
Creutzfeldt-Jakob Disease	A degenerative neurological disorder (brain disease) that is incurable and unfailingly fatal. CJD is at times called a human form of mad cow disease (bovine spongiform encephalopathy or BSE), even though classic CJD is not related to BSE. However, given that BSE is believed to be the cause of variant Creutzfeldt–Jakob (vCJD) disease in humans, the two are usually confused. cellular complex blend, detoxification blend, cardamom, clove, rosemary	Brain pg. 208; Immune & Lymphatic pg. 259
Crohn's Disease	A type of inflammatory bowel disease (IBD), followed by swelling and dysfunction of the intestinal tract. ginger, digestion blend, bergamot, coriander, peppermint	Digestive & Intestinal pg. 235
Croup	A typical childhood ailment. It results from a viral infection of the larynx (voice box) and is associated with mild upper respiratory symptoms such as a cough and runny nose. arborvitae, eucalyptus, lemon, respiration blend, protective blend	Respiratory pg. 307
Crying Baby	A sudden, loud automatic or voluntary vocalization in response to fear, pain, or a startle reflex. calming blend, roman chamomile, grounding blend, protective blend, reassuring blend	Children pg. 225
Cushing's Syndrome	Cushing's syndrome describes the signs and symptoms related to prolonged exposure to inappropriately high levels of the hormone cortisol. This can be caused by taking glucocorticoid drugs, or diseases that result in excess cortisol, CRH levels or adrenocorticotropic hormone (ACTH). frankincense, rosemary, detoxification blend, clove, geranium	Endocrine pg. 244
Cuts	Separation of skin or other tissue created by a sharp edge, generating regular edges. lavender, myrrh, melaleuca, frankincense, protective blend	Integumentary pg. 264
Cyst	An abnormal closed epithelium-lined cavity in the body, containing semisolid material or liquid. cypress, eucalyptus, cardamom, juniper berry, frankincense	Integumentary pg. 264

Diffuse into the air or inhale from cupped hands.
Apply topically directly to affected areas.
Take internally in a capsule or in a glass of water.
TIP For children use 1-2 drops; for adults use 2-4 drops.

AILMENT	RECOMMENDED OILS AND USAGE	BODY SYSTEM/FOCUS AREA
Cystic Fibrosis	An inherited disease that affects the mucus and sweat glands. Cystic fibrosis primarily affects the lungs, pancreas, liver, intestines, sinuses, and sex organs. eucalyptus · lemon · ravensara · respiration blend · frankincense	Respiratory pg. 307
Cystitis	Cystitis is described as inflammation of the urinary bladder. Urethritis is an inflammation of the urethra, which is the passageway that connects the bladder with the exterior of the body. cypress · basil · lemongrass · juniper berry · protective blend	Immune & Lymphatic pg. 259
Cytomegalovirus Infection	A familiar virus that can infect almost anyone. Most people don't know they have CMV because it rarely causes symptoms. However, if someone is pregnant or have a weakened immune system, CMV is cause for concern. cellular complex blend · protective blend · detoxification blend · thyme · oregano	Immune & Lymphatic pg. 259
Dandruff	Dry, scaly material shed from the scalp. cedarwood · cleansing blend · lavender · rosemary · wintergreen	Integumentary pg. 264
Deep Vein Thrombosis	Arises when a blood clot (thrombus) forms in one or more of the deep veins in your body, typically in the legs. DVT can cause leg swelling or pain, but may occur without any symptoms. cellular complex blend · frankincense · tension blend · cypress · massage blend	Cardiovascular pg. 216
Dehydration (heat illness)	Dehydration occurs when more fluid is lost than is consumed, resulting from vigorous exercise, intense diarrhea, fever, vomiting, or even excessive sweating. detoxification blend · lemon · dill · wild orange · metabolic blend	First Aid pg. 251
Dehydrated Skin	Epidermis that lacks sebum or moisture, often identified by a pattern of fine lines, scaling, and itching. sandalwood · myrrh · anti-aging blend · frankincense · lemon	Integumentary pg. 264
Dementia	A collection of symptoms that includes decreased intellectual loss of memory, language, perception, judgment, or reasoning; may involve loss of emotional and behavioral control, personality changes, and reduced problem solving abilities. frankincense · cellular complex blend · clove · melissa · thyme	Brain pg. 208
Dengue Fever	An infectious tropical disease caused by the dengue virus also known as break bone fever. Symptoms include headache, fever, muscle and joint pains, and a distinctive skin rash that is similar to measles. melaleuca · arborvitae · eucalyptus · peppermint · oregano	Immune & Lymphatic pg. 259
Dental Infection	An infection of the jaw, face mouth, or throat that begins as a tooth cavity or infection. protective blend · clove · cinnamon · myrrh · patchouli	Oral Health pg. 291
Depression	A mental state of altered mood associated by feelings of despair, sadness, and discouragement. women's monthly blend · joyful blend · wild orange · uplifting blend · invigorating blend	Brain pg. 208; Limbic pg. 273
Deteriorating Spine	Deterioration of the series of vertebrae that extend from the cranium to the coccyx, providing support and forming a flexible bony case for the spinal cord. helichrysum · cellular complex blend · soothing blend · birch · white fir	Skeletal pg. 313

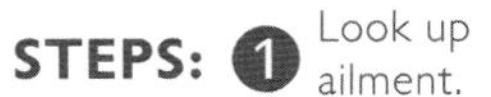

STEPS: 1 Look up ailment. 2 Choose one or more of the recommended oils. (Order of recommendation is left to right.) 3 Use oil(s) as indicated. 4 Learn more: see the corresponding body system/focus area.

AILMENT	RECOMMENDED OILS AND USAGE	BODY SYSTEM/FOCUS AREA
Detoxification	The removal of toxic substances from the body. clove · detoxification blend · lemongrass · helichrysum · rosemary	Detoxification pg. 230
Diabetes	A disease identified by an inability to process sugars in the diet, due to a decrease in or total absence of insulin production. protective blend · metabolic blend · cinnamon · coriander · rosemary	Blood Sugar pg. 205
Diabetes (gestational)	Gestational diabetes (or gestational diabetes mellitus, GDM) is a condition in which women without previously diagnosed diabetes show high blood glucose levels during pregnancy (especially during her third trimester). cinnamon · detoxification blend · coriander · protective blend · juniper berry	Pregnancy, Labor & Nursing pg. 301
Diabetic Sores	Open wounds or sores that normally occur on the bottom of the feet over weight-bearing areas. myrrh · lavender · patchouli · cedarwood · geranium	Integumentary pg. 264
Diaper Rash	Dermatitis of the genitals, buttocks, lower abdomen, or thigh folds of an infant or toddler. lavender · roman chamomile · patchouli · ylang ylang · frankincense	Children pg. 225
Diarrhea	Fast movement of fecal matter through the intestines resulting in poor absorption of nutritive elements, water, and electrolytes and producing abnormally persistent evacuation of watery stools. digestion blend · cardamom · coriander · peppermint · ginger	Digestive & Intestinal pg. 235
Diphtheria	A likely fatal, contagious disease that commonly involves the throat, nose, and air passages, but may also infect the skin. eucalyptus · respiration blend · protective blend · ginger · thyme	Respiratory pg. 307
Diverticulitis	A condition of the diverticulum of the intestinal tract, commonly in the colon, where inflammation may cause distended sacs extending from the colon and pain. digestion blend · ginger · detoxification blend · cilantro · cinnamon	Digestive & Intestinal pg. 235
Dizziness	A disturbed sense of relationship to space; a sensation of unsteadiness and a feeling of movement within the head; disequilibrium, lightheadedness. detoxification blend · cellular complex blend · women's blend · peppermint · grounding blend	Cardiovascular pg. 216
Do Quervain's Tenosynovitis	A painful condition affecting the tendons on the thumb side of the wrist. Commonly causes pain when grasping anything, turning the wrist, or making a fist. lemongrass · cypress · massage blend · soothing blend · birch	Muscular pg. 283; Skeletal pg. 313
Down Syndrome	A genetic disorder and the most common autosomal chromosome abnormality in humans, where extra genetic material from chromosome 21 is transferred to a newly formed embryo. These extra genes and DNA cause changes in development of the embryo and fetus, resulting in physical and mental abnormalities. cellular complex blend · melissa · clove · frankincense · cedarwood	Brain pg. 208
Drug Addiction	An overwhelming desire to continue taking a drug of which one has become habituated through repeated consumption because it produces a particular effect, typically an alteration of mental status. geranium · cassia · detoxification blend · cleansing blend · calming blend	Addictions pg. 190

Diffuse into the air or inhale from cupped hands.
Apply topically directly to affected areas.
Take internally in a capsule or in a glass of water.
TIP For children use 1-2 drops; for adults use 2-4 drops.

AILMENT	RECOMMENDED OILS AND USAGE	BODY SYSTEM/FOCUS AREA
Dumping Syndrome	A condition which occurs after eating in patients with shunts of the upper alimentary canal that includes flushing, sweating, dizziness, weakness, and vasomotor collapse. fennel, ginger, frankincense, helichrysum, digestion blend	Digestive & Intestinal pg. 235
Dysentery	A group of gastrointestinal disorders defined by inflammation of the intestines, particularly the colon. peppermint, ginger, protective blend, myrrh, eucalyptus	Digestive & Intestinal pg. 235
Dysmenorrhea	The existence of painful cramps during menstruation. women's monthly blend, clary sage, cypress, marjoram, thyme	Women's Health pg. 332
Dysphagia	Trouble swallowing. peppermint, ginger, black pepper, fennel, coriander	Digestive & Intestinal pg. 235; Oral Health pg. 291
E. Coli	A Gram-negative, facultative anaerobic, rod-shaped bacterium that is mainly found in the lower intestine of warm-blooded organisms (endotherms). Most E. coli strains are harmless, but some serotypes can cause severe food poisoning in humans, and are at times responsible for product recalls due to food contamination. clove, oregano, arborvitae, protective blend, cassia	Immune & Lymphatic pg. 259
Ear Infection	The existence and growth of bacteria or viruses in the ear. rosemary, basil, melaleuca, helichrysum, lavender	Respiratory pg. 307
Ear Mites	An insect parasite belonging to the order Acarina. focus blend, basil, cedarwood	Respiratory pg. 307; First Aid pg. 251
Earache	A pain in the ear, sensed as dull, sharp, intermittent, burning or constant. helichrysum, basil, soothing blend, ginger, cypress	Respiratory pg. 307
Eczema	Chronic or acute noncontagious inflammation of the skin, defined mainly by itching, redness, and the outbreak of lesions that may discharge serous matter and become scaly and encrusted. geranium, topical blend, helichrysum, roman chamomile, arborvitae	Integumentary pg. 264
Edema	A condition of unusually large fluid volume in the circulatory system or in tissues between the body's cells (interstitial spaces). rosemary, ginger, cypress, lemongrass, basil	Cardiovascular pg. 216; Pregnancy, Labor & Nursing pg. 301
Ehrlichiosis	A bacterial illness transmitted by ticks that causes flu-like symptoms. The symptoms and signs of ehrlichiosis range from mild body aches to severe fever and usually appear within a week or two of a tick bite. cellular complex blend, detoxification blend, frankincense, melissa, clove	Immune & Lymphatic pg. 259
Electrical Hypersensitivity Syndrome	A group of symptoms, caused by exposure to electromagnetic fields, that includes skin itch/rash/flushing/burning, and/or tingling; confusion/poor concentration, and/or memory loss; fatigue and weakness; headache; chest pain and heart problems cellular complex, frankincense, rosemary, lemongrass, helichrysum	Limbic pg. 273

QUICK REFERENCE

STEPS: ❶ Look up ailment. ❷ Choose one or more of the recommended oils. (Order of recommendation is left to right.) ❸ Use oil(s) as indicated. ❹ Learn more: see the corresponding body system/focus area.

AILMENT	RECOMMENDED OILS AND USAGE	BODY SYSTEM/FOCUS AREA
Emotional Trauma	An extremely disturbing experience that leads to lasting emotional impairment or psychological. frankincense, renewing & reassuring blend, cedarwood, grounding blend, melissa	Mood & Behavior pg. 279
Emphysema	A chronic respiratory disease where there is over-inflation of the air sacs (alveoli) in the lungs, which causes a decrease in lung function, and often, breathlessness. black pepper, peppermint, douglas fir, eucalyptus, respiratory blend	Respiratory pg. 307
Endocrine Issues	Group of glands and parts of glands that control metabolic activity. Thyroid, pituitary, ovaries, adrenals, and testes are all part of the endocrine system. frankincense, rosemary, clary sage, detoxification blend, rosemary	Endocrine pg. 244
Endometriosis	A condition in which part of the tissue similar to the lining of the uterus (endometrium) grows in other parts of the body. clary sage, lemon, sandalwood, cypress, geranium	Women's Health pg. 332
Endurance (poor)	Poor strength to continue an activity over a period of time. peppermint, basil, metabolic blend, respiration blend, cinnamon	Energy & Vitality pg. 248
Energy	The fuel for everyday living, essential for health. cinnamon, ginger, peppermint, joyful blend, wild orange	Energy & Vitality pg. 248
Epilepsy	A neurological disorder defined by recurrent seizures with or without a loss of consciousness. frankincense, cellular complex blend, cedarwood, focus blend, clary sage	Brain pg. 208
Epstein-Barr	A herpes virus that is the causative agent of infectious mononucleosis. It is also related to various types of human cancers. detoxification blend, cellular complex blend, basil, respiratory blend, protective blend	Immune & Lymphatic pg. 259
Erectile Dysfunction	The inability to achieve or sustain an erection for satisfactory sexual activity; also known as impotence. cypress, cellular complex, massage blend, clary sage, cassia	Men's Health pg. 276
Esophagitis	Inflammation of the esophagus. peppermint, ginger, lemon, fennel, coriander	Digestive & Intestinal pg. 235
Esophagus (function)	The part of the alimentary canal connecting the throat to the stomach. Esophagus problems can make it painful to eat and swallow. peppermint, lemon, metabolic blend, digestion blend, black pepper	Digestive & Intestinal pg. 235
Estrogen Imbalance	Imbalance in one of a group of hormonal steroid compounds that encourage the development of female secondary sex characteristics. women's blend, clary sage, ginger, geranium, frankincense	Women's Health pg. 332; Detoxification pg. 230
Exhaustion	A state of extreme loss of mental or physical abilities caused by illness or fatigue. detoxification blend, cellular complex blend, cleansing blend, inspiring blend, wild orange	Energy & Vitality pg. 248

Diffuse into the air or inhale from cupped hands.
Apply topically directly to affected areas.
Take internally in a capsule or in a glass of water.
TIP For children use 1-2 drops; for adults use 2-4 drops.

AILMENT	RECOMMENDED OILS AND USAGE	BODY SYSTEM/FOCUS AREA
Eyes (dry)	Dryness of the cornea caused by a deficiency of tear secretion in which the corneal surface appears rough and dull and the eye feels gritty and irritated. wild orange, cellular complex blend, detoxification blend, melaleuca	Respiratory pg. 307
Eyes (swollen)	Transient uncommon enlargement of a body part or area not due to cell proliferation. geranium, patchouli, detoxification blend, cypress, helichrysum	Nervous pg. 287
Fainting (treating)	Loss of consciousness caused by a brief lack of oxygen to the brain. cinnamon, frankincense, cypress, bergamot, peppermint	Cardiovascular pg. 216; First Aid pg. 251
Fatigue	Physical and/or mental exhaustion that can be triggered by stress, overwork, medication, or physical and mental illness or disease. cellular complex blend, detoxification blend, rosemary, cinnamon, thyme	Energy & Vitality pg. 248
Fear	A feeling of dread and agitation caused by the presence or imminence of danger. calming blend, detoxification blend, protective blend, wild orange, grounding blend	Mood & Behavior pg. 279
Fear of Flying	Fear or phobia of flight by vehicle such as a plane or helicopter (aviophobia.) Also fear of heights (acrophobia). Causes great anxiety or even panic attacks, making air travel very challenging. calming blend, vetiver, reassuring blend, focus blend, grounding blend	Mood & Behavior pg. 279
Fever	Any body temperature elevation above 100° F (37.8° C). peppermint, frankincense, eucalyptus, lime, cardamom	Immune & Lymphatic pg. 259
Fibrillation	Fast, uncoordinated contractions of the lower or upper chambers of the heart. marjoram, ginger, lime, massage blend, black pepper	Cardiovascular pg. 216; Muscular pg. 283
Fibrocystic Breasts	Lumpiness in one or both breasts. frankincense, geranium, clary sage, sandalwood, cypress	Endocrine pg. 244; Women's Health pg. 332
Fibroids (uterine)	Growths in the uterus which are non-cancerous (benign). sandalwood, frankincense, lemon, eucalyptus, helichrysum	Immune & Lymphatic pg. 259; Women's Health pg. 332;
Fibromyalgia	A neurosensory disorder defined by widespread joint stiffness, muscle pain, and fatigue. The condition is chronic, but pain comes and goes and moves about the body. soothing blend, cellular complex blend, detoxification blend, birch, wintergreen	Muscular pg. 283 Energy & Vitality pg. 248
Fifth's Disease (Human Parvovirus B19)	A highly contagious and common childhood ailment – sometimes called slapped-cheek disease because of the peculiar face rash that develops. cleansing blend, protective blend, cellular complex blend	Children pg. 225
Floaters	Deposits or condensation in the vitreous jelly of the eye that manifest as floating spots within the vision. Eye floaters may be present in one eye or both eyes. cellular complex blend, detoxification blend, metabolic blend	Nervous pg. 287

STEPS: ❶ Look up ailment. ❷ Choose one or more of the recommended oils. (Order of recommendation is left to right.) ❸ Use oil(s) as indicated. 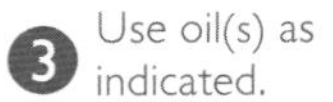 ❹ Learn more: see the corresponding body system/focus area.

AILMENT	RECOMMENDED OILS AND USAGE	BODY SYSTEM/FOCUS AREA
Flu (influenza)	Influenza, commonly known as "the flu", is an infectious disease of birds and mammals caused by RNA viruses of the family Orthomyxoviridae, the influenza viruses. The most common symptoms are chills, fever, runny nose, sore throat, muscle pains, headache, coughing, and weakness/fatigue. protective blend · respiratory blend · oregano · melissa · thyme	Immune & Lymphatic pg. 259
Focal Brain Dysfunction (brain injury)	Injuries confined to one area of the brain, often the result of a severe blow to the head, violent assault, a bullet from a firearm, or a fall. frankincense · helichrysum · cellular complex · sandalwood · grounding blend	Limbic pg. 273; Nervous pg. 287
Follicular Thyroid Cancer	Occurs when cells in the thyroid undergo genetic changes (mutations). The mutations allow the cells to multiply and grow rapidly. rosemary · clary sage · frankincense · lemon · sandalwood	Cellular Health pg. 221
Food Addiction	A person suffering from compulsive overeating has frequent episodes of uncontrolled eating, during which they may feel out of control, often consuming food past the point of being comfortably full. Binging in this way is typically followed by feelings of guilt and depression. grapefruit · metabolic blend · reassuring blend · ginger · basil	Addictions pg. 47
Food Poisoning	Health problems which arising from eating contaminated food. detoxification blend · clove · digestion blend · cinnamon · black pepper	Digestive & Intestinal pg. 235; Immune & Lymphatic pg. 259
Fragile Hair	Damaged or dry hair that is prone to breaking because it is so weak. cedarwood · cellular complex blend · rosemary · women's blend	Integumentary pg. 264
Frozen Shoulder	A condition also known as adhesive capsulitis characterized by stiffness and pain in the shoulder joint. birch · soothing blend · white fir · wintergreen · lemongrass	Muscular pg. 283; Skeletal pg. 313
Fungal Skin Infection	Any inflammatory condition generated by a fungus. frankincense · melaleuca · arborvitae · cedarwood · patchouli	Integumentary pg. 264
Fungus	Any of numerous eukaryotic organisms that duplicate by spores. arborvitae · cinnamon · oregano · clove · melaleuca	Candida pg. 212
Gallbladder	A common term for any condition related to dysfunctional bile ducts, including cholecystitis, cholelithiasis or gallstones, and cancer. detoxification blend · geranium · metabolic blend · grapefruit · rosemary	Digestive & Intestinal pg. 235
Gallbladder Infection	Generally categorized as inflammation in the gallbladder, which can be caused by gallstones (cholelithiasis), excessive alcohol consumption, tumor, or infections that can cause bile to accumulate. clove · protective blend · detoxification blend · coriander · helichrysum	Digestive & Intestinal pg. 235
Gallbladder Stones	A stone-like mass (calculus) in the gallbladder; the existence of gallstones is known medically as cholelithiasis. lemon · cilantro · juniper berry · grapefruit · geranium	Digestive & Intestinal pg. 235

- Diffuse into the air or inhale from cupped hands.
- Apply topically directly to affected areas.
- Take internally in a capsule or in a glass of water.
- TIP: For children use 1-2 drops; for adults use 2-4 drops.

AILMENT	RECOMMENDED OILS AND USAGE	BODY SYSTEM/FOCUS AREA
Ganglion Cyst	Lumps that most frequently develop in the wrist. They're commonly round or oval and are filled with a jelly-like fluid. cellular complex blend (topical, internal); detoxification blend (topical, internal); frankincense (topical, internal); lemongrass (topical, internal); basil (topical, internal)	Skeletal pg. 313
Gangrene	The death or decay of a tissue or an organ caused by a lack of blood supply. melaleuca (topical, internal); melissa (topical, internal); arborvitae (topical); protective blend (topical, internal); lavender (topical, internal)	Cardiovascular pg. 216; Immune & Lymphatic pg. 259
Gas (flatulence)	An overabundance of excessive gas in the digestive tract. fennel (topical, internal); dill (topical, internal); digestion blend (topical, internal); coriander (topical, internal); ginger (topical, internal)	Digestive & Intestinal pg. 235
Gastritis	Inflammation of the lining of the stomach; the term is also commonly used to cover a variety of symptoms resulting from stomach lining inflammation and symptoms of discomfort or burning. ginger (topical, internal); lemongrass (topical, internal); digestion blend (topical, internal); peppermint (topical, internal); coriander (topical, internal)	Digestive & Intestinal pg. 235
Gastroenteritis	Inflammation of the intestines and stomach. clove (internal, topical); bergamot (topical, internal); detoxification blend (topical, internal); protective blend (topical, internal); digestion blend (topical, internal)	Digestive & Intestinal pg. 235
Gastroesophageal Reflux Disease	A condition in which the acidified liquid contents of the stomach backs up into the esophagus. ginger (topical, internal); detoxification blend (topical, internal); lemon (topical, internal); digestion blend (topical, internal); cilantro (topical, internal)	Digestive & Intestinal pg. 235
Genital Warts	Genital warts, which are also called venereal warts or condylomata acuminata, are growths in the genital area generated by a sexually transmitted papillomavirus. lemongrass (topical, internal); arborvitae (topical, internal); detoxification blend (topical, internal); frankincense (topical, internal); thyme (topical, internal)	Women's Health pg. 332; Men's Health pg. 276
Giardia	A typical genus of flagellate protozoans and a major cause of nonbacterial diarrhea in North America and of intestinal disease globally. detoxification blend (topical, internal); cardamom (topical, internal); patchouli (topical, internal); rosemary (topical, internal); lavender (topical, internal)	Digestive & Intestinal pg. 235; Immune & Lymphatic pg. 259
Gingivitis	Inflammation of the gums, identified by redness and swelling. protective blend (topical, internal); clove (topical, internal); myrrh (topical); grapefruit (topical); melaleuca (topical)	Oral Health pg. 291
Glaucoma	A disease associated with elevated intraocular pressure, in which damage to the eye nerve can lead to loss of vision and even blindness. cellular complex blend (topical, internal); arborvitae (topical); frankincense (topical); anti-aging blend (topical); helichrysum (topical)	Nervous pg. 287
Goiter	A goitre or goiter (Latin gutteria, struma), is a swelling of the thyroid gland, sometimes leading to a swelling of the larynx (voice box) or neck. rosemary (topical, internal); detoxification blend (topical, internal); metabolic blend (topical, internal); myrrh (topical, diffuse); lemongrass (topical, internal)	Endocrine pg. 244
Gout	A form of intense arthritis that causes severe swelling and pain in the joints. It most typically affects the big toe, but may also affect the ankle, heel, wrist, hand, or elbow. lemon (topical, internal); wintergreen (topical, internal); douglas fir (topical, internal); massage blend (topical); soothing blend (topical)	Skeletal pg. 313; Pain & Inflammation pg. 294
Grave's Disease	Thyroid dysfunction and all of its clinical associations. metabolic blend (topical, internal); ginger (topical, internal); lemongrass (topical, internal); myrrh (topical, internal); frankincense (topical, internal)	Autoimmune pg. 200

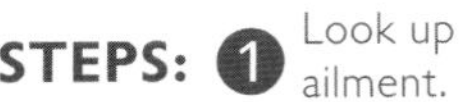

STEPS: 1 Look up ailment. 2 Choose one or more of the recommended oils. (Order of recommendation is left to right.) 3 Use oil(s) as indicated. 4 Learn more: see the corresponding body system/focus area.

AILMENT	RECOMMENDED OILS AND USAGE	BODY SYSTEM/FOCUS AREA
Grief	The commonly emotional response to an external and consciously recognized loss. calming blend · frankincense · comforting blend · bergamot · joyful blend	Mood & Behavior pg. 279
Growing Pains	Pains in the joints and limbs of children or adolescents, frequently appearing at night and often attributed to rapid growth but arising from various unrelated causes. lemongrass · marjoram · soothing blend · white fir · wintergreen	Muscular pg. 283
Gulf War Syndrome	Illnesses experienced by American veterans who were in the Gulf War. Symptoms include fatigue, headache, muscle and/or joint pain, gastrointestinal complaints, neurological problems, and possibly tumors. cellular complex · cedarwood · frankincense · tension blend · patchouli	Limbic pg. 273
Gum Disease	Dentistry Gingival disease, often in the form of gingivitis and bone loss to toxins produced by bacteria in plaque collecting along the gum line. clove · grapefruit · protective blend · myrrh · melaleuca	Oral Health pg. 291
Gums (bleeding)	Gums that bleed during and after tooth brushing. myrrh · helichrysum · clove · frankincense · melaleuca	Oral Health pg. 291
H. Pylori	A type of bacteria called Helicobacter pylori (H. pylori) which infects the stomach. This typically happens during childhood. A common cause of peptic ulcers, H. pylori infection may be present in more than half the people in the world. detoxification blend · patchouli · frankincense · digestion blend · ginger	Immune & Lymphatic pg. 259
Hair (dry)	When the scalp doesn't make enough oil to moisturize the hair, or the hair lets moisture escape. women's blend · patchouli · detoxification blend · geranium · sandalwood	Integumentary pg. 264
Hair Loss	The lack of all or a significant part of the hair on the head or other parts of the body. cellular complex blend · arborvitae · lavender · rosemary · thyme	Integumentary pg. 264
Hair (oily)	cellular complex blend · cleansing blend · rosemary · basil · cypress	Integumentary pg. 264
Halitosis	The condition of having revolting-smelling breath. detoxification blend · metabolic blend · cilantro · peppermint · protective blend	Oral Health pg. 291
Hallucinations	Sensations that appear to be real but are created within the mind. Examples include seeing things that are not there, hearing voices or other sounds, experiencing body sensations like crawling feelings on the skin, or smelling odors that are not there. myrrh · sandalwood · cedarwood · grounding blend · frankincense	Limbic pg. 273
Hands (dry)	An uncomfortable condition marked by scaling, itching, and cracking of the skin on hands. cellular complex blend · oregano · cleansing blend · geranium · sandalwood	Integumentary pg. 264

Diffuse into the air or inhale from cupped hands.
Apply topically directly to affected areas.
Take internally in a capsule or in a glass of water.
TIP For children use 1-2 drops; for adults use 2-4 drops.

AILMENT	RECOMMENDED OILS AND USAGE	BODY SYSTEM/FOCUS AREA
Hand, Foot & Mouth Disease	A mild, contagious viral infection common in young children that is defined by sores in the mouth and a rash on the feet and hands. Hand-foot-and-mouth disease is most normally caused by a coxsackievirus. clove · cellular complex blend · protective blend · melissa · eucalyptus	Immune & Lymphatic pg. 259
Hangover	A group of disagreeable physical effects, including thirst, nausea, headache, fatigue, and irritability, resulting from the heavy consumption of alcohol and/or certain drugs. cinnamon · metabolic blend · detoxification blend · lemon · grapefruit	Detoxification pg. 230
Hardening of Arteries	A chronic condition defined by hardening and thickening of the arteries and the build-up of plaque on the arterial walls. marjoram · basil · lavender · melissa · lemon	Cardiovascular pg. 216
Hashimoto's Disease	An autoimmune disease of the thyroid gland, emerging from diffuse goiter, infiltration of the thyroid gland with lymphocytes, and hypothyroidism. clove · frankincense · myrrh · ginger · peppermint	Endocrine pg. 244; Autoimmune pg. 200
Hay Fever	An allergic condition affecting the mucous membranes of the eyes and upper respiratory tract, typically defined by nasal discharge, sneezing, itchy, watery eyes and normally caused by an abnormal sensitivity to airborne pollen. cilantro · lavender · melaleuca · respiration blend · lemon	Allergies pg. 194
Head Lice	A louse transmitted in crowded conditions – e.g., homeless shelters, day care centers. melaleuca · rosemary · repellent blend · cedarwood · arborvitae	Parasites pg. 298; Integumentary pg. 264; First Aid pg. 251
Headache	Pain in the head which can emerge from many disorders or may be a disorder in and of itself. tension blend · lavender · peppermint · wintergreen · frankincense	Muscular pg. 283; Pain & Inflammation pg. 294
Headaches (blood sugar)	Headaches caused by blood sugar levels being either too high or too low. detoxification blend · cinnamon · cassia · metabolic blend · protective blend	Blood Sugar pg. 205
Headache (sinus)	Pain and headache over the affected sinuses may appear, as well as a feeling of pressure which may worsen when bending over. melissa · cedarwood · rosemary · peppermint · cilantro	Respiratory pg. 307
Headache (tension)	A very typical form of headache that is defined by severe muscle contractions triggered by exertion or stress. frankincense · tension blend · soothing blend · peppermint · tension blend	Muscular pg. 283; Pain & Inflammation pg. 294
Hearing in a Tunnel	The ability to hear only one thing at a time, instead of the culmination of sound from the entire room. helichrysum · lemon · clary sage · cardamom · cleansing blend	Respiratory pg. 307
Hearing Problems	An impairment of any degree of the ability to apprehend sound. frankincense · helichrysum · melaleuca · basil · lemon	Respiratory pg. 307

 Look up ailment. ② Choose one or more of the recommended oils. (Order of recommendation is left to right.) 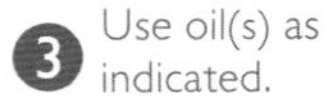 Use oil(s) as indicated. ④ Learn more: see the corresponding body system/focus area.

AILMENT	RECOMMENDED OILS AND USAGE	BODY SYSTEM/FOCUS AREA
Heart Failure	Sudden interruption or inadequate supply of blood to the heart, commonly resulting from occlusion or obstruction of a coronary artery and often defined by severe chest pain. lemongrass, marjoram, rosemary, thyme	Cardiovascular pg. 216
Heartburn	A burning feeling in the chest that can extend to the neck, face, and throat; commonly worsened by bending or lying down. metabolic blend, peppermint, lemon, digestion blend, ginger	Digestive & Intestinal pg. 235
Heat Exhaustion	A condition deriving from exposure to intense heat, defined by dizziness, abdominal cramp, and prostration. Also called heat prostration. peppermint, bergamot, lime, lemon, basil	First Aid pg. 251
Heatstroke	A serious condition caused by impairment of the body's temperature-regulating capabilities, emerging from prolonged exposure to excessive heat and defined by cessation of high fever, sweating, severe headache, hot dry skin, and in serious cases collapse and coma. peppermint, detoxification blend, dill, lemon	Nervous pg. 287
Hematoma	A localized swelling filled with blood emerging from a break in a blood vessel. massage blend, marjoram, cypress, lemongrass, helichrysum	Cardiovascular pg. 216
Hemochromatosis	An inherited blood disorder that causes the body to retain more than normal amounts of iron. This iron excess can lead to serious health consequences, most notably cirrhosis of the liver. detoxification blend, cellular complex blend, arborvitae	Digestive & Intestinal pg. 235
Hemophilia	One of a group of inherited bleeding disorders that cause abnormal or exaggerated bleeding and poor blood clotting. helichrysum, geranium, lavender, vetiver, roman chamomile	Cardiovascular pg. 216
Hemorrhage	Very extreme, massive bleeding that is difficult to control. wild orange, ylang ylang, helichrysum	Cardiovascular pg. 216
Hemorrhoids	Enlarged veins in the lower rectum or anus. helichrysum, detoxification blend, myrrh, digestion blend, cypress	Cardiovascular pg. 216; Digestive & Intestinal pg. 235; Integumentary pg. 264
Hepatitis	An inflammation of the liver, with accompanying liver cell damage or cell death, created frequently by viral infection, but also by certain poisons, drugs, or chemicals. geranium, myrrh, detoxification blend, melaleuca, frankincense	Immune & Lymphatic pg. 259
Hernia, Hiatal	A hiatal hernia happens when part of the stomach pushes upward through the diaphragm. The diaphragm naturally has a small opening (hiatus) through which the food tube (esophagus) passes on its way to connect to the stomach. The stomach can push up through this opening and cause a hiatal hernia. patchouli, cypress, basil, peppermint, ginger	Digestive & Intestinal pg. 235
Hernia, Incisional	Hernia through a previous abdominal incision. melissa, arborvitae, basil, helichrysum, lemongrass	Integumentary pg. 264

Diffuse into the air or inhale from cupped hands. (aromatic)
Apply topically directly to affected areas. (topical)
Take internally in a capsule or in a glass of water. (internal)
TIP For children use 1-2 drops; for adults use 2-4 drops.

AILMENT	RECOMMENDED OILS AND USAGE	BODY SYSTEM/FOCUS AREA
Herniated Disc	Swelling of a fragmented or degenerated intervertebral disc into the intervertebral foramen with likely compression of a nerve root or into the spinal canal with likely compression of the cauda equina in the lumbar region or the spinal cord at higher levels. birch (topical); wintergreen (topical); soothing blend (topical); grounding blend (topical); cypress (topical)	Skeletal pg. 313
Herpes Simplex	A repeated viral disease that is caused by herpes virus type one and is distinct by fluid-containing vesicles on the lips, mouth, or face; cold sore. melissa (topical, internal); clove (topical, internal); peppermint (topical, internal); melaleuca (internal, topical); protective blend (internal, topical)	Immune & Lymphatic pg. 259
Hiccups	The outcome of an involuntary, spasmodic contraction of the diaphragm followed by the closing of the throat. arborvitae (topical, internal); detoxification blend (topical, internal); calming blend (topical, internal); sandalwood (topical, internal); peppermint (internal, topical)	Respiratory pg. 307
Hives	An allergic skin reaction resulting in localized redness, swelling, and itching. roman chamomile (topical); melaleuca (topical, internal); frankincense (topical, internal); peppermint (topical, internal); lavender (internal, topical)	Allergies pg. 194; Integumentary pg. 264
Hoarse Voice	Harsh, raspy, or strained voice. lemon (internal); cinnamon (internal); protective blend (internal); bergamot (internal); frankincense (internal)	Oral Health pg. 291
Hodgkin's Disease	A malignant disease, a form of lymphoma, defined by painless enlargement of the lymph nodes, liver, and spleen. Also called lymphoadenoma or lymphogranulomatosis. rosemary (internal, topical); clove (internal, topical); sandalwood (topical, internal); lemon (internal, topical); frankincense (internal, topical)	Cellular Health pg. 221
Hormonal Imbalance (female)	Subtle changes in the endocrine system resulting in a variety of conditions such as sleep disorders, acne, memory fog, digestive issues, fatigue, persistent hunger, mood swings and depression, weight gain, headaches and migraines, hot flashes, vaginal dryness, breast tenderness, and loss of libido. clary sage (topical, internal); women's monthly blend (topical); frankincense (internal, topical); sandalwood (topical, internal); ylang ylang (topical, internal)	Women's Health pg. 332; Detoxification pg. 230
Hormone Imbalance (male)	Subtle changes in the endocrine system resulting in a variety of conditions such as hot flashes, psychogenic changes, bone mineral loss, decreased libido and/or sexual function, weight gain, depression and other symptoms identical to the female menopause. cleansing blend (topical, aromatic); protective blend (internal, topical); clary sage (topical, internal, aromatic); frankincense (internal, topical, aromatic); ylang ylang (topical, internal, aromatic)	Men's Health pg. 276; Detoxification pg. 230
Hot Flashes	Troublesome warmth beginning in the upper chest, neck, and face followed by chills and sweating. women's blend (topical); women's monthly blend (topical); peppermint (topical, internal); clary sage (topical, internal); grounding blend (topical)	Women's Health pg. 332
Huntington's Disease	A rare hereditary condition that causes mental deterioration and progressive chorea (jerky muscle movements) that ends in dementia. basil (internal, topical); frankincense (internal, topical); geranium (internal, topical); thyme (internal, topical); clove (internal, topical)	Brain pg. 208; Nervous pg. 287
Hydrocephalus	Hydrocephalus is an unusual expansion of cavities (ventricles) within the brain that is caused by the accumulation of cerebrospinal fluid. massage blend (topical); basil (topical, internal); frankincense (topical, internal); cardamom (topical, internal); juniper berry (topical, internal)	Brain pg. 208
Hyperactivity	Excessive or abnormally increased muscular activity or function. cedarwood (topical, aromatic); focus blend (topical, aromatic); vetiver (topical, aromatic); lavender (topical, aromatic); calming blend (topical, aromatic)	Focus & Concentration pg. 255

QUICK REFERENCE

STEPS: 1 Look up ailment. 2 Choose one or more of the recommended oils. (Order of recommendation is left to right.) 3 Use oil(s) as indicated. 4 Learn more: see the corresponding body system/focus area.

AILMENT	RECOMMENDED OILS AND USAGE	BODY SYSTEM/FOCUS AREA
Hyperpnea	Fast and deep respiration that appears normally after exercise or abnormally when associated with fevers or other disorders. peppermint, cardamom, eucalyptus, respiration blend, ylang ylang	Respiratory pg. 307
Hypersomnia	A condition in which a person has trouble staying awake during the day. People who have hypersomnia can fall asleep at any time. This may include a lack of energy and trouble thinking clearly. vetiver, patchouli, marjoram, lavender, cedarwood	Sleep pg. 317
Hyperthyroidism	A medical condition that results from an excess of thyroid hormone in the blood. frankincense, rosemary, myrrh, ginger, lemongrass	Endocrine pg. 244
Hypoglycemia	Low blood sugar which occurs when blood sugar (or blood glucose) concentrations fall below a level necessary to properly support the body's need for energy and stability throughout its cells. metabolic blend, cinnamon, detoxification blend, coriander, juniper berry	Blood Sugar pg. 205
Hypothermia	A condition in which core temperature drops below the needed temperature for normal metabolism and body functions which is defined as 35.0° C (95.0° F). cellular complex blend, patchouli, wild orange	First Aid pg. 251
Hypothyroidism	A state in which thyroid hormone production is below normal. clove, frankincense, myrrh, ginger, peppermint	Endocrine pg. 244
Hysteria	A psychiatric disorder determined by the presentation of a physical ailment without an organic cause. calming blend, frankincense, women's monthly blend, vetiver, grounding blend	Mood & Behavior pg. 279
Ichthyosis Vulgaris	An inherited condition showing up in childhood and defined by fine scales on the trunk and extremities. Also called Ichthyosis simplex. respiration blend, cedarwood, frankincense	Integumentary pg. 264
Immune System	The body's defense that protects against disease (pathogens) and helps to keep the body healthy. protective blend, detoxification blend, clove, melaleuca, oregano	Immune & Lymphatic pg. 259
Impetigo	A localized bacterial infection of the skin. There are two types, epidemic and bullous. geranium, oregano, women's monthly blend, lavender, topical blend	Immune & Lymphatic pg. 259; Integumentary pg. 264
Impotence	Referred to as erectile dysfunction, is the inability to maintain or achieve an erection long enough to engage in sexual intercourse. cleansing blend, geranium, clary sage, massage blend, cassia	Men's Health pg. 276
Incontinence	Loss of bladder control. cypress, massage blend, basil, helichrysum, ylang ylang	Urinary pg. 324
Indigestion	A broad term covering a group of universal symptoms in the digestive tract. It is commonly described as a feeling of bloating, fullness, heartburn, nausea, or gassy discomfort in the chest or abdomen. digestion blend, black pepper, metabolic blend, peppermint, ginger	Digestive & Intestinal pg. 235

Diffuse into the air or inhale from cupped hands.
Apply topically directly to affected areas.
Take internally in a capsule or in a glass of water.
TIP For children use 1-2 drops; for adults use 2-4 drops.

AILMENT	RECOMMENDED OILS AND USAGE	BODY SYSTEM/FOCUS AREA
Infant Reflux	Infant reflux (sometimes called infant acid reflux) is the condition where the contents of the stomach are spit out, commonly shortly after feeding. fennel, digestion blend, peppermint, lavender, dill	Children pg. 225
Infected Wounds	Infiltration and multiplication of microorganisms in body tissues. myrrh, helichrysum, frankincense, melaleuca, lavender	Integumentary pg. 264; First Aid pg. 251
Infection	Infiltration and multiplication of microorganisms in body tissues, commonly causing local cellular injury due to competitive toxins, metabolism, intracellular replication, or antigen-antibody response. protective blend, melissa, clove, oregano, cinnamon	Immune & Lymphatic pg. 259
Infertility	The inability to conceive a pregnancy after trying to do so for at least one full year. clary sage, frankincense, cellular complex blend, ylang ylang, rosemary	Men's Health pg. 276; Women's Health pg. 332
Inflammation	A protective tissue response to destruction of tissues or injury, which serves to dilute, destroy, or wall off both the injurious agent and the injured tissues. wintergreen, birch, soothing blend, frankincense, melaleuca	Pain & Inflammation pg. 294
Inflammatory Bowel Disease	A chronic disorder of the gastrointestinal tract, typically Crohn's disease or an ulcerative form of colitis, defined by inflammation of the intestine and resulting in persistent diarrhea and abdominal cramping. wintergreen, digestion blend, detoxification blend	Autoimmune pg. 200
Inflammatory Myopathies	A group of diseases that involves chronic muscle inflammation, accompanied by muscle weakness. wintergreen, basil, birch, lemongrass, massage blend	Autoimmune pg. 200; Muscular pg. 283
Ingrown Toenail	Abnormal growth of a toenail, with one (usually the outer) edge growing deeply into the nail groove and surrounding tissues. ylang ylang, cellular complex blend, detoxification blend	Integumentary pg. 264
Injury - muscles, bones, connective tissues, bruising/skin	Harm or damage caused to the body, specifically muscular (tear), bone (broken), or other connective tissue trauma. white fir, birch, douglas fir, helichrysum, wintergreen	First Aid pg. 251; Muscular pg. 283; Skeletal pg. 313
Insect Bites	Allergic response of a bite or sting of an insect. Allergic response to a bite or sting of an insect. Commonly, insects which generate allergic responses are either stinging insects such as bees, wasps and hornets or biting insects such as ticks, mosquitoes or even ants. lavender, cleansing blend, roman chamomile, melissa, basil	First Aid pg. 251
Insect Repellent	A substance applied to clothing, skin, or other surfaces which discourages insects from landing or climbing on that surface. There are also insect repellent products available based on sound production, particularly ultrasound. repellent blend, arborvitae, cedarwood, cleansing blend, patchouli	First Aid pg. 251
Insomnia	The inability to access a satisfactory amount or quality of sleep. lavender, vetiver, calming blend, marjoram, roman chamomile	Sleep pg. 317

STEPS: 1 Look up ailment. 2 Choose one or more of the recommended oils. (Order of recommendation is left to right.) 3 Use oil(s) as indicated. 4 Learn more: see the corresponding body system/focus area.

AILMENT	RECOMMENDED OILS AND USAGE	BODY SYSTEM/FOCUS AREA
Insulin Imbalances	A condition in which the cells of the body become resistant to the hormone insulin. Insulin is produced by the pancreas to help the body use sugar (glucose) for storing energy. oregano · metabolic blend · cleansing blend · cinnamon · protective blend	Blood Sugar pg. 205
Insulin Resistance	A physiological condition in which cells fail to respond to the normal actions of the hormone insulin. The body produces insulin, but the cells in the body become resistant to insulin (through changes in their surface receptors) and are unable to use it as effectively. oregano · metabolic blend · ylang ylang · detoxification blend · protective blend	Blood Sugar pg. 205
Iris Inflammation	A condition caused by blunt trauma to the eye. frankincense · helichrysum · cellular complex blend · anti-aging blend · sandalwood	Nervous pg. 287
Irritable Bowel Syndrome	A typical intestinal condition defined by abdominal cramps and pain, changes in bowel movements (diarrhea, constipation, or both), bloating, gassiness, nausea, and other symptoms. digestion blend · ginger · peppermint · cardamom · detoxification blend	Digestive & Intestinal pg. 235
Itching	An acute, disturbing irritation or tickling sensation that may be felt all over the skin's surface or confined to just one area. melaleuca · detoxification blend · metabolic blend · lavender · peppermint	Allergies pg. 194; Integumentary pg. 264
Jaundice	A case in which one's skin and the whites of the eyes are discolored yellow caused by an increased level of bile pigments in the blood resulting from liver disease. detoxification blend · geranium · rosemary · juniper berry · lemongrass	Digestive & Intestinal pg. 235
Jet Lag	A condition marked by insomnia, fatigue, and irritability that is caused by air travel through changing time zones. cellular complex blend · peppermint · reassuring blend · lavender · grounding blend	Sleep pg. 317
Jock Itch	Also known as tinea cruris, jock itch is a growth of fungus in the moist, warm, groin area. melaleuca · thyme · patchouli · myrrh · cedarwood	Men's Health pg. 276; Candida pg. 212
Joint Pain	Severe pain that is sharp, extending along a nerve or group of nerves, experienced in a joint and/or joints. wintergreen · soothing blend · lemongrass · massage blend · roman chamomile	Skeletal pg. 313
Kidney Infection	An inflammation of the kidney and upper urinary tract that commonly results from noncontagious bacterial infection of the bladder. protective blend · cinnamon · juniper berry · coriander · rosemary	Urinary pg. 324
Kidney Stones	A solid build up of material that form in the tubal system of the kidney. lemon · sandalwood · clary sage · wild orange · eucalyptus	Urinary pg. 324
Kidneys	A bean shaped organ primarily responsible for the removal of waste products caused by metabolism. Kidneys serve the body as a natural filter of the blood stream and remove water-soluble wastes, which are diverted to the bladder. juniper berry · lemongrass · thyme · rosemary · coriander	Urinary pg. 324

Diffuse into the air or inhale from cupped hands.
Apply topically directly to affected areas.
Take internally in a capsule or in a glass of water.
TIP For children use 1-2 drops; for adults use 2-4 drops.

AILMENT	RECOMMENDED OILS AND USAGE	BODY SYSTEM/FOCUS AREA
Knee Cartilage Injury	Injury to the cartilage in the knee. lemongrass · white fir · wintergreen · birch · helichrysum	Skeletal pg. 313
Labor	The process during which the uterus contracts and the cervix opens to allow the transition of a baby into the vagina. calming blend · women's monthly blend · ylang ylang · frankincense · clary sage	Pregnancy, Labor & Nursing pg. 301
Lactation Problems	Engorged breasts, sore nipples, and infection that new nursing mothers may experience. fennel · clary sage · dill · coriander · basil	Pregnancy, Labor & Nursing pg. 301
Lactose Intolerance	Failure of the body to digest lactose. cellular complex blend · detoxification blend · dill · coriander · lemongrass	Digestive & Intestinal pg. 235; Immune & Lymphatic pg. 259
Laryngitis	Inflammation of the larynx followed by hoarseness of the voice. lemon · protective blend · myrrh · sandalwood · frankincense	Respiratory pg. 307
Lead Poisoning	A condition caused by a buildup of lead in the body, often over a period of months or years. Even small amounts of lead can cause serious health problems. detoxification blend · cilantro · geranium · grapefruit · black pepper	Detoxification pg. 230
Leaky Gut Syndrome	Gastrointestinal tract dysfunction caused by poor diet, toxins, antibiotics, parasites or infections following increased intestinal wall permeability and absorption of bacteria, fungi, toxins, parasites, etc. digestion blend · dill · ginger · cardamom · lemongrass	Digestive & Intestinal pg. 235
Learning Difficulties	An impairment or significantly reduced ability to learn or understand complex or new information, which translates as underdeveloped language skills, impaired intelligence, and reduced ability to function independently, or impaired social functionality. peppermint · focus blend · vetiver · patchouli · inspiring blend	Brain pg. 208; Focus & Concentration pg. 255
Leg Cramps	An abrupt, involuntary, spasmodic muscular contraction causing severe pain, often existing in the leg or shoulder as the result of chill or strain. wintergreen · massage blend · lemongrass · cypress · soothing blend	Muscular pg. 283
Legg-Calve-Perthes Disease	Occurs when blood supply is temporarily interrupted to the ball part (femoral head) of the hip joint. Without ample blood flow, the bone begins to die therefore breaking more easily and healing poorly melissa · peppermint · ylang ylang	Skeletal pg. 313; Children pg. 225
Legionnaires' Disease	A severe form of pneumonia caused by a bacterium known as legionella. eucalyptus · massage blend · arborvitae · melissa · lemon	Immune & Lymphatic pg. 259
Leukemia	A progressive, malignant disease of the blood-forming organs, distinct by distorted proliferation and development of leukocytes and their precursors in the blood and bone marrow. frankincense · rosemary · cellular complex blend · lemon · sandalwood	Cellular Health pg. 221

QUICK REFERENCE

STEPS: 1 Look up ailment. 2 Choose one or more of the recommended oils. (Order of recommendation is left to right.) 3 Use oil(s) as indicated. 4 Learn more: see the corresponding body system/focus area.

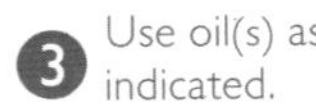

AILMENT	RECOMMENDED OILS AND USAGE	BODY SYSTEM/FOCUS AREA
Libido (low) for Men	A term that envelops disturbances in sexual inclination and psychophysiological changes in the sexual response cycle, which may be accompanied by marked interpersonal difficulty and distress. ylang ylang, women's monthly blend, inspiring blend, cinnamon, ginger	Men's Health pg. 276; Intimacy pg. 270
Libido (low) for Women	The inhibition of the natural arousal aspect of sexual response. ylang ylang, women's monthly blend, roman chamomile, inspiring blend, geranium	Women's Health pg. 332; Intimacy pg. 270
Lichen Nitidus	A skin condition defined by minute, asymptomatic, pinkish or whitish, flat-topped skin papules that may appear in conjunction with lichen planus. cellular complex blend, lemongrass, cleansing blend, douglas fir	Integumentary pg. 264
Limbic System	A complex system of nerves and networks in the brain involving several areas near the edge of the cortex concerned with instinct and mood. It controls the basic emotions (fear, pleasure, anger) and drives (hunger, sex, dominance, care of offspring). melissa, frankincense, sandalwood, bergamot, rose	Limbic pg. 273
Lipoma	A benign, rubbery, soft, encapsulated tumor of adipose tissue, commonly made up of mature fat cells. basil, arborvitae, cellular complex blend, frankincense, clove	Cellular Health pg. 221
Lips (dry)	Lips that have lost moisture and may have become chapped, often due to dehydration or too much sun or wind. cellular complex blend, detoxification blend, women's blend, geranium, lavender	Integumentary pg. 264
Listeria Infection	A food borne bacterial sickness that can be very serious for pregnant women and people with impaired immune systems. Listeria infection is commonly contracted by eating improperly processed deli meats and unpasteurized milk products. detoxification blend, protective blend, melissa, basil, melaleuca	Immune & Lymphatic pg. 259
Liver Disease	Any damage that lowers the functioning of the liver. geranium, clove, frankincense, thyme, lemongrass	Digestive & Intestinal pg. 235
Lockjaw (Tetanus)	A rare but often fatal disease that affects the central nervous system by causing painful muscular contractions. It begins when tetanus bacteria enter the body, typically through a cut or wound exposed to contaminated soil. frankincense, soothing blend, cypress, helichrysum, massage blend	Nervous pg. 287; Muscular pg. 283
Long QT Syndrome	Long QT syndrome (LQTS) is a heart rhythm disorder that can possibly cause fast, chaotic heartbeats. These rapid heartbeats may trigger a seizure or sudden fainting spell. In few cases, the heart may beat erratically for so long that it can cause sudden death. arborvitae, cellular complex blend, detoxification blend	Cardiovascular pg. 216
Lou Gehrig's Disease	A fatal neurological condition in which the motor neurons in the anterior horns of the spinal cord and the corticospinal tracts degenerate. cellular complex blend, oregano, melissa, frankincense, cypress	Nervous pg. 287
Lumbago	An agonizing condition of the lower back, resulting from muscle strain or a slipped disk. detoxification blend, cleansing blend, sandalwood, soothing blend	Muscular pg. 283; Skeletal pg. 313

Diffuse into the air or inhale from cupped hands.
Apply topically directly to affected areas.
Take internally in a capsule or in a glass of water.
TIP For children use 1-2 drops; for adults use 2-4 drops.

AILMENT	RECOMMENDED OILS AND USAGE	BODY SYSTEM/FOCUS AREA
Lupus	A chronic inflammatory autoimmune disorder that may affect many organ systems including the joints, internal organs, and skin. cellular complex blend · detoxification blend · clove · frankincense · protective blend	Autoimmune pg. 200
Lyme Disease	An infection passed on by the bite of ticks carrying the spiral-shaped bacterium Borrelia burgdorferi. thyme · arborvitae · frankincense · black pepper · melissa	Immune & Lymphatic pg. 259
Lymphoma	A type of cancer that affects lymph cells and tissues, including certain white blood cells (T cells and B cells),bone marrow, lymph nodes, and the spleen. wild orange · frankincense · cellular complex blend · thyme · clove	Cellular Health pg. 221
Macular Degeneration	A progressive deterioration of a critical region of the retina called the macula. anti-aging blend * · helichrysum * · coriander * · juniper berry * · frankincense *	Nervous pg. 287
Malabsorption Syndrome	A number of disorders in which the intestine's ability to absorb certain nutrients, such as vitamin B12 and iron, into the bloodstream is negatively affected. invigorating blend · digestion blend · sandalwood · ginger · fennel	Digestive & Intestinal pg. 235
Malaria	A serious infectious disease spread by certain mosquitoes. It is most typical in tropical climates and characterized by recurrent symptoms of fever, chills, and an enlarged spleen. thyme · cinnamon · bergamot · repellent blend (to avoid)	Immune & Lymphatic pg. 259
Marfan Syndrome (Connective Tissue Disorder)	A genetic disorder primarily affecting the connective tissues of the body, manifested in varying degrees by excessive bone elongation and joint flexibility and by abnormalities of the cardiovascular system and eye. lemongrass · helichrysum · massage blend · white fir · basil	Skeletal pg. 313; Muscular pg. 283
Mastitis	An infection of the breast which commonly only occurs in women who are breastfeeding. lavender · women's monthly blend · cellular complex blend · melaleuca · patchouli	Women's Health pg. 332
Measles	A viral infection, which causes an illness displaying a characteristic skin rash known as an exanthem. cellular complex blend · clove · eucalyptus · lavender · melaleuca	Immune & Lymphatic pg. 259
Melanoma	A type of skin cancer that develops in the cells that produce melanin. Melanoma can also form in the eyes and, rarely, in internal organs, such as the intestines. cellular complex blend · sandalwood · frankincense · rosemary · arborvitae	Cellular Health pg. 221
Melatonin Imbalances/ Insufficiencies	Melatonin is a hormone produced at the onset of darkness to aid in sleep. Imbalances or insufficiencies may lead to sleep deprivation or sleeping disorders. patchouli · lavender · roman chamomile · vetiver · sandalwood	Endocrine pg. 244
Meningitis	An inflammation of the membranes surrounding the brain and spinal cord. melaleuca · protective blend · clove · cellular complex blend · basil	Immune & Lymphatic pg. 259

STEPS: ❶ Look up ailment. ❷ Choose one or more of the recommended oils. (Order of recommendation is left to right.) ❸ Use oil(s) as indicated. ❹ Learn more: see the corresponding body system/focus area.

AILMENT	RECOMMENDED OILS AND USAGE	BODY SYSTEM/FOCUS AREA
Menopause	The suspension of menstruation, occurring usually between the ages of 45 and 55. clary sage, women's monthly blend, geranium, thyme, cypress	Women's Health pg. 332
Menorrhagia	Extremely heavy menstrual flow with cycles of normal length. It is also called hypermenorrhea. women's monthly blend, women's blend, rosemary, clary sage, geranium	Women's Health pg. 332
Menstrual Bleeding (excessive)	Heavy or prolonged menstrual periods, or menorrhagia, are the most common type of abnormal bleeding from the uterus. clary sage, women's blend, helichrysum, geranium, frankincense	Women's Health pg. 332
Menstrual Cycle (irregular)	Uncommonly slight or infrequent menstrual flow. clary sage, women's monthly blend, peppermint, frankincense, rosemary	Women's Health pg. 332
Menstrual Pain	A female condition of painful, debilitating menstrual cycles that interfere with daily activities; commonly treated with oral medication. cypress, tension blend, women's monthly blend, clary sage, soothing blend	Women's Health pg. 332
Menstruation (scanty)	Abnormally infrequent or light menstrual flow. ylang ylang, women's monthly blend, peppermint, clary sage, lavender	Women's Health pg. 332
Mental Fatigue	An emotional state associated with extended or extreme exposure to psychic pressure, as in battle or combat fatigue. basil, peppermint, bergamot, invigorating blend, calming blend	Brain pg. 208
Mesenteric Lymphadentis	An inflammation of lymph nodes in a membrane that attaches the intestine to the abdominal wall. rosemary, basil, cypress, melaleuca, lemon	Immune & Lymphatic pg. 259
Mesothelioma	A tumor of the epithelium lining the lungs, heart, or abdomen often associated with exposure to asbestos dust. cellular complex blend, lemongrass, detoxification blend, thyme, basil	Cellular Health pg. 221
Metabolic Muscle Disorders	Related to defects in the enzymes that regulate carbohydrates, lipids, or other metabolic pathways in the muscle fibers, these disorders are caused by a genetic defect that impairs the body's metabolism. ginger, cypress, basil, peppermint, lemongrass	Muscular pg. 283
Metal Toxicity	Heavy metal poisoning is the toxic build up of heavy metals in the soft tissues of the body. cilantro, detoxification blend, frankincense, geranium, juniper berry	Detoxification pg. 230
Migraine	A severe recurring headache, commonly affecting one side of the head, that is determined by sharp pain and is often followed by nausea, vomiting, and visual disturbances. peppermint, marjoram, frankincense, lavender, tension blend	Pain & Inflammation pg. 294; Muscular pg. 283
Miscarriage (afterward)	The spontaneous loss of a pregnancy from conception to 20 weeks' gestation. detoxification blend, cellular complex blend, cleansing blend, frankincense, comforting blend	Pregnancy, Labor & Nursing pg. 301

Diffuse into the air or inhale from cupped hands.
Apply topically directly to affected areas.
Take internally in a capsule or in a glass of water.
TIP For children use 1-2 drops; for adults use 2-4 drops.

AILMENT	RECOMMENDED OILS AND USAGE	BODY SYSTEM/FOCUS AREA
Mitral Valve Prolapse	A heart valve anomaly that involves prolapse of the mitral valve into the left atrium during contraction of the heart's ventricles. This allows leakage of blood through the valve opening. Most people with mitral valve prolapse have no symptoms. However, those who do commonly complain of symptoms such as fatigue, palpitations, chest pain, anxiety, and migraine headaches. cellular complex blend, tension blend, patchouli	Cardiovascular pg. 216
Mold/Mildew	Fungi that grow on damp organic matter, breaking it down. melaleuca, cleansing blend, oregano, thyme	Allergies pg. 194
Moles	A mole (nevus) is a pigmented (colored) blotch on the outer layer of the skin (epidermis). cellular complex blend, detoxification blend, topical blend, frankincense, peppermint	Integumentary pg. 264
Mononucleosis	An infectious disease with symptoms that include severe fatigue, sore throat, swollen lymph nodes, and fever in the armpits and neck. melissa, eucalyptus, protective blend, cinnamon, thyme	Immune & Lymphatic pg. 259
Mood Swings	Alternation of a person's emotional state between periods of depression and euphoria. patchouli, calming blend, focus blend, grounding blend, uplifting blend	Mood & Behavior pg. 279
Morning Sickness	Vomiting and nausea beginning in the morning upon arising, commonly during early pregnancy. ginger, peppermint, digestion blend, bergamot, coriander	Pregnancy, Labor & Nursing pg. 301
Mosquito Bites	Itchy bumps (wheals) that appear after being "bitten" by a mosquito. repellent blend, roman chamomile, cleansing blend, arborvitae, lavender	First Aid pg. 251
Motion Sickness	The uncomfortable nausea, vomiting, and dizziness which people experience when their sense of balance and equilibrium is disturbed by constant motion. digestion blend, ginger, bergamot, metabolic blend, peppermint	Digestive & Intestinal pg. 235
Mouth Ulcers	Ulcers of the oral mucosa commonly caused by a secondary bacterial infection of less severe mucosal lesions caused by an initial disease. protective blend, cinnamon, clove, myrrh, melaleuca	Oral Health pg. 291
MRSA	A strain of Staphylococcus aureus—a commensal which lives harmlessly on the skin and nasal cavity of about one-third of the normal population—which is resistant to methicillin. protective blend, oregano, melissa, thyme, clove	Immune & Lymphatic pg. 259
Mucus	A thick, gel-like, viscous material that functions to protect and moisten inner body surfaces. lemon, fennel, cinnamon, clary sage, digestive blend	Respiratory pg. 307
Multiple Chemical Sensitivity Reaction	A medical condition identified by symptoms that the affected person attributes to low-level chemical exposure. Typically accused substances include pesticides, smoke, plastics, petroleum products, synthetic fabrics, scented products, and paint fumes. ylang ylang, detoxification blend, women's blend	Immune & Lymphatic pg. 259

STEPS: ❶ Look up ailment. ❷ Choose one or more of the recommended oils. (Order of recommendation is left to right.) ❸ Use oil(s) as indicated. ❹ Learn more: see the corresponding body system/focus area.

AILMENT	RECOMMENDED OILS AND USAGE	BODY SYSTEM/FOCUS AREA
Multiple Sclerosis	A chronic autoimmune disorder affecting sensation, movement, and bodily functions, resulting in destruction of the myelin insulation covering nerve fibers (neurons) in the central nervous system (brain and spinal cord). cellular complex blend, frankincense, melissa, clove, sandalwood	Nervous pg. 287
Mumps	A mild short-term viral infection of the salivary glands that commonly occurs during childhood. protective blend, detoxification blend, cellular complex blend, lavender, melaleuca	Immune & Lymphatic pg. 259
Muscle Cramps, Pulls, Strains	Partial (causing pain on muscle stretch but no loss of strength) or total breach (defined by loss of function, pain, and bruising) of muscle fibers due to sudden applied force or overuse. massage blend, marjoram, basil, soothing blend, lemongrass	Athletes pg. 197; Muscular pg. 283; Pain & Inflammation pg. 294
Muscle Pain	Pain in a muscle or a group of muscles that is typically shared by a feeling of unease. peppermint, soothing blend, massage blend, marjoram, wintergreen	Athletes pg. 197; Muscular pg. 283; Pain & Inflammation pg. 294
Muscle Spasms	A quick involuntary contraction of a muscle or group of muscles. basil, coriander, lemongrass, soothing blend, marjoram	Muscular pg. 283; Athletes pg. 197
Muscle Stiffness	Muscles that are halfway to rigidity, tetany; result of inadequate use of the part. massage blend, soothing blend, tension blend, basil, ginger	Muscular pg. 283; Athletes pg. 197
Muscle Strengthening/ Growth	Muscle development from exercise and exertion. When a muscle is pushed to its limits, it will repair and rebuild itself for future exertion. birch, helichrysum, wintergreen, lemongrass, ginger	Muscular pg. 283; Athletes pg. 197
Muscle Weakness	A state of fatigue or loss of strength and/or muscle endurance following strenuous activity in association with the accumulation of lactic acid in muscles. birch, helichrysum, wintergreen, lemongrass, ginger	Muscular pg. 283; Athletes pg. 197
Muscular Dystrophy	A group of inherited disorders in which muscle bulk and strength gradually drop. cellular complex blend, tension blend, lemongrass, frankincense, marjoram	Muscular pg. 283; Athletes pg. 197
Myasthenia Gravis	A chronic autoimmune neuromuscular disease characterized by varying degrees of weakness of the skeletal muscles of the body. helichrysum, ginger, cypress, lemongrass, cellular complex	Muscular pg. 283
Myelofibrosis	Myelofibrosis is a severe bone marrow disorder that disrupts your body's normal production of blood cells. The result is broad scarring in your bone marrow, leading to severe anemia, weakness, fatigue, and often, an enlarged spleen and liver. helichrysum, lemongrass, cellular complex blend, ginger, geranium	Skeletal pg. 313
Myotonic Dystrophy	An inherited disease in which the muscles contract but have decreasing power to relax. The disease leads to a mask-like expressionless face, premature balding, cataracts, and heart arrhythmias. cellular complex, helichrysum, patchouli, ginger, detoxification blend	Muscular pg. 283

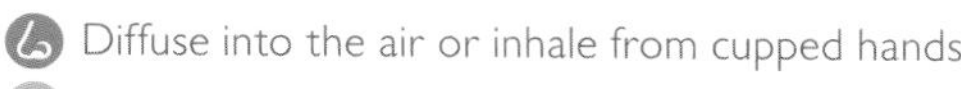
Diffuse into the air or inhale from cupped hands.
Apply topically directly to affected areas.

Take internally in a capsule or in a glass of water.
TIP For children use 1-2 drops; for adults use 2-4 drops.

AILMENT	RECOMMENDED OILS AND USAGE	BODY SYSTEM/FOCUS AREA
Nails	The horny cutaneous plate on the dorsal surface of the distal end of a toe or finger. arborvitae, cellular complex blend, detoxification blend, lemon, frankincense	Integumentary pg. 264
Narcolepsy	A disorder distincted by extreme daytime sleepiness, cataplexy and uncontrollable sleep attacks (a sudden loss of muscle tone, usually lasting up to half an hour). cellular complex blend, detoxification blend, ylang ylang, frankincense, basil	Brain pg. 208
Nasal Polyp	A rounded, stretched piece of pulpy, dependent mucosa that projects into the nasal cavity. eucalyptus, frankincense, rosemary, melissa, respiration blend	Respiratory pg. 307
Nausea	An undesirable sensation vaguely referred to the abdomen and epigastrium, with a tendency to vomit. ginger, detoxification blend, bergamot, basil, peppermint	Digestive & Intestinal pg. 235
Neck Pain	Pain in response to injury or another stimulus that resolves when the injury stimulus is removed or healed. soothing blend, birch, wintergreen, cypress, peppermint	Muscular pg. 283
Nervous Fatigue	Fatigue caused by the central nervous system that cannot be explained by dysfunction of the muscle. arborvitae, cedarwood, basil, patchouli, focus blend	Nervous pg. 287; Energy & Vitality pg. 248
Nervous System	The network of nerve cells and fibers that transmits nerve impulses between parts of the body. cellular complex blend, frankincense, myrrh, peppermint, helichrysum	Nervous pg. 287
Nervousness	A state of concern, with great physical and mental unrest. calming blend, grounding blend, reassuring blend, frankincense, orange	Mood & Behavior pg. 279
Neuralgia	Characterized as an extreme stabbing or burning pain caused by irritation of or damage to a nerve. cellular complex blend, tension blend, ginger, marjoram, eucalyptus	Nervous pg. 287
Neuritis	The inflammation of a nerve or group of nerves that is defined by loss of reflexes, pain and atrophy of the affected muscles. cellular complex blend, frankincense, melissa, eucalyptus, roman chamomile	Nervous pg. 287
Neuromuscular Disorders	A broad term that encompasses many different diseases that affect the function of the skeletal muscles that move the limbs and trunk. massage blend, cypress, tension blend, arborvitae, ginger	Muscular pg. 283
Neuropathy	A condition affecting the nerves supplying the legs and arms. cypress, basil, tension blend, massage blend, wintergreen	Nervous pg. 287
Night Eating Disorder (NED	Sleep-related eating disorders are characterized by abnormal eating patterns during the night. metabolic blend, ginger, cinnamon, cedarwood, joyful blend	Weight pg. 327; Sleep pg. 317; Eating Disorders pg. 240
Night Sweats	Profuse sweating at night, occurring in pulmonary tuberculosis and other continuous crippling affections with low-grade fever. detoxification blend, cellular complex blend, massage blend, lime, ginger	Endocrine pg. 244

QUICK REFERENCE

STEPS: 1 Look up ailment. 2 Choose one or more of the recommended oils. (Order of recommendation is left to right.) 3 Use oil(s) as indicated. 4 Learn more: see the corresponding body system/focus area.

AILMENT	RECOMMENDED OILS AND USAGE	BODY SYSTEM/FOCUS AREA
Nose (dry)	Irritation caused from insufficient mucus in the nasal cavity. Moist noses are optimal for catching airborne pollutants that can cause infections. cellular complex blend, cleansing blend, protective blend, geranium, lavender	Respiratory pg. 307
Nose bleed	Caused most frequently by picking but can occur as a result of vigorous trauma, sneezing, irritated mucous membranes, vitamin K deficiency, leukemia, hypertension, and other conditions. geranium, helichrysum, soothing blend, myrrh, cypress	Respiratory pg. 307
Numbness	Loss of sensation or feeling. frankincense, arborvitae, basil, massage blend, ginger	Nervous pg. 287
Obesity	Obesity is an uncommon quantity of body fat, usually 20% or more over an individual's ideal body weight. metabolic blend, ginger, cinnamon, grapefruit	Weight pg. 327
Obsessive Compulsive Disorder (OCD)	A type of anxiety disorder, which one can experience a prolonged, excessive worry about circumstances in one's life. OCD is defined by distressing repetitive thoughts, impulses, or images that are intense, frightening, absurd, or unusual. These thoughts are followed by ritualized actions that are usually bizarre and irrational. focus blend, frankincense, calming blend, cedarwood, comforting blend	Brain pg. 208
Ocular Rosacea	Inflammation that causes redness, burning, and itching of the eyes. It often develops in people who have rosacea, a chronic skin condition that affects the face. cellular complex blend, cardamom, tension blend, frankincense, anti-aging blend	Nervous pg. 287
Olfactory Loss	The loss of the sense of smell cellular complex blend, soothing blend, helichrysum, peppermint, basil	Allergies pg. 194
Oppositional Defiant Disorder	A childhood disorder described by the Diagnostic and Statistical Manual of Mental Disorders (DSM) as an ongoing pattern of anger-guided hostility, disobedience, and defiant behavior toward authority figures which goes beyond the bounds of normal childhood behavior. cellular complex blend, calming blend, grounding blend, wild orange	Mood & Behavior pg. 279
Osgood-Schlatter Disease	An irritation of the patellar ligament at the tibial tuberosity which is defined by painful lumps just below the knee and is often seen in young adolescents. Risk factors may include excess weight and overzealous conditioning (running and jumping), but adolescent bone growth is at the root of it. massage blend, cypress, arborvitae, coriander, eucalyptus	Skeletal pg. 313
Osteoarthritis	A form of arthritis, occurring commonly in older persons, that is defined by chronic degeneration of the cartilage of the joints. white fir, birch, wintergreen, peppermint, soothing blend	Skeletal pg. 313; Pain & Inflammation pg. 294
Osteomyelitis	A bone infection, usually caused by a bacteria. Over time, the result can be destruction of the bone itself. helichrysum, birch, white fir, lemongrass, clove	Skeletal pg. 313

Diffuse (diffuse) into the air or inhale from cupped hands.
Apply (topical) topically directly to affected areas.
Take (internal) internally in a capsule or in a glass of water.
TIP For children use 1-2 drops; for adults use 2-4 drops.

AILMENT	RECOMMENDED OILS AND USAGE	BODY SYSTEM/FOCUS AREA
Osteoporosis	A disease defined by loss in bone mass and density, occurring commonly in postmenopausal women, resulting in a predisposition to fractures and bone deformities such as vertebral collapse. lemongrass (topical, internal); helichrysum (topical, internal); cypress (topical); clove (topical); geranium (topical)	Skeletal pg. 313
Ovarian Cyst	A cystic tumor of the ovary, which is commonly benign. frankincense (topical, internal); detoxification blend (topical, internal); cellular complex blend (topical, internal); clary sage (topical, internal); basil (topical, diffuse)	Women's Health pg. 332
Over Exercised	Overuse of muscle and connective tissue that may cause injury or exhaustion. lime (topical, internal); marjoram (topical); peppermint (topical); soothing blend (topical); birch (topical)	Muscular pg. 283; Athletes pg. 197
Overactive Bladder (OAB)	Overactive bladder is the leakage of urine in large amounts at unexpected times, including during sleep. detoxification blend (topical, internal); cypress (topical); massage blend (topical); juniper berry (topical, internal); ginger (topical, internal)	Urinary pg. 324
Overeating	Uncontrolled ingestion of sizable quantities of food in a discrete interval, usually with a lack of control over the activity. ginger (topical, internal); cinnamon (topical, internal); metabolic blend (topical, internal); coriander (topical, internal); grapefruit (topical, internal)	Eating Disorders pg. 240
Overwhelmed	cellular complex blend (internal, diffuse, topical); frankincense (diffuse, topical); reassuring blend (diffuse, topical); grounding blend (diffuse, topical); calming blend (diffuse, topical)	Mood & Behavior pg. 279
Ovulation (lack of)	Ovulation problems can develop from dysfunction of the part of the glands and brain that control ovulation or dysfunction of the ovaries. frankincense (topical, diffuse); myrrh (topical, diffuse); clary sage (topical, diffuse); ylang ylang (topical, diffuse); jasmine (topical, diffuse)	Women's Health pg. 332
Paget's Disease	A disease in which the bones become enlarged and weakened, resulting in fracture or deformation. Also, a rare form of breast cancer involving the areola and nipple. cellular complex blend (internal, topical); white fir (topical); birch (topical); cypress (topical); basil (topical)	Skeletal pg. 313
Pain	An undesirable sensation occurring in varying degrees of severity as a consequence of disease, injury, or emotional disorder. soothing blend (topical); peppermint (topical); birch (topical); wintergreen (topical); eucalyptus (topical)	Pain & Inflammation pg. 294
Palpitations	A sensitivity in which a person is aware of an intermittent, hard, or rapid heartbeat. frankincense (internal, topical); lavender (internal, topical); thyme (internal, topical); orange (internal, topical); ylang ylang (topical)	Cardiovascular pg. 216
Pancreatitis	An inflammation of the pancreas, an organ that is essential in digestion. detoxification blend (internal, topical); cellular complex blend (internal, topical); marjoram (internal, topical); protective blend (internal, topical); lemon (internal, topical)	Endocrine pg. 244
Panic Attacks	Periods of intense apprehension or fear that occur suddenly and of variable duration from minutes to hours. Panic attacks usually begin abruptly, may reach a peak within 10 minutes, but may continue for much longer if the sufferer had the attack triggered by a situation from which they are not able to escape. frankincense (topical, diffuse); reassuring blend (topical, diffuse); calming blend (topical, diffuse); grounding blend (topical, diffuse); wild orange (topical, diffuse)	Mood & Behavior pg. 279

STEPS: ❶ Look up ailment. ❷ Choose one or more of the recommended oils. (Order of recommendation is left to right.) ❸ Use oil(s) as indicated. ❹ Learn more: see the corresponding body system/focus area.

AILMENT	RECOMMENDED OILS AND USAGE	BODY SYSTEM/FOCUS AREA
Paralysis	Paralysis is defined as complete loss of strength in an affected limb or muscle group. cellular complex blend, ginger, lemongrass, sandalwood, melissa	Nervous pg. 287
Parasites	An organism that feeds, grows, and is sheltered on or in a different organism while contributing nothing to the survival of its host. detoxification blend, clove, oregano, protective blend, roman chamomile	Parasites pg. 298
Parathyroid Dis-order	An imbalance of parathyroid hormone (PTH), which helps the body maintain the right balance of calcium and phosphorous. melissa, detoxification blend, women's monthly blend, ginger, invigorating blend	Endocrine pg. 244
Parkinson's Disease	A gradual nervous disease appearing most often after the age of 50, associated with the ruin of brain cells that produce dopamine. cellular complex blend, detoxification blend, marjoram, frankincense, cinnamon	Nervous pg. 287; Brain pg. 208
Pelvic Pain Syndrome	Pain in the pelvis that arises in endometritis, appendicitis, and oophoritis. The character and onset of pelvic pain and any factors that aggravate or alleviate it are important in making a diagnosis. women's monthly blend, tension blend, cypress, geranium, ginger	Digestive & Intestinal pg. 235
Perforated Ear Drum	A perforated eardrum happens when there is a rupture or hole in the eardrum, the thin membrane that separates the outer ear canal from the middle ear. arborvitae, cellular complex blend, detoxification blend, ylang ylang, patchouli	Respiratory pg. 307
Pericardial Disease	Occurs when there is too much fluid buildup around the heart. detoxification blend, marjoram, protective blend, juniper berry, lemongrass	Cardiovascular pg. 216
Perimenopause	The 3- to 5- year period before menopause during which progesterone and estrogen levels decline and symptoms of hormone deprivation begin. women's blend, cellular complex blend, detoxification blend, clary sage, rosemary	Women's Health pg. 332
Periodic Limb Movement Disorder	Repetitive cramping or jerking of the legs during sleep. massage blend, tension blend, basil, marjoram, lavender	Sleep pg. 317
Pernicious Anemia	A severe anemia associated with poor intake or absorption of vitamin B12, defined by defective production of red blood cells. detoxification blend, cleansing blend, women's blend	Autoimmune pg. 200; Cardiovascular pg. 216
Perspiration (excessive)	An inherited disorder of the eccrine sweat glands in which emotional stimuli cause volar or axillary sweating. detoxification blend, cilantro, coriander, lemon, geranium	Endocrine pg. 244
Phantom Pains	Pain, itching, tingling, or numbness in the place where the amputated part used to be. helichrysum, basil, lavender, soothing blend, massage blend	Nervous pg. 287
Phlebitis	A vein that is inflamed. detoxification blend, basil, lemon, helichrysum, lavender	Cardiovascular pg. 216

(Diffuse icon) Diffuse into the air or inhale from cupped hands.
(Topical icon) Apply topically directly to affected areas.
(Internal icon) Take internally in a capsule or in a glass of water.
TIP For children use 1-2 drops; for adults use 2-4 drops.

AILMENT	RECOMMENDED OILS AND USAGE	BODY SYSTEM/FOCUS AREA
Pica	A craving for something that is not normally regarded as nutritive, such as dirt, clay, paper, or chalk. Pica is a classic clue to iron deficiency in children, and it may also occur with zinc deficiency. multivitamin supplements (internal); cinnamon (internal); clove (internal); cilantro (internal); detoxification blend (internal)	Eating Disorders pg. 240
Pinkeye	Redness and swelling of the conjunctiva, the mucous membrane that lines the eyelid and eye surface, causing the lining of the eye to become pink and swollen. melaleuca (topical); frankincense (topical); ravensara (topical); clary sage (topical); melissa (topical)	
Pinworms	A parasitic nematode worm, Enterobius vermicularis, infecting the rectum, colon, and anus of humans. clove (internal, topical); oregano (internal, topical); thyme (internal, topical); digestive blend (internal, topical); protective blend (internal, topical)	Parasites pg. 298
Pituitary	An endocrine gland about the size of a pea. It is a protrusion off the bottom of the hypothalamus at the base of the brain. The anterior pituitary (or adenohypophysis) is a lobe of the gland that regulates several physiological processes (including stress, growth, reproduction, and lactation). Hormones secreted from the pituitary gland help control: growth, blood pressure, certain functions of the sex organs, thyroid glands and metabolism as well as some aspects of pregnancy, childbirth, nursing, water/salt concentration and the kidneys, temperature regulation and pain relief. cellular complex blend (internal, topical); ginger (internal, topical, diffuse); patchouli (internal, topical, diffuse); frankincense (topical, diffuse); sandalwood (internal, topical, diffuse)	Endocrine pg. 244
Plague	Plague is a severe, possibly life-threatening infectious disease that is commonly transmitted to humans by the bites of rodent fleas. detoxification blend (internal, topical); cellular complex blend (internal, topical); cleansing blend (topical); protective blend (topical, internal, diffuse); clove (internal, topical, diffuse)	Immune & Lymphatic pg. 259
Plantar Fasciitis	Inflammation to the plantar fascia ligament most commonly caused by strain or injury, causing micro-tears to the ligament as it attaches to the heel bone or other areas of tightness on the sole of the foot. basil (topical); arborvitae (topical); white fir (topical); eucalyptus (topical); soothing blend (topical)	Skeletal pg. 313
Plantar Warts	An unpleasant verrucous lesion on the sole of the foot. cellular complex blend (topical); ylang ylang (topical); cleansing blend (topical); oregano (topical); protective blend (topical)	Integumentary pg. 264
Plaque	An semi-hardened accumulation of substances from fluids that surround an area. Examples include dental plaque and cholesterol plaque. protective blend (topical); clove (topical); thyme (topical); myrrh (topical); lemon (topical)	Oral Health pg. 291
Pleurisy	An infection of the membrane that surrounds and protects the lungs (the pleura). rosemary (topical, internal, diffuse); eucalyptus (topical, internal, diffuse); cinnamon (topical, internal, diffuse); cypress (topical, diffuse); thyme (topical, diffuse)	Respiratory pg. 307
Pneumonia	An infection in the lungs that can be caused by almost any class of organism known to cause human infections. eucalyptus (topical, diffuse); protective blend (topical, internal, diffuse); arborvitae (topical, diffuse); ravensara (topical, diffuse); respiratory blend (topical, diffuse)	Respiratory pg. 307
Poison Ivy	A North American vine or shrub that has compound leaves with three leaflets, small green flowers, and whitish berries which causes a rash on contact. frankincense (topical); lavender (topical, internal); geranium (topical); cleansing blend (topical); roman chamomile (topical)	First Aid pg. 251; Integumentary pg. 264

STEPS: 1 Look up ailment. 2 Choose one or more of the recommended oils. (Order of recommendation is left to right.) 3 Use oil(s) as indicated. 4 Learn more: see the corresponding body system/focus area.

AILMENT	RECOMMENDED OILS AND USAGE	BODY SYSTEM/FOCUS AREA
Polio	A highly infectious viral disease that may attack the central nervous system and is defined by symptoms that range from a mild non-paralytic infection to total paralysis in a matter of hours. sandalwood, cellular complex blend, detoxification blend, frankincense, wild orange	Immune & Lymphatic pg. 259; Nervous pg. 287
Polymyositis	A disease featuring inflammation of the muscle fibers. The cause of the disease is not known. cellular complex, cypress, ginger, basil, soothing blend	Muscular pg. 283; Pain & Inflammation pg. 294
Polyps	A tumor with a small flap that attaches itself to the wall of different vascular organs such as the rectum, uterus and nose. lemongrass, basil, eucalyptus, peppermint, frankincense	Cellular Health pg. 221
Polycystic Ovary Syndrome (PCOS)	A common endocrine system disorder among women of reproductive age. Women with PCOS may have enlarged ovaries that consist of small collections of fluid, called follicles which are located in each ovary as seen during an ultrasound exam. cellular complex blend, women's monthly blend, frankincense, clary sage, ginger	Women's Health pg. 332
Porphyria	Any group of disturbances of porphyrin metabolism defined by excess porphyrins (various biologically active compounds with a distinct structure) in the urine and by extreme sensitivity to light. cellular complex blend, detoxification blend, cardamom, ginger, basil	Nervous pg. 287
Postpartum Depression	An emotional disorder that starts after childbirth and typically lasts beyond six weeks. detoxification blend, frankincense, wild orange, clary sage, joyful blend	Pregnancy, Labor & Nursing pg. 301
Post Traumatic Stress Disorder	A common anxiety disorder that develops after exposure to a terrifying event or ordeal in which grave physical harm occurred or was threatened. cedarwood, frankincense, reassuring blend, sandalwood, grounding blend	Limbic pg. 273
Pre-Workout Muscle Prep	To help insure a good workout and decrease chance of injury, preparation or stretching should be implemented before a workout. soothing blend, massage blend, marjoram, lime, coriander	Athletes pg. 197
Precocious Puberty	Puberty appearing at an unusually early age. In most children, the process is normal in every respect except the uncommon early age. In a minority of children, the early development is triggered by a disease such as a tumor or injury of the brain. detoxification blend, women's blend, women's monthly blend	Endocrine pg. 244
Preeclampsia	A condition during pregnancy that results in high blood pressure, large amounts of protein in the urine. and swelling that doesn't go away. Also called toxemia. marjoram, lavender, calming blend, roman chamomile, cypress	Pregnancy, Labor & Nursing pg. 301
Pregnancy	The time from conception to birth. cellular complex blend, metabolic blend, clary sage, geranium, ylang ylang	Pregnancy, Labor & Nursing pg. 301
Pregnancy (post-term)	Delivery on or after 41 weeks plus three days of gestation, 10 days over the estimated date of delivery." frankincense, women's blend, detoxification blend, clary sage, rosemary	Pregnancy, Labor & Nursing pg. 301

Diffuse into the air or inhale from cupped hands.
Apply topically directly to affected areas.
Take internally in a capsule or in a glass of water.
TIP For children use 1-2 drops; for adults use 2-4 drops.

AILMENT	RECOMMENDED OILS AND USAGE	BODY SYSTEM/FOCUS AREA
Premenstrual Syndrome	A combination of emotional, physical, psychological, and mood disturbances that occur after a woman's ovulation and typically ending with the onset of her menstrual flow. The most common mood-related symptoms are irritability, depression, crying, oversensitivity, and mood swings. women's monthly blend, geranium, cellular complex blend, clary sage, women's blend	Women's Health pg. 332
Preterm Labor	Labor before the thirty-seventh week of pregnancy. arborvitae, detoxification blend, cleansing blend, lavender	Pregnancy, Labor & Nursing pg. 301
Prostatitis	Enlargement or inflammation of the prostate gland which is relatively typical in adult males. detoxification blend, tension blend, cleansing blend, thyme, cypress	Men's Health pg. 276
Psoriasis	A continual, non-contagious skin disease defined by inflamed lesions covered with silvery-white scabs of dead skin. geranium, clary sage, thyme, helichrysum, roman chamomile	Integumentary pg. 264
Purging Disorder	An eating disorder characterized by recurrent purging (self-induced vomiting and misuse of laxatives, diuretics, or enemas) to control weight or body shape. food enzymes, metabolic blend, grounding blend, ginger, fennel	Eating Disorders pg. 240
Pyorrhea	Purulent inflammation of the tooth sockets and gums, usually leading to loosening of the teeth. clove, myrrh, rosemary, protective blend, helichrysum	Oral Health pg. 291
Q Fever	A sickness caused by a type of bacteria, Coxiella burnetii, resulting in a rash and fever. arborvitae, detoxification blend, cellular complex blend, clove, protective blend	Immune & Lymphatic pg. 259
Radiation Damage	Malignant skin lesions and premalignant (e.g. Bowen's disease, squamous cell carcinoma, and basal cell carcinoma during later adult life) developing after long-term exposure to ultraviolet radiation. arborvitae, cellular complex blend, detoxification blend, peppermint, sandalwood	Immune & Lymphatic pg. 259
Rashes	A spotted, pink or red skin outbreak that may be followed by itching and is caused by contact with an allergen, disease, drug reaction, or food ingestion. detoxification blend, arborvitae, roman chamomile, melaleuca, lavender	Allergies pg. 194; Integumentary pg. 264
Raynaud's Disease	A disorder in which the toes or fingers (digits) suddenly experience reduced blood circulation. cellular complex blend, cypress, arborvitae, protective blend, rosemary	Cardiovascular pg. 216
Reiter's Arthritis	A type of reactive arthritis caused by a reaction to a bacterial infection, generally in the intestines, genitals, or urinary tract. May also include redness, joint swelling, and pain in the knees, ankles, and feet. basil, cypress, soothing blend, massage blend, wintergreen	Skeletal pg. 313
Renal Artery Stenosis	The narrowing of one or both arteries that carry blood to your kidneys (renal arteries). Narrowing of the arteries prevents normal amounts of oxygen-rich blood from reaching your kidneys. Reduced blood flow may increase blood pressure and injure kidney tissue. rosemary, detoxification blend, lemon, basil, marjoram	Cardiovascular pg. 216

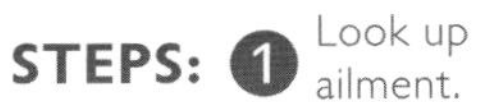

STEPS: 1 Look up ailment. 2 Choose one or more of the recommended oils. (Order of recommendation is left to right.) 3 Use oil(s) as indicated. 4 Learn more: see the corresponding body system/focus area.

AILMENT	RECOMMENDED OILS AND USAGE	BODY SYSTEM/FOCUS AREA
Reproductive System	A system of sex organs that work together for the purpose of sexual reproduction, also known as the genital system. clary sage · ylang ylang · women's monthly blend · ginger · metabolic blend	Men's Health pg. 276; Women's Health pg. 332
Restless Leg Syndrome	A condition defined as a troublesome urge or need to move the legs (or arms)–akathisia–commonly followed by an uncomfortable deep-seated feeling in the legs that is brought on by rest. massage blend · soothing blend · wintergreen · cypress · basil	Nervous pg. 287
Restlessness	A failure to achieve relaxation; a feeling of mild mental discomfort. grounding blend · lavender · joyful blend · bergamot · calming blend	Stress pg. 321; Sleep pg. 317; Mood & Behavior pg. 279
Retinitis Pigmentosa	A group of inherited disorders that slowly leads to blindness due to abnormalities of the photoreceptors in the retina. cellular complex blend · frankincense · helichrysum · juniper berry · cardamom	Nervous pg. 287
Rheumatic Fever	A sickness which emerges as a complication of untreated or inadequately treated strep throat infection. arborvitae · melissa · wintergreen · basil · ginger	Pain & Inflammation pg. 294
Rheumatism	Inflammation, degeneration, or metabolic derangement of connective tissue structures, with pain, stiffness, or limitation of motion; it includes such disorders as arthritis, osteoarthritis, bursitis, and sciatica. basil · detoxification blend · soothing blend · massage blend · birch	Skeletal pg. 313
Rheumatoid Arthritis	A chronic disease of the musculoskeletal system, defined by swelling and inflammation of joints (in the hands, knees, wrists, and feet), fatigue, and muscle weakness. basil · soothing blend · massage blend · cypress · marjoram	Pain & Inflammation pg. 294; Skeletal pg. 313
Rhinitis	An infection of the mucous lining of the nose. metabolic blend · respiration blend · oregano · eucalyptus · peppermint	Respiratory pg. 307
Ringworm	A fungal infection of the skin. melaleuca · thyme · cardamom · lemongrass · oregano	Integumentary pg. 264
Rosacea	A skin disease typically appearing in people during their 30s and 40s. It is marked by redness of the face, flushing of the skin, and the presence of hard pimples (papules) or pus-filled pimples (pustules), and small, visible, spider-like veins called telangiectasias. cellular complex blend · roman chamomile · helichrysum · clary sage · rosemary	Integumentary pg. 264
Roseola	A feverish condition of young children that lasts around five days during the last two of which the patient has a rose-colored rash. Roseola is caused by the human herpes virus. melissa · protective blend · oregano · black pepper · coriander	Children pg. 225
RSV (respiratory syncytial virus)	A virus that causes infections of the lungs and respiratory tract. The virus is so common that most children have been infected by age two. eucalyptus · melissa · rosemary · ravensara · respiration blend	Children pg. 225

[diffuse] Diffuse into the air or inhale from cupped hands.
[topical] Apply topically directly to affected areas.
[internal] Take internally in a capsule or in a glass of water.
TIP For children use 1-2 drops; for adults use 2-4 drops.

AILMENT	RECOMMENDED OILS AND USAGE	BODY SYSTEM/FOCUS AREA
Rubella	An extremely contagious viral disease, spread through contact with discharges from the throat and nose of an infected person. basil [topical] [internal]; lemon [topical] [internal] [diffuse]; melaleuca [topical] [internal] [diffuse]; metabolic blend [internal] [topical]; coriander [internal] [topical]	Immune & Lymphatic pg. 259
Rumination Disorder	The regurgitation of food after almost every meal, part of it being vomited and the rest swallowed; this is sometimes seen in infants. frankincense [diffuse] [topical]; grounding blend [diffuse] [topical]; digestion blend [topical] [diffuse]; ginger [topical] [internal]; peppermint [internal] [diffuse]	Eating Disorders pg. 240
Scabies	A somewhat contagious infection caused by a tiny mite (Sarcoptes scabiei). repellent blend [topical]; arborvitae [topical]; protective blend [internal] [topical]; topical blend [internal] [topical]; melaleuca [internal] [topical]	Integumentary pg. 264
Scarlet Fever	An acute contagious disease caused by a hemolytic streptococcus, occurring mainly among children and defined by a scarlet skin eruption and high fever. melissa [topical] [internal] [diffuse]; eucalyptus [topical] [internal] [diffuse]; ravensara [topical] [diffuse]; melaleuca [topical] [internal] [diffuse]; thyme [topical] [internal] [diffuse]	Children pg. 225
Scarring	The fibrous tissue that replaces normal tissue ruined by disease or injury. anti-aging blend [topical]; lavender [topical]; sandalwood [topical]; frankincense [topical]; helichrysum [topical]	Integumentary pg. 264
Schizophrenia	A psychotic disorder (or a group of disorders) distinct by extremely impaired emotions, thinking, and behaviors. cellular complex blend [internal]; patchouli [topical] [diffuse]; frankincense [topical] [internal] [diffuse]; bergamot [topical] [internal] [diffuse]; sandalwood [topical] [internal] [diffuse]	Brain pg. 208
Schmidt's Syndrome	Paralysis on one side, affecting the soft palate, vocal cord, sternocleidomastoid muscle, and trapezius muscle, by cause of a lesion of the nucleus ambiguous and the nucleus accessorius. ginger [internal] [topical]; cardamom [internal] [topical]; rosemary [internal] [topical]; frankincense [internal] [topical]; basil [internal] [topical]	Autoimmune pg. 200
Sciatica	An inflammation of the sciatic nerve, commonly defined by pain and tenderness along the course of the nerve through the leg and thigh. helichrysum [topical]; birch [topical]; wintergreen [topical]; peppermint [topical]; roman chamomile [topical]	Nervous pg. 287
Scleroderma	A gradual disease that affects the skin and connective tissue (including fat, bone, cartilage, and the tissue that supports the blood vessels and nerves throughout the body). massage blend [topical]; douglas fir [topical] [internal]; patchouli [topical] [internal]; wintergreen [topical]; helichrysum [topical] [internal]	Autoimmune pg. 200;
Scoliosis	A side-to-side curve of the spine. helichrysum [topical]; wintergreen [topical]; soothing blend [topical]; lemongrass [topical]; massage blend [topical]	Skeletal pg. 313
Scurvy	A lack of vitamin C (ascorbic acid) in the diet. helichrysum [topical] [internal]; cypress [topical]; lemon [internal] [topical]; geranium [topical] [internal]; ginger [topical] [internal]	Energy & Vitality pg. 248
Seasonal Affective Disorder (SAD)	A type of depression that tends to occur as the days grow shorter in the fall and winter. bergamot [topical] [diffuse]; clary sage [topical] [diffuse]; joyful blend [topical] [diffuse]; invigorating blend [topical] [diffuse]; wild orange [topical] [diffuse]	Mood & Behavior pg. 279
Sebaceous Cyst	Noncancerous small bumps beneath the skin that can appear anywhere on the skin, but are most common on the face, neck and trunk. grounding blend [topical]; cedarwood [topical] [internal]; fennel [topical] [internal]; clary sage [topical] [internal]; basil [topical] [internal]	Integumentary pg. 264

QUICK REFERENCE

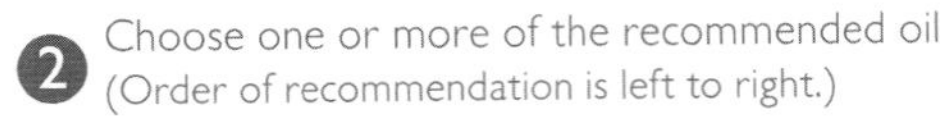

STEPS: ❶ Look up ailment. ❷ Choose one or more of the recommended oils. (Order of recommendation is left to right.) ❸ Use oil(s) as indicated. ❹ Learn more: see the corresponding body system/focus area.

AILMENT	RECOMMENDED OILS AND USAGE	BODY SYSTEM/FOCUS AREA
Seizures	A convulsion or attack of epilepsy. frankincense, cedarwood, peppermint, grounding blend, sandalwood	Brain pg. 208; Nervous pg. 287
Sepsis	A bacterial infection in the body tissues or bloodstream. This is a very broad term covering the presence of many types of microscopic disease-causing organisms. basil, protective blend, detoxification blend, thyme, massage blend	Immune & Lymphatic pg. 259
Sex Drive/Hyper-sexuality (excessive)	An obsession with sexual thoughts, urges, or behaviors that may cause distress and negatively affect one's health, job, relationships, or other parts of life. marjoram, arborvitae	Limbic pg. 273
Shigella Infection	An intestinal disease caused by a family of bacteria known as shigella. The main sign of shigella infection is bloody diarrhea. eucalyptus, black pepper, clove, basil, arborvitae	Immune & Lymphatic pg. 259
Shin Splints	A typical injury that affects athletes who engage in running sports or physical activity. This condition is defined by pain in the lower part of the leg between the ankle and knee. massage blend, soothing blend, lemongrass, wintergreen, basil	Skeletal pg. 313
Shingles	A painful, girdle-like skin outbreak that may occur on the trunk of the body; also called herpes zoster or zona. black pepper, frankincense, detoxification blend, melissa, melaleuca	Immune & Lymphatic pg. 259
Shock	A medical emergency in which the tissues and organs of the body are not receiving a sufficient flow of blood. frankincense, focus blend, geranium, helichrysum, peppermint	Nervous pg. 287; First Aid pg. 251
Sickle Cell Anemia	A disorder of the blood caused by an inherited abnormal hemoglobin that causes distorted red blood cells. The sickled red blood cells are fragile and prone to rupture. When the number of red blood cells decreases from rupture, anemia is the result. geranium, arborvitae, cardamom, detoxification blend, cinnamon	Cardiovascular pg. 216
Silent Thyroiditis	Swelling (inflammation) of the thyroid gland. The disorder can cause hyperthyroidism, followed by hypothyroidism. detoxification blend, wild orange, rosemary, ginger, coriander	Endocrine pg. 244
Sinus Congestion	An inflammation of the sinuses, air spaces within the bones of the face. Sinusitis is commonly due to an infection within these spaces. lemon, peppermint, lemongrass, cinnamon, protective blend	Respiratory pg. 307
Sinusitis	An inflammation of the sinuses, air spaces within the bones of the face, typically due to an infection within these spaces. melissa, cardamom, eucalyptus, respiratory blend, rosemary	Respiratory pg. 307

Diffuse into the air or inhale from cupped hands.
Apply topically directly to affected areas.
Take internally in a capsule or in a glass of water.
TIP For children use 1-2 drops; for adults use 2-4 drops.

AILMENT	RECOMMENDED OILS AND USAGE	BODY SYSTEM/FOCUS AREA
Sjogren's Syndrome	A chronic autoimmune disease appearing mostly in older women, defined by dryness of mucous membranes, keratoconjunctivitis, telangiectasias on the face, and enlargement of both parotid glands. It is often associated with rheumatoid arthritis, Raynaud's phenomenon, and dental caries. detoxification blend, lemon, protective blend, lavender, cellular complex blend	Autoimmune pg. 200
Skin (dry)	Chapped or flaky skin caused from dehydration, lack of omega 3s, or sun or wind damage. myrrh, arborvitae, melaleuca, lavender, geranium	Integumentary pg. 264
Skin (oily)	A skin condition that may be caused from hormones, climate, gentics, or from cosmetics and lotions used. cellular complex blend, cleansing blend, skin clearing blend, lemon	Integumentary pg. 264
Skin Ulcers	A lesion of a mucous membrane or the skin. cellular complex blend, arborvitae, myrrh, lavender	Integumentary pg. 264
Sleep Apnea	A disorder characterized by a reduction or pause of breathing (airflow) during sleep, common among adults but rare among children. Although a diagnosis of sleep apnea often will be suspected on the basis of a person's medical history, several tests can be used to confirm the diagnosis. Treatment can be either surgical or nonsurgical. respiration blend, eucalyptus, peppermint, rosemary, wintergreen	Sleep pg. 317; Respiratory pg. 307
Sleepwalking	Purposeful moving or walking while in a deep stage of sleep. grounding blend, vetiver, lavender, geranium, black pepper	Sleep pg. 317
Smell (loss of)	The inability to smell; may be short-term, selective (only affecting certain aromas), or permanent and total. helichrysum, sandalwood, arborvitae, peppermint, basil	Immune & Lymphatic pg. 259
Smoking Addiction	A physical addiction to tobacco products. Nicotine dependence is an addiction to tobacco products caused by the drug nicotine. Nicotine reliance means you can't stop using the substance, even though it's causing you harm. black pepper, clove, cilantro, detoxification blend, cinnamon	Addictions pg. 190
Snake Bites	A bite from a snake which may be nonpoisonous or poisonous—which may cause envenomation and, if extreme can be fatal. sandalwood, geranium, cypress, basil, melaleuca	First Aid pg. 251
Snoring	A sound achieved during sleep by vibration of loose tissue in the upper airway. To breathe during sleep with harsh, snorting noises caused by pulsing of the soft palate. eucalyptus, respiration blend, peppermint, rosemary	Respiratory pg. 307
Social Anxiety Disorder	Social anxiety is a discomfort or a fear when a person is in social interactions that involve a concern about being evaluated by others or being judged. It is typically defined by an intense fear of what others are thinking about them (specifically fear of embarrassment, criticism, or rejection). grounding blend, wild orange, bergamot, reassuring blend, lime	Brain pg. 208; Mood & Behavior pg. 279
Sore Feet	Painful; tender; aching. basil, ginger, soothing blend, massage blend, wintergreen	Muscular pg. 283; Skeletal pg. 313

STEPS: 1 Look up ailment. 2 Choose one or more of the recommended oils. (Order of recommendation is left to right.) 3 Use oil(s) as indicated. 4 Learn more: see the corresponding body system/focus area.

AILMENT	RECOMMENDED OILS AND USAGE	BODY SYSTEM/FOCUS AREA
Sore Muscles	Limited range of motion, muscle weakness, and tenderness on palpation, occurring 24 to 48 hours after excessive or prolonged muscular activity. massage blend, tension blend, marjoram, peppermint, lime	Muscular pg. 283; Pain & Inflammation pg. 294
Sore Throat	Any of various inflammations of the pharynx, tonsils, or larynx defined by pain in swallowing. lemon, protective blend, thyme, melaleuca, cinnamon	Respiratory pg. 307; Oral Health pg. 291
Spina Bifida	An extreme birth abnormality in which the spinal cord is malformed and lacks its common protective soft tissue and skeletal coverings. cellular complex blend, white fir, soothing blend, eucalyptus, lavender	Nervous pg. 287; Skeletal pg. 313
Sprains	An injury to a ligament when the joint is carried through a range of motion larger than its normal range without dislocation or fracture. soothing blend, lemongrass, massage blend, marjoram, wintergreen	Muscular pg. 283; Pain & Inflammation pg. 294
Staph Infection	Staphylococcus is a group of bacteria found on the skin or nose of many healthy individuals. Generally a localized staph infection can include of collection of pus, such as a boil or abscess. The area is typically tender or painful and may be reddened and swollen. oregano, cinnamon, protective blend, eucalyptus, melaleuca	Immune & Lymphatic pg. 259
Stevens-Johnson Syndrome	A serious form of erythema multiforme in which the systemic symptoms are serious and the lesions vast, involving multiple body areas, typically the mucous membranes. arborvitae, myrrh, detoxification blend, melaleuca, cedarwood	Integumentary pg. 264
Stomach Ache	Pain in the abdomen or stomach area. ginger, detoxification blend, digestion blend, peppermint, coriander	Digestive & Intestinal pg. 235
Strep Throat	An infection of the mucous membranes lining the pharynx; occasionally the tonsils are also infected. protective blend, lemon, melaleuca, cinnamon, oregano	Immune & Lymphatic pg. 259
Stress	An organism's total response to environmental pressures or demands. joyful blend, wild orange, reassuring blend, lavender, calming blend	Limbic pg. 273; Stress pg. 321
Stress Fractures	A fracture of bone caused by replicated application of a heavy load, such as the constant pounding on a surface by runners, dancers, and gymnasts. soothing blend, white fir, birch, wintergreen, helichrysum	Skeletal pg. 313
Stretch Marks	Purplish 'stripes' on the thighs, lower abdomen, breasts, and iliac crests in pregnancy and after corticosteroid excess, which whiten over time (some stretch marks caused by obesity), but do not disappear. anti-aging blend, geranium, sandalwood, frankincense, lavender	Integumentary pg. 264; Pregnancy, Labor & Nursing pg. 301
Stroke	The sudden death of brain cells in a localized area due to insufficient blood flow. basil, fennel, bergamot, cypress, helichrysum	Brain pg. 208; Cardiovascular pg. 216

Diffuse into the air or inhale from cupped hands.

Apply topically directly to affected areas.

Take internally in a capsule or in a glass of water.

TIP For children use 1-2 drops; for adults use 2-4 drops.

AILMENT	RECOMMENDED OILS AND USAGE	BODY SYSTEM/FOCUS AREA
Stye	Infection of the sebaceous gland of an eyelash. melaleuca *, frankincense *, cellular complex blend *, rosemary *, sandalwood *	Respiratory pg. 307
Sunburn	Overexposure to the sun that causes redness and inflammation. lavender, frankincense, helichrysum, anti-aging blend, peppermint	Integumentary pg. 264; First Aid pg. 251
Swimmer's Itch	An allergic skin infection caused by a sensitivity to flatworms that die under the skin, causing an itchy rash. detoxification blend, cleansing blend, frankincense	Integumentary pg. 264; Candida pg. 212
Tachycardia	A fast heart rate which is above 100 beats per minute in an adult. frankincense, helichrysum, grounding blend, lavender, ylang ylang	Cardiovascular pg. 216
Taste, Loss	Because the sensations of taste and smell are related, often taste loss may be associated with sinus or olfactory blockages. The taste sensation often decreases with age. helichrysum, detoxification blend, cleansing blend, peppermint, melissa	Nervous pg. 287
Tear Duct (blocked)	A blocked nasolacrimal duct which typically moves tears from the eyes to the nose. lemongrass *, melaleuca *, cleansing blend *, eucalyptus *, lavender *	Respiratory pg. 307
Teeth Grinding	The habit of grinding and clenching one's teeth occurring at night during sleep. wild orange, geranium, roman chamomile, lavender, calming blend	Oral Health pg. 291
Teething Pain	Flare up or, colloquially, cutting of the teeth, commonly of the deciduous teeth; inflammation of the gingival tissues during this period may cause a brief painful condition. clove, lavender, myrrh, grapefruit, helichrysum	Oral Health pg. 291; Children pg. 225
Tendonitis	The inflammation of a tendon, a hard rope-like tissue that connects muscle to bone. lemongrass, cardamom, massage blend, cypress, marjoram	Muscular pg. 283
Tennis Elbow	An inflammation of many structures of the elbow characterized by tenderness, soreness and/or pain. lemongrass, ginger, massage blend, soothing blend, peppermint	Muscular pg. 283; Skeletal pg. 313
Tension (muscle)	Pain caused by muscle tightness, usually in the neck, shoulders, back or head. lemongrass, wintergreen, tension blend, ginger, peppermint	Muscular pg. 283
Testosterone (low)	A hormone required for male development; appropriate levels in both men and women help lead to optimal functioning. Symptoms of low testosterone in men include excessive fatigue, weakness, depression and drop in sex drive. Symptoms for low testosterone in women include depression, feelings of apathy or disconnectedness, low libido and reduced cognitive ability ("fuzzy" brain). detoxification blend, sandalwood, cleansing blend	Men's Health pg. 276
Thrush	A contagious disease caused by a Candida albicans, fungus that appears most often in children and infants, defined by small whitish outbreaks on the mouth, throat, and tongue. lemon, wild orange, fennel, melaleuca, lavender	Candida pg. 212; Children pg. 225

* For oil usage with eyes, apply oils to temples and around eyes. Dilute as necessary. Do NOT place oils in eyes or even touch eyes when oils are on your fingers

QUICK REFERENCE

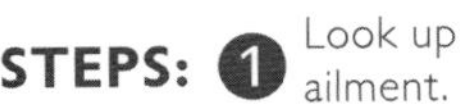

STEPS: 1 Look up ailment. 2 Choose one or more of the recommended oils. (Order of recommendation is left to right.) 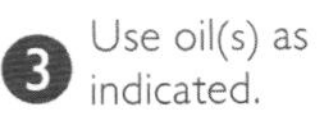 3 Use oil(s) as indicated. 4 Learn more: see the corresponding body system/focus area.

AILMENT	RECOMMENDED OILS AND USAGE	BODY SYSTEM/FOCUS AREA
Tick Bites	Bites from any of numerous small bloodsucking parasitic arachnids of the group Ixodidae and Argasidae, many of which spread febrile diseases. melaleuca, repellent blend, cleansing blend, myrrh, lavender	Parasites pg. 298 First Aid pg. 251;
Tinnitis	Hearing buzzing, ringing, or other sounds without an external cause. helichrysum, basil, melaleuca, frankincense, juniper berry	Respiratory pg. 307
Tissue Pain	Unpleasant physical sensation conveyed to the brain by sensory nerves. soothing blend, tension blend, lemongrass, massage blend, helichrysum	Muscular pg. 283
Tissue Regeneration	The correct registration of the shape of tissues under any condition by means of a sufficient material. cellular complex blend, lemongrass, patchouli, myrrh, helichrysum	Muscular pg. 283; Integumentary pg. 264
Temporomandibular Joint Dysfunction (TMJ)	A disorder of the jaw muscles and nerves caused by injury to the temporomandibular joint. The injured temporomandibular joint leads to pain with chewing, clicking, and popping of the jaw; swelling on the sides of the face; nerve inflammation; headaches; tooth grinding; Eustachian tube dysfunction; and sometimes dislocation of the temporomandibular joint. helichrysum, soothing blend, calming blend, grounding blend, wintergreen	Skeletal pg. 313
Tonsillitis	A swelling and infection of the tonsils, which are oval-shaped masses of lymph gland tissue located on both sides of the back of the throat. protective blend, lemon, cinnamon, eucalyptus, melaleuca	Oral Health pg. 291
Toothache	A soreness or pain around or within a tooth, indicating inflammation and possible infection. clove, melaleuca, helichrysum, protective blend, cinnamon	Oral Health pg. 291
Tourette Syndrome	An inherited disorder of the nervous system, defined by a variable expression of unwanted movements and noises (tics). frankincense, cellular complex blend, cedarwood, patchouli, bergamot	Nervous pg. 287; Brain pg. 208
Toxemia	The condition arising from the escalation of bacterial products (toxins) by the bloodstream. cellular complex blend, detoxification blend, metabolic blend, patchouli, cypress	Pregnancy, Labor & Nursing pg. 301
Transverse Myelitis	An unusual neurological syndrome caused by inflammation (a protective response which includes pain, swelling, heat, and redness) of the spinal cord, defined by back pain, weakness, and bowel and bladder problems. cellular complex blend, thyme, soothing blend, arborvitae, basil	Brain pg. 208
Trigeminal Neuralgia	A disorder of the trigeminal nerve that causes episodes of stabbing, sharp pain in the lips, cheek, gums, or chin on one side of the face. frankincense, helichrysum, myrrh, bergamot, basil	Nervous pg. 287
Tuberculosis	A probable fatal contagious disease that can affect almost any part of the body, but is mainly an infection of the lungs. eucalyptus, melissa, lemon, protective blend, respiratory blend	Respiratory pg. 307

Diffuse into the air or inhale from cupped hands.
Apply topically directly to affected areas.
Take internally in a capsule or in a glass of water.
TIP For children use 1-2 drops; for adults use 2-4 drops.

AILMENT	RECOMMENDED OILS AND USAGE	BODY SYSTEM/FOCUS AREA
Tularemia	A sickness caused by a bacterium. It results in rash, fever, and greatly enlarged lymph nodes. thyme · rosemary · detoxification blend · oregano · coriander	Immune & Lymphatic pg. 259
Tumor	An uncommon growth of tissue resulting from uncontrolled, continuous multiplication of cells. cellular complex blend · frankincense · detoxification blend · rosemary · clove	Cellular Health pg. 221
Turner Syndrome	A condition that affects only women and girls, resulting when a sex chromosome (the X chromosome) is missing or partially missing. Turner syndrome can cause a variety of medical and developmental problems, including failure to start puberty, short height, infertility, heart defects, certain learning disabilities, and social adjustment problems. myrrh · frankincense · clary sage · thyme · sandalwood	Endocrine pg. 244
Typhoid	Many different sicknesses are called "typhus," all of them caused by one of the bacteria in the family Rickettsiae. Each sickness appears when the bacteria is passed to a human through contact with an infected insect. basil · protective blend · detoxification blend · cinnamon · peppermint	Immune & Lymphatic pg. 259
Ulcers, Duodenal	An ulcer of the duodenum, one of the two most typical types of peptic ulcers. detoxification blend · ginger · digestion blend · frankincense · myrrh	Digestive & Intestinal pg. 235
Ulcers, Gastric	An ulcer of the inner wall of the stomach, one of the two most typical kinds of peptic ulcers. cellular complex blend · digestion blend · detoxification blend · geranium · peppermint	Digestive & Intestinal pg. 235
Ulcers, Leg	A site of damage to the mucous membrane or skin that is portrayed by the formation of pus, death of tissue, and is frequently accompanied by an inflammatory reaction. metabolic blend · cellular complex blend · detoxification blend · cleansing blend · lavender	Integumentary pg. 264
Ulcers, Peptic	Ulcers in the upper duodenum and stomach (first portion of the small intestine) caused by a bacterium and stomach acid called Helicobacter pylori. ginger · geranium · cinnamon · fennel · juniper berry	Digestive & Intestinal pg. 235
Ulcers, Varicose	Loss of skin surface in the drainage area of a varicose vein, typically in the leg, emerging from stasis and infection. detoxification blend · helichrysum · tension blend · melaleuca · geranium	Cardiovascular pg. 216; Integumentary pg. 264
Ureter Infection	Infection in the tube that transfers urine from the kidney to the bladder, with each kidney having one ureter. cinnamon · lemongrass · cedarwood · protective blend · cleansing blend	Urinary pg. 324
Urine Flow (poor)	Abnormally slight or infrequent urination. bergamot · metabolic blend · detoxification blend · basil · juniper berry	Urinary pg. 324
Urinary Tract Infection (UTI)	An infection in any part of the urinary system, ureters, kidneys, bladder and urethra. protective blend · thyme · basil · lemongrass · cleansing blend	Urinary pg. 324

STEPS: ❶ Look up ailment. ❷ Choose one or more of the recommended oils. (Order of recommendation is left to right.) ❸ Use oil(s) as indicated. ❹ Learn more: see the corresponding body system/focus area.

AILMENT	RECOMMENDED OILS AND USAGE	BODY SYSTEM/FOCUS AREA
Urination (Painful/ Frequent)	The painful or abnormally frequent ejection of urine. detoxification blend, protective blend, cinnamon, basil, massage blend	Urinary pg. 324
Uterine Bleeding	Any loss of blood from the uterus. helichrysum, frankincense, myrrh, clary sage, roman chamomile	Pregnancy, Labor & Nursing pg. 301
Uvetitis	An infection of the uveal tract, which lines the inside of the eye behind the cornea. cellular complex blend, frankincense, detoxification blend, coriander, anti-aging blend	Nervous pg. 287
Vaginal Yeast Infection	Inflammation of the vagina, defined by vaginal irritation, intense itchiness, and vaginal discharge. Yeast infections occur when there is an overgrowth of fungus in the vaginal area. melissa, melaleuca, rosemary, cinnamon, protective blend (dilute heavily)	Candida pg. 212; Women's Health pg. 332
Vaginitis	Vaginal inflammation. melaleuca, detoxification blend, melissa, basil, rosemary	Women's Health pg. 332
Varicose Veins	Tortuous, dilated, elongated superficial veins that are commonly seen in the legs. helichrysum, cypress, cardamom, peppermint, lemongrass	Cardiovascular pg. 216; Integumentary pg. 264
Vertigo	A feeling of whirling or irregular motion, either of oneself or of external objects, generally caused by inner ear disease. cellular complex blend, invigorating blend, geranium, ginger, helichrysum	Cardiovascular pg. 216
Virus	Specifically, a term for a group of infectious agents, which, with few exceptions, are capable of passing through fine filters that retain most bacteria, are usually not visible through the light microscope, lack independent metabolism, and are incapable of growth or reproduction apart from living cells oregano, protective blend, arborvitae, melaleuca, cinnamon	Immune & Lymphatic pg. 259
Vision (poor)	Deterioration of vision such that there is compelling visual handicap but also significant usable residual vision. anti-aging blend, lemongrass, cellular complex blend, sandalwood, frankincense	Nervous pg. 287
Vitiligo	A condition in which a decrease of cells that give color to the skin (melanocytes) results in smooth, white patches in the midst of ordinary pigmented skin. cellular complex blend, detoxification blend, women's blend, vetiver, sandalwood	Autoimmune pg. 200; Integumentary pg. 264
Vomiting	Forcible elimination of contents of stomach through the mouth. digestion blend, cellular complex blend, detoxification blend, ginger, peppermint	Digestive & Intestinal pg. 235; Detoxification pg. 230
Warts	Small, benign growths generated by a viral infection of the mucous or skin membrane. oregano, lemongrass, thyme, frankincense, protective blend	Integumentary pg. 264

Diffuse into the air or inhale from cupped hands.

Apply topically directly to affected areas.

Take internally in a capsule or in a glass of water.

TIP For children use 1-2 drops; for adults use 2-4 drops.

AILMENT	RECOMMENDED OILS AND USAGE		BODY SYSTEM/FOCUS AREA
Wasp Sting	Painful stings or bites from the hymenoptera family which includes bees, yellow jackets, hornets, wasps, and ants. These stings are generally harmless; however, more serious allergic reactions may occur which can be deadly.	lavender, myrrh, cleansing blend, roman chamomile	First Aid pg. 251
Water Retention	When too much fluid is released into tissue spaces between cells, causing swelling.	detoxification blend, metabolic blend, grapefruit, lemon, cypress	Pregnancy, Labor & Nursing pg. 301
Whiplash	An abrupt, moderate-to-severe strain affecting the discs, muscles, bones, nerves, or tendons of the neck.	tension blend, helichrysum, white fir, soothing blend, lemongrass	Muscular pg. 283
Withdrawal Symptoms	A group of mental or physical symptoms that may appear when a person abruptly or gradually stops using a drug to which he or she has become dependent.	cellular complex blend, cilantro, cinnamon, juniper berry	Addictions pg. 190; Mood & Behavior pg. 279; Focus & Concentration pg. 255
Workout Recovery	The period of time directly following sustained exercise that the body returns to resting metabolic rate and muscles strengthened through the process of tearing and rebuilding lose their soreness.	massage blend, soothing blend, marjoram, tension blend, lime	Athletes pg. 197
Worms	A family of parasites defined by a long body, either round (nematodes) or flat (platyhelminthes). They mainly reside in the intestinal tract, but some types can also live in other major organs and tissue, such as the brain or muscles, respectively.	clove, oregano, thyme, lemongrass, protective blend	Digestive & Intestinal pg. 235
Wounds	Occurs when the integrity of any tissue is compromised.	myrrh, helichrysum, lavender, cleansing blend, douglas fir	Integumentary pg. 264
Wrinkles	A by-product of the aging course. Skin cells divide more slowly, and the inner layer, called the dermis, begins to thin with age.	sandalwood, anti-aging blend, geranium, frankincense, roman chamomile	Integumentary pg. 264
Xenoestrogens	A type of xenohormone that imitates estrogen and creates byproduct estrogen metabolites as it is utilized by the body.	detoxification blend, basil, ginger, women's monthly blend, clary sage	Detoxification pg. 230
Xerophthalmia	Dry eyes.	cellular complex blend, detoxification blend, lemon, cilantro, anti-aging blend	Nervous pg. 287
Yeast	Candidiasis is a common type of yeast infection caused by the candida fungi, which live on the surface of the body. Several types of yeast infection are possible including thrush, candidal rashes (diaper rash), and more severe systemic candidal infections.	melaleuca, lemongrass, thyme, oregano, protective blend	Candida pg. 212

SECTION 3

NATURAL SOLUTIONS

Becoming familiar with the qualities and common benefits of essential oils is a key part of living THE ESSENTIAL LIFE. As you become versed in the powerful qualities of each oil, blend, and supplement, you will find confidence in turning to nature as your first resource for wellness. Nature's vast diversity provides answers to any health interest, be it physical, mental, or emotional.

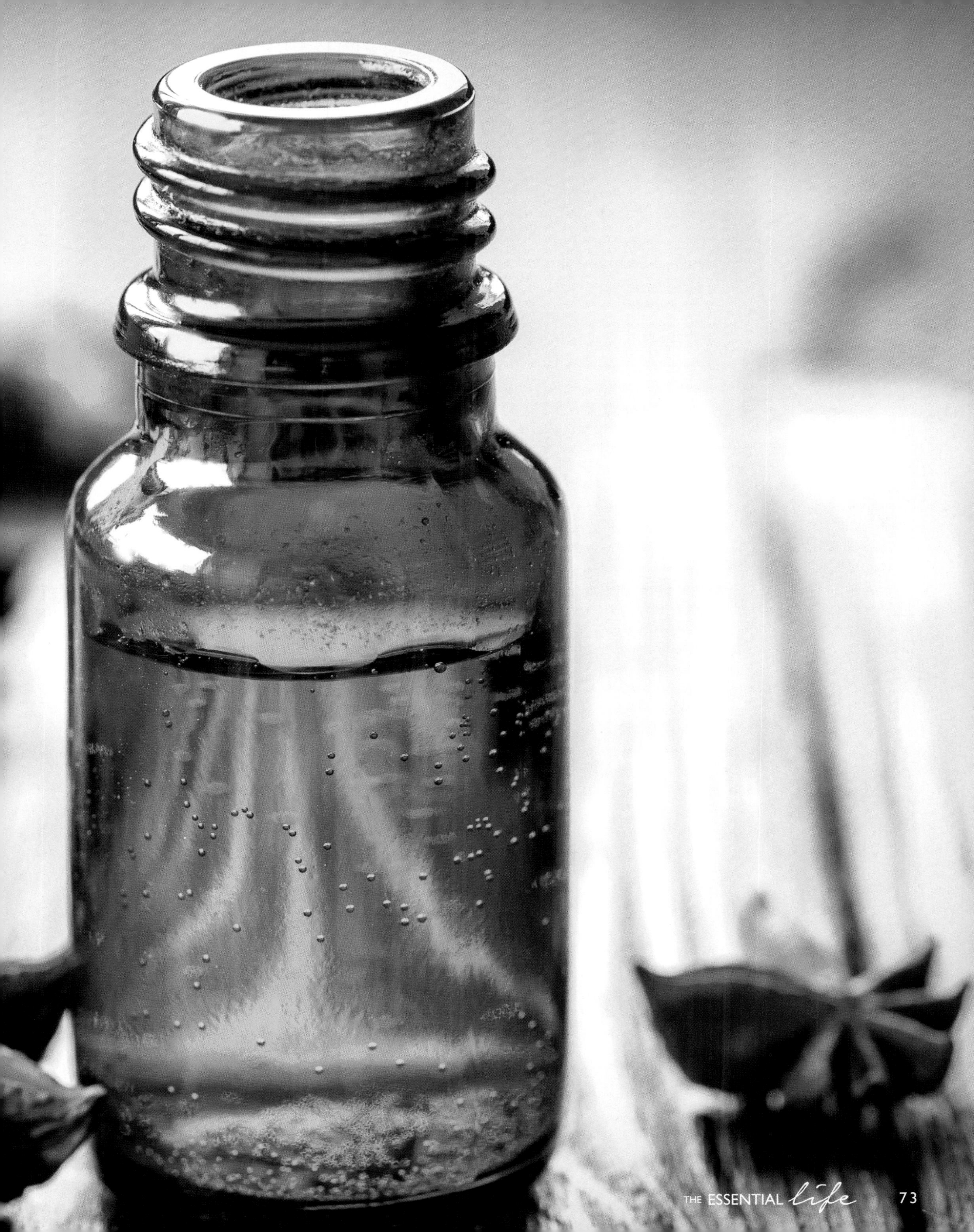

SINGLE OILS

This section provides a detailed reference for the origins, qualities, purposes, and safety of individual essential oils. The top uses of each oil are intended to be a succinct guide, as more detailed uses are highlighted in *Body Systems*.

Please note the symbols =aromatic =topical =internal that specify recommended usage. While all oils are meant to be used aromatically and most topically, only verified pure therapeutic essential oils are intended for internal use. (See *Why Quality Matters* and *How to Use Essential Oils* for further detail.)

ARBORVITAE

THUJA PLICATA

woody
majestic
strong

TOP USES

CANDIDA & FUNGAL ISSUES
Apply topically or diffuse to fight fungal issues and candida.

VIRUSES
Apply topically to bottoms of feet.

RESPIRATORY ISSUES
Apply topically with fractionated coconut oil to chest.

REPELLENT
Diffuse , spray on surfaces, or apply topically repel bugs and insects.

CANCER
Apply topically to bottoms of feet to assist with proper cellular function and processes.

STIMULANT
Apply topically under nose and back of neck to stimulate nervous system and awareness.

BACTERIAL SUPPORT
Apply topically to bottoms of feet or spine with fractionated coconut oil. Spray diluted in water on surfaces or diffuse to kill airborne pathogens.

SKIN COMPLAINTS
Apply topically with lavender to troubled skin.

SUN
Apply topically with helichrysum or lavender to protect against sun exposure.

MEDITATION
Diffuse to enhance spiritual awareness and state of calm.

EMOTIONAL BALANCE
Use aromatically and topically to get from Overzealous ⟶ Composed.

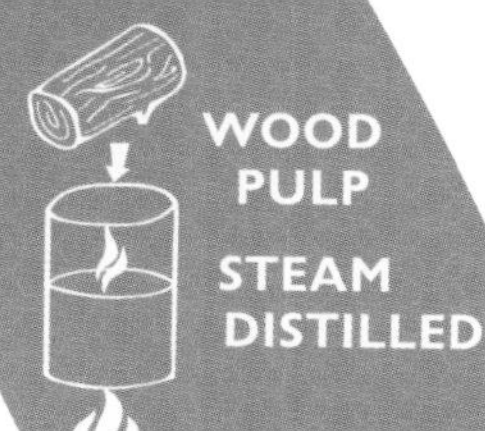

WOOD PULP

STEAM DISTILLED

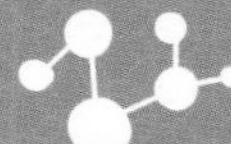

MAIN CONSTITUENTS
Methyl thujate
Hinokitiol
Thujic acid

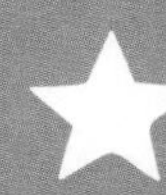

TOP PROPERTIES
Antiviral
Antifungal
Antibacterial
Stimulant

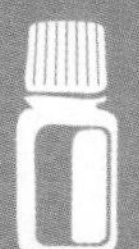

BLENDS WELL WITH
Cedarwood
Frankincense
Birch

SAFETY
Dilution recommend. Possible skin sensitivity.

SINGLE OILS

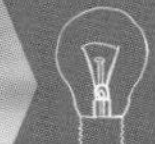

Arborvitae trees can live for over 800 years. It's no surprise that Arborvitae means "Tree of Life."

RESEARCH: Effect of arborvitae seed on cognitive function and a-7nAChR protein expression of hippocampus in model rats with Alzheimer's disease, Cheng XL, Xiong XB, Xiang MQ, *Cell Biochem Biophys*, 2013

Conservative surgical management of stage IA endometrial carcinoma for fertility preservation, Mazzon I, Corrado G, Masciullo V, Morricone D, Ferrandina G, Scambia G., *Fertil Steril*, 2010

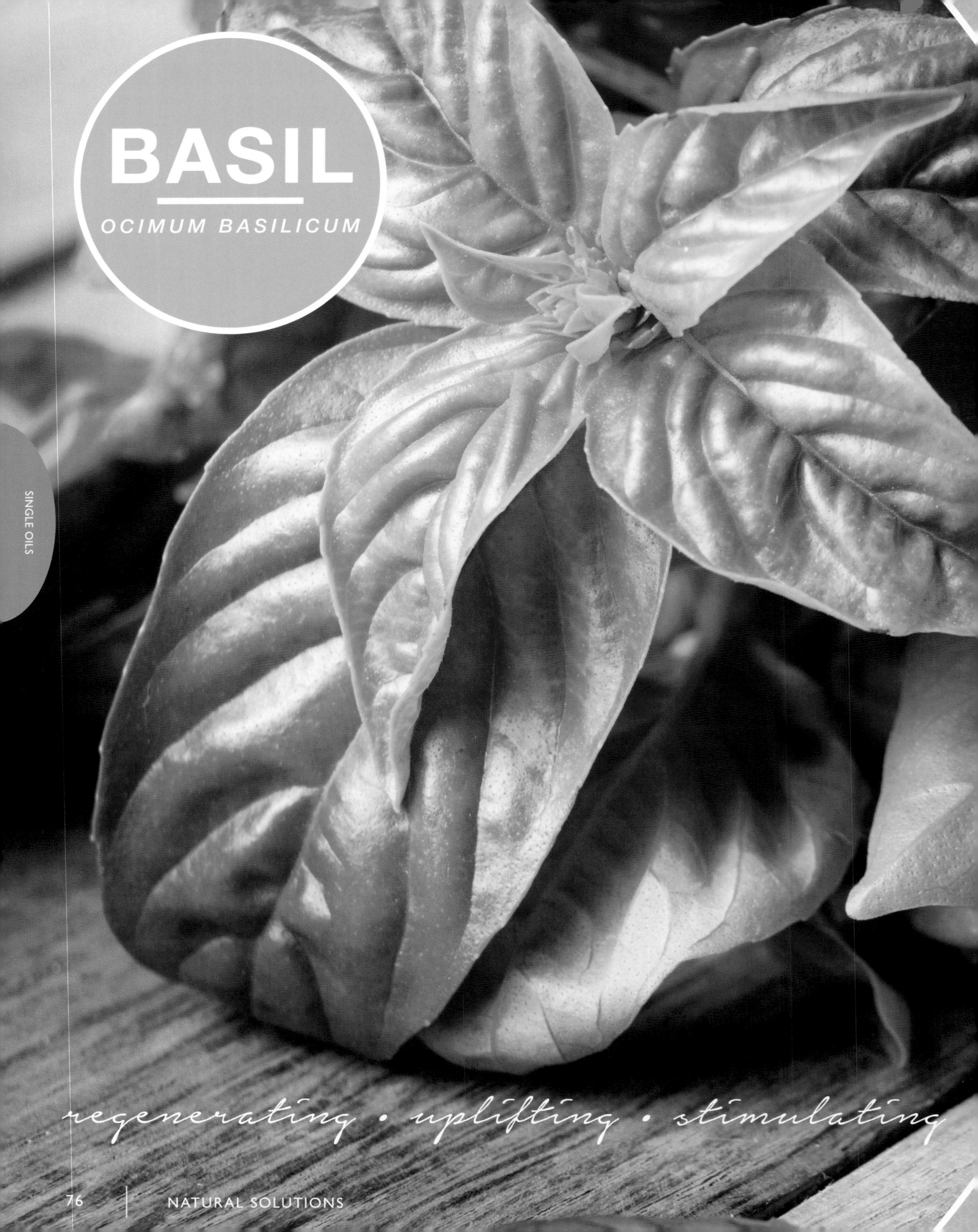

BASIL

OCIMUM BASILICUM

SINGLE OILS

regenerating • uplifting • stimulating

LEAVES

STEAM DISTILLED

MAIN CONSTITUENTS
Linalool
Methylchavicol
Eugenol

TOP PROPERTIES
Stimulant
Neurotonic
Steroidal
Regenerative
Antispasmodic
Anti-inflammatory
Antibacterial
Digestive

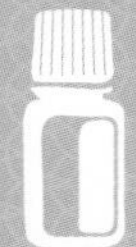

FOUND IN
Massage blend
Tension blend

BLENDS WELL WITH
Lime
Peppermint
Bergamot

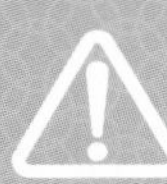

SAFETY
Dilution recommend. Possible skin sensitivity. Caution with pregnancy & epilepsy. Can act as relaxant if overused.

TOP USES

ADRENAL FATIGUE
Apply topically under nose, to bottoms of feet, and/or adrenals to wake up body's electrical system.

EARACHE
Apply topically on and around ear to relieve pain and infection.

MIGRAINE
Apply with wintergreen or peppermint topically to temples and back of neck to assist with migraines and dizziness.

MENTAL FATIGUE
Diffuse aromatically and apply topically to energize the mind.

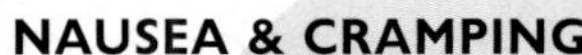

NAUSEA & CRAMPING
Take internally in a capsule or apply to abdomen to ease discomfort.

GOUT & RHEUMATISM
Apply topically to spine, bottoms of feet, ears, ankles, or area over heart.

MENSTRUAL ISSUES
Apply topically to lower abdomen to stimulate menstrual flow & assist with PMS cramping.

EMOTIONAL BALANCE
Use aromatically and topically to get from Inundated ⟶ Relieved.

MUSCLE SPASMS
Apply topically to spine or bottoms of feet, or take internally in a capsule to decrease inflammation.

BITES
Diffuse aromatically or spray diluted in water to repel insects. Apply topically for bug, snake, or spider bites.

One of the most universally applicable oils, basil is from the Greek word meaning "king." Ancient Greeks believed it opened the gateways to heaven.

RESEARCH: Cyclodextrin-Complexed Ocimum basilicum Leaves Essential Oil Increases Fos Protein Expression in the Central Nervous System and Produces an Antihyperalgesic Effect in Animal Models for Fibromyalgia, Nascimento SS, *International Journal of Molecular Sciences*, 2014
Central Properties and Chemical Composition of Ocimum basilicum Essential Oil, Ismail M, *Pharmaceutical Biology*, 2006
A comparative study of antiplaque and antigingivitis effects of herbal mouthrinse containing tea tree oil, clove, and basil with commercially available essential oil mouthrinse, Kothiwale SV, Patwardhan V, Gandhi M, Sohoni R, Kumar A, *Journal of Indian Society of Periodontology*, 2014
Protective effect of basil (Ocimum basilicum L.) against oxidative DNA damage and mutagenesis, BeriĐ T, *Food and Chemical Toxicology*, 2008
Biological effects, antioxidant and anticancer activities of marigold and basil essential oils, Mahmoud GI, *Journal of Medicinal Plants Research*, 2013
Increased seizure latency and decreased severity of pentylenetetrazol-induced seizures in mice after essential oil administration, Koutroumanidou E, *Epilepsy Research and Treatment*, 2013
Antigiardial activity of Ocimum basilicum essential oil, de Almeida I, *Parasitology Research*, 2007
Antibacterial Effects of the Essential Oils of Commonly Consumed Medicinal Herbs Using an In Vitro Model, SokoviĐ M, *Molecules*, 2010

SINGLE OILS

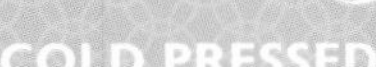

RIND

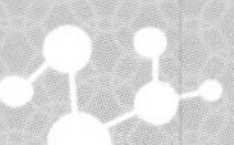

COLD PRESSED

MAIN CONSTITUENTS
Limonene
Linalyl formate
Linalol

TOP PROPERTIES
Neurotonic
Anti-inflammatory
Antidepressant
Antibacterial
Antifungal
Digestive

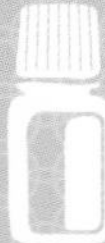

FOUND IN
Invigorating blend
Women's monthly blend

BLENDS WELL WITH
Ylang ylang
Lavender
Patchouli

SAFETY
Avoid direct sunlight or UV rays to applied area for 12 hours. Possible skin sensitivity.

RESEARCH: Neuropharmacology of the essential oil of bergamot, Bagetta G, Morrone LA, Rombolà L, Amantea D, Russo R, Berliocchi L, Sakurada S, Sakurada T, Rotiroti D, Corasaniti MT, *Fitoterapia*, 2010
The effects of the inhalation method using essential oils on blood pressure and stress responses of clients with essential hypertension, Hwang JH, *Korean Society of Nursing Science*, 2006
The physical effects of aromatherapy in alleviating work-related stress on elementary school teachers in Taiwan, Liu SH, Lin TH, Chang KM, *Evidence-Based Complementary and Alternative Medicine*, 2013
The Essential Oil of Bergamot Stimulates Reactive Oxygen Species Production in Human Polymorphonuclear Leukocytes, Cosentino M, Luini A, Bombelli R, Corasaniti MT, Bagetta G, Marino F, *Phytotherapy Research*, 2014

BERGAMOT

CITRUS BERGAMIA

uplifting • assuring • restoring

SINGLE OILS

TOP USES

INSOMNIA
Apply topically or diffuse aromatically before bed.

STRESS
Apply topically to back of neck & bottoms of feet or diffuse.

JOINT ISSUES & MUSCLE CRAMPS
Apply topically to affected area or take internally in a capsule.

FUNGUS ISSUES
Apply topically to affected areas.

COUGHS, INFECTIONS & BRONCHITIS
Apply topically to chest.

ACNE, OILY SKIN, ECZEMA & PSORIASIS
Apply topically to affected area.

APPETITE LOSS
Diffuse aromatically and take internally in a capsule.

SELF-WORTH ISSUES
Apply topically to support feeling comfortable in own skin.

EMOTIONAL BALANCE
Use aromatically and topically to get from Inadequate→Worthy.

Bergamot was used in the first eau de cologne & is used to flavor Earl Grey tea.

RESEARCH: Anticancer activity of liposomal bergamot essential oil (BEO) on human neuroblastoma cells, Celia C, Trapasso E, Locatelli M, Navarra M, Ventura CA, Wolfram J, Carafa M, Morittu VM, Britti D, Di Marzio L, Paolino D, *Colloids and Surfaces*, 2013

The essential oil of bergamot enhances the levels of amino acid neurotransmitters in the hippocampus of rat: implication of monoterpene hydrocarbons, Morrone LA, Rombolà L, Pelle C, Corasaniti MT, Zappettini S, Paudice P, Bonanno G, Bagetta G, *Pharmacological Research*, 2007

The effects of inhalation of essential oils on the body weight, food efficiency rate and serum leptin of growing SD rats, Hur MH, Kim C, Kim CH, Ahn HC, Ahn HY, *Korean Society of Nursing Science*, 2006

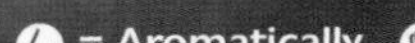 = Aromatically 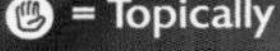 = Topically 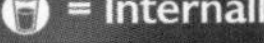 = Internally

BIRCH

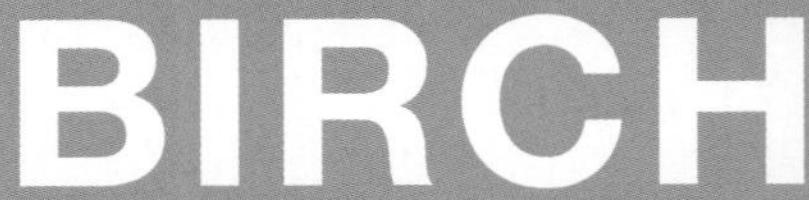

BETULA LENTA

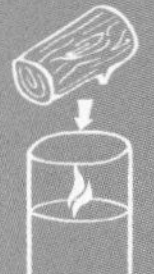

WOOD

STEAM DISTILLED

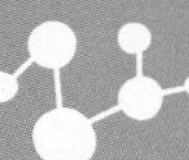

MAIN CONSTITUENT
Methyl salicylate
Betulene
Butulinol

TOP PROPERTIES
Analgesic
Tonic
Anti-rheumatic
Stimulant
Steroidal
Warming

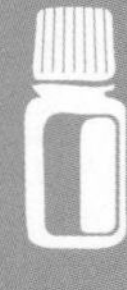

BLENDS WELL WITH
Peppermint
Lavender
Cypress

invigorate · activate · soothe

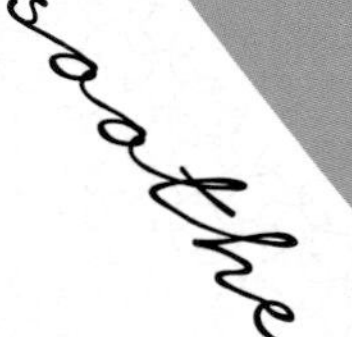

SAFETY
Not for internal use. Avoid during pregnancy. Not for use by epileptics.

TOP USES

CONNECTIVE TISSUE & MUSCLE INJURIES
Apply topically to affected area.

ARTHRITIS, RHEUMATISM & GOUT
Apply topically to affected area.

MUSCLE PAIN & SPASMS
Apply topically to area of concern for cortisone-like action.

FEVER
Apply topically on spine.

BONE SPURS, GALL & KIDNEY STONES & CATARACTS
Apply topically to bottoms of feet or areas of concern.

ULCERS & CRAMPS
Apply topically to abdomen as needed.

EMOTIONAL BALANCE
Use aromatically and topically to get from Cowardly→Courageous.

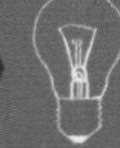

Birch is used to make root beer.

RESEARCH: Repelling properties of some plant materials on the tick Ixodes ricinus L., Thorsell W, Mikiver A, Tunón H, *Phytomedicine*, 2006 *spicy • warming • circulating*

BLACK PEPPER

PIPER NIGRUM

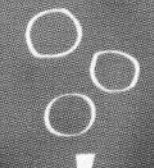

BERRIES

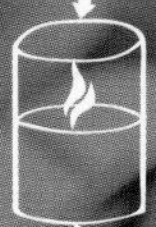

STEAM DISTILLED

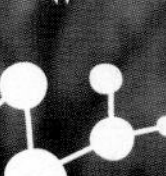

MAIN CONSTITUENTS
Caryophyllene
Limonene
Carene

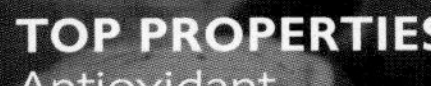

TOP PROPERTIES
Antioxidant
Antispasmodic
Digestive
Expectorant
Neorotonic
Stimulant
Rubefacient

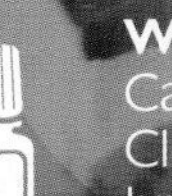

BLENDS WELL WITH
Cardamom
Clove
Juniper berry

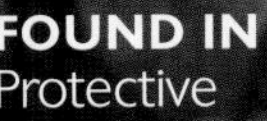

FOUND IN
Protective blend softgels

SAFETY
Dilution recommended. Possible skin sensitivity if old or oxidized.

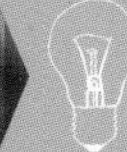

Black pepper shares a similar chemical structure to melissa essential oil

SINGLE OILS

TOP USES

CONSTIPATION, DIARRHEA & GAS
Take internally in capsule or apply topically to abdomen.

DRAINING & CLEANSING RESPIRATORY & LYMPHATIC
Use internally by placing a drop under tongue and inhale.

CIRCULATION ISSUES
Apply topically with a warm compress to increase circulation and blood flow to muscles and nerves.

COLD & FLU
For seasonal threats use internally in a capsule or apply topically to bottoms of feet.

CONGESTED AIRWAYS
Diffuse or apply topically to chest with white fir to clear airways.

FOOD FLAVOR
Enhance your favorite foods by adding 1 drop as seasoning while also assisting digestion.

ANXIETY
Diffuse aromatically or apply topically under nose or on bottoms of feet.

CRAMPS, SPRAINS & MUSCLE SPASMS
Apply topically to affected area.

SMOKING
Use 1 drop under tongue & inhale aromatically to assist with cigarette cravings and associated anxiety.

EMOTIONAL BALANCE
Use aromatically and topically to get from Repressed ⟶ Honest.

RESEARCH: Black pepper and piperine reduce cholesterol uptake and enhance translocation of cholesterol transporter proteins, Duangjai A, *Journal of Natural Medicine*, 2013
Growth inhibition of pathogenic bacteria and some yeasts by selected essential oils and survival of L. monocytogenes and C. albicans in apple-carrot juice., Irkin R, *Foodborne Pathogens and Disease*, 2009
Antioxidative Properties and Inhibition of Key Enzymes Relevant to Type-2 Diabetes and Hypertension by Essential Oils from Black Pepper, Oboh G, *Advances in Pharmacological Sciences*, 2013
Black pepper essential oil to enhance intravenous catheter insertion in patients with poor vein visibility: a controlled study, Kristiniak S, *Journal of Alternative and Complementary Medicine*, 2012
Olfactory stimulation using black pepper oil facilitates oral feeding in pediatric patients receiving long-term enteral nutrition, Munakata M, *The Tohoku Journal of Experimental Medicine*, 2008
The effects of aromatherapy on nicotine craving on a U.S. campus: a small comparison study, Cordell B, Buckle J, *The Journal of Alternative and Complementary Medicine*, 2013
A randomized trial of olfactory stimulation using black pepper oil in older people with swallowing dysfunction, Ebihara T, *Journal of the American Geriatrics Society*, 2009

= Aromatically = Topically = Internally

CARDAMOM

ELETTARIA CARDAMOMUM

invigorate
relax
cleanse

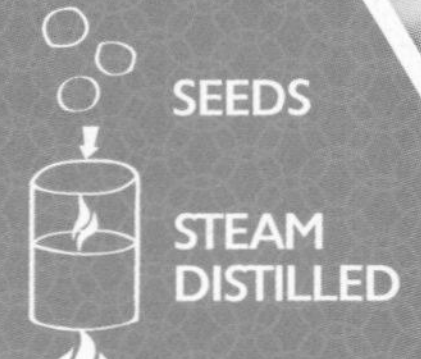

SEEDS

STEAM DISTILLED

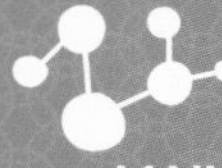

MAIN CONSTITUENTS
Terpinyl acetate
1,8-cineole
Linalool

TOP PROPERTIES
Digestive
Antispasmodic
Anti-inflammatory
Decongestant
Expectorant
Tonic
Stomachic
Carminative

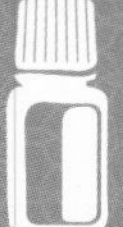

FOUND IN
Respiration blend
Respiration blend lozenge

BLENDS WELL WITH
Peppermint
Lavender
Clove

TOP USES

CONGESTION
Apply topically to chest or diffuse aromatically.

STOMACHACHE & CONSTIPATION
Use internally in a capsule or apply topically to calm and promote digestion.

MENSTRUAL & DIGESTIVE ISSUES
Apply topically to abdomen.

GASTRITIS & STOMACH ULCERS
Use internally in a capsule.

MUSCLE PAIN
Apply topically to relieve pain and inflammation.

SORE THROAT & FEVERS
Protect against seasonal threats by diffusing aromatically or apply topically.

MENTAL FATIGUE & CONFUSION
Clear your mind and ease fatigue by applying topically under nose and to back of neck.

PANCREATITIS
Apply topically to area over pancreas to cleanse and restore pancreatic function.

BAD BREATH & HOUSEHOLD ODORS
Use internally in a capsule for breath or diffuse aromatically to clear air of odors.

COOKING
Use to season your favorite foods and enhance flavors.

EMOTIONAL BALANCE
Use aromatically and topically to get from Self-centered⟶Charitable.

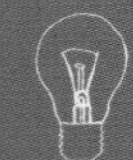

Known as the most expensive cooking spice, cardamom is also a close relative of ginger.

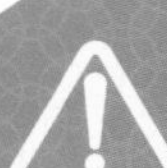

SAFETY
Safe for NEAT application.

RESEARCH: Antimicrobial activity of the bioactive components of essential oils from Pakistani spices against Salmonella and other multi-drug resistant bacteria., Naveed R, Hussain I, *BMC Complementary and Alternative Medicine*, 2013
Gastroprotective effect of cardamom, Elettaria cardamomum Maton, fruits in rats, Jamal A, *Journal of Ethnopharmacology*, 2006
Aromatherapy as a Treatment for Postoperative Nausea: A randomized trial, Hunt R, *Anesthesia and Analgesia*, 2013
Treatment of irritable bowel syndrome with herbal preparations: results of a double-blind, randomized, placebo-controlled, multi-centre trial, Madisch A, *Alimentary Pharmacology and Therapeutics*, 2004
Identification of proapoptopic, anti-inflammatory, anti-proliferative, anti-invasive and anti-angiogenic targets of essential oils in cardamom by dual reverse virtual screening and binding pose analysis, Bhattacharjee B, Asian Pacific *Journal of Cancer Prevention*, 2013
Activity of Essential Oils Against Bacillus subtilis Spores, Lawrence HA, *Journal of Microbiology and Biotechnology*, 2009

CASSIA

CINNAMOMUM CASSIA

spicy • strong • warming

TOP USES

COLD EXTREMITIES
Apply topically diluted to increase blood flow and bring warmth to skin and limbs.

UPSET STOMACH & VOMITING
Use internally in a capsule to stimulate digestion.

DETOX FOR EAR, NOSE, THROAT, LUNGS
Use internally in a capsule to clear yeast, phlegm & plaque.

WATER RETENTION
Use internally in a capsule or apply topically to bottoms of feet with fractionated coconut oil.

BLOOD SUGAR BALANCE
Use internally in a capsule with meals to support balanced blood sugar levels.

METABOLISM BOOST
Use internally in a capsule to increase metabolism.

SEXUAL DRIVE
Diffuse aromatically or inhale aroma from bottle to increase sexual desire.

COOKING
Add to your favorite recipe for a sweet cinnamon-like flavor.

EMOTIONAL BALANCE
Use aromatically and topically to get from Uncertain ⟶ Bold.

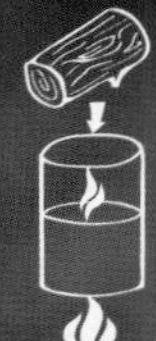

BARK

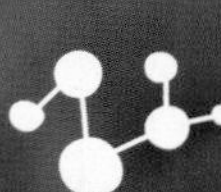

STEAM DISTILLED

MAIN CONSTITUENTS
Cinnamaldehyde
Eugenol
Chavicol

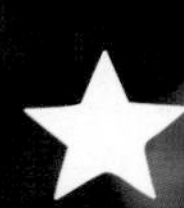

TOP PROPERTIES
Decongestant
Carminative
Detoxifier
Cardiotonic
Antimicrobial
Antiviral
Antifungal
Antispasmodic

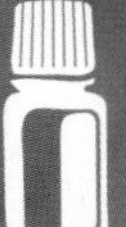

BLENDS WELL WITH
Wild orange
Ginger
White fir

SAFETY
Dilute heavily for topical use. May cause skin irritation. Can reduce milk supply in lactating women.

Make cinnamon sweet candy water by adding 1 drop of cassia with 2 drops of grapefruit.

RESEARCH: Anti-inflammatory effects of essential oil from the leaves of Cinnamomum cassia and cinnamaldehyde on lipopolysaccharide-stimulated J774A.1 cells., Pannee C, *Journal of Advanced Pharmaceutical Technology & Research*, 2014
From type 2 diabetes to antioxidant activity: a systematic review of the safety and efficacy of common and cassia cinnamon bark., Dugoua JJ, Seely D, Perri D, Cooley K, Forelli T, Mills E, Koren G, *Canadian Journal of Physiology and Pharmacology*, 2007
A review on anti-inflammatory activity of monoterpenes, de Cássia da Silveira e Sá R, Andrade LN, de Sousa DP, *Molecules*, 2013
Cinnamomum cassia essential oil inhibits MSH-induced melanin production and oxidative stress in murine B16 melanoma cells, Chou ST, Chang WL, Chang CT, Hsu SL, Lin YC, Shih Y, *International Journal of Molecular Sciences*, 2013
Randomized clinical trial of a phytotherapic compound containing Pimpinella anisum, Foeniculum vulgare, Sambucus nigra, and Cassia augustifolia for chronic constipation, Picon PD, Picon RV, Costa AF, Sander GB, Amaral KM, Aboy AL, Henriques AT, *BMC Complementary and Alternative Medicine*, 2010
Antimicrobial activities of cinnamon oil and cinnamaldehyde from the Chinese medicinal herb Cinnamomum cassia Blume, Ooi LS, Li Y, Kam SL, Wang H, Wong EY, Ooi VE, *The American Journal of Chinese Medicine*, 2006

CEDARWOOD

JUNIPERUS VIRGINIANA

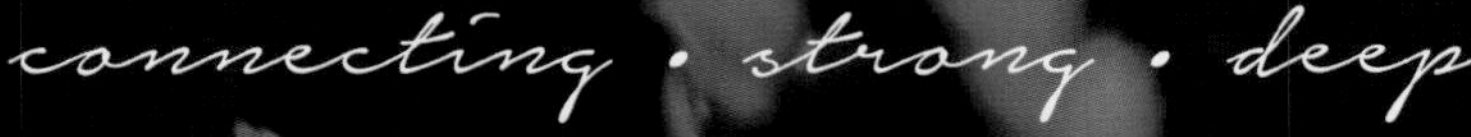

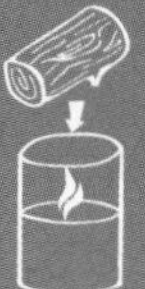

WOOD

STEAM DISTILLED

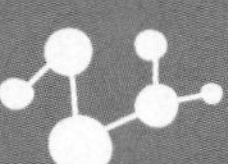

MAIN CONSTITUENTS
Alpha cedrene
Cedrol

TOP PROPERTIES
Anti-inflammatory
Diuretic
Astringent
Antiseptic
Insecticidal
Sedative

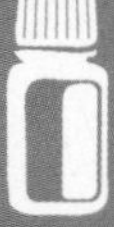

FOUND IN
Repellent blend
Women's monthly blend

BLENDS WELL WITH
Bergamot
Juniper berry
Cypress

SAFETY
Dilution recommended.
Possible skin sensitivity.

TOP USES

ADD & ADHD
Apply topically over chest, on bottoms of feet and/or inhale deeply aromatically to soothe anxious feelings.

PSORIASIS & ECZEMA
Apply 1 drop topically with 1 drop lavender to affected area.

CALMING & ANXIETY
Put on the palm of hands and inhale or apply topically to bottoms of feet.

COUGH & SINUS ISSUES
Apply topically to chest and forehead and then cup hands over nose to inhale aromatically.

STROKE
Apply topically on back of neck and bottoms of feet.

URINARY TRACT, BLADDER & VAGINAL INFECTION
Apply topically to lower abdomen for infection support.

GUMS
Apply topically to gums.

INSECT REPELLENT
Dilute topically with fractionated coconut oil and apply to skin or use aromatically in diffuser to deter insects.

ACNE
Apply with 1 drop melaleuca topically to blemishes.

EMOTIONAL BALANCE
Use aromatically and topically to get from Alone ——→ Connected.

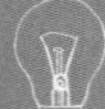

Cedarwood can grow to over 100 feet tall and is mentioned several times in the Bible.

RESEARCH: Repellency of Essential Oils to Mosquitoes (Diptera: Culicidae), Barnard DR, *Journal of Medical Entomology*, 1999
Repellency of essential oils to mosquitoes (Diptera: Culicidae), Barnard DR, *Journal of Medical Entomology*, 1999
Fumigant toxicity of plant essential oils against Camptomyia corticalis (Diptera: Cecidomyiidae), Kim JR, Haribalan P, Son BK, Ahn YJ, *Journal of Economic Entomology*, 2012
Bactericidal activities of plant essential oils and some of their isolated constituents against Campylobacter jejuni, Escherichia coli, Listeria monocytogenes, and Salmonella enterica, Friedman M, Henika PR, Mandrell RE, *Journal of Food Protection*, 2002
Chemical composition and antibacterial activity of selected essential oils and some of their main compounds, Wanner J, Schmidt E, Bail S, Jirovetz L, Buchbauer G, Gochev V, Girova T, Atanasova T, Stoyanova A, *Natural Product Communications*, 2010
Randomized trial of aromatherapy: successful treatment for alopecia areata, Hay IC, Jamieson M, Ormerod AD, *Archives of Dermatology*, 1998

fresh • awakening • cleansing

CILANTRO

CORIANDRUM SATIVUM

TOP USES

HEAVY METAL DETOX & ANTIOXIDANT ISSUES
Use internally in a capsule to detox heavy metals and free radicals from the body.

GAS, INDIGESTION & BLOATING
Apply topically over stomach for digestion support.

ALLERGIES
Apply topically over liver or on bottoms of feet to ease allergies by reducing toxic load in liver.

LIVER & KIDNEY SUPPORT
Use internally in a capsule or apply topically over liver.

FUNGAL INFECTIONS
Use internally in a capsule and apply topically to infected area.

COOKING
Dip toothpick and add internally to your favorite salad, dip, or guacamole recipe.

BODY ODOR
Combine with peppermint internally in a capsule to diminish strong body odor.

ANXIETY
Use aromatically in a diffuser to ease anxious feelings.

EMOTIONAL BALANCE
Use aromatically and topically to get from Obsessed ⟶ Expansive.

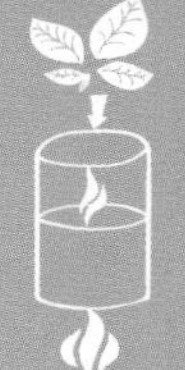

LEAVES

STEAM DISTILLED

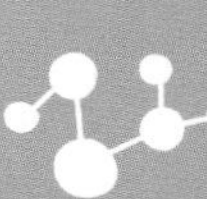

MAIN CONSTITUENTS
Decenal
Dodecenal

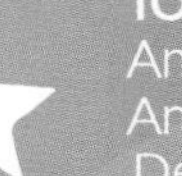

TOP PROPERTIES
Antioxidant
Antifungal
Detoxifying
Antibacterial

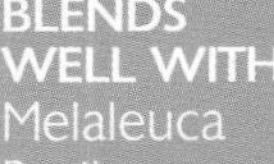

BLENDS WELL WITH
Melaleuca
Basil
Lemon

FOUND IN
Detoxification blend
Tension blend
Cleansing blend

SAFETY
Safe to apply NEAT.

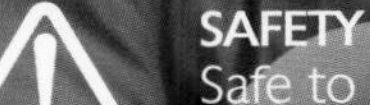

Relatives of parsley, cilantro and coriander essential oils are from the same plant. Cilantro is extracted from the leaf and coriander from the seed.

RESEARCH: Antimicrobial activity of individual and mixed fractions of dill, cilantro, coriander and eucalyptus essential oils, Delaquis PJ, Stanich K, Girard B, Mazza G, *International Journal of Food Microbiology*, 2002

CINNAMON BARK

CINNAMOMUM ZEYLANICUM

protecting • spicy • awakening

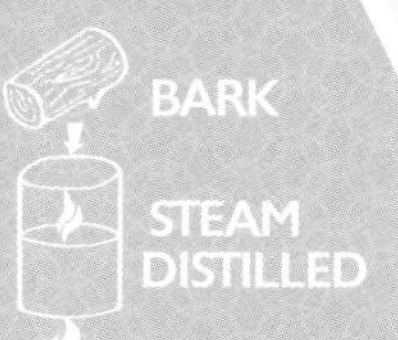

BARK

STEAM DISTILLED

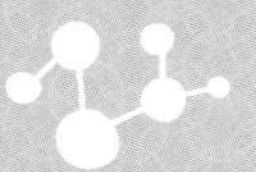

MAIN CONSTITUENTS
Cinnamaldehyde
Eugenol
Phenol

TOP PROPERTIES
Antiseptic
Antimicrobial
Antioxidant
Antifungal
Antiviral
Aphrodisiac

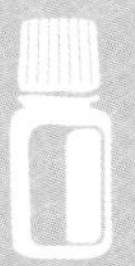

FOUND IN
Women's monthly blend
Metabolic blend
Protective blend

BLENDS WELL WITH
Wild orange
Patchouli
Myrrh

SAFETY
Dilute for topical application. Can cause skin irritation.

TOP USES

PANCREAS & BLOOD SUGAR
Use internally in a capsule to balance blood sugar.

COLD & FLU
Take internally in a capsule or topically on bottoms of feet for immune support. Diffuse aromatically to cleanse air.

CHOLESTEROL & HEART ISSUES
Apply 1 drop topically diluted to limbs for warming & increased blood flow.

ORAL HEALTH
Gargle 1 drop in water to combat oral infection.

GERMS & BACTERIA
Use internally in a capsule or add in a glass spray bottle and use to clean surfaces to combat germs and bacteria.

VAGINAL HEALTH
Use internally in a capsule.

MALE & FEMALE SEXUAL ISSUES
Use internally in a capsule for hormone support and balance.

MUSCLE STRAIN & PAIN
Apply topically diluted to soothe.

COOKING
Add internally to your favorite baking recipe for a spicy twist.

EMOTIONAL BALANCE
Use aromatically and topically to get from Denied ⟶ Receptive.

SINGLE OILS

Used in biblical times and by the ancient Egyptians, cinnamon was often traded, but its origin was a closely guarded secret.

RESEARCH: Some evidences on the mode of action of Cinnamomum verum bark essential oil, alone and in combination with piperacillin against a multi-drug resistant Escherichia coli strain., Yap PS, Krishnan T, Chan KG, Lim SH, *Journal of Microbiology and Biotechnology*, 2014

In-vitro and in-vivo anti-Trichophyton activity of essential oils by vapour contact, Inouye S, Uchida K, Yamaguchi H, *Mycoses*, 2001

Ameliorative effect of the cinnamon oil from Cinnamomum zeylanicum upon early stage diabetic nephropathy, Mishra A, Bhatti R, Singh A, Singh Ishar MP, *Planta Medica*, 2010

Cinnamon bark extract improves glucose metabolism and lipid profile in the fructose-fed rat, Kannappan S, Jayaraman T, Rajasekar P, Ravichandran MK, *Anuradha CV*, 2006

The cinnamon-derived dietary factor cinnamic aldehyde activates the Nrf2-dependent antioxidant response in human epithelial colon cells, Wondrak GT, Villeneuve NF, Lamore SD, Bause AS, Jiang T, Zhang DD, *Molecules*, 2010

Antibacterial activity of essential oils and their major constituents against respiratory tract pathogens by gaseous contact, Inouye S, Takizawa T, Yamaguchi H, *The Journal of Antimicrobial Chemotherapy*, 2001

CLARY SAGE

SALVIA SCLAREA

balancing • musky • feminine

FLOWER

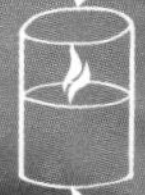

STEAM DISTILLED

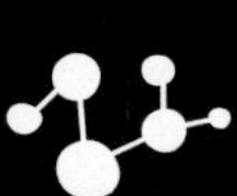

MAIN CONSTITUENT
Linalyl acetate

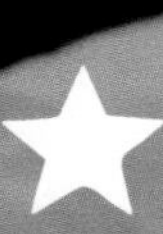

TOP PROPERTIES
Emmenagogue
Galactagogue
Neurotonic
Mucolytic
Anticoagulant
Sedative
Antispasmodic

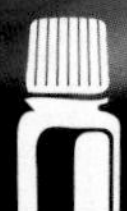

FOUND IN
Women's monthly blend

BLENDS WELL WITH
Lavender
Ylang ylang
Geranium

SAFETY
Caution during early stages of pregnancy.

TOP USES

ENDOMETRIOSIS & BREAST CANCER
Apply topically to breasts or take internally in capsule to regulate estrogen and promote healthy cells.

LOW MILK SUPPLY
For increased lactation apply topically to each breast.

BREAST ENLARGEMENT
Apply topically to each breast for natural enlargement.

PARKINSON'S, SEIZURES & CONVULSIONS
Apply topically to back of neck to support healthy brain function.

CHILD BIRTH
Apply topically down spine or on abdomen to help bring on labor.

PMS & MENOPAUSE
Use internally in a capsule or apply topically on abdomen.

POSTPARTUM DEPRESSION & ANXIETY
Diffuse aromatically or apply topically to the bottoms of feet.

HOT FLASHES
Combine with peppermint in a spray bottle and spritz topically for cooling relief.

INSOMNIA
Take under the tongue or topically on the bottoms of the feet.

EMOTIONAL BALANCE
Use aromatically and topically to get from Limited ⟶ Enlightened.

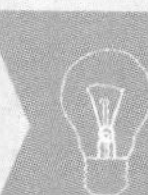

Clary sage is derived from Latin meaning "clear eyes." Medieval monks favored it for eye troubles.

RESEARCH : Changes in 5-hydroxytryptamine and Cortisol Plasma Levels in Menopausal Women After Inhalation of Clary Sage Oil, Lee KB, Cho E, Kang YS, *Phytotherapy Research*, 2014

Randomized controlled trial for Salvia sclarea or Lavandula angustifolia: differential effects on blood pressure in female patients with urinary incontinence undergoing urodynamic examination, Seol GH, Lee YH, Kang P, You JH, Park M, Min SS, *The Journal of Alternative and Complementary Medicine*, 2013

Antidepressant-like effect of Salvia sclarea is explained by modulation of dopamine activities in rats, Seol GH, Shim HS, Kim PJ, Moon HK, Lee KH, Shim I, Suh SH, Min SS, *Journal of Ethnopharmacology*, 2010

Aromatherapy massage on the abdomen for alleviating menstrual pain in high school girls: a preliminary controlled clinical study, Hur MH, Lee MS, Seong KY, Lee MK, *Evidence-Based Complementary and Alternative Medicine*, 2012

Pain relief assessment by aromatic essential oil massage on outpatients with primary dysmenorrhea: a randomized, double-blind clinical trial, Ou MC, Hsu TF, Lai AC, Lin YT, Lin CC, *The Journal of Obstetrics and Gynecology Research*, 2012

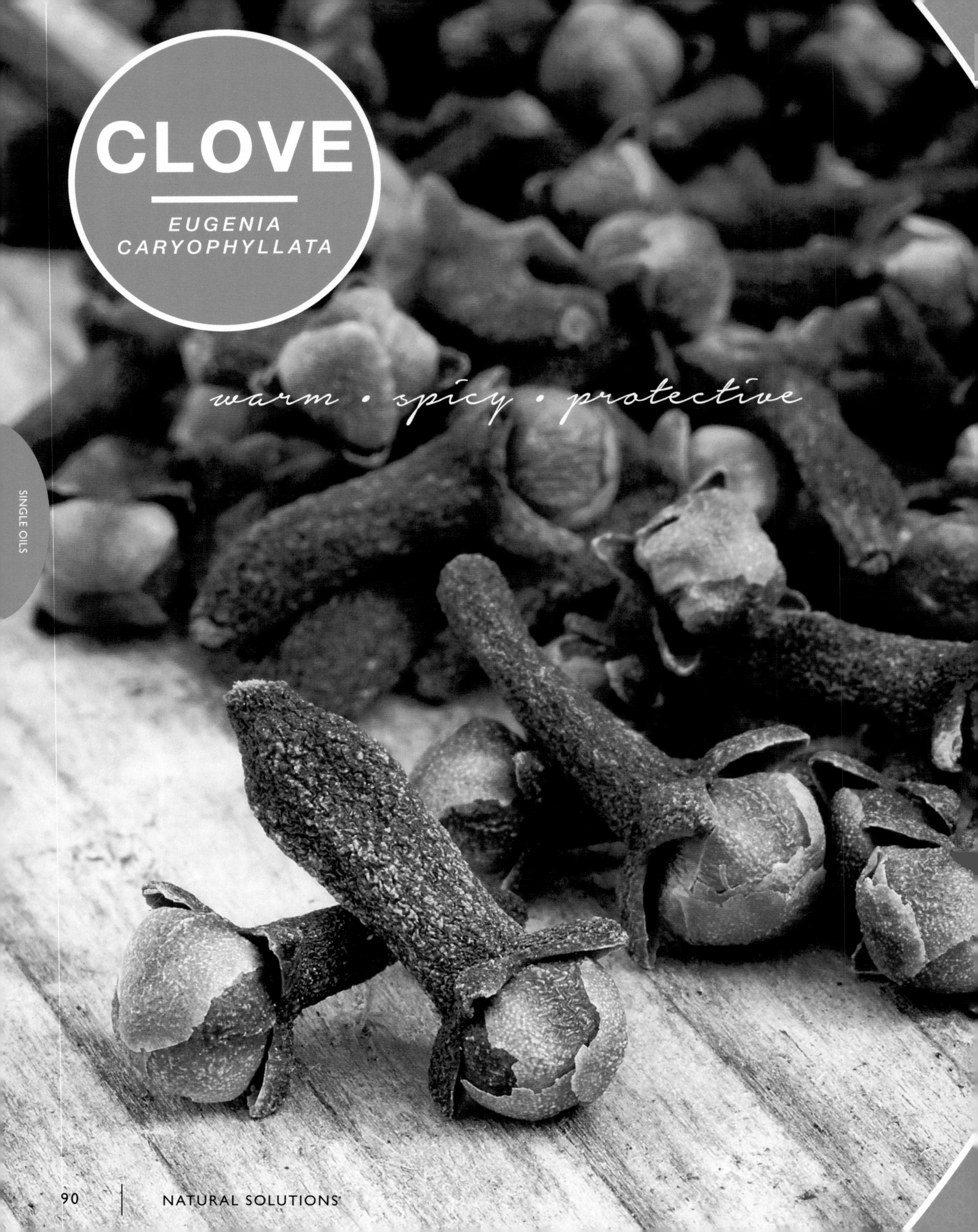

CLOVE

EUGENIA CARYOPHYLLATA

warm • spicy • protective

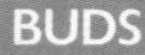

BUDS

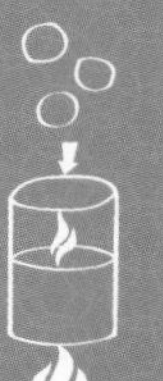

STEAM DISTILLED

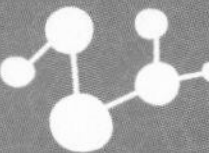

MAIN CONSTITUENT
Eugenol

TOP PROPERTIES
Antioxidant
Antiviral
Antibacterial
Antifungal
Expectorant
Nervine
Anti-parasitic
Regenerative
Vermicide

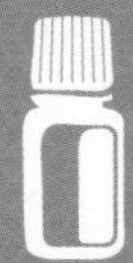

FOUND IN
Protective blend
Cellular complex blend

BLENDS WELL WITH
Cinnamon
Rosemary
Wild orange

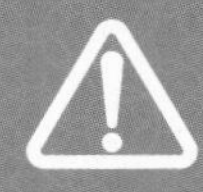

SAFETY
Dilute for topical application. Can cause skin irritation.

TOP USES

LIVER & BRAIN SUPPORT
Dilute topically and apply to bottoms of feet or take internally in a capsule.

IMMUNE BOOST
Use topically diluted on bottoms of feet or internally in a capsule.

CIRCULATION & HYPERTENSION
Apply topically diluted to limbs to increase blood flow and move blood clots and plaque.

TOOTH PAIN & CAVITIES
Dilute and apply topically to area to ease pain.

THYROID ISSUES & METABOLISM SUPPORT
Apply diluted topically over thyroid or use internally in a capsule.

INFECTION
Dilute topically over affected area, internally in a capsule to combat infection.

SMOKING ADDICTION
Apply topically with black pepper along tongue to subdue smoking cravings.

VIRUS & COLD
Apply topically along spine or use internally in a capsule.

EMOTIONAL BALANCE
Use aromatically and topically to get from Dominated ⟶ Supported.

Clove is a powerful antioxidant. As a dried spice it measures 300,000 on the ORAC scale and as an essential oil, measures over 1 million.

RESEARCH: Antimicrobial Activities of Clove and Thyme Extracts, Nzeako BC, Al-Kharousi ZS, Al-Mahrooqui Z, *Sultan Qaboos University Medical Journal*, 2006
Antimicrobial activity of clove oil and its potential in the treatment of vaginal candidiasis, Ahmad N, Alam MK, Shehbaz A, Khan A, Mannan A, Hakim SR, Bisht D, Owais M, *Journal of Drug Targeting*, 2005
Eugenol (an essential oil of clove) acts as an antibacterial agent against Salmonella typhi by disrupting the cellular membrane, Devi KP, Nisha SA, Sakthivel R, Pandian SK, *Journal of Ethnopharmacology*, 2010
The effect of clove and benzocaine versus placebo as topical anesthetics, Alqareer A, Alyahya A, Andersson L, *Journal of Dentistry*, 2006
Synergistic effect between clove oil and its major compounds and antibiotics against oral bacteria, Moon SE, Kim HY, Cha JD, *Archives of Oral Biology*, 2011
Antifungal activity of clove essential oil and its volatile vapour against dermatophytic fungi, Chee HY, Lee MH, *Mycobiology*, 2007
Microbicide activity of clove essential oil (Eugenia caryophyllata), Nuñez L, Aquino MD, *Brazilian Journal of Microbiology*, 2011
Anti-arthritic effect of eugenol on collagen-induced arthritis experimental model, Grespan R, Paludo M, Lemos Hde P, Barbosa CP, Bersani-Amado CA, Dalalio MM, Cuman RK, *Biological and Pharmaceutical Bulletin*, 2012
A novel aromatic oil compound inhibits microbial overgrowth on feet: a case study, Misner BD, *Journal of the International Society of Sports Nutrition*, 2007

SINGLE OILS

CORIANDER

CORIANDRUM SATIVUM

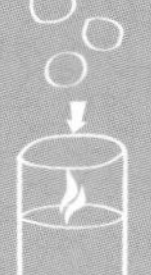

SEEDS

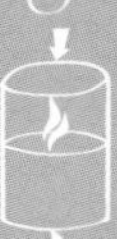

STEAM DISTILLED

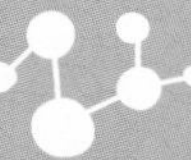

MAIN CONSTITUENTS
Linalool
Terpenes

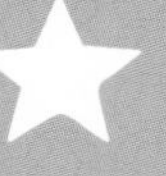

TOP PROPERTIES
Analgesic
Antioxidant
Anti-inflammatory
Digestive
Antibacterial
Antispasmodic

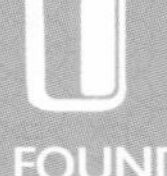

FOUND IN
Digestion blend

BLENDS WELL WITH
Ginger
Clove
Peppermint

SAFETY
Safe for NEAT application.

calming · green · stimulating

TOP USES

GAS & NAUSEA
Rub topically over abdomen or take internally in a glass of water.

BLOOD SUGAR
Use with cinnamon internally in a capsule with meals to help regulate blood sugar.

ITCHY SKIN & RASHES
Apply topically to area of concern.

JOINT PAIN
Apply topically directly to area of concern for soothing relief.

NO APPETITE
Take internally in a capsule or aromatically in palms of hands and inhale.

FOOD POISONING
Use internally in a capsule or rub topically on abdomen.

BODY ODOR
Take internally in a capsule.

LOW ENERGY & NERVOUS EXHAUSTION
Put in palms of hands and inhale aromatically or apply topically to bottoms of feet.

EMOTIONAL BALANCE
Use aromatically and topically to get from Apprehensive ⟶ Participating.

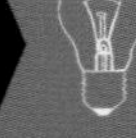

Coriander comes from the seeds of the cilantro herb; cilantro is from the leaf of the same plant.

RESEARCH: Coriandrum sativum L. protects human keratinocytes from oxidative stress by regulating oxidative defense systems., Park G, Kim HG, Kim YO, Park SH, Kim SY, Oh MS, *Skin Pharmacology and Physiology*, 2012

Antioxidant and Hepatoprotective Potential of Essential Oils of Coriander (Coriandrum sativum L.) and Caraway (Carum carvi L.) (Apiaceae), Samojlik I, Lakic N, Mimica-Dukic N, Dakovic-Svajcer K, Bozin B, *Journal of Agricultural and Food Chemistry*, 2010

Inhalation of coriander volatile oil increased anxiolytic-antidepressant-like behaviors and decreased oxidative status in beta-amyloid (1-42) rat model of Alzheimer's disease., Cioanca O, Hritcu L, Mihasan M, Trifan A, Hancianu M, *Physiology & Behavior*, 2014

Coriandrum sativum L. (Coriander) Essential Oil: Antifungal Activity and Mode of Action on Candida spp., and Molecular Targets Affected in Human Whole-Genome Expression, Freires Ide A, Murata RM, Furletti VF, Sartoratto A, Alencar SM, Figueira GM, de Oliveira Rodrigues JA, Duarte MC, Rosalen PL, *PLoS One*, 2014

Antimicrobial activity against bacteria with dermatological relevance and skin tolerance of the essential oil from Coriandrum sativum L. fruits, Casetti F, Bartelke S, Biehler K, Augustin M, Schempp CM, Frank U, *Phytotherapy Research*, 2012

Coriander (Coriandrum sativum L.) essential oil: its antibacterial activity and mode of action evaluated by flow cytometry, Silva F, Ferreira S, Queiroz JA, Domingues FC, *Journal of Medical Microbiology*, 2011 *lively • clean • energizing*

CYPRESS

CUPRESSUS SEMPERVIRENS

TOP USES

BED WETTING & INCONTINENCE
Apply topically over bladder and/or bladder reflex point on foot.

RESTLESS LEG, CARPAL TUNNEL & ARTHRITIS
Apply topically to area(s) of concern to promote circulation and ease chronic pain.

VARICOSE VEINS & HEMORRHOIDS
Rub topically over area of concern.

CELLULITE
Rub topically over area followed by a hot compress to assist with penetration through cellulite layers to release cellulite.

WHOOPING & SPASTIC COUGH
Apply topically over lungs followed by a hot compress to support healthy respiratory function.

PROSTATE, PANCREAS & OVARY ISSUES
Massage topically over the area of concern or the corresponding reflex point.

LIVER & GALLBLADDER DECONGESTANT
Apply topically to liver reflex point on foot and over area of liver.

HEAVY PERIODS, ENDOMETRIOSIS & FIBROIDS
Gently massage topically on abdomen over area of uterus, ovaries, or area of concern.

CALMING & ENERGIZING
Inhale or use aromatically in a diffuser.

EDEMA & TOXEMIA
Apply topically to clear lymph, promote blood flow, and circulation.

EMOTIONAL BALANCE
Use aromatically and topically to get from Stalled → Progressing.

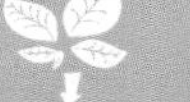

LEAVES

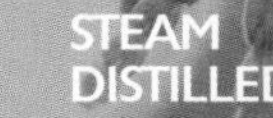

STEAM DISTILLED

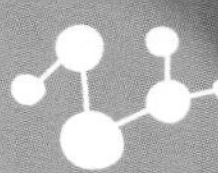

MAIN CONSTITUENTS
Alpha-pinene
Carene
Limonene

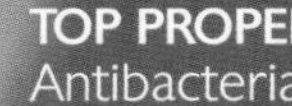

TOP PROPERTIES
Antibacterial
Antiseptic
Anti-rheumatic
Stimulant
Vasoconstrictor
Tonifying

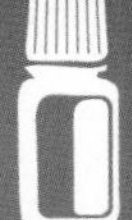

FOUND IN
Massage blend

BLENDS WELL WITH
Basil
Lavender
Bergamot

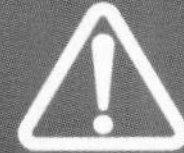

SAFETY
Not for internal use.

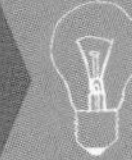

The ancient Greeks loved cypress so much they dedicated it to Pluto, the god of Hades.

RESEARCH: Immunological and Psychological Benefits of Aromatherapy Massage, Kuriyama H, Watanabe S, Nakaya T, Shigemori I, Kita M, Yoshida N, Masaki D, Tadai T, Ozasa K, Fukui K, Imanishi J, *Evidence-based Complementary and Alternative Medicine*, 2005

Chemical composition, bio-herbicidal and antifungal activities of essential oils isolated from Tunisian common cypress (Cupressus sempervirens L.), Ismail A, Lamia H, Mohsen H, Samia G, Bassem J, *Journal of Medicinal Plants Research*, 2013

Immunological and Psychological Benefits of Aromatherapy Massage, Kuriyama H, Watanabe S, Nakaya T, Shigemori I, Kita M, Yoshida N, Masaki D, Tadai T, Ozasa K, Fukui K, Imanishi J, *Evidence-Based Complementary and Alternative Medicine*, 2005

Effect of aromatherapy massage on abdominal fat and body image in post-menopausal women, Kim HJ, *Taehan Kanho Hakhoe Chi*, 2007

Evaluation of the Effects of Plant-derived Essential Oils on Central Nervous System Function Using Discrete Shuttle-type Conditioned Avoidance Response in Mice, Umezu T., *Phytotherapy Research*, 2012

DILL

ANETHUM GRAVEOLENS

detoxing · disinfecting · cleansing

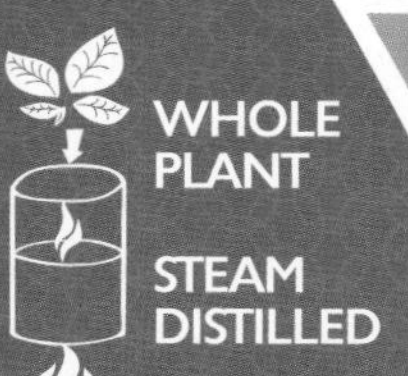

WHOLE PLANT

STEAM DISTILLED

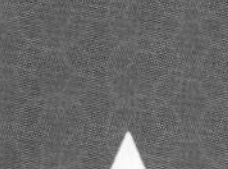

MAIN CONSTITUENTS
Monoterpenes
D'Limonene
Alpha & Beta Pinenes

TOP PROPERTIES
Antispasmodic
Expectorant
Stimulant
Galactagogue
Carminative
Emmenagogue
Hypertensive
Antibacterial

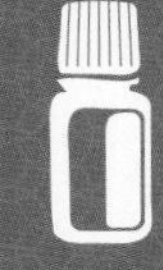

BLENDS WELL WITH
Citrus oils

SAFETY
Safe for NEAT application.

TOP USES

MUSCLE SPASMS
Apply topically to calm muscles.

NERVOUSNESS
Diffuse aromatically or apply topically with roman chamomile to calm nervousness.

SUGAR ADDICTION & PANCREAS SUPPORT
Take internally to decrease addiction and lower glucose levels.

DETOX & ELECTROLYTE BALANCE
Take internally.

CHOLESTEROL & HIGH BLOOD PRESSURE
Take internally.

RESPIRATORY ISSUES
Apply topically to chest or take internally to break up and move mucus.

GAS, BLOATING & INDIGESTION
Take internally to support healthy digestion.

LACK OF MENSTRUATION
Apply topically on abdomen.

COLIC
Apply topically on abdomen with fractionated coconut oil or bottoms of feet for colicky baby.

EMOTIONAL BALANCE
Use aromatically and topically to get from Avoiding ⟶ Intentional.

SINGLE OILS

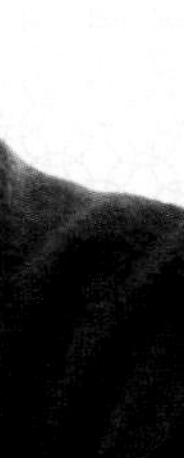

Used extensively in soft drinks and alcoholic beverages.

RESEARCH: Effects of Cd, Pb, and Cu on growth and essential oil contents in dill, peppermint, and basil, Zheljazkov VD, Craker LE, Xing B, *Environmental and Experimental Botany*, 2006
Dill (Anethum graveolens L.) seed essential oil induces Candida albicans apoptosis in a metacaspase-dependent manner, Chen Y, Zeng H, Tian J, Ban X, Ma B, Wang Y, *Fungal Biology*, 2014
Anethum graveolens: An Indian traditional medicinal herb and spice, Jana S, Shekhawat GS, *Pharmacognosy Review*, 2010
Hypolipidemic activity of Anethum graveolens in rats, Hajhashemi V, Abbasi N, *Phytotherapy Research*, 2008
Antifungal mechanism of essential oil from Anethum graveolens seeds against Candida albicans, Chen Y, Zeng H, Tian J, Ban X, Ma B, Wang Y, *Journal of Medical Microbiology*, 2013

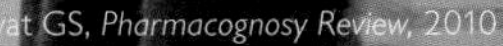

DOUGLAS FIR

PSEUDOTSUGA MENZIESII

cleansing
promoting
grounding

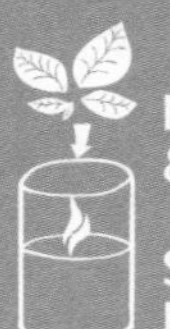

NEEDLES & BRANCH

STEAM DISTILLED

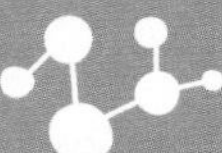

MAIN CONSTITUENTS
Beta-pinene
Alpha-pinene
3-carvene
Sabinene

TOP PROPERTIES
Antioxidant
Analgesic
Antimicrobial
Antiseptic
Anti-catarrhal
Astringent
Diuretic
Expectorant
Laxative
Sedative
Stimulant
Tonic

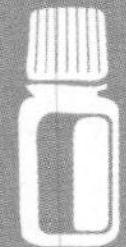

BLENDS WELL WITH
Cedarwood
Vetiver
Bergamot
Wild orange

SAFETY
Dilute to minimize skin sensitivity. Not for internal use.

TOP USES

CONSTRICTED AIRWAYS & SINUS ISSUES
Apply topically to chest or bridge of nose.

RESPIRATORY INFECTION
Apply topically to chest or bridge of nose.

COUGH
Apply topically to throat and chest or diffuse to prevent or relieve a cough.

MENTAL FOG
Apply topically to temples and forehead or diffuse.

MUSCLE & JOINT SORENESS
Massage topically with wintergreen to affected area for soothing relief.

RHEUMATIC & ARTHRITIC CONDITIONS
Apply topically to affected areas.

DEPRESSION & TENSION
Apply topically to temples, forehead, and back of neck or diffuse to relax and ground.

CONSTIPATION
Apply topically to abdomen.

SKIN IRRITATIONS & ABRASIONS
Apply topically to affected areas.

CELLULITE & SKIN CLEANSING
Massage topically with grapefruit to desired area.

Considered to be the classic Christmas tree, the Douglas Fir tree was used by Native Americans in the Pacific Northwest to heal a wide variety of ailments.

RESEARCH: Antimicrobial activity of some Pacific Northwest woods against anaerobic bacteria and yeast. Johnston WH, Karchesy JJ, Constantine GH, Craig AM. Phytother Res. 2001 Nov;15(7):586-8.
Douglas-fir root-associated microorganisms with inhibitory activity towards fungal plant pathogens and human bacterial pathogens. Axelrood PE, Clarke AM, Radley R, Zemcov SJ. Can J Microbiol. 1996 Jul;42(7):690-700.
Food-related odor probes of brain reward circuits during hunger: a pilot FMRI study. Bragulat V, Dzemidzic M, Bruno C, Cox CA, Talavage T, Considine RV, Kareken DA. Obesity (Silver Spring). 2010 Aug;18(8):1566-71. doi: 10.1038/oby.2010.57. Epub 2010 Mar 25.
Contemporary use of bark for medicine by two Salishan native elders of southeast Vancouver Island, Canada. Turner NJ, Hebda RJ. J Ethnopharmacol. 1990 Apr;29(1):59-72.

enlivening • fresh • clearing

EUCALYPTUS

EUCALYPTUS RADIATA

LEAVES

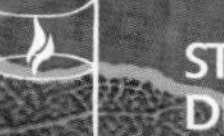

STEAM DISTILLED

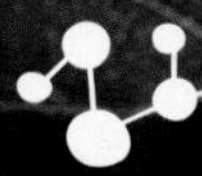

MAIN CONSTITUENTS
Eucalyptol
Alpha-terpineol

TOP PROPERTIES
Antiviral
Antibacterial
Expectorant
Analgesic
Insecticidal
Hypotensive
Disinfectant
Catalyst

FOUND IN
Protective blend
Skin clearing blend
Respiration blend
Repellent blend

BLENDS WELL WITH
Rosemary
Peppermint
Cardamom

SAFETY
Dilution recommended. Possible skin sensitivity.

TOP USES

EARACHES
Dilute and apply topically to outer ear and bone behind the ear or on chest.

CONGESTION, COUGH, BRONCHITIS & PNEUMONIA
Dilute and apply topically to chest or use in a diffuser.

ASTHMA & SINUSITIS
Put in palms of hands and inhale aromatically or apply diluted to chest and feet.

FEVER
Apply topically with peppermint down the spine to help lower fevers.

SHINGLES, MALARIA, COLD & FLU
Diffuse aromatically or apply topically to bottoms of feet or along the spine.

MUSCLE FATIGUE & PAIN
Dilute and gently massage topically over area to ease overused muscles.

MENTAL SLUGGISHNESS
Use aromatically with rosemary in palms and inhale deeply to improve bloodflow to the brain.

CLEANING DISINFECTANT
Add 10-15 drops to a spray bottle for a quick-drying disinfecting cleaner.

DUST MITES
Apply 10-15 drops to a spray bottle and use as a dust mite deterrent.

EMOTIONAL BALANCE
Use aromatically and topically to get from Congested ——→ Stimulated.

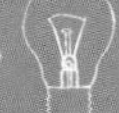

Eucalyptus was widely used in World War I to control infections and influenza.

RESEARCH: Remedies for common family ailments: 10. Nasal decongestants, Sinclair A, *Professional Care of Mother and Child*, 1996
Immune-Modifying and Antimicrobial Effects of Eucalyptus Oil and Simple Inhalation Devices, Sadlon AE, Lamson DW, *Alternative Medicine Review: A Journal of Clinical Therapeutic*, 2010
Effect of inhaled menthol on citric acid induced cough in normal subjects, Morice AH, Marshall AE, Higgins KS, Grattan TJ, *Thorax*, 1994
The effects of aromatherapy on pain, depression, and life satisfaction of arthritis patients, Kim MJ, Nam ES, Paik SI, *Taehan Kanho Hakhoe Chi*, 2005
In vitro antagonistic activity of monoterpenes and their mixtures against 'toe nail fungus' pathogens, Ramsewak RS, Nair MG, Stommel M, Selanders L, *Phytotherapy Research*, 2003
Antibacterial, antifungal, and anticancer activities of volatile oils and extracts from stems, leaves, and flowers of Eucalyptus sideroxylon and Eucalyptus torquata, Ashour HM, *Cancer Biology and Therapy*, 2008

FENNEL

FOENICULUM VULGARE

strong • purifying • supporting

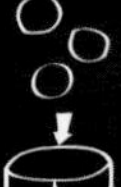
SEEDS

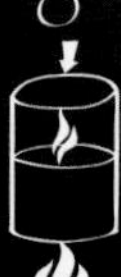
STEAM DISTILLED

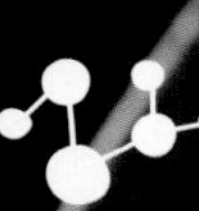
MAIN CONSTITUENTS
Benzene
Anethole
Limonene

TOP PROPERTIES
Antispasmodic
Emmenagogue
Galactagogue
Diuretic
Mucolytic
Digestive
Anti-inflammatory

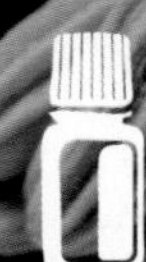
FOUND IN
Women's monthly blend
Digestion blend

BLENDS WELL WITH
Lavender
Peppermint
Basil

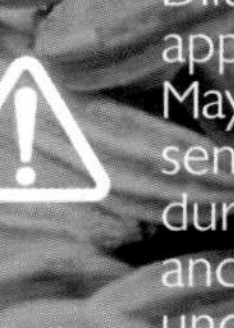
SAFETY
Dilute for topical application. May cause skin sensitivity. Caution during pregnancy and with children under 5 years old. Not for use with epileptics.

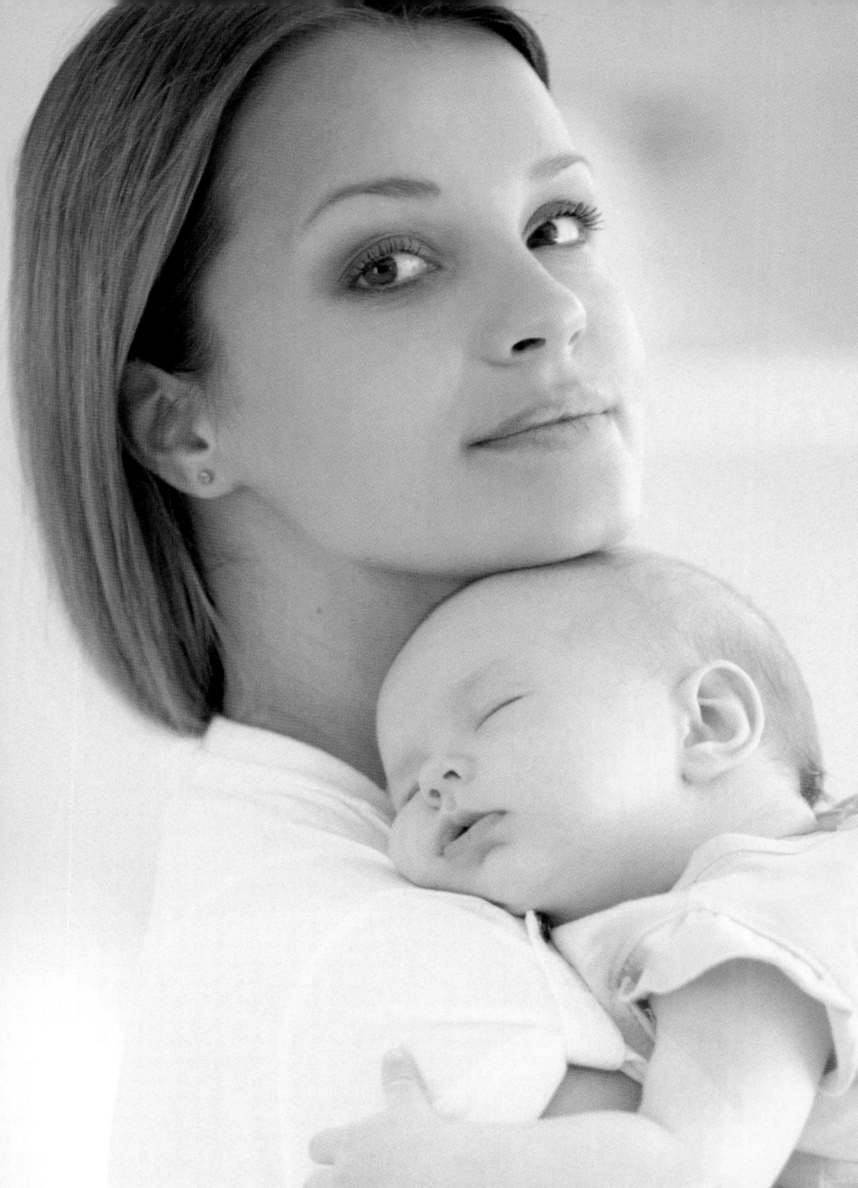

TOP USES

NAUSEA, COLIC & FLATULENCE
Take internally in a glass or rub topically on abdomen.

MENSTRUAL ISSUES & PMS
Take internally in a capsule or apply topically on abdomen to tone female organs and support healthy menstruation.

MENOPAUSE & PREMENOPAUSE ISSUES
Take internally in a capsule or gently massage topically over abdomen.

CRAMPS & SPASMS
Dilute and rub topically onto distressed muscles for relief.

BREAST FEEDING OR LOW MILK SUPPLY
Use internally in a capsule to increase milk supply.

EDEMA & FLUID RETENTION
Massage topically with grapefruit over affected areas or take internally of each in a capsule.

COUGH & CONGESTION
Apply diluted topically to chest and throat.

INTESTINAL PARASITES & SLUGGISH BOWELS
Take internally with lemon in a capsule.

HUNGER PAINS
Use internally to curb hunger as needed.

EMOTIONAL BALANCE
Use aromatically and topically to get from Unproductive ⟶ Flourishing.

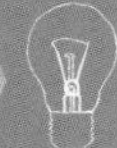

Ancient Roman warriors used fennel because it was believed it gave them strength during battle.

RESEARCH: In vitro antifungal activity and mechanism of essential oil from fennel (Foeniculum vulgare L.) on dermatophyte species, Zeng H, Chen X, Liang J, *Journal of Medical Microbiology*, 2014
Antinociceptive activity of alpha-pinene and fenchone, Him A, Ozbek H, Turel I, Oner AC, *Pharmacology Online*, 2008
The palliation of nausea in hospice and palliative care patients with essential oils of Pimpinella anisum (aniseed), Foeniculum vulgare var. dulce (sweet fennel), Anthemis nobilis (Roman chamomile) and Mentha x piperita (peppermint), Gilligan NP, *International Journal of Aromatherapy*, 2005
Comparison of fennel and mefenamic acid for the treatment of primary dysmenorrhea, Namavar Jahromi B, Tartifizadeh A, Khabnadideh S, *International Journal of Gynaecology and Obstetrics: the Official Organ of the International Federation of Gynaecology and Obstetrics*, 2003
Carvacrol, a component of thyme oil, activates PPAR alpha and gamma and suppresses COX-2 expression, Hotta M, Nakata R, Katsukawa M, Hori K, Takahashi S, Inoue H., *Journal of Lipid Research*, 2010.
Effects of herbal essential oil mixture as a dietary supplement on egg production in quail, Çabuk M, Eratak S, Alçicek A, Bozkurt M., *The Scientific World Journal*, 2014
Antimicrobial and antiplasmid activities of essential oils, Schelz Z, Molnar J, Hohmann J, *Fitoterapia*, 2006
Chemical composition, antimicrobial and antioxidant activities of anethole-rich oil from leaves of selected varieties of fennel [Foeniculum vulgare Mill. ssp. vulgare var. azoricum (Mill.) Thell], Senatore F, Oliviero F, Scandolera E, Taglialatela-Scafati O, Roscigno G, Zaccardelli M, De Falco E, *Fitoterapia*, 2013
Salinity impact on yield, water use, mineral and essential oil content of fennel (Foeniculum vulgare Mill.), Semiz GD, Unlukara A, Yurtseven E, Suarez DL, Telci I, *Journal of Agricultural Science*, 2012
Efficacy of plant essential oils on postharvest control of rots caused by fungi on different stone fruits in vivo, Lopez-Reyes JG, Spadaro D, Prelle A, Garibaldi A, Gullino ML, *Journal of Food Protection*, 2013

FRANKINCENSE

BOSWELLIA FREREANA

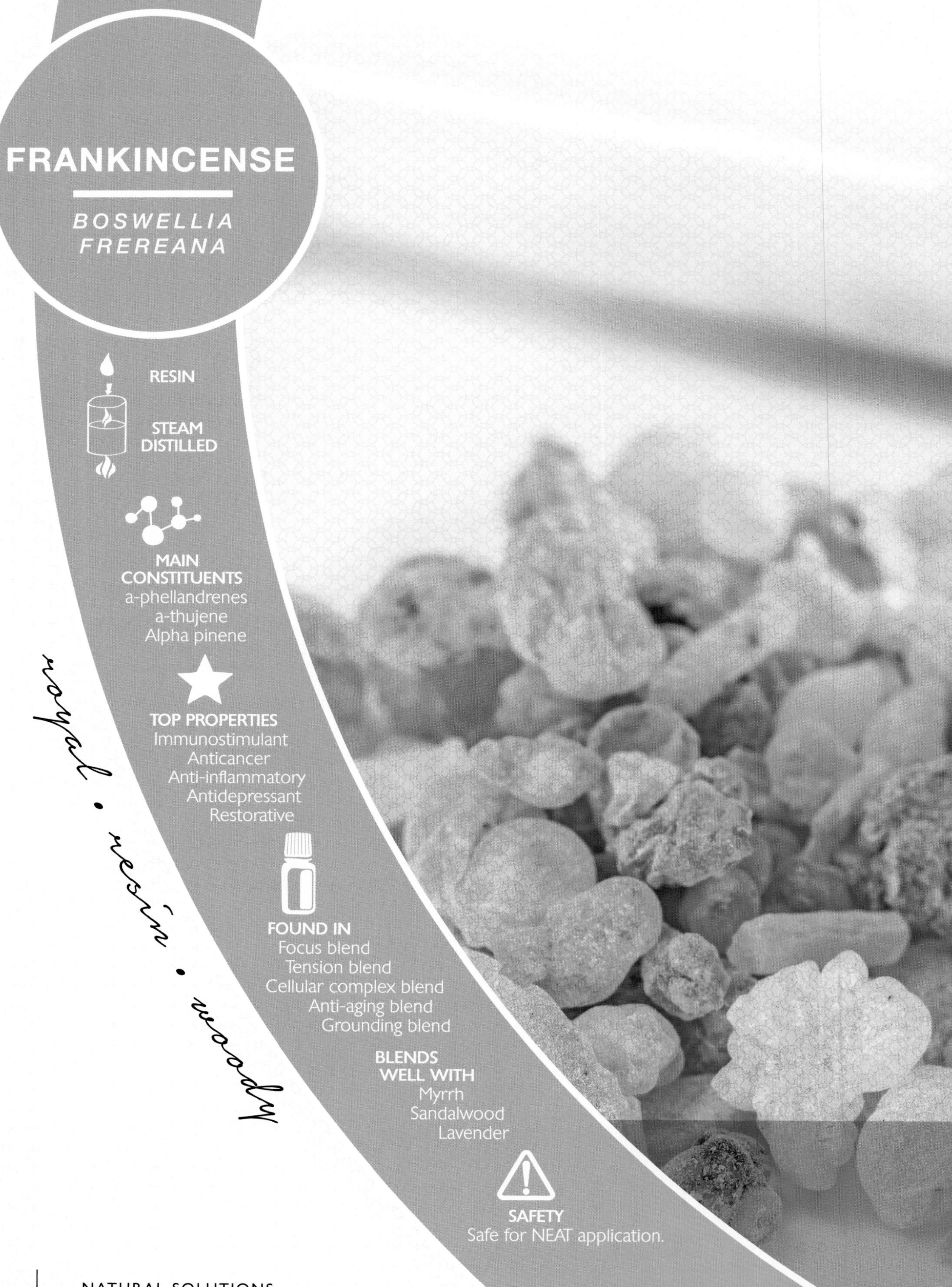

RESIN

STEAM DISTILLED

MAIN CONSTITUENTS
a-phellandrenes
a-thujene
Alpha pinene

TOP PROPERTIES
Immunostimulant
Anticancer
Anti-inflammatory
Antidepressant
Restorative

FOUND IN
Focus blend
Tension blend
Cellular complex blend
Anti-aging blend
Grounding blend

BLENDS WELL WITH
Myrrh
Sandalwood
Lavender

SAFETY
Safe for NEAT application.

royal • resin • woody

TOP USES

CANCER & TUMORS
Use internally in a capsule with lavender, grapefruit, and clove or massage topically over affected area to support healthy tumor and cancer response.

SEIZURES & TRAUMA
Put 1 drop internally under the tongue and apply topically along hairline to help lessen seizures and relieve trauma.

ALZHEIMER'S DISEASE, DYMENTIA & BRAIN INJURY
Use internally or apply topically under nose and back of neck, or in a diffuser.

DEPRESSION
Diffuse aromatically or put under the tongue to ease depression symptoms.

WOUND HEALING & WRINKLES
Apply topically to wounds or wrinkles to support skin regeneration.

SCARS & STRETCH MARKS
Combine with myrrh and apply topically to help reduce the appearance of scars and stretch marks.

SCIATICA & BACK PAIN
Use topically over affected area or internally in a capsule to reduce inflammation. Dilute to cover more surface area.

IMMUNE SYSTEM & CELLULAR HEALTH
Take internally in a capsule or apply on the bottoms of feet.

WARTS
Apply topically with oregano diluted to combat warts.

CONGESTION, COUGH & ALLERGIES
For gentle relief inhale and apply topically with peppermint and rosemary to chest and throat.

MEDITATION, PRAYER & FOCUS
Apply topically under nose and back of neck or aromatically in a diffuser to ease tension and bring focus.

EMOTIONAL BALANCE
Use aromatically and topically to get from Separated ⟶ Unified.

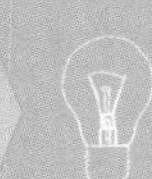

Nearly all ancient religions have used frankincense in their spiritual practices including ancient Egyptians, Greeks, Romans, Christians, Jews, Muslims, Hindus, and Buddhists.

RESEARCH: Frankincense oil derived from Boswellia carteri induces tumor cell specific cytotoxicity, Frank MB, Yang Q, Osban J, Azzarello JT, Saban MR, Saban R, Ashley RA, Welter JC, Fung KM, Lin HK, *BMC Complementary and Alternative Medicine*, 2009
Differential effects of selective frankincense (Ru Xiang) essential oil versus non-selective sandalwood (Tan Xiang) essential oil on cultured bladder cancer cells: a microarray and bioinformatics study, Dozmorov MG, Yang Q, Wu W, Wren J, Suhail MM, Woolley CL, Young DG, Fung KM, Lin HK, 2014
Composition and potential anticancer activities of essential oils obtained from myrrh and frankincense, Chen Y, Zhou C, Ge Z, Liu Y, Liu Y, Feng W, Li S, Chen G, Wei T, *Oncology Letters*, 2013
Volatile composition and antimicrobial activity of twenty commercial frankincense essential oil samples, Van Vuurena SF, Kamatoub GPP, Viljoenb, AM, *South African Journal of Botany*, 2010
Effects of Aroma Hand Massage on Pain, State Anxiety and Depression in Hospice Patients with Terminal Cancer, Chang SY, *Journal of Korean Academy of Nursing*, 2008
Evaluation of the Effects of Plant-derived Essential Oils on Central Nervous System Function Using Discrete Shuttle-type Conditioned Avoidance Response in Mice, Umezu T., *Phytotherapy Research*, 2012
Chemistry and immunomodulatory activity of frankincense oil, Mikhaeil BR, Maatooq GT, Badria FA, Amer MM, *Zeitschrift fur Naturforschung C*, 2003
Boswellia frereana (frankincense) suppresses cytokine-induced matrix metalloproteinase expression and production of pro-inflammatory molecules in articular cartilage, Blain EJ, Ali AY, Duance VC, *Phytotherapy Research*, 2012
The additive and synergistic antimicrobial effects of select frankincense and myrrh oils--a combination from the pharaonic pharmacopoeia, de Rapper S, Van Vuuren SF, Kamatou GP, Viljoen AM, Dagne E, *Letters in Applied Microbiology*, 2012

GERANIUM

PELARGONIUM GRAVEOLENS

strengthening
releasing
stabilizing

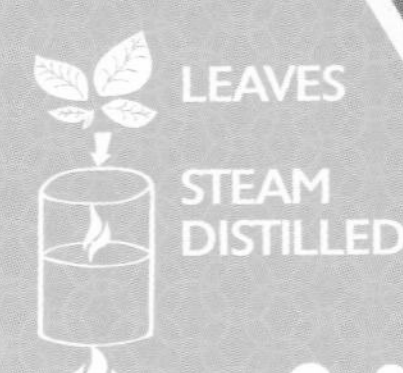

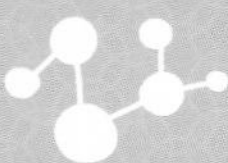

MAIN CONSTITUENTS
Citronellol
Geraniol

TOP PROPERTIES
Haemostatic
Detoxifier
Regenerative
Anti-allergenic
Antihemorrhagic
Antitoxic

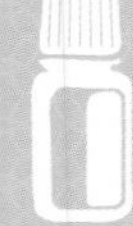

FOUND IN
Women's monthly blend
Detoxification blend

BLENDS WELL WITH
Lavender
Sandalwood
Patchouli

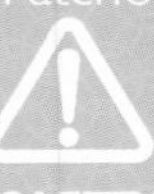

SAFETY
Dilution recommended, possible skin sensitivity.

TOP USES

LIVER, GALL BLADDER, PANCREAS & KIDNEY SUPPORT
Apply topically over area of concern or take internally in a capsule.

CUTS & WOUNDS
To help keep wounds clean and promote healing apply topically for tissue regeneration.

PMS & HORMONE BALANCING
Massage topically on abdomen or take internally under the tongue.

LOW LIBIDO
Massage topically diluted over abdomen or take 1 drop internally under the tongue to increase sexual drive.

DRY OR OILY HAIR & SKIN
Apply topically to scalp or troubled skin to retain oil balance.

MOISTURIZER
Dilute topically with fractionated coconut oil and use as a moisturizer for skin hydration and balance.

BODY ODOR
Apply topically under arms to decrease unpleasant body odor.

EMOTIONAL BALANCE
Use aromatically and topically to get from Neglected ⟶ Mended.

A powerful floral oil often referred to as the "poor man's rose." If you don't have rose, reach for geranium!

RESEARCH: Bioactivity-guided investigation of geranium essential oils as natural tick repellents, Tabanca N, Wang M, Avonto C, Chittiboyina AG, Parcher JF, Carroll JF, Kramer M, Khan IA, *Journal of Agricultural and Food Chemistry*, 2013

The antibacterial activity of geranium oil against Gram-negative bacteria isolated from difficult-to-heal wounds, Sienkiewicz M, Poznacska-Kurowska K, Kaszuba A, Kowalczyk E, *Burns*, 2014

Suppression of neutrophil accumulation in mice by cutaneous application of geranium essential oil, Maruyama N, Sekimoto Y, Ishibashi H, Inouye S, Oshima H, Yamaguchi H, Abe S, *Journal of Inflammation (London, England)*, 2005

Hypoglycemic and antioxidant effects of leaf essential oil of Pelargonium graveolens, L'Hér. in alloxan induced diabetic rats, Boukhris M, Bouaziz M, Feki I, Jemai H, El Feki A, Sayadi S, *Lipids in Health and Disease*, 2012

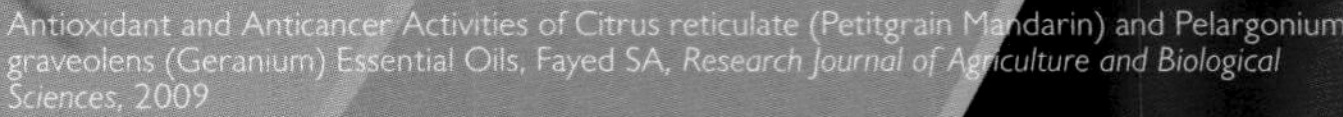

Antioxidant and Anticancer Activities of Citrus reticulate (Petitgrain Mandarin) and Pelargonium graveolens (Geranium) Essential Oils, Fayed SA, *Research Journal of Agriculture and Biological Sciences*, 2009

Aromatherapy Massage Affects Menopausal Symptoms in Korean Climacteric Women: A Pilot-Controlled Clinical Trial, Myung-HH, Yun Seok Y, Myeong SL, *Evidence-based Complementary and Alternative Medicine*, 2008

GINGER

ZINGIBER OFFICINALE

warming
accelerating
stimulating

TOP USES

NAUSEA, MORNING SICKNESS & LOSS OF APPETITE
Diffuse aromatically or take internally in a glass with warm water or apply topically to wrists.

MOTION SICKNESS & VERTIGO
Inhale aroma from palms or take internally in a capsule.

MEMORY & BRAIN SUPPORT
Inhale aroma from palms or take internally in a capsule.

HEARTBURN & REFLUX
Take internally in a capsule with lemon to calm heart-burn & reflux.

SPASMS & CRAMPS
Dilute topically and apply to area of discomfort for warming relief.

COLIC & CONSTIPATION
Rub topically diluted over intestines or take internally in a glass of warm water to ease constipation and promote healthy digestion.

CONGESTION & SINUSITIS
Dilute and apply topically and gently rub over chest and throat or add aromatically to a diffuser to relieve congestion symptoms.

COLD, FLU & SORE THROAT
Use internally in a capsule, or gargle or apply topically to bottoms of feet to strengthen immunity.

ALCOHOL ADDICTION
Take internally in a capsule as needed for cravings.

SPRAINS & BROKEN BONES
Dilute topically and apply to area of concern to promote healing.

EMOTIONAL BALANCE
Use aromatically and topically to get from Apathetic ⟶ Activated.

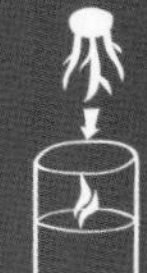

ROOT

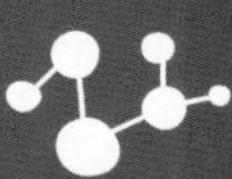

STEAM DISTILLED

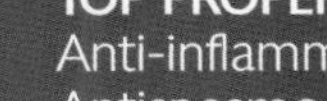

MAIN CONSTITUENT
Alpha-zingiberene

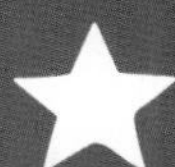

TOP PROPERTIES
Anti-inflammatory
Antispasmodic
Digestive
Laxative
Analgesic
Stimulant
Decongestant
Neurotonic

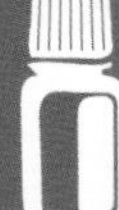

FOUND IN
Metabolic blend
Digestion blend

BLENDS WELL WITH
Frankincense
Cinnamon
Grapefruit

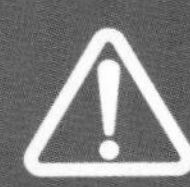

SAFETY
Dilution recommended. May cause skin sensitivity.

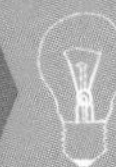

Has been used as a medicinal herb for centuries.

RESEARCH: Gastroprotective activity of essential oils from turmeric and ginger, Liju VB, Jeena K, Kuttan R., *Journal of Basic and Clinical Physiology and Pharmacology*, 2014
Reversal of pyrogallol-induced delay in gastric emptying in rats by ginger (Zingiber officinale), Gupta YK, Sharma M, *Methods and Findings in Experimental and Clinical Pharmacology*, 2001
The essential oil of ginger, Zingiber officinale, and anaesthesia, Geiger JL, *International Journal of Aromatherapy*, 2005
Effectiveness of aromatherapy with light thai massage for cellular immunity improvement in colorectal cancer patients receiving chemotherapy, Khiewkhern S, Promthet S, Sukprasert A, Eunhpinitpong W, Bradshaw P, *Asian Pacific Journal of Cancer Prevention*, 2013
Antioxidant, anti-inflammatory and antinociceptive activities of essential oil from ginger, Jeena K, Liju VB, Kuttan R, *Indian Journal of Physiology and Pharmacology*, 2013
A brief review of current scientific evidence involving aromatherapy use for nausea and vomiting, Lua PL, Zakaria NS, *The Journal of Alternative and Complementary Medicine*, 2012
Anti-inflammatory effects of ginger and some of its components in human bronchial epithelial (BEAS-2B) cells, Podlogar JA, Verspohl EJ, *Phytotherapy Research*, 2012
Medicinal plants as antiemetics in the treatment of cancer: a review, Haniadka R, Popouri S, Palatty PL, Arora R, Baliga MS, *Integrative Cancer Therapies*, 2012
Inhibitory potential of ginger extracts against enzymes linked to type 2 diabetes, inflammation and induced oxidative stress, Rani MP, Padmakumari KP, Sankarikutty B, Cherian OL, Nisha VM, Raghu KG, *International Journal of Food Sciences and Nutrition*, 2011
Ginger: An herbal medicinal product with broad anti-inflammatory actions, Grzanna R, Lindmark L, Frondoza CG, *Journal of Medicinal Food*, 2005

GRAPEFRUIT

CITRUS X PARADISI

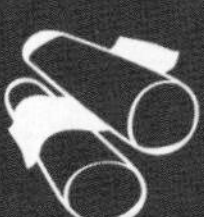

RIND

COLD PRESSED

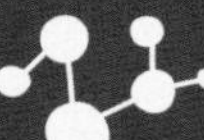

MAIN CONSTITUENTS
d - limonene
Myrcene

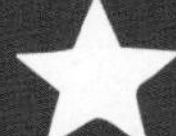

TOP PROPERTIES
Diuretic
Antioxidant
Antiseptic
Astringent
Antitoxic
Purifier
Expectorant

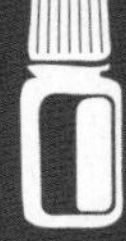

FOUND IN
Massage blend
Invigorating blend
Metabolic blend

BLENDS WELL WITH
Basil
Peppermint
Rosemary

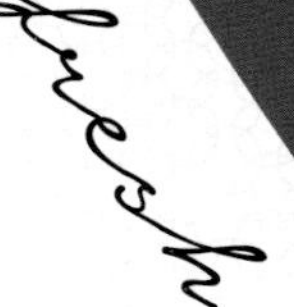

SAFETY
Avoid direct sun or UV exposure for 12 hours after topical application.

citrus • detoxifying • fresh

SINGLE OILS

TOP USES

WEIGHT LOSS & CELLULITE
Take internally in water or in a capsule or apply topically to areas of concern to break down and wash away fat. Tip: hydrate well.

ADDICTIONS & SUGAR CRAVINGS
Diffuse aromatically or take in a capsule.

OILY SKIN & ACNE
Dilute topically and apply to areas of concern to better manage breakouts.

DETOXIFICATION
Rub topically on bottoms of feet or take internally in drinking water for an overall detox.

LYMPHATIC & KIDNEY CLEANSING
Use internally in water or apply topically over lymphatic system and kidneys to cleanse and improve function.

BREAST & UTERINE HEALTH & PROGESTERONE BALANCE
Use internally in a capsule or apply topically to area of concern.

ADRENAL FATIGUE
Use topically with basil over adrenals and on bottoms of feet or take internally in a capsule to support adrenal recovery.

GALLSTONES & GALLBLADDER SUPPORT
Take internally with geranium in a capsule.

HANGOVER
Take internally in a capsule to ease symptoms.

EMOTIONAL BALANCE
Use aromatically and topically to get from Divided ⟶ Validated.

Many prescription drugs contain a warning against grapefruit, however the essential oil is very different and very safe.

RESEARCH: Olfactory stimulatory with grapefruit and lavender oils change autonomic nerve activity and physiological function, Nagai K, Niijima A, Horii Y, Shen J, Tanida M, *Autonomic Neuroscience: basic & clinical*, 2014
Minor Furanocoumarins and Coumarins in Grapefruit Peel Oil as Inhibitors of Human Cytochrome P450 3A4, César TB, Manthey JA, Myung K, *Journal of Natural Products*, 2009
Antimicrobial effects of essential oils in combination with chlorhexidine digluconate, Filoche SK, Soma K, Sissons CH, *Oral Microbiology and Immunology*, 2005
Inhibition of acetylcholinesterase activity by essential oil from Citrus paradisi, Miyazawa M, Tougo H, Ishihara M, *Natural Product Letters*, 2001
Olfactory stimulation with scent of essential oil of grapefruit affects autonomic neurotransmission and blood pressure, Tanida M, Niijima A, Shen J, Nakamura T, Nagai K, *Brian Research*, 2005
Mechanism of changes induced in plasma glycerol by scent stimulation with grapefruit and lavender essential oils, Shen J, Niijima A, Tanida M, Horii Y, Nakamura T, Nagai K, *Neuroscience Letters*, 2007
Olfactory stimulation with scent of grapefruit oil affects autonomic nerves, lipolysis and appetite in rats, Shen J, Niijima A, Tanida M, Horii Y, Maeda K, Nagai K, *Neuroscience Letters*, 2005
Effects of fragrance inhalation on sympathetic activity in normal adults, Haze S, Sakai K, Gozu Y, *The Japanese Journal of Pharmacology*, 2002
Effect of olfactory stimulation with flavor of grapefruit oil and lemon oil on the activity of sympathetic branch in the white adipose tissue of the epididymis, Niijima A, Nagai K, *Experimental Biology and Medicine*, 2003
Effect of aromatherapy massage on abdominal fat and body image in post-menopausal women, Kim HJ, *Taehan Kanho Hakhoe Chi*, 2007

healing • fusing • regenerating

HELICHRYSUM

HELICHRYSUM ITALICUM

TOP USES

WRINKLES & STRETCH MARKS
Rub topically with myrrh onto wrinkles and stretch marks. Dilute if using on face.

NOSE BLEEDS
Apply topically over bridge of nose to stop bleeding.

SCARS & WOUNDS
Apply topically to scars and wounds to support skin renewal.

SHOCK & PAIN RELIEF
Apply topically on back of neck or area of pain.

PSORIASIS & SKIN CONDITIONS
Apply topically with lavender over areas of concern.

VARICOSE VEINS
Apply topically with cypress and gently massage into affected areas.

BLEEDING & HEMORRHAGING
Apply topically where needed to help blood to coagulate.

TINNITIS & EARACHE
Massage topically behind the ears to calm spasms or inflammation.

COUGH & CONGESTION
Combine with sandalwood and lemon and rub topically along throat and chest to ease coughs and congestion.

ALCOHOL & HEAVY METAL TOXICITY
Take internally in a capsule to promote healthy liver and pancreas function and heavy metal chelation.

EMOTIONAL BALANCE
Use aromatically and topically to get from Wounded ⟶ Reassured.

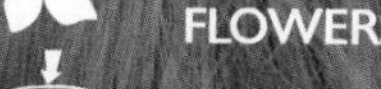

FLOWERS

STEAM DISTILLED

MAIN CONSTITUENTS
Neryl acetate
Italidione
y-curcumene
l-limonene

TOP PROPERTIES
Antispasmodic
Anticatarrhal
Neuroprotective
Neurotonic
Vasoconstrictor
Haemostatic
Nervine
Analgesic

FOUND IN
Soothing blend
Anti-aging blend

BLENDS WELL WITH
Lavender
Clary Sage
Rose

SAFETY
Safe for NEAT application.

This precious oil is often hand picked on the island of Corsica and used as "liquid stitches."

SINGLE OILS

RESEARCH: Chemical composition and biological activity of the essential oil from Helichrysum microphyllum Cambess. ssp. tyrrhenicum Bacch., Brullo e Giusso growing in La Maddalena Archipelago, Sardinia., Ornano L, Venditti A, Sanna C, Ballero M, Maggi F, Lupidi G, Bramucci M, Quassinti L, Bianco A, *Journal of Oleo Science*, 2014

Arzanol, an anti-inflammatory and anti-HIV-1 phloroglucinol alpha-Pyrone from Helichrysum italicum ssp. microphyllum, Appendino G, Ottino M, Marquez N, Bianchi F, Giana A, Ballero M, Sterner O, Fiebich BL, Munoz E, *Journal of Natural Products*, 2007

Protective role of arzanol against lipid peroxidation in biological systems, Rosa A, Pollastro F, Atzeri A, Appendino G, Melis MP, Deiana M, Incani A, Loru D, Dessì MA, *Chemical and Physics of Lipids*, 2011

Arzanol, a prenylated heterodimeric phloroglucinyl pyrone, inhibits eicosanoid biosynthesis and exhibits anti-inflammatory efficacy in vivo, Bauer J, Koeberle A, Dehm F, Pollastro F, Appendino G, Northoff H, Rossi A, Sautebin L, Werz O, *Biochemical Pharmacology*, 2011

Anti-inflammatory and antioxidant properties of Helichrysum italicum, Sala A, Recio M, Giner RM, Máñez S, Tournier H, Schinella G, Ríos JL, *The Journal of Pharmacy and Pharmacology*, 2002

Effects of Helichrysum italicum extract on growth and enzymatic activity of Staphylococcus aureus, Nostro A, Bisignano G, Angela Cannatelli M, Crisafi G, Paola Germanò M, Alonzo V, *International Journal of Antimicrobial Agents*, 2001

Helichrysum italicum extract interferes with the production of enterotoxins by Staphylococcus aureus., Nostro A, Cannatelli MA, Musolino AD, Procopio F, Alonzo V, *Letters in Applied Microbiology*, 2002

Assessment of the anti-inflammatory activity and free radical scavenger activity of tiliroside., Sala A, Recio MC, Schinella GR, Máñez S, Giner RM, Cerdá-Nicolás M, Rosí JL, *European Journal of Pharmacology*, 2003

JASMINE

JASMINUM GRANDIFLORUM

euphoria
splendor
joy

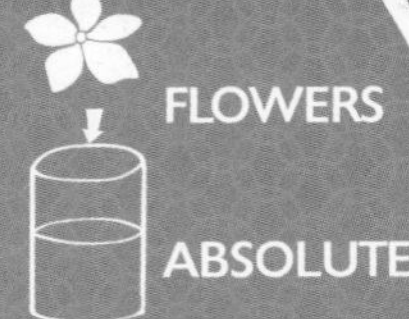

FLOWERS

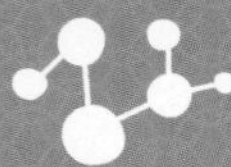

ABSOLUTE

MAIN CONSTITUENTS
Benzyl acetate
Benzyl benzoate
phytol

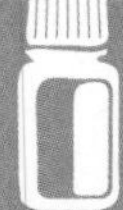

TOP PROPERTIES
Antidepressant
Aphrodisiac
Antispasmodic
Calming
Regenerative
Carminative

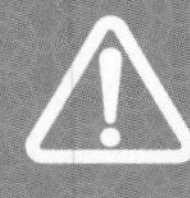

FOUND IN
Women's monthly blend

BLENDS WELL WITH
Lavender
Sandalwood
Rose

SAFETY
Safe for NEAT application.

TOP USES

DEPRESSION & ANXIETY
Diffuse aromatically and apply topically under nose and to back of neck.

LOW LIBIDO
Apply topically to reflex points or diffuse aromatically.

FINE LINES & WRINKLES
Apply topically to skin nightly.

PINKEYE
Apply topically around eye.

EXHAUSTION
Apply topically to back of neck and bottoms of feet.

IRRITATED & DRY SKIN
Apply topically with fractionated coconut oil to affected area.

PMS & HORMONAL BALANCE
Apply topically to back of neck or bottoms of feet.

PERFUME
Combine with sandalwood and a carrier oil and apply topically as desired.

EMOTIONAL BALANCE
Use aromatically and topically to get from Hampered ⟶ Liberated.

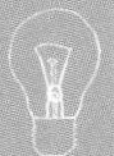

In India jasmine is known as "Queen of the Night" because it typically blossoms in the night.

RESEARCH: The influence of essential oils on human attention and alertness, Ilmberger J, Heuberger E, Mahrhofer C, Dessovic H, Kowarik D, Buchbauer G, *Chemical Senses*, 2001
The influence of essential oils on human vigilance, Heuberger E, Ilmberger J, *Natural Product Communications*, 2010
Effects of Aromatherapy Massage on Blood Pressure and Lipid Profile in Korean Climacteric Women, Myung-HH , Heeyoung OH, Myeong SL , Chan K, Ae-na C, Gil-ran S, *International Journal of Neuroscience*, 2007
Sedative effects of the jasmine tea odor and (R)-(-)-linalool, one of its major odor components, on autonomic nerve activity and mood states, Kuroda K, Inoue N, Ito Y, Kubota K, Sugimoto A, Kakuda T, Fushiki T, *European Journal of Applied Physiology*, 2005
Aromatherapy Massage Affects Menopausal Symptoms in Korean Climacteric Women: A Pilot-Controlled Clinical Trial, Myung-HH, Yun Seok Y, Myeong SL, *Evidence-based Complementary and Alternative Medicine*, 2008
Stimulating effect of aromatherapy massage with jasmine oil, Hongratanaworakit T, *Natural Product Communications*, 2010
Activities of Ten Essential Oils towards Propionibacterium acnes and PC-3, A-549 and MCF-7 Cancer Cells, Zu Y, Yu H, Liang L, Fu Y, Efferth T, Liu X, Wu N, *Molecules*, 2010

detoxing
revitalizing
toning

JUNIPER BERRY

JUNIPERUS COMMUNIS

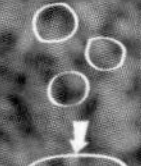
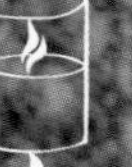

BERRIES

STEAM DISTILLED

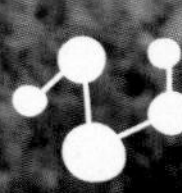

MAIN CONSTITUENTS
Alpha pinene
Sabinene

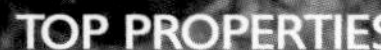

TOP PROPERTIES
Detoxifier
Diuretic
Antiseptic
Antispasmodic
Astringent
Anti-rheumatic
Carminative
Anti-parasitic

FOUND IN
Detoxification blend

BLENDS WELL WITH
Grapefruit
Bergamot
Cypress

SAFETY
Safe for NEAT application.

A favorite oil for its fragrance, Juniper berries are also used for making gin.

SINGLE OILS

TOP USES

LIVER ISSUES
Use internally in a capsule to support cleansing.

DETOX
Take internally in a capsule to detox.

ACNE & PSORIASIS
Dilute and apply topically to area of concern.

URINARY HEALTH & WATER RETENTION
Rub topically with grapefruit over abdomen or needed area or use internally in a capsule with grapefruit to promote healthy urination.

PLAGUES & EPIDEMICS
Apply topically along spine or to bottoms of feet or internally.

CHOLESTEROL & BLOOD SUGAR SUPPORT
Take internally in a capsule to help manage cholesterol levels.

TENSION & STRESS
Put in palms and inhale deeply or apply topically under nose or to bottoms of feet.

DEPRESSION
Diffuse or use topically under nose or on bottoms of feet.

EMOTIONAL BALANCE
Use aromatically and topically to get from Denying ⟶ Insightful.

RESEARCH: Fumigant toxicity of plant essential oils against Camptomyia corticalis (Diptera: Cecidomyiidae), Kim JR, Haribalan P, Son BK, Ahn YJ, *Journal of Economic Entomology*, 2012
Antimicrobial activity of juniper berry essential oil (Juniperus communis L., Cupressaceae), Pepeljnjak S, Kosalec I, Kalodera Z, Blazevic N, *Acta Pharmaceutica*, 2005
Antioxidant activities and volatile constituents of various essential oils, Wei A, Shibamoto T, *Journal of Agriculture and Food Chemistry*, 2007

LAVENDER

LAVANDULA ANGUSTIFOLIA

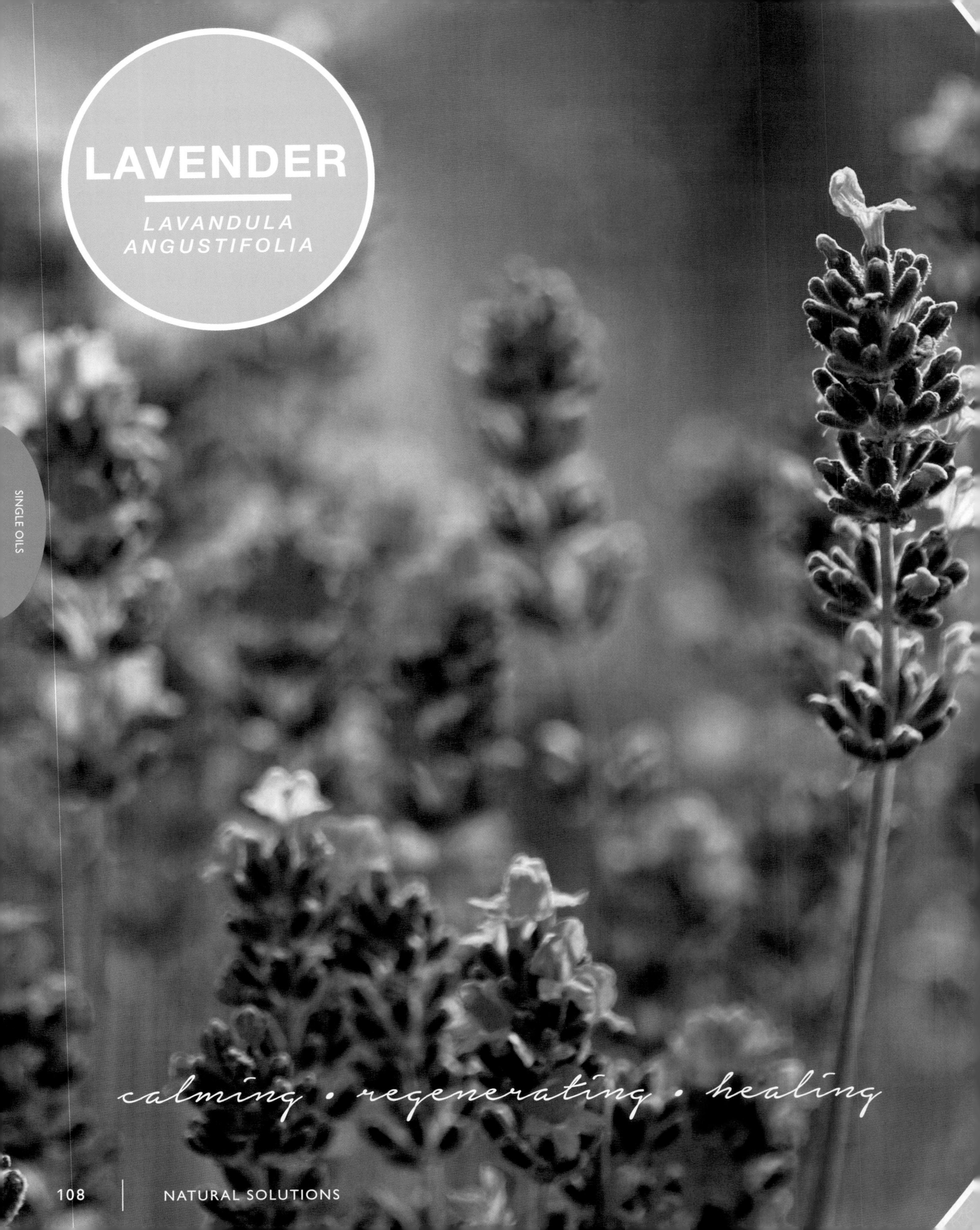

calming • regenerating • healing

SINGLE OILS

FLOWERS

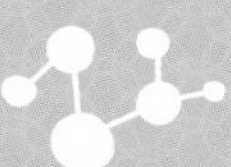

STEAM DISTILLED

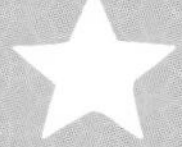

MAIN CONSTITUENTS
Linalool
a-terpineol
Linalyl acetate
b-ocimene

TOP PROPERTIES
Sedative
Astringent
Antihistamine
Cytophylactic
Antispasmodic
Antidepressant
Analgesic
Hypotensive
Nervine
Relaxing
Soothing
Antispasmodic
Antibacterial
Regenerative
Cardiotonic

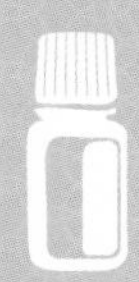

FOUND IN
Tension blend
Calming blend
Women's monthly blend
Anti-aging blend
Massage blend

BLENDS WELL WITH
Clary sage
Wild orange
Frankincense

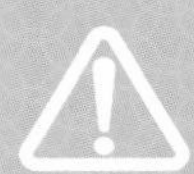

SAFETY
When in doubt use lavender! Safe for NEAT application.

TOP USES

SLEEP ISSUES
Apply topically to bottoms of feet or put aromatically in a diffuser to induce sleep.

STRESS, ANXIETY & TEETH GRINDING
Rub topically over heart and on back of neck or inhale aromatically from palms of hands.

FOCUS & CONCENTRATION
Apply 1 drop topically with with vetiver or diffuse to uplift mood.

SUNBURNS, BURNS & SCARS
Use topically on area of concern tissue to soothe and promote skin healing.

ALLERGIES & HAY FEVER
Take internally with lemon and peppermint in a capsule, or use each aromatically in palms and inhale.

PAINS & SPRAINS
Massage topically onto area of discomfort.

CUTS, WOUNDS & BLISTERS
Put topically on wounds on sites to comfort, cleanse and help heal.

HIGH BLOOD PRESSURE
Use topically on pulse points and over heart or internally in a capsule.

MIGRAINES & HEADACHES
Inhale aromatically or apply topically on temples and back of neck.

EMOTIONAL BALANCE
Use aromatically and topically to get from Unheard ⟶ Expressed.

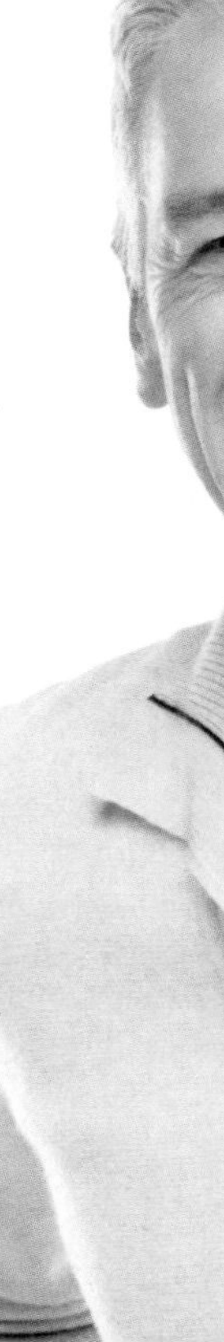

SINGLE OILS

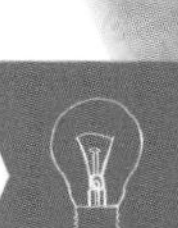

Lavender means "to wash" in Latin. It is likely the most used essential oil globally, and for good reason, as it serves in all things calming!

RESEARCH: An olfactory stimulus modifies nighttime sleep in young men and women, Goel N, Kim H, Lao RP, *Chronobiology International*, 2005

Effects of lavender aromatherapy on insomnia and depression in women college students, Lee IS, Lee GJ, *Taehan Kanho Hakhoe Chi*, 2006

Effects of lavender (lavandula angustifolia Mill.) and peppermint (Mentha cordifolia Opiz.) aromas on subjective vitality, speed, and agility, Cruz AB, Lee SE, Pagaduan JC, Kim TH, *The Asian International Journal of Life Sciences*, 2012

Topical lavender oil for the treatment of recurrent aphthous ulceration, Altaei DT, *American Journal of Dentistry*, 2012

Lavender essential oil inhalation suppresses allergic airway inflammation and mucous cell hyperplasia in a murine model of asthma, Ueno-Iio T, Shibakura M, Yokota K, Aoe M, Hyoda T, Shinohata R, Kanehiro A, Tanimoto M, Kataoka M, *Life Sciences*, 2014

Lavender essential oil in the treatment of migraine headache: a placebo-controlled clinical trial, Sasannejad P, Saeedi M, Shoeibi A, Gorji A, Abbasi M, Foroughipour M, *European Neurology*, 2012

Effect of aromatherapy on symptoms of dysmenorrhea in college students: A randomized placebo-controlled clinical trial, Han SH, Hur MH, Buckle J, Choi J, Lee MS, *The Journal of Alternative and Complementary Medicine*, 2006

The effects of aromatherapy on pain, depression, and life satisfaction of arthritis patients, Kim MJ, Nam ES, Paik SI, *Taehan Kanho Hakhoe Chi*, 2005

Effect of lavender oil (Lavandula angustifolia) on cerebral edema and its possible mechanisms in an experimental model of stroke,Vakili A, Sharifat S, Akhavan MM, Bandegi AR, *Brain Research*, 2014

Two US practitioners' experience of using essential oils for wound care, Hartman D, Coetzee JC, *Journal of Wound Care*, 2002

Lavender and the nervous system, Koulivand PH, Khaleghi Ghadiri M, Gorji A, *Evidence-Based Complementary and Alternative Medicine*, 2013

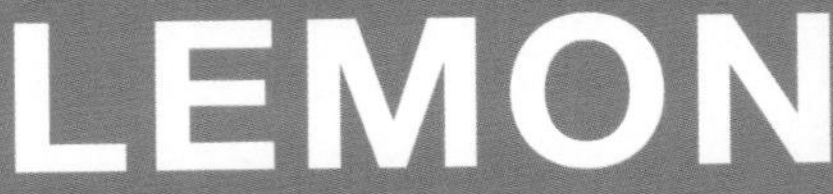

LEMON

CITRUS LIMON

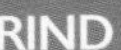

RIND

COLD PRESSED

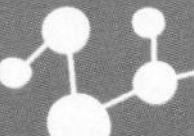

MAIN CONSTITUENTS
d-limonene
Alpha pinenes
Beta pinenes

TOP PROPERTIES
Antiseptic
Diuretic
Antioxidant
Antibacterial
Detoxification
Disinfectant
Mucolytic
Astringent
Degreaser

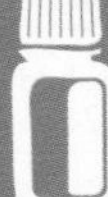

FOUND IN
Respiration blend
Invigorating blend
Cleansing blend
Metabolic blend

BLENDS WELL WITH
Basil
Peppermint
Rosemary

SAFETY
Avoid exposure of affected area to sunlight or UV rays for 12 hours after direct topical application..

uplifting • invigorating • refreshing

TOP USES

KIDNEY & GALL STONES
Take internally in water to detoxify the body.

DETOX & LYMPHATIC CLEANSING
Take internally in a glass of water or apply topically to ears and ankles to cleanse and balance pH.

HEARTBURN & REFLUX
Use internally with ginger essential oil in a glass of water to help relieve heartburn and reflux symptoms.

CONGESTION & MUCUS
Rub topically over chest or use aromatically in a diffuser.

STRESS
Diffuse aromatically.

RUNNY NOSE & ALLERGIES
Inhale or apply topically over bridge of nose to slow a runny nose. Take 2-4 drops internally with lavender and peppermint for allergy relief.

GOUT, RHEUMATISM & ARTHRITIS
Take internally in a glass of water.

DEGREASER & FURNITURE POLISH
Use 10-15 drops mixed with water in a glass spray bottle.

VARICOSE VEINS
Apply topically with cypress.

CONCENTRATION
Inhale aromatically with rosemary.

EMOTIONAL BALANCE
Use aromatically and topically to get from Mindless ⟶ Energized.

SINGLE OILS

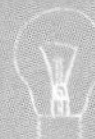

It takes approximately 45 lemons to produce a 15 ml bottle of lemon essential oil.

RESEARCH: Screening of the antibacterial effects of a variety of essential oils on respiratory tract pathogens, using a modified dilution assay method, Inouye S, Yamaguchi H, Takizawa T, *Journal of Infection and Chemotherapy: Official Journal of the Japan Society of Chemotherapy*, 2001

Antioxidative effects of lemon oil and its components on copper induced oxidation of low density lipoprotein, Grassmann J, Schneider D, Weiser D, Elstner EF, *Arzneimittel-Forschung*, 2001

The effect of lemon inhalation aromatherapy on nausea and vomiting of pregnancy: a double-blinded, randomized, controlled clinical trial, Yavari Kia P, Safajou F, Shahnazi M, Nazemiyeh H, *Iranian Red Crescent Medical Journal*, 2014

Chemical composition of the essential oils of variegated pink-fleshed lemon (Citrus x limon L. Burm. f.) and their anti-inflammatory and antimicrobial activities, Hamdan D, Ashour ML, Mulyaningsih S, El-Shazly A, Wink M, *Zeitschrift Fur Naturforschung C-A Journal of Biosciences*, 2013

Essential oil from lemon peels inhibit key enzymes linked to neurodegenerative conditions and pro-oxidant induced lipid peroxidation, Oboh G, Olasehinde TA, Ademosun AO, *Journal of Oleo Science*, 2014

Effect of flavour components in lemon essential oil on physical or psychological stress, Fukumoto S, Morishita A, Furutachi K, Terashima T, Nakayama T, Yokogoshi H, *Stress and Health*, 2008

Cytological aspects on the effects of a nasal spray consisting of standardized extract of citrus lemon and essential oils in allergic rhinopathy, Ferrara L, Naviglio D, Armone Caruso A, *ISRN Pharmaceutics*, 2012

Aromatherapy as a safe and effective treatment for the management of agitation in severe dementia: the results of a double-blind, placebo-controlled trial with Melissa, Ballard CG, O'Brien JT, Reichelt K, Perry EK, *The Journal of Clinical Psychiatry*, 2002

SINGLE OILS

LEMONGRASS

CYMBOPOGON FLEXUOSUS

electrifying
regenerating
purifying

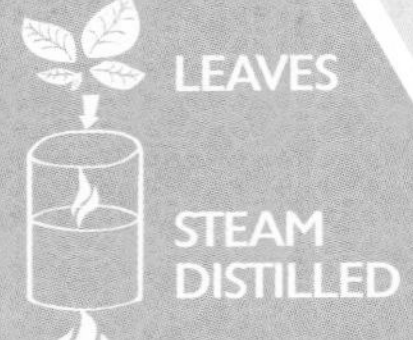

LEAVES

STEAM DISTILLED

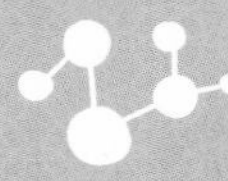

MAIN CONSTITUENTS
Geranial
Neral
Geraniol
Farnesol

TOP PROPERTIES
Anti-inflammatory
Antimicrobial
Analgesic
Anti-carcinoma
Anti-mutagenic
Decongestant
Regenerative
Anti-rheumatic

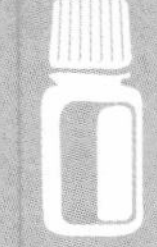

FOUND IN
Cellular complex blend

BLENDS WELL WITH
Basil
Ginger
Peppermint

SAFETY
Dilute for topical application as can cause skin sensitivity.

TOP USES

CANCER & TUMORS
Use internally in a capsule.

BLOOD PRESSURE & CHOLESTEROL
Take internally in a capsule.

HYPO- & HYPERTHYROID
Take internally in a capsule.

BLADDER & KIDNEY INFECTION & STONES
Use internally in a capsule or dilute and apply topically over abdomen.

DIGESTIVE ISSUES
Combine with peppermint and apply diluted topically over abdomen or internally in a capsule.

EMOTIONAL BALANCE
Use aromatically and topically to get from Obstructed ⟶ Flowing.

JOINT, TENDON & LIGAMENT PAIN
Apply topically to affected area to soothe and regenerate.

INSECT & PARASITE REPELLENT
Combine 10-15 drops with water or fractionated coconut oil in a spray bottle and apply topically or put 3-6 drops in a diffuser.

COOKING
Add 1 drop to your favorite recipes for more flavorful dishes.

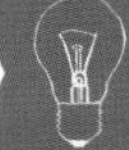

Lemongrass essential oil is used in the pharmaceutical industry for the synthesis of Vitamin A.

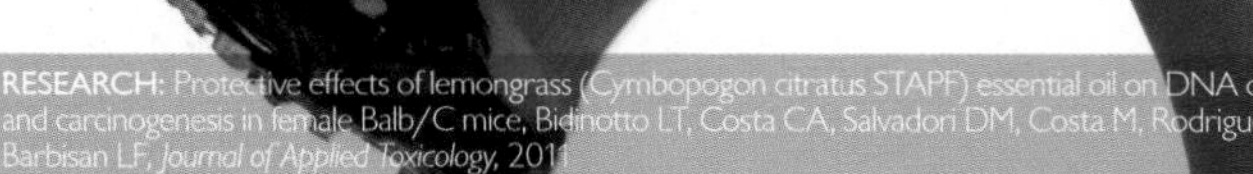

RESEARCH: Protective effects of lemongrass (Cymbopogon citratus STAPF) essential oil on DNA damage and carcinogenesis in female Balb/C mice, Bidinotto LT, Costa CA, Salvadori DM, Costa M, Rodrigues MA, Barbisan LF, *Journal of Applied Toxicology*, 2011

The anti-biofilm activity of lemongrass (Cymbopogon flexuosus) and grapefruit (Citrus paradisi) essential oils against five strains of Staphylococcus aureus, Adukwu EC, Allen SC, Phillips CA, *Journal of Applied Microbiology*, 2012

Protective effect of lemongrass oil against dexamethasone induced hyperlipidemia in rats: possible role of decreased lecithin cholesterol acetyl transferase activity, Kumar VR, Inamdar MN, Nayeemunnisa, Viswanatha GL, *Asian Pacific Journal of Tropical Medicine*, 2011

The GABAergic system contributes to the anxiolytic-like effect of essential oil from Cymbopogon citratus (lemongrass), Costa CA, Kohn DO, de Lima VM, Gargano AC, Flório JC, Costa M, *Journal of Ethnopharmacology*, 2011

The effect of lemongrass EO highlights its potential against antibiotic resistant Staph. aureus in the healthcare environment., Adukwu EC, Allen SC, Phillips CA, *Journal of Applied Microbiology*, 2012

Anticancer activity of an essential oil from Cymbopogon flexuosus (lemongrass), Sharma PR, Mondhe DM, Muthiah S, Pal HC, Shahi AK, Saxena AK, Qazi GN, *Chemico-Biological Interactions*, 2009

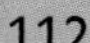

LIME

CITRUS AURANTIFOLIA

renewing · energizing · purifying

TOP USES

SORE THROAT
Gargle internally with water.

RESPIRATORY, LYMPH & LIVER CONGESTION
Use internally in a capsule or apply topically over area of concern.

URINARY & DIGESTIVE ISSUES
Use internally in a glass of water.

MEMORY & CLARITY
Inhale or diffuse aromatically.

EXHAUSTION & DEPRESSION
Apply topically or diffuse aromatically to energize and uplift.

HERPES & COLD SORES
Take internally in a capsule or apply topically to outbreaks.

CHICKEN POX
Use internally in a capsule or dilute topically and apply on spots.

HEAD LICE
Use topically with melaleuca on scalp.

PAIN & INFLAMMATION
Massage topically over area of discomfort or use internally in a capsule to decrease inflammation and increase antioxidants.

EMOTIONAL BALANCE
Use aromatically and topically to get from Faint ⟶ Enlivened.

RIND

COLD PRESSED

MAIN CONSTITUENTS
Limonene
Beta-pinene
Gamma terpinene

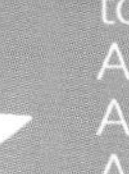

TOP PROPERTIES
Anti-inflammatory
Antiseptic
Antioxidant
Antibacterial
Tonic
Uplifting
Detoxifier
Disinfectant
Diuretic

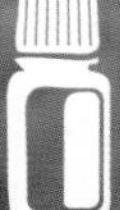

FOUND IN
Focus blend
Cleansing blend

BLENDS WELL WITH
Bergamot
Black pepper
Rosemary

SAFETY
Avoid sunlight and UV ray exposure on affected area for 12 hours after direct topical application. Can cause skin sensitivity.

A popular oil in perfumery for men. In times past British sailors drank lime juice to prevent scurvy.

SINGLE OILS

RESEARCH: Protective effects of lemongrass (Cymbopogon citratus STAPF) essential oil on DNA damage and carcinogenesis in female Balb/C mice, Bidinotto LT, Costa CA, Salvadori DM, Costa M, Rodrigues MA, Barbisan LF, *Journal of Applied Toxicology*, 2011
The anti-biofilm activity of lemongrass (Cymbopogon flexuosus) and grapefruit (Citrus paradisi) essential oils against five strains of Staphylococcus aureus, Adukwu EC, Allen SC, Phillips CA, *Journal of Applied Microbiology*, 2012
Protective effect of lemongrass oil against dexamethasone induced hyperlipidemia in rats: possible role of decreased lecithin cholesterol acetyl transferase activity, Kumar VR, Inamdar MN, Nayeemunnisa, Viswanatha GL, *Asian Pacific Journal of Tropical Medicine*, 2011
The GABAergic system contributes to the anxiolytic-like effect of essential oil from Cymbopogon citratus (lemongrass), Costa CA, Kohn DO, de Lima VM, Gargano AC, Flório JC, Costa M, *Journal of Ethnopharmacology*, 2011
The effect of lemongrass EO highlights its potential against antibiotic resistant Staph. aureus in the healthcare environment, Adukwu EC, Allen SC, Phillips CA, *Journal of Applied Microbiology*, 2012
Anticancer activity of an essential oil from Cymbopogon flexuosus (lemongrass), Sharma PR, Mondhe DM, Muthiah S, Pal HC, Shahi AK, Saxena AK, Qazi GN, *Chemico-Biological Interactions*, 2009

MARJORAM

ORIGANUM MAJORANA

LEAVES

STEAM DISTILLED

MAIN CONSTITUENTS
Linalool
Terpinen-4-ol

TOP PROPERTIES
Vasodilator
Antispasmodic
Digestive Stimulant
Antibacterial
Antifungal
Hypotensive
Sedative

FOUND IN
Massage blend
Tension blend

BLENDS WELL WITH
Lavender
Rosemary
Ylang Ylang

SAFETY
Use with caution in first trimester of pregnancy.

relaxing • connecting • pleasing

TOP USES

CARPAL TUNNEL, TENDONITIS & ARTHRITIS
Use topically on area of discomfort to soothe and calm.

MUSCLE CRAMPS & SPRAINS
Massage topically over cramps or sprains to calm.

HIGH BLOOD PRESSURE
Apply topically over heart and to pulse points or take internally with 2 drops lemongrass in a capsule.

CROUP & BRONCHITIS
Apply topically to neck, chest, and upper back.

PANCREATITIS
Apply 1 or 2 drops topically over pancreas.

OVERACTIVE SEX DRIVE
Apply topically to abdomen.

BOILS, COLD SORES & RINGWORM
Take internally in a capsule or apply topically to affected area.

MIGRAINES & HEADACHES
Massage topically onto back of neck, over headache and along hairline.

COLIC & CONSTIPATION
Take internally in a capsule or rub topically over abdomen and on lower back to improve peristalsis.

CALMING & ANXIETY
Rub topically on back of neck and on bottoms of feet or diffuse to relieve stress.

EMOTIONAL BALANCE
Use aromatically and topically to get from Doubtful ⟶ Trusting.

Also known as "Joy of the Mountains," marjoram symbolized happiness to the ancient Greeks and Romans.

RESEARCH: Comparative effects of Artemisia dracunculus, Satureja hortensis and Origanum majorana on inhibition of blood platelet adhesion, aggregation and secretion, Yazdanparast R, Shahriyary L, *Vascular Pharmacology*, 2008
The effects of aromatherapy on pain, depression, and life satisfaction of arthritis patients, Kim MJ, Nam ES, Paik SI, *Taehan Kanho Hakhoe Chi*, 2005
Immunological and Psychological Benefits of Aromatherapy Massage, Kuriyama H, Watanabe S, Nakaya T, Shigemori I, Kita M, Yoshida N, Masaki D, Tadai T, Ozasa K, Fukui K, Imanishi J, *Evidence-Based Complementary and Alternative Medicine*, 2005
Ovicidal and adulticidal activities of Origanum majorana essential oil constituents against insecticide-susceptible and pyrethroid/malathion-resistant Pediculus humanus capitis (Anoplura: Pediculidae), Yang YC, Lee SH, Clark JM, Ahn YJ, *Journal of Agricultural and Food Chemistry*, 2009
Essential oil inhalation on blood pressure and salivary cortisol levels in prehypertensive and hypertensive subjects, Kim IH, Kim C, Seong K, Hur MH, Lim HM, Lee MS, *Evidence-Based Complementary and Alternative Medicine*, 2012
Free radical scavenging and antiacetylcholinesterase activities of Origanum majorana L. essential oil, Mossa AT, Mawwar GA, *Human & Experimental Toxicology*, 2011
Pain relief assessment by aromatic essential oil massage on outpatients with primary dysmenorrhea: a randomized, double-blind clinical trial, Ou MC, Hsu TF, Lai AC, Lin YT, Lin CC, *The Journal of Obstetrics and Gynecology Research*, 2012

MELALEUCA

MELALEUCA ALTERNIFOLIA

powerful • cleansing • resolving

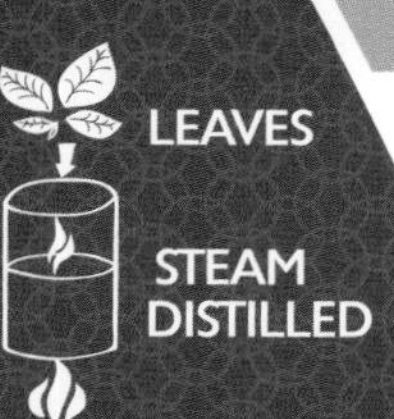

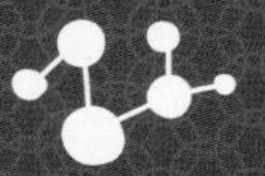

MAIN CONSTITUENTS
a- & y-terpinenes
Terpinen-4-ol
p-cymene

TOP PROPERTIES
Antiseptic
Antibacterial
Antifungal
Anti-parasitic
Antiviral
Analgesic
Decongestant

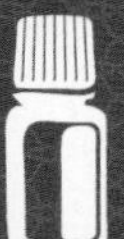

FOUND IN
Respiration blend
Cleansing blend

BLENDS WELL WITH
Cypress
Thyme
Lavender

SAFETY
Safe for NEAT application.

TOP USES

ECZEMA, ATHLETE'S FOOT & CANDIDA
Use internally in a capsule or dilute and apply topically on affected area.

BRONCHITIS, COLD & FLU
Use internally in a capsule, rub topically on throat or diffuse.

CUTS & WOUNDS
Use topically with lavender to clean and disinfect wounds.

ACNE, PINKEYE, STAPH INFECTION & MRSA
Use internally in a capsule or topically on affected area.

SORE THROAT & TONSILITIS
Take internally in a capsule or in warm water and gargle.

DANDRUFF, SCABIES, LICE
Add topically to shampoo. Leave the lather on your head for a few minutes.

HIVES, RASHES & ITCHY EYES
Use internally in a capsule or dilute and use topically on affected area. For eyes, apply to bottoms of second and third toes.

CAVITIES & GUM DISEASE
Use internally in a capsule or topically on affected area.

SHOCK
Apply topically under nose or along spine.

EMOTIONAL BALANCE
Use aromatically and topically to get from Unsure ⟶ Collected.

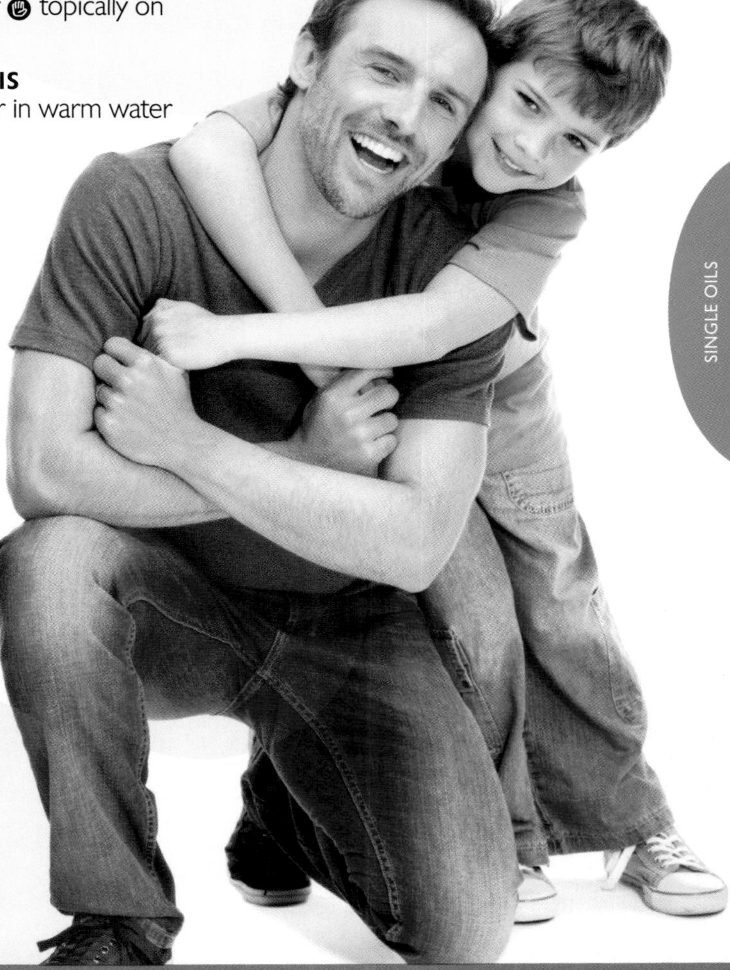

With 12 times the antiseptic power of a phenol, Australian Aborigines have used "Tea Tree" for centuries, often crushing leaves in their hands and inhaling the aroma for colds and illnesses.

RESEARCH: Essential oil of Melaleuca alternifolia for the treatment of oral candidiasis induced in an immunosuppressed mouse model, de Campos Rasteiro VM, da Costa AC, Araújo CF, de Barros PP, Rossoni RD, Anbinder AL, Jorge AO, Junqueira JC, *BMC Complementary and Alternative Medicine*, 2014

Tea tree oil-induced transcriptional alterations in Staphylococcus aureus., Cuaron JA, Dulal S, Song Y, Singh AK, Montelongo CE, Yu W, Nagarajan V, Jayaswal RK, Wilkinson BJ, Gustafson JE, *Phytotherapy Research*, 2013

Susceptibility to Melaleuca alternifolia (tea tree) oil of yeasts isolated from the mouths of patients with advanced cancer, Bagg J, Jackson MS, Petrina Sweeney M, Ramage G, Davies AN, *Oral Oncology*, 2006

Cooling the burn wound: evaluation of different modalites., Jandera V, Hudson DA, de Wet PM, Innes PM, Rode H, *Burns : Journal of the International Society for Burn Injuries*, 2000

Anti-inflammatory effects of Melaleuca alternifolia essential oil on human polymorphonuclear neutrophils and monocytes, Caldefie-Chézet F, Guerry M, Chalchat JC, Fusillier C, Vasson MP, Guillot J, *Free Radical Research*, 2004

Tea tree oil reduces histamine-induced skin inflammation, Koh KJ, Pearce AL, Marshman G, Finlay-Jones JJ, Hart PH, *British Journal of Dermatology*, 2002

Terpinen-4-ol, the main component of Melaleuca alternifolia (tea tree) oil inhibits the in vitro growth of human melanoma cells, Calcabrini A, Stringaro A, Toccacieli L, Meschini S, Marra M, Colone M, Salvatore G, Mondello F, Arancia G, Molinari A, *Journal of Investigative Dermatology*, 2004

A comparative study of tea-tree oil versus benzoylperoxide in the treatment of acne, Bassett IB, Pannowitz DL, Barnetson RS, *Medical Journal of Australia*, 1990

Topically applied Melaleuca alternifolia (tea tree) oil causes direct anti-cancer cytotoxicity in subcutaneous tumour bearing mice, Ireland DJ, Greay SJ, Hooper CM, Kissick HT, Filion P, Riley TV, Beilharz MW, *Journal of Dermatological Science*, 2012

Tea tree oil as a novel anti-psoriasis weapon, Pazyar N, Yaghoobi R, *Skin Pharmacology and Physiology*, 2012

MELISSA

MELISSA OFFICINALIS

awakening • authentic • restorative

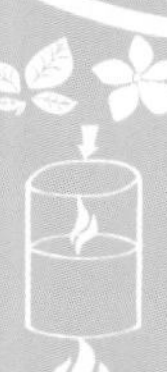

LEAVES & FLOWERS

STEAM DISTILLED

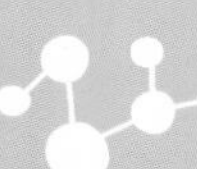

MAIN CONSTITUENTS
Geranial
Germacrene
Neral
B- Caryophyllene

TOP PROPERTIES
Antidepressant
Antiviral
Hypotensive
Sedative
Nervine
Antispasmodic
Antihistamine
Antibacterial

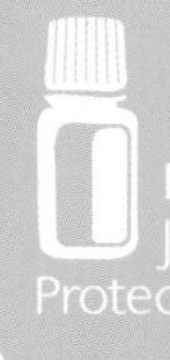

FOUND IN
Joyful blend
Protective blend softgels

BLENDS WELL WITH
Geranium
Lemon
Lavender

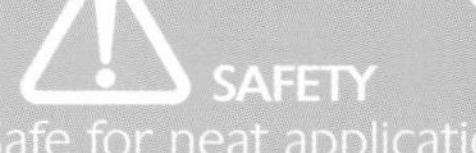

SAFETY
Safe for neat application.

TOP USES

COLDS, COLD SORES, HERPES & FEVER BLISTERS
Apply on sores or use internally in a capsule for support with cold sores or herpes.

DEPRESSION, ANXIETY & SHOCK
Apply topically to back of neck and ears or diffuse or apply topically to roof of mouth and hold for 5-10 seconds.

HYPERTENSION & PALPITATIONS
Apply topically to back of neck or over heart or diffuse.

VERTIGO
Apply topically behind ears and back of neck or internally.

ECZEMA
Massage diluted topically over area of discomfort for calming relief.

INFERTILITY, STERILITY & MENSTRUAL ISSUES
Gently rub topically over abdomen or take internally in a capsule to regulate hormones.

HIGH BLOOD PRESSURE
Use internally in a capsule or apply topically over heart and back of neck.

DYSENTERY & INDIGESTION
Use internally in a capsule or apply topically over abdomen.

FEVERS & VIRAL INFECTIONS
Apply topically along spine or bottoms of feet or take internally in a capsule.

EMOTIONAL BALANCE
Use aromatically and topically to get from Depressed ⟶ Light-filled.

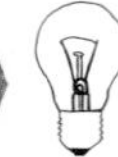

Also known as "Lemon Balm." To make this precious essential oil 66 lbs (30 kgs) are needed to fill one 5ml bottle.

RESEARCH: Low level of Lemon Balm (Melissa officinalis) essential oils showed hypoglycemic effects by altering the expression of glucose metabolism genes in db/db mice, Mi Ja Chung, Sung-Yun Cho and Sung-Joon Lee, *The Journal of the Federation of American Societies for Experimental Biology*, 2008

Apoptosis-Inducing Effects of Melissa officinalis L. Essential Oil in Glioblastoma Multiforme Cells, Queiroz RM, Takiya CM, Guimarães LP, Rocha Gda G, Alviano DS, Blank AF, Alviano CS, Gattass CR, *Cancer Investigation*, 2014

In Vivo Potential Anti-Inflammatory Activity of Melissa officinalis L. Essential Oil, Bounihi A, Hajjaj G, Alnamer R, Cherrah Y, Zellou A, *Advances in Pharmacological Sciences*, 2013

Antiviral activity of the volatile oils of Melissa officinalis L. against Herpes simplex virus type-2, Allahverdiyev A, Duran N, Ozguven M, Koltas S, *Phytomedicine*, 2004

Aromatherapy as a safe and effective treatment for the management of agitation in severe dementia: the results of a double-blind, placebo-controlled trial with Melissa, Ballard CG, O'Brien JT, Reichelt K, Perry EK, *The Journal of Clinical Psychiatry*, 2002

Chemical composition and in vitro antimicrobial activity of essential oil of Melissa officinalis L. from Romania, Hăncianu M, Aprotosoaie AC, Gille E, Poiată A, Tuchiluş C, Spac A, Stănescu U, *Revista Medico-Chirurgicala a Societatii de Medici si Naturalisti din Iasi*, 2008

Chemical composition and larvicidal evaluation of Mentha, Salvia, and Melissa essential oils against the West Nile virus mosquito Culex pipiens, Koliopoulos G, Pitarokili D, Kioulos E, Michaelakis A, Tzakou O, *Parasitology Research*, 2010

MYRRH

COMMIPHORA MYRRHA

drying • healing • nurturing

TOP USES

GUM DISEASE & BLEEDING
Apply topically to gums to soothe complaints.

FINE LINES
Apply topically to area of concern.

THYROID HEALTH & IMMUNE SYSTEM
Apply topically over thyroid and bottoms of feet.

DIGESTIVE UPSET & CRAMPING
Apply topically to abdomen or take in capsule.

ECZEMA & WOUNDS
Apply to affected area, especially to weeping areas.

INFECTION & VIRUS
Take internally in a capsule or apply to bottoms of feet.

CONGESTION & MUCUS
Apply topically to chest and diffuse aromatically to clear airways and dry up congestion.

MEDITATION
Diffuse aromatically to create a sense of calm.

DEPRESSION & ANXIETY
Apply topically to flex points or diffuse.

EMOTIONAL BALANCE
Use aromatically and topically to get from Disconnected ⟶ Nurtured.

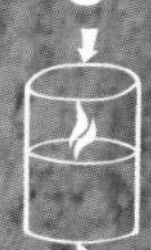

RESIN

STEAM DISTILLED

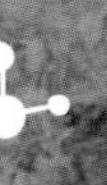

MAIN CONSTITUENTS
Myrrh sesquiter-penoid
Curzerene

TOP PROPERTIES
Anti-inflammatory
Antiviral
Antimicrobial
Expectorant
Anti-infectious
Carminative
Antifungal

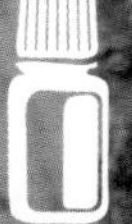

FOUND IN
Anti-aging blend

BLENDS WELL WITH
Frankincense
Sandalwood
Lavender

SAFETY
Safe for NEAT application.

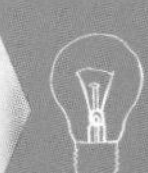

Myrrh means "bitter" and was referred to in the Bible as the balm of Gilead. It was given as a gift to the Christ Child and also presented at his death to be used prior to burial.

RESEARCH: Systematic Review of Complementary and Alternative Medicine Treatments in Inflammatory Bowel Diseases., Langhorst J, Wulfert H, Lauche R, Klose P, Cramer H, Dobos GJ,Korzenik,J, *Journal of Crohn's & Colitis*, 2015

Clinical trial of aromatherapy on postpartum mother's perineal healing, Hur MH, Han SH, *Journal of Korean Academy of Nursing*, 2004

Composition and potential anticancer activities of essential oils obtained from myrrh and frankincense, Chen Y, Zhou C, Ge Z, Liu Y, Liu Y, Feng W, Li S, Chen G, Wei T, *Oncology Letters*, 2013

In vitro cytotoxic and anti-inflammatory effects of myrrh oil on human gingival fibroblasts and epithelial cells, Tipton DA, Lyle B, Babich H, Dabbous MKh, Toxicology in Vitro, 2003

Anti-inflammatory and analgesic activity of different extracts of Commiphora myrrha, Su S, Wang T, Duan JA, Zhou W, Hua YQ, Tang YP, Yu L, Qian DW, *Journal of Ethnopharmacology*, 2011

Myrrh: Medical Marvel or Myth of the Magi?, Nomicos EY, *Holistic Nursing Practice*, 2007

Chemical composition and antibacterial activity of selected essential oils and some of their main compounds, Wanner J, Schmidt E, Bail S, Jirovetz L, Buchbauer G, Gochev V, Girova T, Atanasova T, Stoyanova A, *Natural Product Communications*, 2010

The Effect of Commiphora molmol (Myrrh) in Treatment of Trichomoniasis vaginalis infection, El-Sherbiny GM, El Sherbiny ET, *Iranian Red Crescent Medical Journal*, 2011

Sesquiterpenoids from myrrh inhibit androgen receptor expression and function in human prostate cancer cells, Wang XL, Kong F, Shen T, Young CY, Lou HX, Yuan HQ, *Acta Pharmacologica Sinica*, 2011

OREGANO

ORIGANUM VULGARE

strong
resolving
powerful

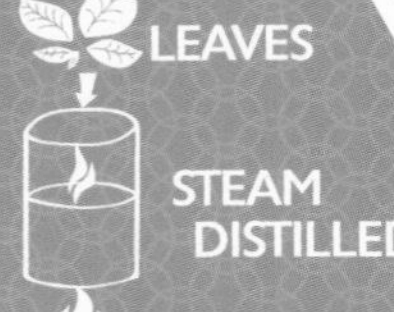

STEAM DISTILLED

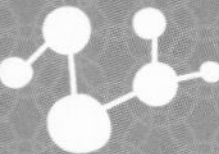

MAIN CONSTITUENTS
Carvacrol
Thymol

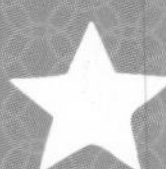

TOP PROPERTIES
Antibacterial
Antifungal
Anti-parasitic
Antiviral
Immunostimulant

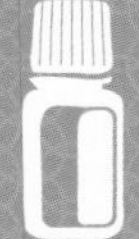

FOUND IN
Protective blend softgels

BLENDS WELL WITH
Thyme
Basil
Clove

SAFETY
Small dosage recommended. Dilute for topical application as can cause sensitive skin. Caution during pregnancy.

TOP USES

VIRUSES
Take internally in a capsule.

STREP THROAT & TONSILITIS
Gargle 1 drop diluted in water as needed.

STAPH INFECTION & MRSA
Apply topically to affected area or take internally in a capsule.

INTESTINAL WORMS & PARASITES
Take internally in a capsule.

WARTS, CALLOUSES & CANKER SORES
Apply topically 1 drop diluted with fractionated coconut oil and 2 drops frankincense directly to affected areas.

PNEUMONIA & TUBERCULOSIS
Apply topically 1 drop diluted with fractionated coconut oil to bottoms of feet to boost immunity.

URINARY INFECTION
Take internally with lemongrass in a capsule.

ATHLETE'S FOOT, RINGWORM & CANDIDA
To stimulate digestion take in a capsule.

CARPAL TUNNEL & RHEUMATISM
Apply topically diluted to painful area for comfort.

EMOTIONAL BALANCE
Use aromatically and topically to get from Obstinate ⟶ Unattached.

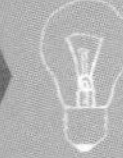

This powerful and potent essential oil packs a punch. It is helpful against antibiotic-resistant bacteria

RESEARCH: Antiviral efficacy and mechanisms of action of oregano essential oil and its primary component carvacrol against murine norovirus, Gilling DH, Kitajima M, Torrey JR, Bright KR, *Journal of Applied Microbiology*, 2014
Origanum vulgare subsp. hirtum Essential Oil Prevented Biofilm Formation and Showed Antibacterial Activity against Planktonic and Sessile Bacterial Cells, Schillaci D, Napoli EM, Cusimano MG, Vitale M, Ruberto A, *Journal of Food Protection*, 2013
Oregano essential oil as an antimicrobial additive to detergent for hand washing and food contact surface cleaning, Rhoades J, Gialagkolidou K, Gogou M, Mavridou O, Blatsiotis N, Ritzoulis C, Likotrafiti E, *Journal of Applied Microbiology*, 2013
Evaluation of bacterial resistance to essential oils and antibiotics after exposure to oregano and cinnamon essential oils, Becerril R, Nerín C, Gómez-Lus R, *Foodborne Pathogens and Disease*, 2012
Supercritical fluid extraction of oregano (Origanum vulgare) essentials oils: anti-inflammatory properties based on cytokine response on THP-1 macrophages, Ocaña-Fuentes A, Arranz-Gutiérrez E, Señorans FJ, Reglero G, *Food and Chemical Toxicology*, 2010
Antioxidant and antimicrobial activities of essential oils obtained from oregano, Karakaya S, El SN, Karagözlü N, Sahin S, *Journal of Medicinal Food*, 2011
Anti-inflammatory and anti-ulcer activities of carvacrol, a monoterpene present in the essential oil of oregano, Silva FV, Guimarães AG, Silva ER, Sousa-Neto BP, Machado FD, Quintans-Júnior LJ, Arcanjo DD, Oliveira FA, Oliveira RC, *Journal of Medicinal Food*, 2012

PATCHOULI

POGOSTEMON CABLIN

calming · recovering · stabilizing

TOP USES

ANXIETY & DOPAMINE ISSUES
Diffuse or apply topically under nose and back of neck to calm emotions.

OILY HAIR & IMPETIGO
Apply topically to troubled area.

SORES & INFECTIONS
Apply topically to area of concern or bottoms of feet.

BODY ODOR
Apply topically as a deodorant where needed.

FLUID RETENTION
Take internally with grapefruit.

INSECT & MOSQUITO REPELLENT
Diffuse or apply to repel pests.

INSECTS BITES, SNAKE BITES & STINGS
Apply with lavender to soothe bites.

DIGEST TOXIC MATERIAL
Take internally in a capsule with ginger.

APPETITE & WEIGHT ISSUES
Take internally in a capsule with ginger.

STRETCH MARKS & SKIN ISSUES
Apply topically with myrrh to soothe troubled skin.

EMOTIONAL BALANCE
Use aromatically and topically to get from Degraded ⟶ Enhanced.

LEAVES

STEAM DISTILLED

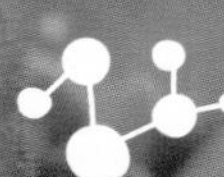

MAIN CONSTITUENTS
Alpha pinene
Sabinene

TOP PROPERTIES
Aphrodisiac
Sedative
Diuretic
Antifungal
Antispasmodic
Insecticide
Antidepressant

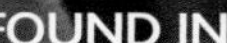

FOUND IN
Women's blend
Focus blend

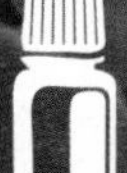

BLENDS WELL WITH
Grapefruit
Bergamot
Cypress
Sandalwood
Vetiver
Clary sage

SAFETY
Safe for NEAT application.

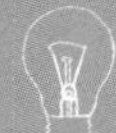

Patchouli has a long history in the perfume trade, but became famous from the 1960 hippie movement.

RESEARCH: Repellency to Stomoxys calcitrans (Diptera: Muscidae) of Plant Essential Oils Alone or in Combination with Calophyllum inophyllum Nut Oil, Hieu TT, Kim SI, Lee SG, Ahn YJ, *Journal of Medical Etomology*, 2010
Immunologic mechanism of Patchouli alcohol anti-H1N1 influenza virus may through regulation of the RLH signal pathway in vitro, Wu XL, Ju DH, Chen J, Yu B, Liu KL, He JX, Dai CQ, Wu S, Chang Z, Wang YP, Chen XY, *Current Microbiology*, 2013
The effects of inhalation of essential oils on the body weight, food efficiency rate and serum leptin of growing SD rats, Hur MH, Kim C, Kim CH, Ahn HC, Ahn HY, *Korean Society of Nursing Science*, 2006
Oral administration of patchouli alcohol isolated from Pogostemonis Herba augments protection against influenza viral infection in mice, Li YC, Peng SZ, Chen HM, Zhang FX, Xu PP, Xie JH, He JJ, Chen JN, Lai XP, Su ZR, *International Immunopharmacology*, 2012
Anti-inflammatory activity of patchouli alcohol in RAW264.7 and HT-29 cells, Jeong JB, Shin YK, Lee SH, *Food and Chemical Toxicology*, 2013
Evaluation of the Effects of Plant-derived Essential Oils on Central Nervous System Function Using Discrete Shuttle-type Conditioned Avoidance Response in Mice, Umezu T., *Phytotherapy Research*, 2012

PEPPERMINT

MENTA PIPERITA

adaptive • invigorating • cooling

LEAVES

STEAM DISTILLED

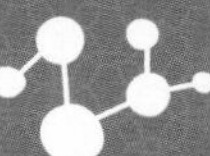

MAIN CONSTITUENTS
Menthol
Menthone
a- & b- pinenes
Menthyl acetate

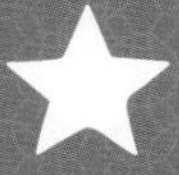

TOP PROPERTIES
Anti-inflammatory
Analgesic
Antispasmodic
Warming
Invigorating
Cooling
Expectorant
Vasoconstrictor
Stimulating

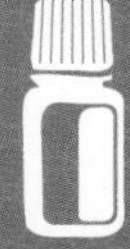

FOUND IN
Tension blend
Metabolic blend
Soothing blend
Digestion blend
Massage blend
Respiration blend

BLENDS WELL WITH
Wild orange
Grapefruit

SAFETY
Dilute for topical application as may cause skin sensitivity. Avoid at night as it is a stimulant.

TOP USES

HEADACHES & MIGRAINES
Apply topically to temples, above ears, and back of neck.

BAD BREATH
Gargle 1 drop internally with water.

ASTHMA & SINUSITIS
Apply topically to chest and back or bottoms of feet.

DECREASE MILK SUPPLY
Apply topically to breasts with fractionated coconut oil or take internally in a capsule or water.

LOSS OF SENSE OF SMELL
Inhale or apply diluted topically over bridge of the nose.

GASTRITIS & DIGESTIVE DISCOMFORT
Take internally in a capsule or cup of water or apply topically over abdomen.

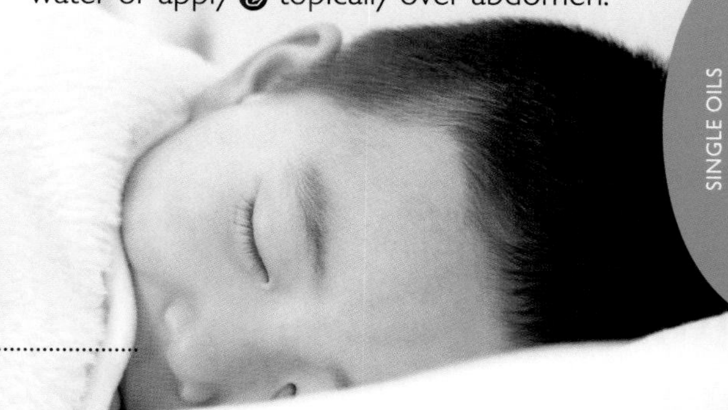

ALERTNESS
Inhale or apply topically under nose and/or back of neck.

FEVERS & HOT FLASHES
Apply topically on back of neck, spine, or bottoms of feet.

AUTISM
Apply topically on back of neck, spine, or bottoms of feet.

CRAVINGS
Inhale or apply topically under nose before or in between meals to suppress appetite.

ALLERGIES & HIVES
Take internally in a capsule or with water or apply topically under nose or to bottoms of feet.

GAMMA RADIATION EXPOSURE
Take internally in a capsule or water for antioxidant support.

EMOTIONAL BALANCE
Use aromatically and topically to get from Hindered⟶Invigorated.

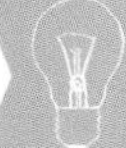

Peppermint, with its stimulant qualities, and lavender, with its sedative qualities, make a great combination.

RESEARCH: Screening of the antibacterial effects of a variety of essential oils on respiratory tract pathogens, using a modified dilution assay method, Inouye S, Yamaguchi H, Takizawa T, *Journal of Infection and Chemotherapy: Official Journal of the Japan Society of Chemotherapy*, 2001

The influence of essential oils on human attention and alertness, Ilmberger J, Heuberger E, Mahrhofer C, Dessovic H, Kowarik D, Buchbauer G, *Chemical Senses*, 2001

Enteric-coated, pH-dependent peppermint oil capsules for the treatment of irritable bowel syndrome in children, Kline RM, Kline JJ, Di Palma J, Barbero GJ, *The Journal of Pediatrics*, 2001

Cutaneous application of menthol 10% solution as an abortive treatment of migraine without aura: a randomised, double-blind, placebo-controlled, crossed-over study, Borhani Haghighi A, Motazedian S, Rezaii R, Mohammadi F, Salarian L, Pourmokhtari M, Khodaei S, Vossoughi M, Miri R, *The International Journal of Clinical Practice*, 2010

Peppermint oil for the treatment of irritable bowel syndrome: a systematic review and meta-analysis, Khanna R, MacDonald JK, Levesque BG, *Journal of Clinical Gastroenterology*, 2014

Effects of Peppermint and Cinnamon Odor Administration on Simulated Driving Alertness, Mood and Workload, Raudenbush B, Grayhem R, Sears T, Wilson I., *North American Journal of Psychology*, 2009

Preliminary investigation of the effect of peppermint oil on an objective measure of daytime sleepiness, Norrish MI, Dwyer KL, *International journal of psychophysiology: official journal of the International Organization of Psychophysiology*, 2005

Controlled breathing with or without peppermint aromatherapy for postoperative nausea and/or vomiting symptom relief: a randomized controlled trial, Sites DS, Johnson NT, Miller JA, Torbush PH, Hardin JS, Knowles SS, Nance J, Fox TH, Tart RC, *Journal of PeriAnesthesia Nursing*, 2014

Antioxidant components of naturally-occurring oils exhibit marked anti-inflammatory activity in epithelial cells of the human upper respiratory system, Gao M, Singh A, Macri K, Reynolds C, Singhal V, Biswal S, Spannhake EW, *Respiratory Research*, 2011

The effects of peppermint on exercise performance, Meamarbashi A, Rajabi A, *Journal of International Society of Sports Nutrition*, 2013

RAVENSARA

RAVENSARA AROMATICA

reviving
clearing
relaxing

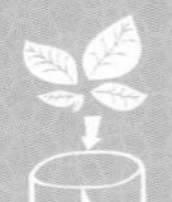
LEAVES

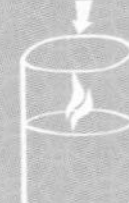
STEAM DISTILLED

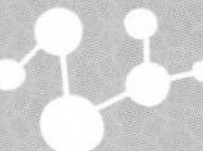
MAIN CONSTITUENTS
1,8-cineole

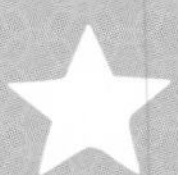
TOP PROPERTIES
Antiviral
Antibacterial
Immunostimulant
Expectorant
Analgesic
Muscle Relaxant
Stimulant

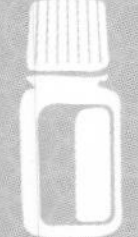
FOUND IN
Protective blend softgels

BLENDS WELL WITH
Lavender
White fir
Cedarwood

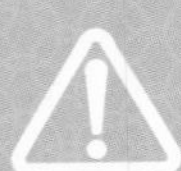
SAFETY
Safe for NEAT application on all ages.

TOP USES

CHILLS & FLU
Apply topically to affected area & bottoms of feet.

WHOOPING COUGH & BRONCHITIS
Apply topically to chest & bottoms of feet. Diffuse.

NERVOUS & MENTAL FATIGUE
Apply topically over adrenal glands & pulse points.

GERMS & BUGS
Diffuse to cleanse air.

MUSCLE & JOINT PAIN
Apply topically to affected area.

EMOTIONAL BALANCE
Use aromatically and topically to get from Uncommitted ——→ Resolute.

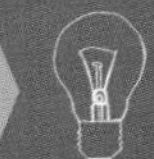
Ravensara is indigenous to Madagascar and has grown in popularity since the '80s.

ROMAN CHAMOMILE

ANTHEMIS NOBILIS

bright • calming • sweet

TOP USES

STRESS & SHOCK
Diffuse or apply topically to back of neck.

DRY & IRRITATED SKIN
Apply topically to area of concern.

LOWER BLOOD PRESSURE
Apply topically over heart or on back of neck or take in a capsule.

SCIATICA & LOWER BACK PAIN
Apply topically to area of concern.

INSOMNIA & OVEREXCITEMENT
Diffuse or apply topically to back of neck and forehead.

PMS & CRAMPS
Apply topically to abdomen.

FEVERS & EARACHES
Apply topically to bottoms of feet and to ears as needed.

ANGER & IRRITABILITY
Diffuse or apply topically under nose or back of neck.

PARASITES & WORMS
Apply topically to abdomen or take internally in a capsule to promote expulsion.

ANOREXIA
Apply topically to back of neck or take internally in a capsule.

INSECT BITES, BEE & HORNET STINGS
Apply topically to area of concern or take internally in a capsule.

EMOTIONAL BALANCE
Use aromatically and topically to get from Frustrated ⟶ Purposeful.

FLOWERS

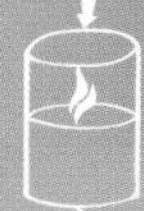

STEAM DISTILLED

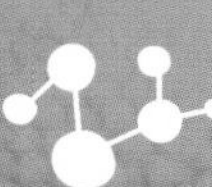

MAIN CONSTITUENTS
Geranial
Germacrene
Neral
Caryophyllene

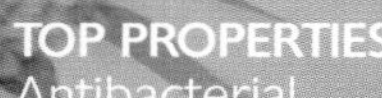

TOP PROPERTIES
Antibacterial
Antifungal
Sedative
Antiviral
Immunostimulant
Hypnotonic

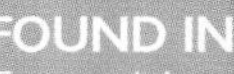

FOUND IN
Focus blend
Tension blend
Calming blend
Women's monthly blend

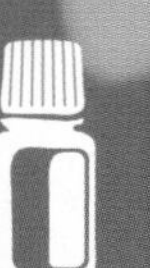

BLENDS WELL WITH
Lavender

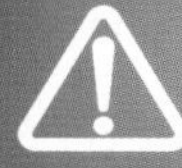

SAFETY
Safe for NEAT application.

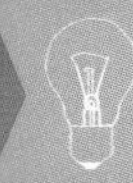

Ancient Romans used roman chamomile before battle to empower them with courage and clear minds.

SINGLE OILS

RESEARCH: Cytological aspects on the effects of a nasal spray consisting of standardized extract of citrus lemon and essential oils in allergic rhinopathy, Ferrara L, Naviglio D, Armone Caruso A, *ISRN Pharm*, 2012

Volatiles from steam-distilled leaves of some plant species from Madagascar and New Zealand and evaluation of their biological activity, Costa R, Pizzimenti F, Marotta F, Dugo P, Santi L, Mondello L., *Nat Prod Commun*, 2010 Nov

Application of near-infrared spectroscopy in quality control and determination of adulteration of African essential oils, Juliani HR, Kapteyn J, Jones D, Koroch AR, Wang M, Charles D, Simon JE, *Phytochem Anal*, 2006 Mar-Apr

Determination of the absolute configuration of 6-alkylated alpha-pyrones from Ravensara crassifolia by LC-NMR, Queiroz EF, Wolfender JL, Raoelison G, Hostettmann K, *Phytochem Anal*, 2003 Jan-Feb

Antiviral activities in plants endemic to madagascar, Hudson JB, Lee MK, Rasoanaivo P, *Pharm Biol*, 2000

Two 6-substituted 5,6-dihydro-alpha-pyrones from Ravensara anisata, Andrianaivoravelona JO, Sahpaz S, Terreaux C, Hostettmann K, Stoeckli-Evans H, Rasolondramanitra J, *Phytochemistry 1999* Sep

Study of the antimicrobial action of various essential oils extracted from Malagasy plants. II: Lauraceae, Raharivelomanana PJ, Terrom GP, Bianchini JP, Coulanges P, *Arch Inst Pasteur Madagascar*, 1989

ROSE

ROSA DAMASCENA

FLOWERS

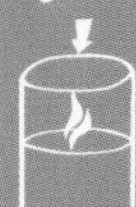
STEAM DISTILLED

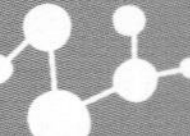
MAIN CONSTITUENTS
Cirronellol
Geranol
Nerol

TOP PROPERTIES
Antidepressant
Aphrodisiac
Antispasmodic
Emmenagogue
Sedative
Tonic

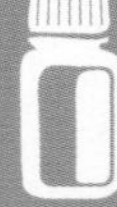
FOUND IN
Anti-aging blend
Women's blend
Repellent blend

BLENDS WELL WITH
Sandalwood
Lavender
Geranium

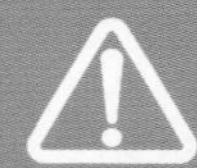
SAFETY
Safe for NEAT application.

intimate • connecting • radiant

TOP USES

LOW LIBIDO
Diffuse and apply topically over navel and heart.

SCARS, WOUNDS & WRINKLES
Apply topically to area of concern.

GRIEF & DEPRESSION
Diffuse and apply topically to back of neck and over heart.

IRREGULAR OVULATION
Apply topically to abdomen.

SEIZURES
Apply topically to back of neck.

FACIAL CAPILLARIES & REDNESS
Apply topically to area of concern.

SEMEN PRODUCTION & IMPOTENCY
Apply topically to navel.

EMOTIONAL BALANCE
Use aromatically and topically to get from Isolated ⟶ Loved.

Known as the "Queen of Flowers," it takes about 12,000 rose blossoms to make a single 5mL bottle.

refreshing • cooling • clearing

ROSEMARY

ROSMARINUS OFFICINALIS

TOP USES

RESPIRATORY INFECTIONS
Apply topically to chest and diffuse aromatically.

CANCER
Take internally in a capsule.

HAIR LOSS
Apply topically to scalp.

MEMORY
Apply topically under nose and across forehead or diffuse.

BELL'S PALSY & MULTIPLE SCLEROSIS
Apply topically to bottoms of feet and internally in a capsule.

MENTAL, ADRENAL & CHRONIC FATIGUE
Diffuse with basil to combat fatigue.

JAUNDICE & LIVER CONDITION
Take internally in a capsule.

NERVOUSNESS & DEPRESSION
Diffuse to de-stress.

TIRED & STIFF MUSCLES
Apply topically with wintergreen.

CELLULITE
Take internally in a capsule and diffuse

FAINTING
Apply topically to skin with geranium.

EMOTIONAL BALANCE
Use aromatically and topically to get from Confused⟶Open-minded.

LEAVES

STEAM DISTILLED

MAIN CONSTITUENTS
Linalool
Terpinen-4-ol

TOP PROPERTIES
Analgesic
Thins mucus
Improves brain function
Stimulant

FOUND IN
Detoxification blend
Tension blend

BLENDS WELL WITH
Peppermint
Basil
Lavender

SAFETY
Caution against high use during pregnancy, people with epilepsy and high blood pressure.

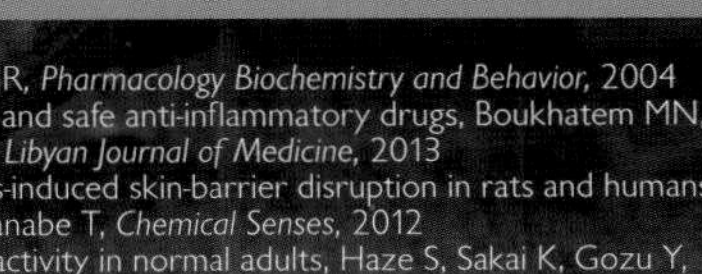
In ancient times, rosemary was a favorite oil to drive away evil spirits.

SINGLE OILS

RESEARCH: The effects of prolonged rose odor inhalation in two animal models of anxiety, Bradley BF, Starkey NJ, Brown SL, Lea RW, *Physiology & Behavior*, 2007
The metabolic responses to aerial diffusion of essential oils, Wu Y, Zhang Y, Xie G, Zhao A, Pan X, Chen T, Hu Y, Liu Y, Cheng Y, Chi Y, Yao L, Jia W, *PLOS One*, 2012
Essential oils and anxiolytic aromatherapy, Setzer WN, *Natural Product Communications*, 2009
The effects of clinical aromatherapy for anxiety and depression in the high risk postpartum woman – a pilot study, Conrad P, Adams C, *Complementary Therapies in Clinical Practice*, 2012
Anxiolytic-like effects of rose oil inhalation on the elevated plus-maze test in rats, de Almeida RN, Motta SC, de Brito Faturi C, Catallani B, Leite JR, *Pharmacology Biochemistry and Behavior*, 2004
Rose geranium essential oil as a source of new and safe anti-inflammatory drugs, Boukhatem MN, Kameli A, Ferhat MA, Saidi F, Mekarnia M, *The Libyan Journal of Medicine*, 2013
Effect of "rose essential oil" inhalation on stress-induced skin-barrier disruption in rats and humans, Fukada M, Kano E, Miyoshi M, Komaki R, Watanabe T, *Chemical Senses*, 2012
Effects of fragrance inhalation on sympathetic activity in normal adults, Haze S, Sakai K, Gozu Y, *The Japanese Journal of Pharmacology*, 2002
Relaxing effect of rose oil on humans, Hongratanaworakit T, *Natural Product Communications*, 2009

SANDALWOOD

SANTALUM ALBUM

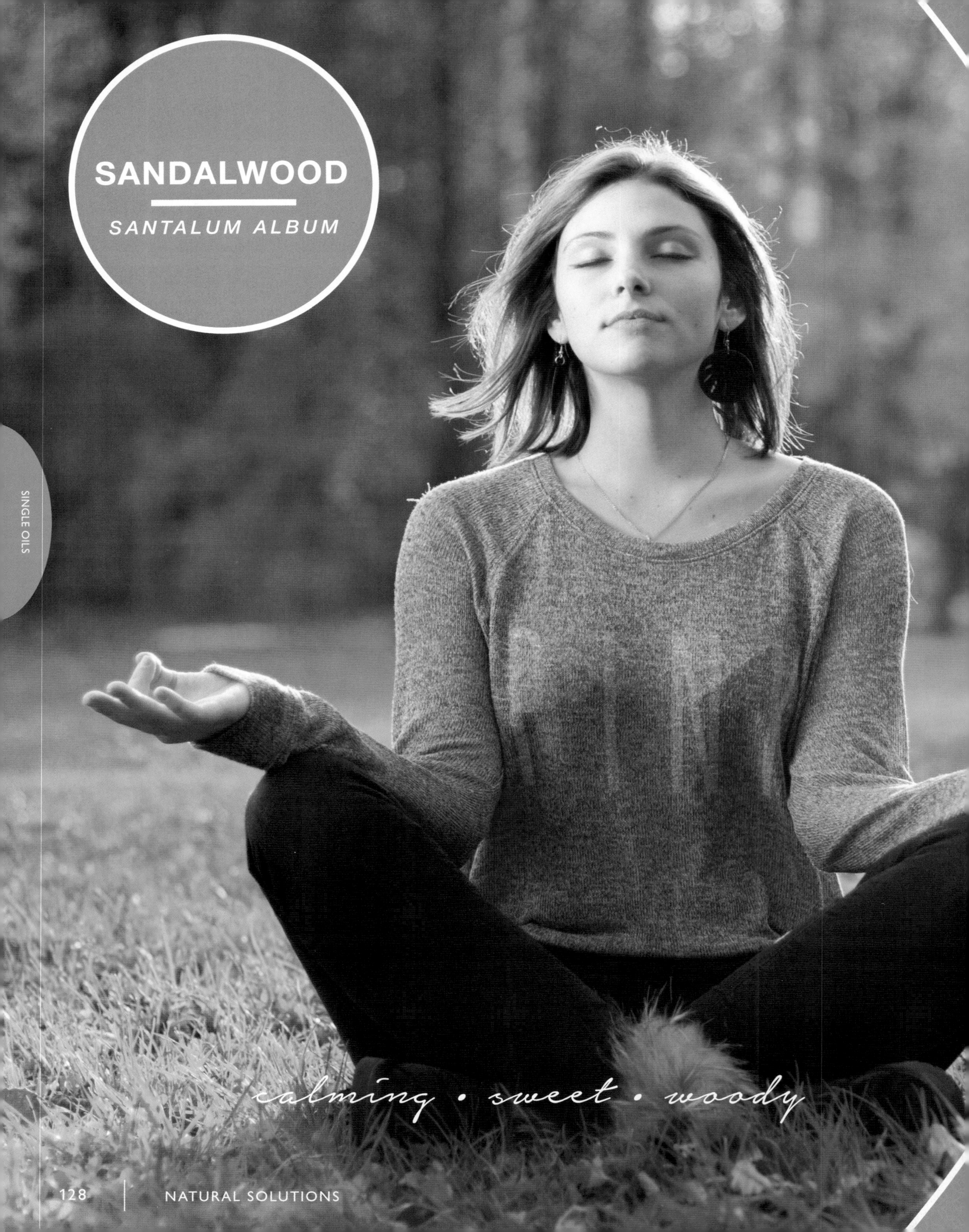

SINGLE OILS

calming • sweet • woody

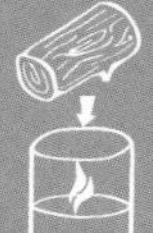

WOOD

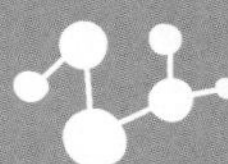

STEAM DISTILLED

MAIN CONSTITUENTS
a- & b-santalols
a- & b-santalenes

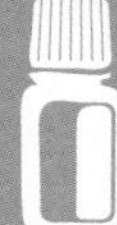

TOP PROPERTIES
Anti-inflammatory
Anti-carcinoma
Astringent
Antidepressant
Calming
Sedative

FOUND IN
Repellent blend
Women's blend
Anti-aging blend
Focus blend
Calming blend

BLENDS WELL WITH
Frankincense
Lavender
White Fir

SAFETY
Safe for NEAT application.

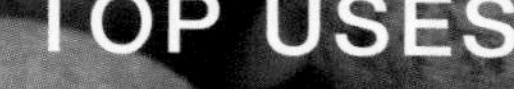

TOP USES

DRY SKIN & SCALP
Use topically or in shampoo.

CALMING & RELAXING
Diffuse in air and apply topically under nose.

SCARS & BLEMISHES
Apply topically directly to affected area.

WOUND CARE & SKIN INFECTIONS
Apply topically to heal skin.

SPASMS & CRAMPS
Apply topically over area of concern.

CANCER & TUMORS
Take internally to protect against tumors.

ALZHEIMER'S DISEASE
Take internally to support immune system.

INSOMNIA & RESTLESSNESS
Apply topically to bottoms of feet and inhale for a restful night.

MEDITATION & YOGA
Enjoy sandalwood in diffuser to enhance meditation.

EMOTIONAL BALANCE
Use aromatically and topically to get from Uninspired → Devoted.

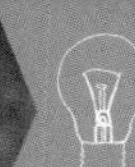

Sandalwood has been used for various spiritual and religious uses. Today Hindus still anoint the temple floor and walls to enhance spiritual ambiance.

RESEARCH: Olfactory receptor neuron profiling using sandalwood odorants, Bieri S, Monastyrskaia K, Schilling B, *Chemical Senses*, 2004

Differential effects of selective frankincense (Ru Xiang) essential oil versus non-selective sandalwood (Tan Xiang) essential oil on cultured bladder cancer cells: a microarray and bioinformatics study, Dozmorov MG, Yang Q, Wu W, Wren J, Suhail MM, Woolley CL, Young DG, Fung KM, Lin HK, *Chinese Medicine*, 2014

Sandalwood oil prevent skin tumour development in CD1 mice, Dwivedi C, Zhang Y, *European Journal of Cancer Prevention*, 1999

Chemopreventive effects of α-santalol on skin tumor development in CD-1 and SENCAR mice, Dwivedi C, Guan X, Harmsen WL, Voss AL, Goetz-Parten DE, Koopman EM, Johnson KM, Valluri HB, Matthees DP, Cancer Epidemiology, *Biomarkers and Prevention*, 2003

Alpha-santalol, a chemopreventive agent against skin cancer, causes G2/M cell cycle arrest in both p53-mutated human epidermoid carcinoma A431 cells and p53 wild-type human melanoma UACC-62 cells, Zhang X, Chen W, Guillermo R, Chandrasekher G, Kaushik RS, Young A, Fahmy H, Dwivedi C, *BMC Research Notes*, 2010

α-santalol, a derivative of sandalwood oil, induces apoptosis in human prostate cancer cells by causing caspase-3 activation, Bommareddy A, Rule B, VanWert AL, Santha S, Dwivedi C, *Phytomedicine*, 2012

Skin cancer chemopreventive agent, α-santalol, induces apoptotic death of human epidermoid carcinoma A431 cells via caspase activation together with dissipation of mitochondrial membrane potential and cytochrome c release, Kaur M, Agarwal C, Singh RP, Guan X, Dwivedi C, Agarwal R, *Carcinogenesis*, 2005

Evaluation of in vivo anti-hyperglycemic and antioxidant potentials of α-santalol and sandalwood oil, Misra BB, Dey S, *Phytomedicine*, 2013

SPEARMINT

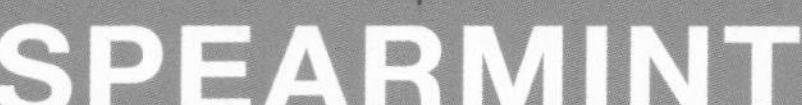

MENTHA SPICATA

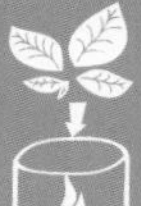

WHOLE PLANT

STEAM DISTILLED

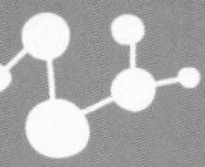

MAIN CONSTITUENTS
Carvone
Limonene
Beta-myrcene

TOP PROPERTIES
Anti-inflammatory
Digestive
Stimulant
Carminative
Antiseptic

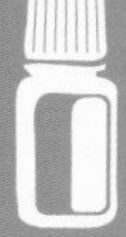

BLENDS WELL WITH
Peppermint
Wintergreen
Ginger

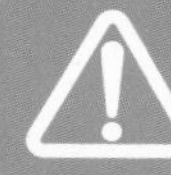

SAFETY
Safe for neat application.

relieving · uplifting · promoting

TOP USES

INDIGESTION, NAUSEA & COLIC
Apply topically to affected area or take internally in a capsule.

BAD BREATH
Swish and swallow 1 drop diluted in water.

BRONCHITIS & RESPIRATORY ISSUES
Apply topically to chest and back or diffuse.

ACNE, SORES & SCARS
Apply topically to area of concern.

DEPRESSION & FATIGUE
Diffuse and apply topically to back of neck.

STRESS & NERVOUS ISSUES
Diffuse apply topically to back of neck.

SLOW OR HEAVY MENSTRUATION
Diffuse and apply topically to back of neck.

HEADACHES & MIGRAINES
Diffuse and apply topically to back of neck.

EMOTIONAL BALANCE
Use aromatically and topically to get from Weary ⟶ Refreshed.

A common flavor for toothpaste & candy, the ancient Greeks enjoyed bathing with spearmint.

RESEARCH: Aromatherapy as a Treatment for Postoperative Nausea: A randomized Trial, Hunt R, Dienemann J, Norton HJ, Hartley W, Hudgens A, Stern T, Divine G, *Anesthesia and Analgesia*, 2013
Inhibition by the essential oils of peppermint and spearmint of the growth of pathogenic bacteria, Imai H, Osawa K, Yasuda H, Hamashima H, Arai T, Sasatsu M, *Microbios*, 2001
Influence of the chirality of (R)-(-)- and (S)-(+)-carvone in the central nervous system: a comparative study, de Sousa DP, de Farias Nóbrega FF, de Almeida RN, Chirality, 2007
Comparison of essential oils from three plants for enhancement of antimicrobial activity of nitrofurantoin against enterobacteria, Rafii F, Shahverdi AR, *Chemotherapy*, 2007
Botanical perspectives on health peppermint: more than just an after-dinner mint, Spirling LI, Daniels IR, *Journal for the Royal Society for the Promotion of Health*, 2001
The effect of gender and ethnicity on children's attitudes and preferences for essential oils: a pilot study, Fitzgerald M, Culbert T, Finkelstein M, Green M, Johnson A, Chen S, *Explore (New York, N.Y.)*, 2007

healing · rejuvenating · uplifting

SPIKENARD

NARDOSTACHYS JATAMANSI

TOP USES

AGING SKIN
Apply topically as need to affected area.

INSOMNIA, STRESS & TENSION
Diffuse and apply topically to bottoms of feet before bed.

PMS & MENSTRUAL ISSUES
Apply topically to affected area & pulse points.

NAUSEA & DIGESTIVE DISCOMFORT
Apply topically to affected area & bottoms of feet.

ANXIETY & DEPRESSION
Apply topically to pulse points & diffuse.

MUSCLE SPASMS
Apply topically to affected area.

ULCERS, GAS & INDIGESTION
Apply topically to abdomen or to affected area.

PINKEYE & RASHES
Apply topically to affected area.

EMOTIONAL BALANCE
Use aromatically and topically to get from Agitated ⟶ Tranquil.

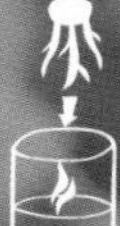

ROOTS

STEAM DISTILLED

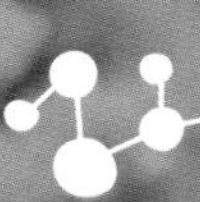

MAIN CONSTITUENTS
a-patchoulene
Bornyl acetate
Valeranone

TOP PROPERTIES
Anti-inflammatory
Antispasmodic
Sedative
Antibacterial
Antifungal
Deodorant
Laxative
Tonic

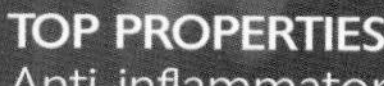

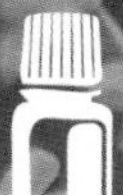

BLENDS WELL WITH
Ginger
Cassia
Myrrh

SAFETY
Safe for NEAT application.

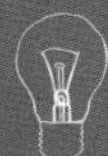

Spikenard, one of the Romans' favorite perfumes, is featured in the Bible several times.

SINGLE OILS

RESEARCH: Aromatherapy as a Treatment for Postoperative Nausea: A randomized Trial, Hunt R, Dienemann J, Norton HJ, Hartley W, Hudgens A, Stern T, Divine G, *Anesthesia and Analgesia*, 2013
Inhibition by the essential oils of peppermint and spearmint of the growth of pathogenic bacteria, Imai H, Osawa K, Yasuda H, Hamashima H, Arai T, Sasatsu M, *Microbios*, 2001
Influence of the chirality of (R)-(-)- and (S)-(+)-carvone in the central nervous system: a comparative study, de Sousa DP, de Farias Nóbrega FF, de Almeida RN, *Chirality*, 2007
Comparison of essential oils from three plants for enhancement of antimicrobial activity of nitrofurantoin against enterobacteria, Rafii F, Shahverdi AR, *Chemotherapy*, 2007
Botanical perspectives on health peppermint: more than just an after-dinner mint, Spirling LI, Daniels IR, *Journal for the Royal Society for the Promotion of Health*, 2001
The effect of gender and ethnicity on children's attitudes and preferences for essential oils: a pilot study, Fitzgerald M, Culbert T, Finkelstein M, Green M, Johnson A, Chen S, *Explore (New York, N.Y.)*, 2007

TANGERINE

CITRUS RETICULATA

balancing • cleansing • uplifting

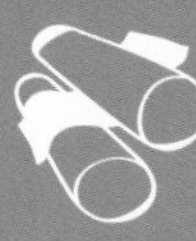

RIND

COLD PRESSED

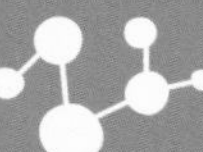

MAIN CONSTITUENTS
a-pinene
Limonene

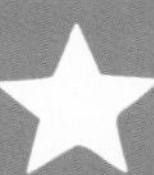

TOP PROPERTIES
Antioxidant
Anticoagulant
Anti-inflammatory
Laxative
Sedative
Mucolytic

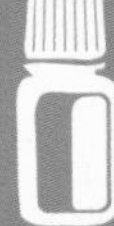

FOUND IN
Cellular complex blend

BLENDS WELL WITH
Bergamot
Clary sage
Lavender

SAFETY
Dilute for topical application, may cause skin sensitivity.

TOP USES

ACHY FATIGUED MUSCLES & LIMBS
Apply topically to affected areas.

CONGESTION
Take internally with peppermint in a capsule.

POOR CIRCULATION
Apply topically diluted with ginger to affected areas.

ARTHRITIS & MUSCLE PAIN
Apply topically diluted to problematic area.

PARASITES
Take internally with clove in a capsule.

WATER RETENTION
Take internally in a capsule.

SADNESS & IRRITABILITY
Diffuse or apply topically under nose and back of neck.

EMOTIONAL BALANCE
Use aromatically and topically to get from Oppressed ⟶ Restored.

RESEARCH: Evaluation of the chemical constituents and the antimicrobial activity of the volatile oil of Citrus reticulata fruit (Tangerine fruit peel) from South West Nigeria, Ayoola GA, Johnson OO, Adelowotan T, Aibinu IE, Adenipekun E, Adepoju AA, Coker HAB, Odugbemi TO, *African Journal of Biotechnology*, 2008

In-vitro and in-vivo anti-Trichophyton activity of essential oils by vapour contact, Inouye S, Uchida K, Yamaguchi H, *Mycoses*, 2001

Antidepressant-like effect of carvacrol (5-Isopropyl-2-methylphenol) in mice: involvement of dopaminergic system, Melo FH, Moura BA, de Sousa DP, de Vasconcelos SM, Macedo DS, Fonteles MM, Viana GS, de Sousa FC, *Fundamental and Clinical Pharmacology*, 2011

Atomic force microscopy analysis shows surface structure changes in carvacrol-treated bacterial cells, La Storia A, Ercolini D, Marinello F, Di Pasqua R, Villani F, Mauriello G, *Research in Microbiology*, 2011

Screening of the antibacterial effects of a variety of essential oils on microorganisms responsible for respiratory infections, Fabio A, Cermelli C, Fabio G, Nicoletti P, Quaglio P, *Phytotherapy Research*, 2007

Stimulative and sedative effects of essential oils upon inhalation in mice, Lim WC, Seo JM, Lee CI, Pyo HB, Lee BC, *Archives of Pharmacal Research*, 2005 *resolving · powerful · expelling*

THYME

THYMUS VULGARIS

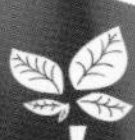

LEAVES

STEAM DISTILLED

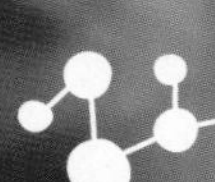

MAIN CONSTITUENTS
Thymol
Terpinen-4-ol

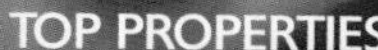

TOP PROPERTIES
Analgesic
Mucolytic
Stimulant
Antioxidant
Anti-rheumatic
Antiviral
Expectorant

FOUND IN
Detoxification blend
Tension blend

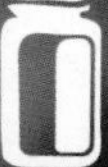

BLENDS WELL WITH
Rosemary
Basil
Lavender

SAFETY
Caution against high use during pregnancy, in people with epilepsy and high blood pressure.

Thyme means "to fumigate" in Greek, and is one of the most potent antioxidant essential oils.

TOP USES

ASTHMA & CROUP
Dilute and massage topically onto chest and diffuse aromatically.

COLDS & FLU
Take in a capsule internally and diffuse aromatically to support the immune system.

HAIR LOSS
Apply topically to stimulate hair growth.

MEMORY & CONCENTRATION
Diffuse aromatically to increase alertness and memory.

LOW BLOOD PRESSURE
Apply topically to bottoms of feet and pulse points.

FATIGUE
Diffuse aromatically with basil to combat fatigue.

STRESS & DEPRESSION
Diffuse aromatically to de-stress.

PAIN & SORE MUSCLES
Apply topically with wintergreen.

MRSA, ILLNESS RECOVERY, INCONTINENCE & BLADDER INFECTION
Apply topically to skin with geranium.

EMOTIONAL BALANCE
Use aromatically and topically to get from Unyielding⟶Yielding.

RESEARCH: Antimicrobial Activities of Clove and Thyme Extracts, Nzeako BC, Al-Kharousi ZS, Al-Mahrooqui Z, *Sultan Qaboos University Medical Journal*, 2006
Antimicrobial activity of clove oil and its potential in the treatment of vaginal candidiasis, Ahmad N, Alam MK, Shehbaz A, Khan A, Mannan A, Hakim SR, Bisht D, Owais M, *Journal of Drug Targeting*, 2005
Eugenol (an essential oil of clove) acts as an antibacterial agent against Salmonella typhi by disrupting the cellular membrane, Devi KP, Nisha SA, Sakthivel R, Pandian SK, *Journal of Ethnopharmacology*, 2010
The effect of clove and benzocaine versus placebo as topical anesthetics, Alqareer A, Alyahya A, Andersson L, *Journal of Dentistry*, 2006
Synergistic effect between clove oil and its major compounds and antibiotics against oral bacteria, Moon SE, Kim HY, Cha JD, *Archives of Oral Biology*, 2011
Antifungal activity of clove essential oil and its volatile vapour against dermatophytic fungi, Chee HY, Lee MH, *Mycobiology*, 2007
Microbicide activity of clove essential oil (Eugenia caryophyllata), Nuñez L, Aquino MD, *Brazilian Journal of Microbiology*, 2012
Anti-arthritic effect of eugenol on collagen-induced arthritis experimental model, Grespan R, Paludo M, Lemos Hde P, Barbosa CP, Bersani-Amado CA, Dalalio MM, Cuman RK, *Biological and Pharmaceutical Bulletin*, 2012
A novel aromatic oil compound inhibits microbial overgrowth on feet: a case study, Misner BD, *Journal of the International Society of Sports Nutrition*, 2007

VETIVER

VETIVERIA ZIZANIOIDES

regenerating • reassuring • enduring

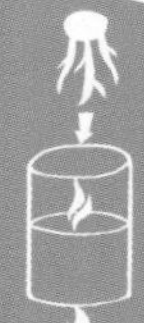

ROOTS

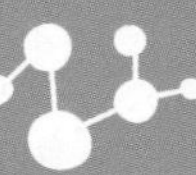

STEAM DISTILLED

MAIN CONSTITUENTS
a- & b-vetivones
Isovalencenol

TOP PROPERTIES
Stimulant
Tonic
Sedative
Antiseptic
Immunostimulant
Vermifuge
Antispasmodic
Rubaficient

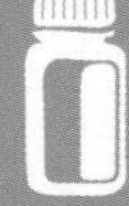

FOUND IN
Women's blend
Focus blend

BLENDS WELL WITH
Lavender
Sandalwood
Ylang ylang

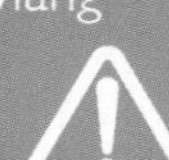

SAFETY
Safe for NEAT application.

TOP USES

ADD, ADHD, FOCUS & CONCENTRATION
Combine with lavender and apply topically to feet, spine, and back of neck just under skull, and diffuse aromatically.

ANOREXIA
Apply topically to feet and spine and diffuse aromatically.

VITILIGO
Apply topically to affected areas of the skin.

TUBURCULOSIS
Apply topically to feet and spine and diffuse aromatically.

INSOMNIA
Apply topically to bottoms of feet or to the spine and diffuse aromatically for a more restful sleep.

BREAST ENLARGEMENT
Dilute and apply topically to breasts.

PTSD, DEPRESSION & ANXIETY
Combine with melissa and diffuse aromatically and apply topically to pulse points.

POSTPARTUM DEPRESSION
Diffuse aromatically and apply topically to pulse points.

STRETCH MARKS, DISCOLORATION & SCARS
Apply topically to affected areas for reduced scarring.

EMOTIONAL BALANCE
Use aromatically and topically to get from Ungrounded ⟶ Rooted.

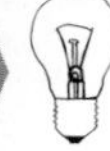

Vetiver is a natural tranquilizer, and in Ayurvedic medicine is known as the oil of "Tranquility."

RESEARCH: Effect of calcium on growth performance and essential oil of vetiver grass (Chrysopogon zizanioides) grown on lead contaminated soils, Danh LT, Truong P, Mammucari R, Foster N, *International Journal of Phytoremediation*, 2011
Effect of Vetiveria zizanioides Essential Oil on Melanogenesis in Melanoma Cells: Downregulation of Tyrosinase Expression and Suppression of Oxidative Stress, Peng HY, Lai CC, Lin CC, Chou ST, *The Scientific World Journal*, 2014
Constituents of south Indian vetiver oils, Mallavarapu GR, Syamasundar KV, Ramesh S, Rao BR, *Natural Product Communications*, 2012
In Vitro Antioxidant Activities of Essential Oils, Veerapan P, Khunkitti W, Isan *Journal of Pharmaceutical Sciences*, 2011
Antioxidant potential of the root of Vetiveria zizanioides (L.) Nash, Luqman S, Kumar R, Kaushik S, Srivastava S, Darokar MP, Khanuja SP, *Indian Journal of Biochemistry and Biophysics*, 2009
Volatiles emitted from the roots of Vetiveria zizanioides suppress the decline in attention during a visual display terminal taskvi, Matsubara E, Shimizu K, Fukagawa M, Ishizi Y, Kakoi C, Hatayama T, Nagano J, Okamoto T, Ohnuki K, Kondo R, *Biomedical Research*, 2012
Evaluation of the Effects of Plant-derived Essential Oils on Central Nervous System Function Using Discrete Shuttle-type Conditioned Avoidance Response in Mice, Umezu T, *Phytotherapy Research*, 2012

stimulating · clearing · calming

WHITE FIR

ABIES ALBA

TOP USES

SINUSITIS & ASTHMA
Dilute and apply topically to chest & diffuse aromatically to ease breathing.

MUSCLE & JOINT PAIN
Massage topically to affected area for soothing relief.

MUSCLE FATIGUE & REGENERATION
Apply topically to soothe tired muscles.

BURSITIS & RHEUMATICA
Apply topically to affected areas.

AIRBORNE PATHOGENS
Diffuse aromatically to fight germs.

CIRCULATION ISSUES
Massage topically to affected area to help increase circulation.

STRESS & FOGGY MIND
Diffuse aromatically with frankincense for better focus and clarity of thought.

BRONCHITIS & CONGESTION
Apply topically to chest or bridge of nose.

COLDS & FLU
Apply topically to chest & diffuse aromatically.

URINARY INFECTION & EDEMA
Apply topically over bladder.

FURNITURE POLISH
Apply to surface using a cloth.

EMOTIONAL BALANCE
Use aromatically and topically to get from Blocked ⟶ Receiving.

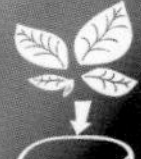

NEEDLES

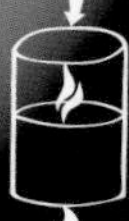

STEAM DISTILLED

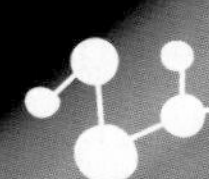

MAIN CONSTITUENTS
l-limonene
b-pinene
Camphene

TOP PROPERTIES
Analgesic
Antiarthritic
Antiseptic
Stimulant
Antioxidant

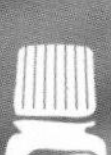

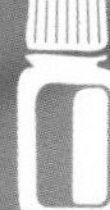

FOUND IN
Repellent blend

BLENDS WELL WITH
Lavender
Frankincense
Bergamot

SAFETY
Safe for NEAT application.

Used to decorate homes as Christmas trees. Native Americans used this tree to clear respiratory problems.

SINGLE OILS

RESEARCH: Repellency to Stomoxys calcitrans (Diptera: Muscidae) of Plant Essential Oils Alone or in Combination with Calophyllum inophyllum Nut Oil, Hieu TT, Kim SI, Lee SG, Ahn YJ, *Journal of Medical Etomology*, 2010

The battle against multi-resistant strains: Renaissance of antimicrobial essential oils as a promising force to fight hospital-acquired infections, Warnke PH, Becker ST, Podschun R, Sivananthan S, Springer IN, Russo PA, Wiltfang J, Fickenscher H, Sherry E, *Journal of Cranio-Maxillo-Facial Surgery*, 2009

WILD ORANGE

CITRUS SINENSIS

uplifting
invigorating
renewing

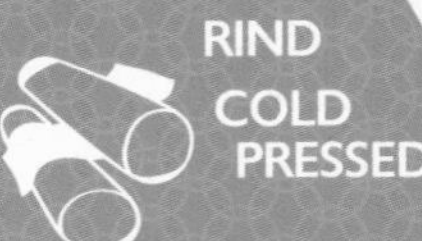

RIND

COLD PRESSED

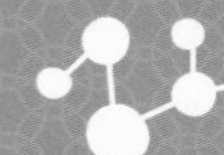

MAIN CONSTITUENTS
d-limonene
Terpinolene
Myrcene

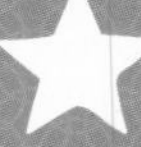

TOP PROPERTIES
Energizing
Sedative
Anti-carcinoma
Carminative
Antiseptic
Antidepressant
Immunostimulant

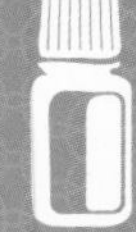

FOUND IN
Invigorating blend
Repellent blend
Cellular complex blend
Protective blend

BLENDS WELL WITH
Cinnamon
Lavender
Peppermint

SAFETY
Avoid direct sunlight for up to 12 hours after topical application.

TOP USES

INSOMNIA & STRESS
Diffuse aromatically or inhale from palms of hand to balance energy and uplift mood.

HEARTBURN & SLUGGISH BOWELS
Take internally in a capsule with ginger.

SCURVY & COLDS
Diffuse aromatically or apply topically on bottoms of feet.

ANXIETY & NERVOUSNESS
Diffuse aromatically or apply topically to pulse points.

MENOPAUSE
Apply topically to pulse points as needed and diffuse.

ANXIETY & FEAR, CONCENTRATION
Diffuse aromatically with peppermint or inhale both from palms of hands.

DETOX
Use internally in a glass of water or capsule to assist with cleansing.

COOKING
Add 1 drop to dishes, frostings, and smoothies for a sweet, rich citrus flavor.

EMOTIONAL BALANCE
Use aromatically and topically to get from Drained ⟶ Productive.

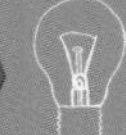

The Chinese first recognized the value of the peel of an orange for treating coughs and colds.

RESEARCH: Antimicrobial Effect and Mode of Action of Terpeneless Cold Pressed Valencia Orange Essential Oil on Methicillin-Resistant Staphylococcus aureus, Muthaiyan A, Martin EM, Natesan S, Crandall PG, Wilkinson BJ, Ricke SC, Journal of Applied Microbiology, 2012
Insecticidal properties of volatile extracts of orange peels, Ezeonu FC, Chidume GI, Udedi SC, Bioresource Technology, 2001
An experimental study on the effectiveness of massage with aromatic ginger and orange essential oil for moderate-to-severe knee pain among the elderly in Hong Kong, Yip YB, Tam AC, Complementary Therapies in Medicine, 2008
Oil of bitter orange: new topical antifungal agent, Ramadan W, Mourad B, Ibrahim S, Sonbol F, International Journal of Dermatology, 1996
Ambient odor of orange in a dental office reduces anxiety and improves mood in female patients, Lehrner J, Eckersberger C, Walla P, Pötsch G, Deecke L, Physiology and Behavior, 2000
Effect of sweet orange aroma on experimental anxiety in humans., Goes TC, Antunes FD, Alves PB, Teixeira-Silva F, The Journal of Alternative and Complementary Medicine
Effect of aromatherapy on patients with Alzheimer's disease, Jimbo D, Kimura Y, Taniguchi M, Inoue M, Urakami K, Psychogeriatrics, 2009

WINTERGREEN

GAULTHERIA PROCUMBENS

warming • relieving • repairing

TOP USES

GOUT & RHEUMATISM
Dilute and apply topically to affected area to sooth discomfort.

ARTHRITIS
Dilute and apply topically to ease the pain.

NEURALGIA & CRAMPS
Dilute and apply topically to reduce cramps.

BONE SPURS & PAIN
Dilute and apply topically to affected area.

CARTILAGE INJURY
Dilute and apply topically to reduce inflammation.

ROTATOR CUFF ISSUES & FROZEN SHOULDER
Dilute and apply topically to ease pain and inflammation.

DANDRUFF
Mix 1-2 drops with shampoo and apply topically to scalp.

DERMATITIS
Dilute and apply topically to reduce irritation to affected areas.

BLADDER INFECTION
Dilute and apply topically as needed to reduce symptoms and clear congestion.

EMOTIONAL BALANCE
Use aromatically and topically to get from Stubborn ——→ Accepting.

LEAVES

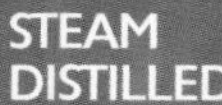

STEAM DISTILLED

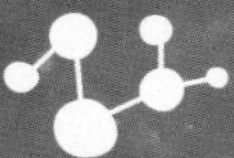

MAIN CONSTITUENT
Methyl salicylate

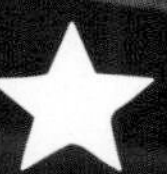

TOP PROPERTIES
Anti-inflammatory
Analgesic
Anti-rheumatic

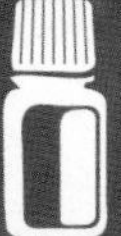

FOUND IN
Soothing blend
Tension blend

SAFETY
Dilute for topical application. May cause skin sensitivity.

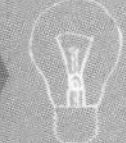

A naturally occurring compound found in wintergreen, "methyl salicylate" is related to the chemical that makes aspirin.

RESEARCH: Comparison of oral aspirin versus topical applied methyl salicylate for platelet inhibition, Tanen DA, Danish DC, Reardon JM, Chisholm CB, Matteucci MJ, Riffenburgh RH, *Annals of Pharmacotherapy*, 2008
Fumigant toxicity of plant essential oils against Camptomyia corticalis (Diptera: Cecidomyiidae), Kim JR, Haribalan P, Son BK, Ahn YJ, *Journal of Economic Entomology*, 2012
Field evaluation of essential oils for reducing attraction by the Japanese beetle (Coleoptera: Scarabaeidae), Youssef NN, Oliver JB, Ranger CM, Reding ME, Moyseenko JJ, Klein MG, Pappas RS, *Journal of Economic Entomology*, 2009
Essential oils and their compositions as spatial repellents for pestiferous social wasps, Zhang QH, Schnidmiller RG, Hoover DR, *Pest Management Science*, 2013

YARROW

ACHILLEA MILLEFOLIUM

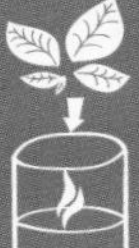
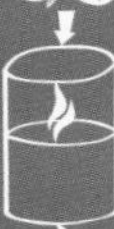

LEAVES

STEAM DISTILLED

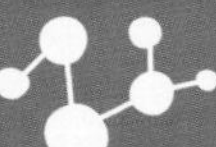

MAIN CONSTITUENTS
a-pinene
b-pinene
1,8 cineole

TOP PROPERTIES
Anti-inflammatory
Anti-rheumatic
Antispasmodic
Cicatrisant

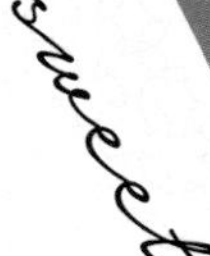

relieving • sweet • repairing

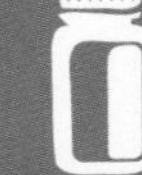

BLENDS WELL WITH
Lavender
Black pepper
Cedarwood
Cypress

SAFETY
Dilute with topical application.
May cause skin sensitivity.

TOP USES

VARICOSE VEINS
Apply topically daily to affected area.

PMS & MENSTRUAL PAIN
Apply topically to affected area and pulse points.

HEMORRHOIDS
Dilute and apply to affected area.

CRAMPS & DIGESTIVE UPSET
Apply topically to affected area.

WOUNDS & BITES
Apply topically to wounds or cuts.

GALL BLADDER ISSUES
Apply topically to affected area and bottoms of feet.

SKIN ISSUES & ECZEMA
Apply topically with lavender to affected area.

EMOTIONAL BALANCE
Use aromatically and topically to get from Erratic ⟶ Balanced.

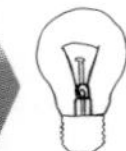

In ancient Greece, Achilles was said to use yarrow to ease a painful achilles tendon.

RESEARCH: Chamazulene carboxylic acid and matricin: a natural profen and its natural prodrug, identified through similarity to synthetic drug substances, Ramadan M, Goeters S, Watzer B, Krause E, Lohmann K, Bauer R, Hempel B, Imming P, *Journal of Natural Products*, 2006

Comparative evaluation of 11 essential oils of different origin as functional antioxidants, antiradicals and antimicrobials in foods, Sacchetti G, Maietti S, Muzzoli M, Scaglianti M, Manfredini S, Radice M, Bruni R, *Food Chemistry*, 2005

YLANG YLANG

CANANGA ODORATA

calming • floral • soothing

TOP USES

HORMONE IMBALANCE
Apply to bottoms of feet and pulse points, take internally under tongue or in capsule, or diffuse.

LOW LIBIDO & IMPOTENCE
Diffuse and apply topically to pulse points.

EQUILIBRIUM & MENTAL FATIGUE
Apply topically to back of neck just under skull, top of forehead, and behind ears. Inhale from palms of hands.

HIGH BLOOD PRESSURE & HEARTBEAT ISSUES
Apply topically to bottoms of feet and over the heart. Inhale from palms of hands.

ANXIETY, FRUSTRATION, STRESS & FEAR
Diffuse or inhale from palms of hands and apply topically to pulse points.

STIMULATES HAIR GROWTH
Apply topically directly to affected area.

COLIC & STOMACH ACHE
Apply topically on area of concern or take in a capsule.

OILY SKIN
Apply topically on affected area or take in a capsule.

EMOTIONAL BALANCE
Use aromatically and topically to get from Burdened ⟶ Exuberant.

FLOWERS

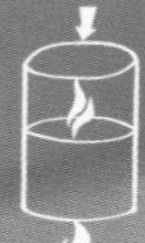

STEAM DISTILLED

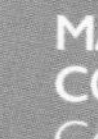

MAIN CONSTITUENTS
Germacrene
Caryophyllene
a-farnesene

TOP PROPERTIES
Hypotensive
Aphrodisiac
Antispasmodic
Sedative

FOUND IN
Focus blend
Calming blend
Joyful blend
Womens monthly blend
Women's blend

BLENDS WELL WITH
Sandalwood
Bergamot
Frankincense

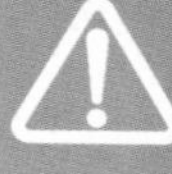

SAFETY
Safe for NEAT application.

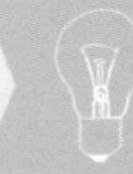

In Java, ylang ylang flowers adorn the newlyweds' bed and is often used as an aphrodisiac.

RESEARCH: Relaxing Effect of Ylang ylang Oil on Humans after Transdermal Absorption, Hongratanaworakit T, Buchbauer G, *Phytotherapy Research*, 2006
Safety assessment of Ylang-Ylang (Cananga spp.) as a food ingredient., Burdock GA, Carabin IG, *Food and Chemical Toxicology*, 2008
Effects of Ylang-Ylang aroma on blood pressure and heart rate in healthy men, Jung DJ, Cha JY, Kim SE, Ko IG, Jee YS, *Journal of Exercise Rehabilitation*, 2013
Evaluation of the harmonizing effect of ylang-ylang oil on humans after inhalation, Hongratanaworakit T, Buchbauer G, *Planta Medica*, 2004
Essential oil inhalation on blood pressure and salivary cortisol levels in prehypertensive and hypertensive subjects, Kim IH, Kim C, Seong K, Hur MH, Lim HM, Lee MS, *Evidence-Based Complementary and Alternative Medicine*, 2012
The Effects of Herbal Essential Oils on the Oviposition-deterrent and Ovicidal Activities of Aedes aegypti (Linn.), Anopheles dirus (Peyton and Harrison) and Culex quinquefasciatus (Say), Siriporn P, Mayura S, *Tropical Biomedicine*, 2012
Evaluation of the Effects of Plant-derived Essential Oils on Central Nervous System Function Using Discrete Shuttle-type Conditioned Avoidance Response in Mice, Umezu T., *Phytotherapy Research*, 2012
Effects of aromatherapy on changes in the autonomic nervous system, aortic pulse wave velocity and aortic augmentation index in patients with essential hypertension, Cha JH, Lee SH, Yoo YS, *Journal of Korean Academy of Nursing*, 2010

OIL BLENDS

While many companies provide blends of essential oils, the proprietary blends found in this book have been carefully and artistically crafted to offer superior efficacy and therapeutic benefits. Because natural chemistry is a crucial point of attention in the art of blending essential oils, it is important to turn to blends that possess qualities of highest purity, potency, and complementary relationships between the individual oils that comprise the blend.

Please note the symbols (=aromatic =topical =internal) that specify recommended usage. While all oils are meant to be used aromatically, and most topically, only verified pure therapeutic essential oils are intended for internal use. (See "Why Quality Matters," pg. 9 and "How to Use Essential Oils" pg. 11 for further detail.)

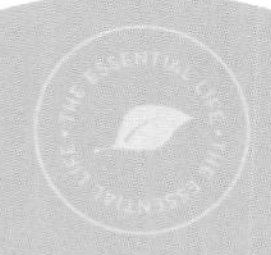

regenerating • youthful • replenishing

ANTI-AGING

BLEND

TOP USES

WRINKLES
Apply topically to face, neck, and hands.

FINE LINES
Apply topically daily.

SUN DAMAGE
Apply topically to assist healing.

SCARS
Apply topically to problematic areas.

STRETCH MARKS
Apply topically to affected area.

BLEMISHES
Apply topically to affected area.

TENSION & MOOD BALANCE
Apply topically to pulse points or diffuse.

SKIN CANCER
Apply topically to affected area.

MEDITATION
Diffuse and apply topically to pulse points.

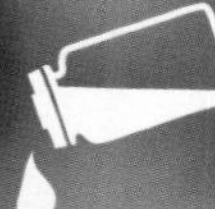

MAIN INGREDIENTS
Frankincense
Hawaiian sandalwood
Lavender
Myrrh
Helichrysum
Rose

SAFETY
Safe for NEAT application.

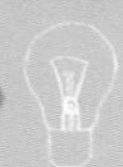

A beautiful blend with time-honored essential oils for radiant skin.

OIL BLENDS

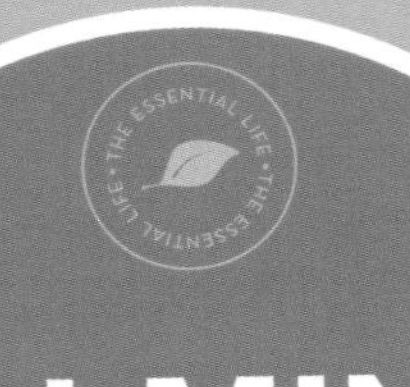

CALMING

BLEND

sweet
warm
calming

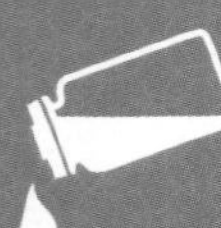

MAIN INGREDIENTS
Lavender
Sweet marjoram
Roman chamomile
Ylang ylang
Sandalwood
Vanilla

TOP USES

INSOMNIA & SLEEP ISSUES
Diffuse aromatically or apply topically under nose or to bottoms of feet.

STRESS & ANXIETY
Apply topically to back of neck or diffuse.

ADD/ADHD & HYPERACTIVITY
Diffuse or apply topically on back of neck.

TENSION & MOOD SWINGS
Diffuse aromatically or apply topically to back of neck.

SKINCARE
Apply topically to area of concern.

MUSCLE TENSION
Apply topically to area of concern.

PERFUME
Apply topically.

ANGER
Diffuse aromatically or apply topically under nose or to bottoms of feet.

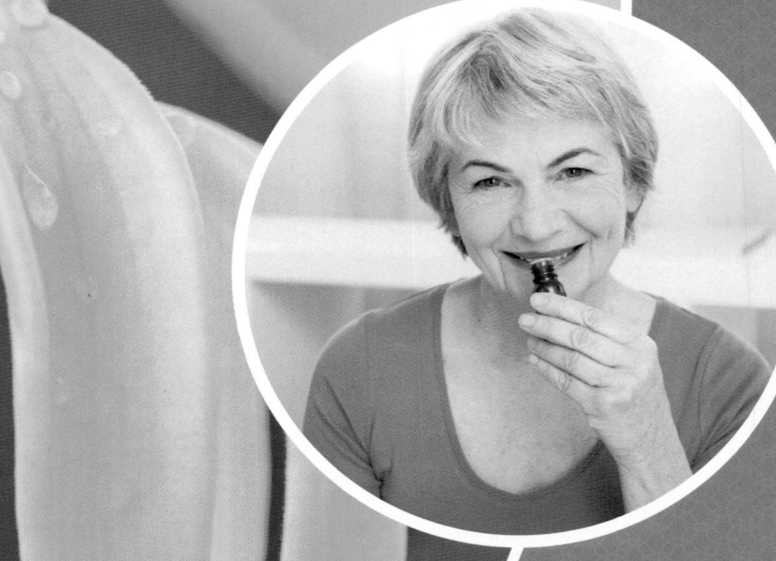

SAFETY
Safe for NEAT application.

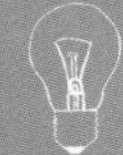

Create a moment of peace and calm anywhere, anytime. Calming blend soothes the soul and calms the mind.

regenerating
corrective
repairing

CELLULAR

COMPLEX BLEND

OIL BLENDS

MAIN INGREDIENTS
Frankincense
Wild orange
Lemongrass
Thyme
Summer savory
Clove
Niaouli

SAFETY
Dilution recommended for topical application, may cause skin sensitivity.

TOP USES

TOP USES

NERVE DAMAGE
Apply topically to bottoms of feet or diluted to spine. Take internally in a capsule.

CANCER & TUMORS
Apply topically to bottoms of feet or diluted to spine. Take internally in a capsule.

THYROID & CELLULAR REPAIR
Apply topically to bottoms of feet or diluted to spine. Take internally in a capsule.

AUTOIMMUNE DISORDERS
Apply topically to bottoms of feet or take internally in a capsule.

VIRUSES
Apply topically to bottoms of feet or take internally in a capsule.

FUNGAL CONDITIONS
Apply topically to bottoms of feet or take internally in a capsule.

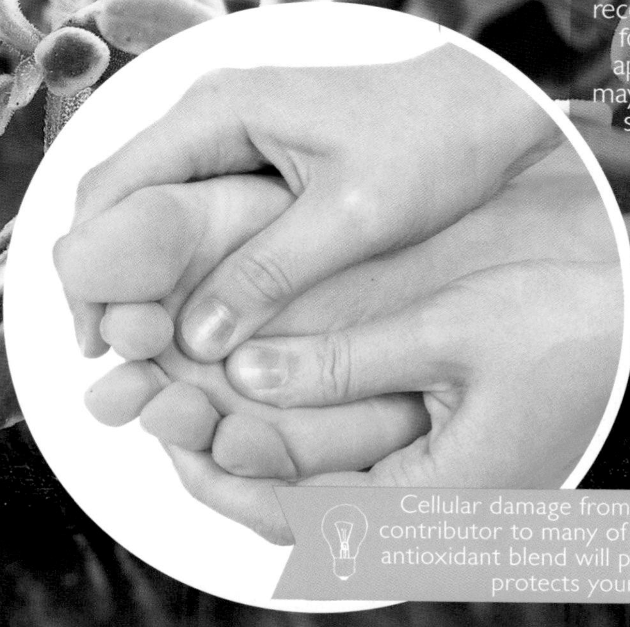

Cellular damage from free radicals is an underlying contributor to many of today's illnesses. This powerful antioxidant blend will protect your cellular health as it protects your long-term wellness.

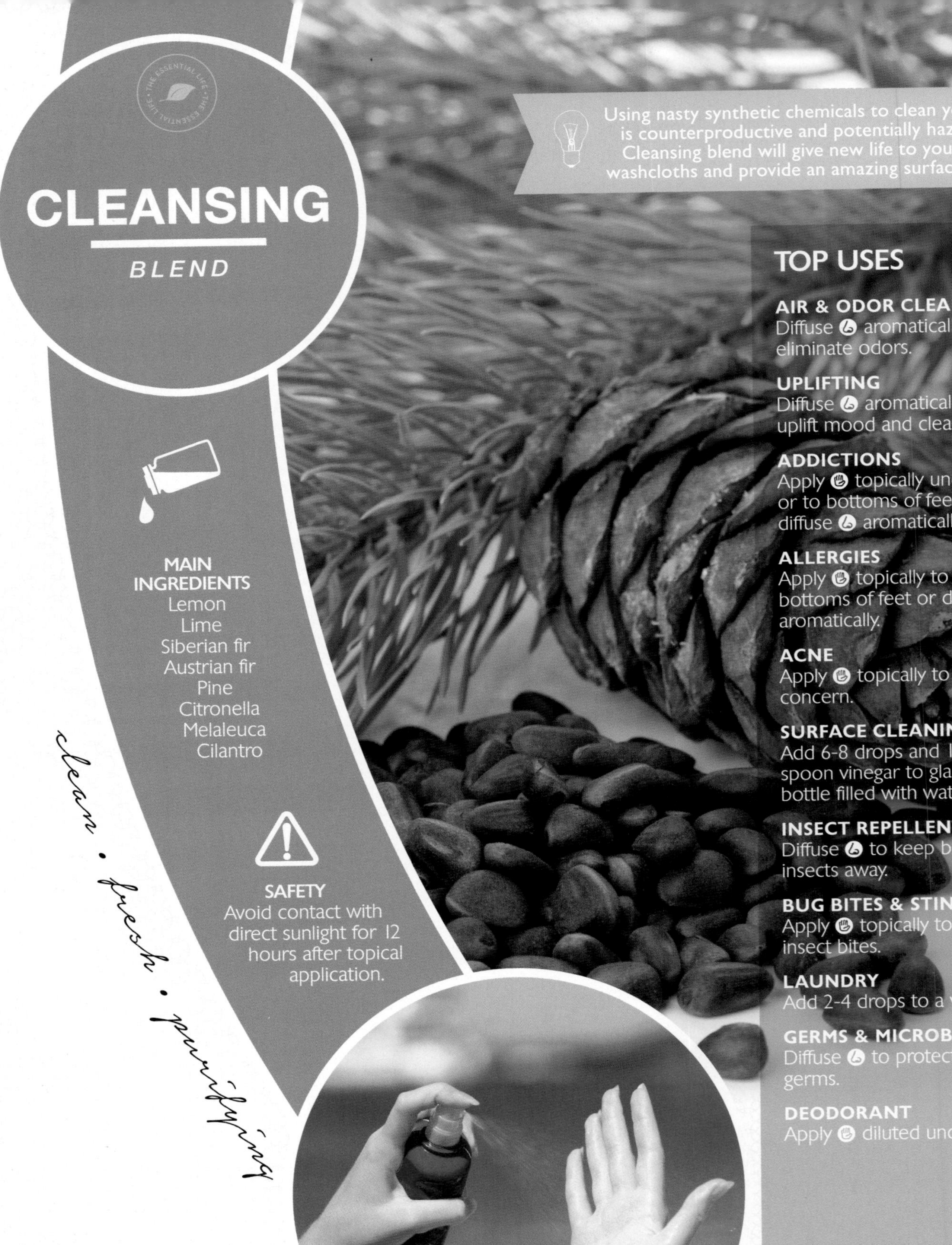

Using nasty synthetic chemicals to clean your home is counterproductive and potentially hazardous. Cleansing blend will give new life to your stinky washcloths and provide an amazing surface cleaner.

CLEANSING

BLEND

MAIN INGREDIENTS
Lemon
Lime
Siberian fir
Austrian fir
Pine
Citronella
Melaleuca
Cilantro

clean • fresh • purifying

SAFETY
Avoid contact with direct sunlight for 12 hours after topical application.

TOP USES

AIR & ODOR CLEANSING
Diffuse aromatically to eliminate odors.

UPLIFTING
Diffuse aromatically to uplift mood and clear mind.

ADDICTIONS
Apply topically under nose or to bottoms of feet or diffuse aromatically.

ALLERGIES
Apply topically to chest or bottoms of feet or diffuse aromatically.

ACNE
Apply topically to area of concern.

SURFACE CLEANING
Add 6-8 drops and 1 table-spoon vinegar to glass spray bottle filled with water.

INSECT REPELLENT
Diffuse to keep bugs and insects away.

BUG BITES & STINGS
Apply topically to bug and insect bites.

LAUNDRY
Add 2-4 drops to a wash.

GERMS & MICROBES
Diffuse to protect against germs.

DEODORANT
Apply diluted under arms.

COMFORTING
BLEND

soothe • mend • alleviate

TOP USES

BRAIN IMPAIRMENT
Apply topically to forehead, back of neck, and toes.

EMOTIONAL RELEASE & REASSURANCE
Diffuse aromatically and apply topically to the chest.

SPIRITUAL CONNECTIVITY & MEDITATION
Apply topically to forehead and chest and inhale.

LOW LIBIDO
Diffuse aromatically and apply topically to bottoms of feet.

SKIN REPAIR & ANTI-AGING
Apply topically to affected area with carrier oil.

GRIEF & SADNESS
Diffuse aromatically and apply topically on chest.

LUNG & BRONCHIAL INFECTION
Apply topically on chest and bottoms of feet and diffuse aromatically.

URINARY INFECTION & EDEMA
Apply topically to bottoms of feet.

IRREGULAR & RACING HEARTBEAT
Inhale aromatically and apply topically to chest.

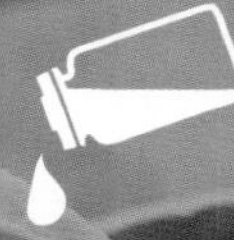

MAIN INGREDIENTS
Frankincense
Patchouli
Ylang ylang
Laudanum
Sandalwood
Rose

SAFETY
Safe for NEAT application.

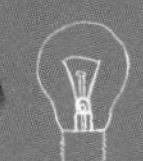

When the loss of something loved or treasured occurs, use this blend to comfort through sadness or grief and move forward in life.

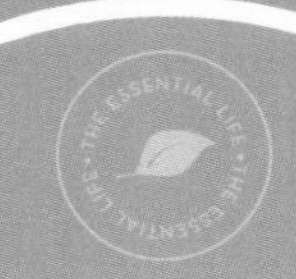

DETOXIFICATION

BLEND

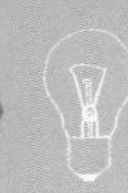

A regular cleansing regime helps ensure healthy kidney and liver function. Take 1-3 drops in a capsule, juice, or tea during first week of weight loss program.

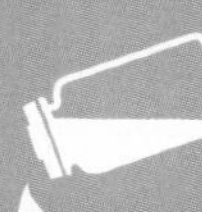

MAIN INGREDIENTS
Tangerine
Rosemary
Geranium
Juniper berry
Cilantro

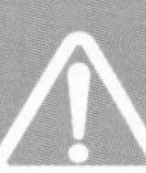

SAFETY
Avoid direct sunlight for 12 hours after topical application.

refreshing · detoxing · cleaning

TOP USES

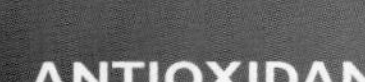

ANTIOXIDANT
Take internally in a capsule.

URINARY TRACT & DIGESTIVE ISSUES
Take internally or apply topically over liver and kidneys.

KIDNEY & LIVER CLEANSING
Take internally in a capsule or apply topically to lower abdomen.

HEAVY METAL DETOXIFICATION
Take internally in a capsule.

WEIGHT LOSS & DETOXIFICATION
Take internally in a capsule.

ENDOCRINE CLEANSING
Take internally in a capsule or apply topically to abdomen or bottoms of feet.

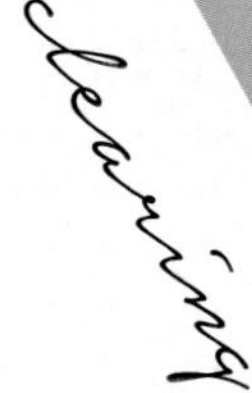

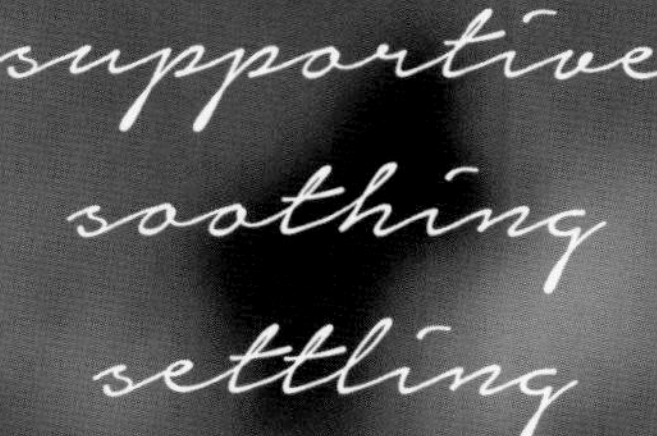

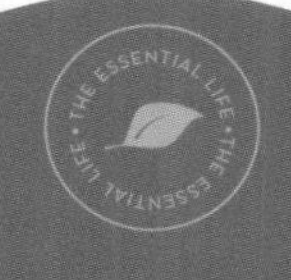

DIGESTION

BLEND

TOP USES

BLOATING, GAS & NAUSEA
Apply over stomach and take internally in a capsule.

REFLUX & INDIGESTION
Take internally with lemon in water.

DRY, SORE THROAT
Take internally directly into back of throat.

MORNING SICKNESS
Apply topically to pulse points and stomach.

MOTION & TRAVEL SICKNESS
Inhale aromatically or apply topically under nose or drink internally.

COLITIS
Take internally daily in capsule.

DIARRHEA & CONSTIPATION
Take as needed in capsule or in water.

CROHN'S DISEASE & CHRONIC FATIGUE
Take internally in a capsule.

FOOD POISONING
Take internally in a capsule.

SINUS ISSUES
Apply topically diluted over bridge and side of nose and navel.

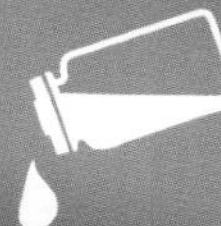

MAIN INGREDIENTS
Ginger
Peppermint
Caraway
Coriander
Anise
Tarragon
Fennel

SAFETY
Safe for NEAT application. Dilute if necessary.

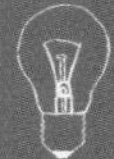

Many essential oils aid digestion. Peppermint is a well-known digestive aid and a primary ingredient in this blend.

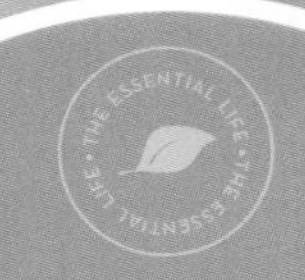

ENCOURAGING

BLEND

motivate
invigorate
stimulate

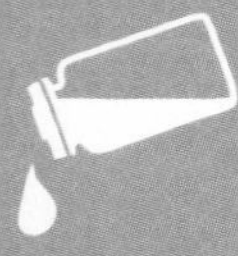

MAIN INGREDIENTS
Peppermint
Clementine
Coriander
Basil
Melissa
Rosemary

TOP USES

MENTAL FATIGUE & EXHAUSTION
Diffuse aromatically or apply topically to temples and back of neck.

PHYSICAL EXHAUSTION
Inhale aromatically and apply topically over adrenal glands and on bottoms of feet to enhance endurance.

DIGESTIVE ISSUES
Apply topically over abdomen, on pulse points, or on bottoms of feet.

BRONCHITIS & ASTHMA
Diffuse aromatically and apply topically to neck and chest.

DEPRESSION
Diffuse or apply topically to chest, forehead, and back of neck.

ACHES & PAINS
Apply topically to affected area.

DEPLETION & STAGNATION
Inhale from palms of hands and apply topically to pulse points to renew & refresh.

CONFUSION & OVERWHELM
Inhale or apply topically under nose, on forehead, back of neck, or chest.

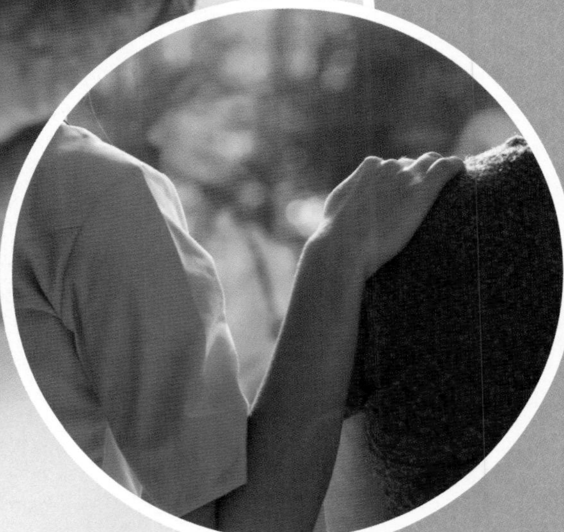

SAFETY
Dilute for skin sensitivity. If pregnant or nursing, consult your physician. Avoid exposure to direct sunlight or UV rays for up to 12 hours after topical use.

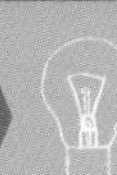

Squelch the frustration and doubt that can halt progress with this blend's ability to encourage productivity, creativity, and confidence.

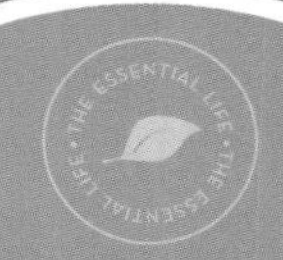

FOCUS

OR ATTENTION BLEND

grounding
earthy
clarifying

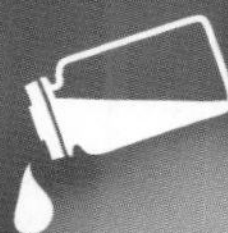

MAIN INGREDIENTS
Amyris
Patchouli
Frankincense
Lime
Ylang ylang
Sandalwood
Roman chamomile

SAFETY
Caution with sun/UV exposure for 12 hours after direct topical application.

TOP USES

ADD/ADHD
Apply topically to back of neck, spine, or bottoms of feet.

CONCENTRATION & FOCUS
Apply topically to back of neck or diffuse.

NERVOUSNESS & ANXIETY
Apply topically to pulse points and inhale.

CALMING & GROUNDING
Apply topically to pulse points and inhale.

DEPRESSION
Diffuse aromatically or apply topically to bottoms of feet and back of neck.

STRESS & HYPERACTIVITY
Apply topically to back of neck and pulse points.

MENTAL CLARITY
Diffuse and apply topically to back of neck.

MID-AFTERNOON SLUMP
Diffuse and apply topically to back of neck.

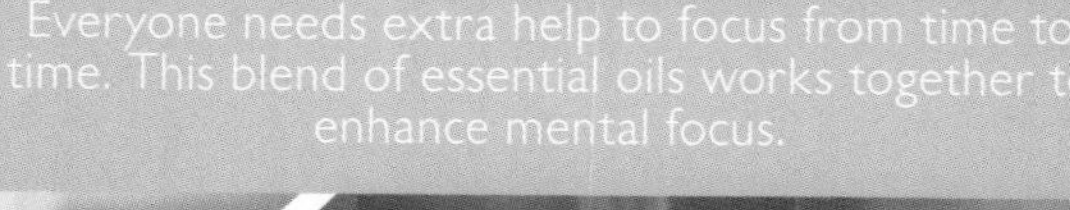

Everyone needs extra help to focus from time to time. This blend of essential oils works together to enhance mental focus.

OIL BLENDS

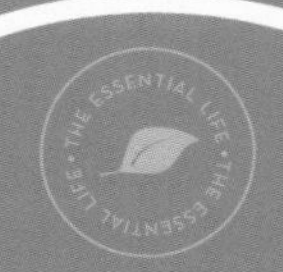

GROUNDING

BLEND

Life's little surprises and stress can leave us off guard and unbalanced. This blend helps to restore and ground us.

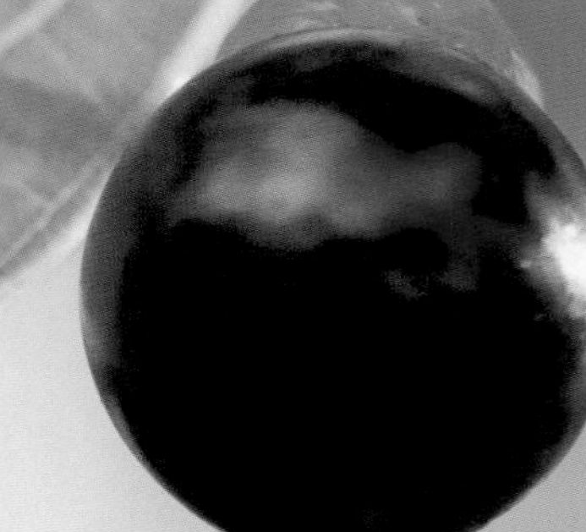

MAIN INGREDIENTS
Spruce
Ho wood
Frankincense
Blue tansy
Blue chamomile

stabilizing • centering • sweet

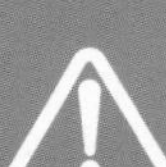

SAFETY
Safe for NEAT application.

TOP USES

STRESS & ANXIETY
Apply topically to bottoms of feet daily.

JET LAG & TRAVEL ANXIETY
Inhale aromatically.

MOOD SWINGS & STRESS
Apply topically to the back of neck.

NEUROLOGICAL CONDITIONS
Apply topically to back of neck and pulse points.

CONVULSIONS, EPILEPSY & PARKINSON'S
Apply topically to back of neck or along spine.

TRANQUILITY & MEDITATION
Apply topically under nose and across forehead or inhale aromatically.

ANGER & RAGE
Inhale aromatically or apply topically under nose or bottoms of feet.

FEAR, GRIEF & TRAUMA
Inhale aromatically or apply topically under nose or on bottoms of feet.

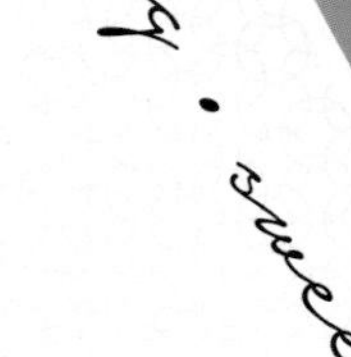

festive · warming · spicy

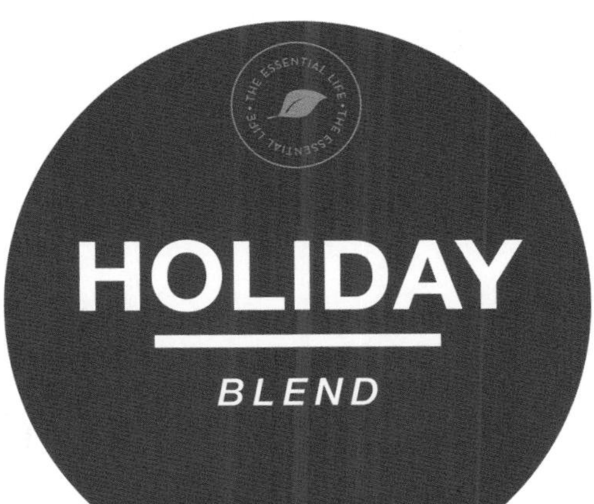

HOLIDAY

BLEND

TOP USES

HEADACHE & MIGRAINE
Apply topically to temples and back of neck.

TENSION & STRESS
Apply topically to pulse points and inhale.

NECK & SHOULDER DISCOMFORT
Apply topically to area of discomfort.

ARTHRITIS
Apply topically to area of discomfort.

RESTFUL SLEEP
Apply topically to back of neck.

BLOOD SUGAR
Apply topically to bottoms of feet or drink internally a drop in water.

MAIN INGREDIENTS
Wild orange
Pine
Cassia
Cinnamon bark
Vanilla

SAFETY
Dilute for topical application.

This blend inspires the joy of the holidays while also stimulating immunity.

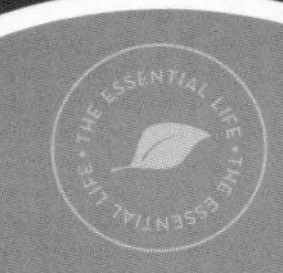

INSPIRING

BLEND

excite
enliven
elevate

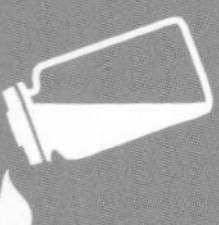

MAIN INGREDIENTS
Cardamom
Cinnamon
Ginger
Clove
Sandalwood
Jasmine

TOP USES

SLUGGISH DIGESTION & ELIMINATION
Apply topically to lower abdomen with carrier oil.

LUNG & SINUS CONGESTION
Diffuse aromatically or inhale from hands.

DEPRESSION & ENERGY ISSUES
Diffuse aromatically or inhale from cupped hands to energize and uplift.

CIRCULATION
Apply to bottoms of feet to warm and stimulate movement.

LOW LIBIDO & SEXUAL PERFORMANCE
Diffuse aromatically or apply to bottoms of feet.

MENSTRUATION & MENOPAUSE ISSUES
Apply topically to lower abdomen with carrier oil or pressure points below inside and outside of ankles.

MENTAL FOG & MEMORY ISSUES
Apply topically to toes or diffuse.

INFECTIONS
Apply topically to bottoms of feet.

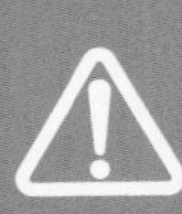

SAFETY
Dilute for skin sensitivity. If pregnant or nursing, consult your physician.

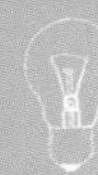

This blend can nurture the natural desire to embrace new and exciting experiences in life with passion and courage.

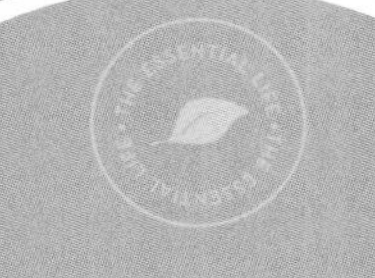

INVIGORATING

BLEND

citrus • sweet • uplifting

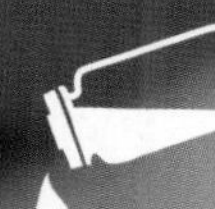

MAIN INGREDIENTS
Bergamot
Clementine
Grapefruit
Lemon
Mandarin
Tangerine
Vanilla
Wild orange

SAFETY
Caution with sun/UV exposure for 12 hours after direct topical application.

TOP USES

DEPRESSION, STRESS & ANXIETY
Diffuse aromatically or apply topically under nose and back of neck to both uplift and calm.

AIR FRESHENER
Diffuse aromatically to clear air and odors.

ANTISEPTIC CLEANER
Mix with water in a glass bottle and apply to surfaces.

EATING DISORDERS
Diffuse aromatically or inhale from bottle.

PERFUME & DEODORANT
Apply topically as desired.

LAUNDRY
Add 2-4 drops to rinse cycle to freshen and kill germs.

LYMPHATIC & IMMUNE BOOST
Diffuse aromatically or apply topically under nose and back of neck.

When you pause to uplift and invigorate your senses with this blend of citrus essential oils, you will find increased energy and zest for life.

JOYFUL

BLEND

happy
citrus
sweet

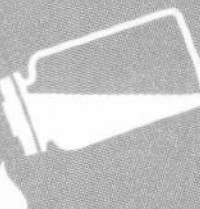

MAIN INGREDIENTS
Lavandin
Lavender
Sandalwood
Tangerine
Melissa
Ylang ylang
Elemi

TOP USES

ELEVATE MOOD & MIND
Diffuse aromatically and apply topically to pulse points.

ENERGIZE & REFRESH
Diffuse aromatically and apply topically to pulse points.

STRESS & ANXIETY
Apply topically to back of neck and inhale.

DEPRESSION & MOOD DISORDERS
Apply topically to back of neck and inhale.

GRIEF & SORROW
Diffuse aromatically and apply topically to pulse points.

STIMULATING & UPLIFTING
Apply topically to back of neck and inhale.

IMMUNITY
Apply topically to bottoms of feet.

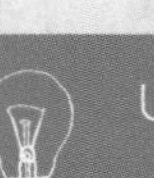

Use this blend to energize both body and mind.

SAFETY
Avoid sunlight/UV rays for 12 hours after topical application.

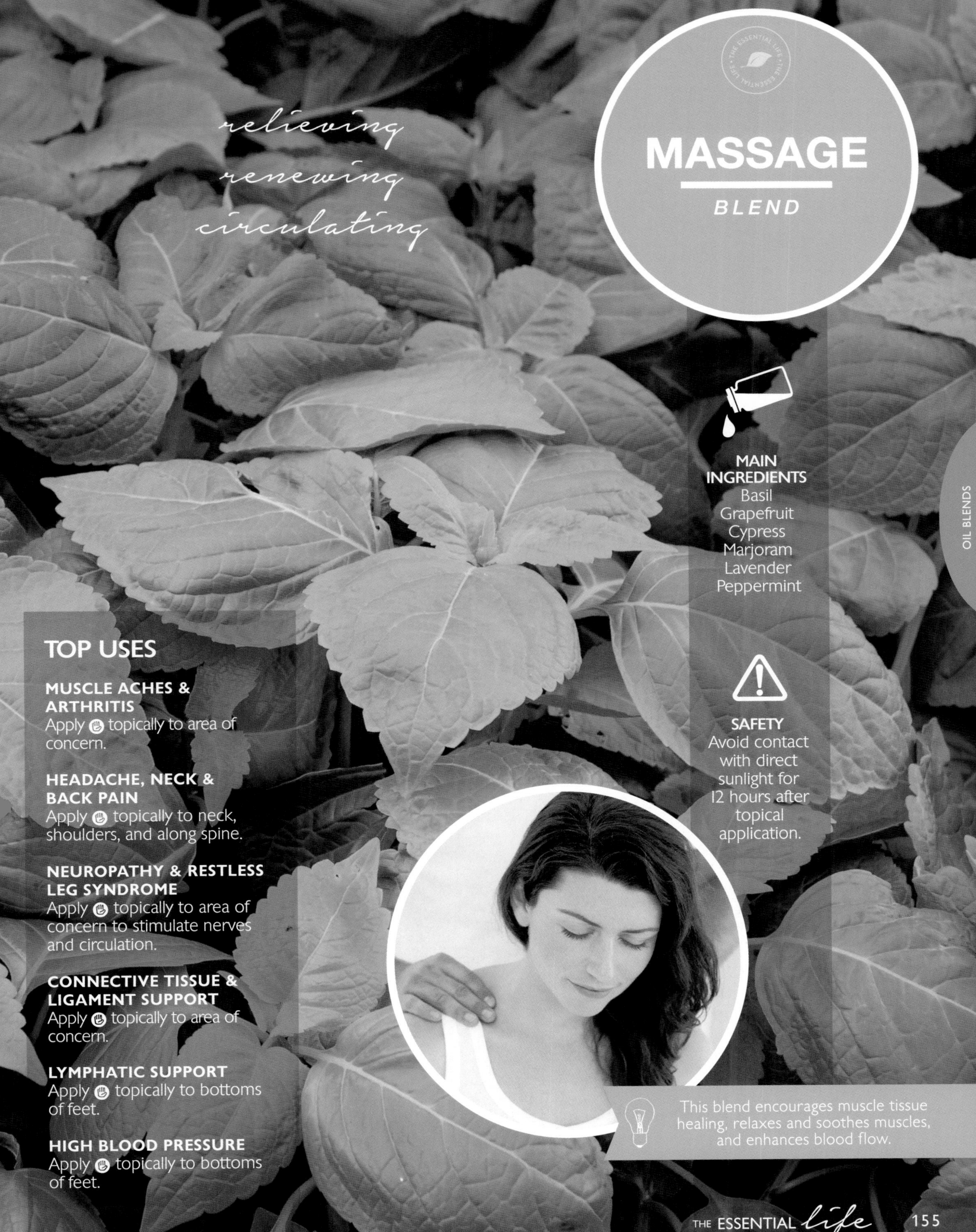

relieving
renewing
circulating

MASSAGE

BLEND

MAIN INGREDIENTS
Basil
Grapefruit
Cypress
Marjoram
Lavender
Peppermint

SAFETY
Avoid contact with direct sunlight for 12 hours after topical application.

TOP USES

MUSCLE ACHES & ARTHRITIS
Apply topically to area of concern.

HEADACHE, NECK & BACK PAIN
Apply topically to neck, shoulders, and along spine.

NEUROPATHY & RESTLESS LEG SYNDROME
Apply topically to area of concern to stimulate nerves and circulation.

CONNECTIVE TISSUE & LIGAMENT SUPPORT
Apply topically to area of concern.

LYMPHATIC SUPPORT
Apply topically to bottoms of feet.

HIGH BLOOD PRESSURE
Apply topically to bottoms of feet.

This blend encourages muscle tissue healing, relaxes and soothes muscles, and enhances blood flow.

MEN'S

BLEND

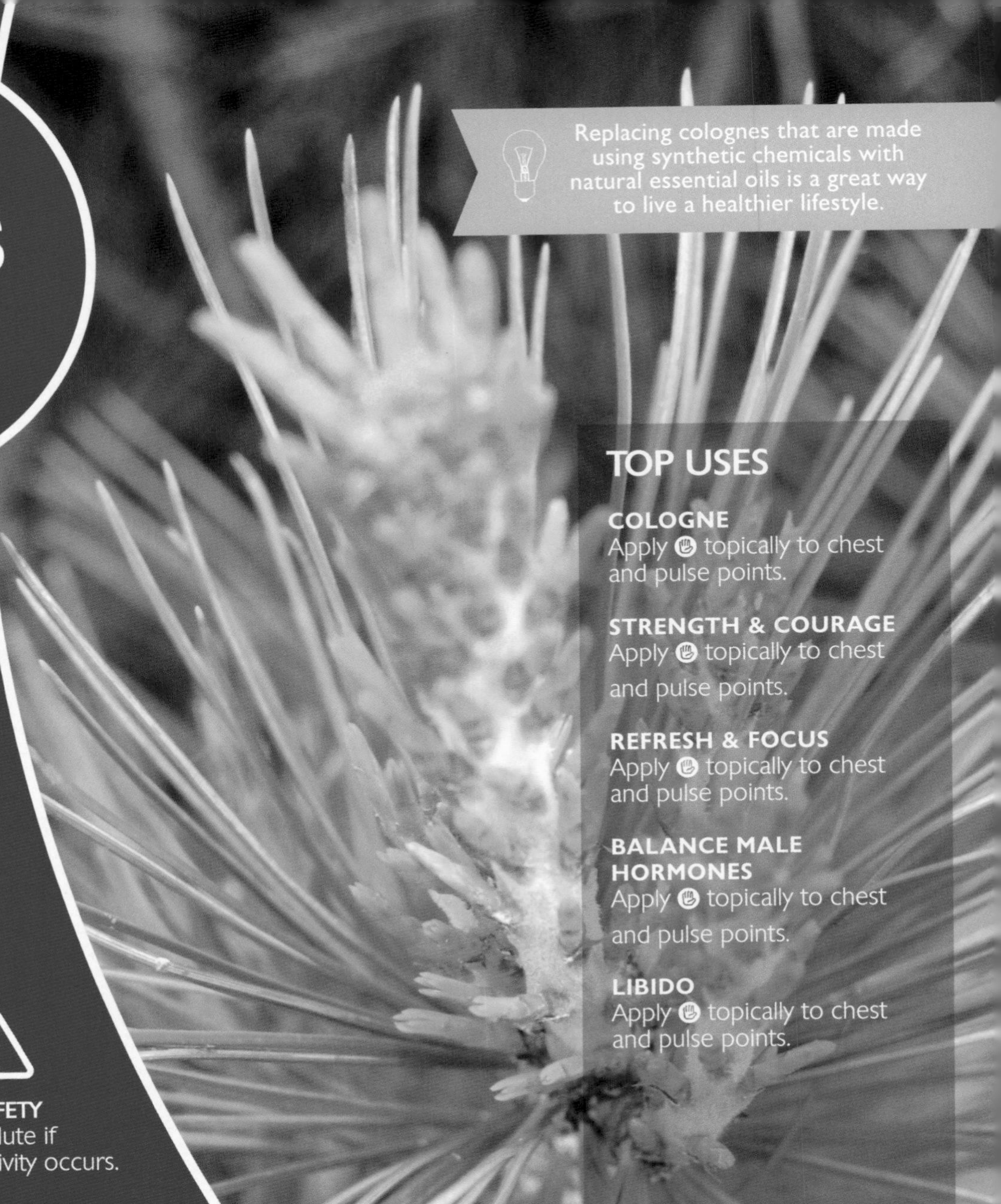

Replacing colognes that are made using synthetic chemicals with natural essential oils is a great way to live a healthier lifestyle.

MAIN INGREDIENTS
White fir
Pine
Blue spruce
Cedarwood
Juniper

SAFETY
Dilute if sensitivity occurs.

fresh · grounding · woody

TOP USES

COLOGNE
Apply topically to chest and pulse points.

STRENGTH & COURAGE
Apply topically to chest and pulse points.

REFRESH & FOCUS
Apply topically to chest and pulse points.

BALANCE MALE HORMONES
Apply topically to chest and pulse points.

LIBIDO
Apply topically to chest and pulse points.

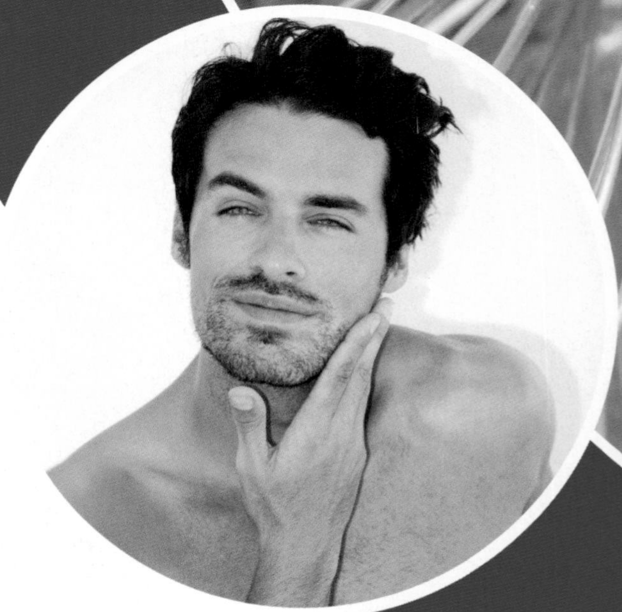

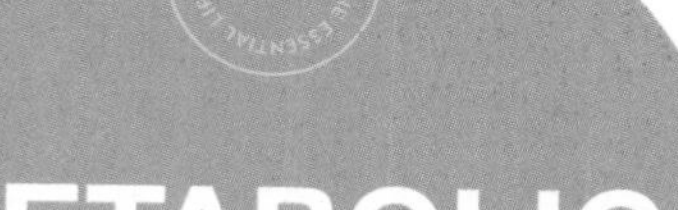

METABOLIC

OR WEIGHT LOSS BLEND

cleansing • spicy • refreshing

TOP USES

WEIGHT LOSS & OBESITY
Take 6-8 drops internally up to 25 drops daily in capsule or water.

INFLAMMATION
Apply topically to bottoms of feet or take internally in capsule.

OVER-FATIGUE & EATING DISORDERS
Take internally in a capsule or with water or apply topically to bottoms of feet and inhale from bottle.

APPETITE & CRAVINGS
Take 1 drop internally under tongue and inhale from bottle to suppress appetite.

LYMPHATIC STIMULANT/SUPPORT
Diffuse aromatically or apply topically to bottoms of feet.

CONGESTION & COLDS
Take internally in a capsule or water.

URINARY TRACT SUPPORT
Take internally in a capsule or water.

BLOOD SUGAR BALANCE
Take internally in a capsule or water.

CELLULITE
Apply topically to area of concern.

STIMULATE METABOLISM
Take internally in a capsule or water.

DETOXIFICATION & CLEANSING
Take internally in a capsule or water.

DIGESTIVE STIMULANT & CALMING
Take internally in a capsule or water.

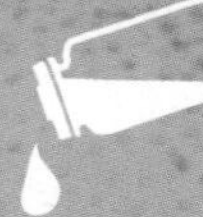

MAIN INGREDIENTS
Grapefruit
Lemon
Peppermint
Ginger
Cinnamon

SAFETY
Avoid sunlight/UV rays for 12 hours after direct topical application.

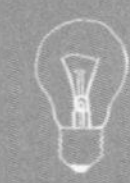

Reducing cravings and balancing blood sugar are important steps for weight loss.

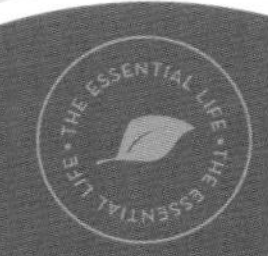

PROTECTIVE

OR IMMUNITY BLEND

spicy
supportive
warming

TOP USES

COLDS & FLU
Take internally in a capsule or apply topically to bottoms of feet.

STAPH, STREP THROAT & COUGHS
Gargle 1 drop in water and swallow. Apply topically to chest and throat or take internally in a capsule or with water.

ANTISEPTIC CLEANER
Diffuse aromatically or dilute with water and apply to surfaces.

URINARY TRACT SUPPORT
Take internally in capsule or apply topically to lower abdomen.

COLD SORES, WARTS & INFECTED WOUNDS
Apply topically diluted to affected area.

ORAL HEALTH
Gargle 1 drop in water.

FUNGAL & PARASITE ISSUES
Apply to affected area or take internally in a capsule.

CHRONIC FATIGUE & AUTOIMMUNE DISEASE
Take internally in capsule or apply topically to bottoms of feet.

KILLING GERMS & AIRBORNE PATHOGENS
Take internally in capsule or apply topically to bottoms of feet.

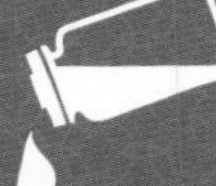

MAIN INGREDIENTS
Wild orange
Clove
Cinnamon
Eucalyptus
Rosemary

SAFETY
Dilute for topical application and avoid sunlight/UV rays for 12 hours after direct topical application.

A strong immunity combats viral and bacterial threats to the body. Use this blend to keep your family healthy.

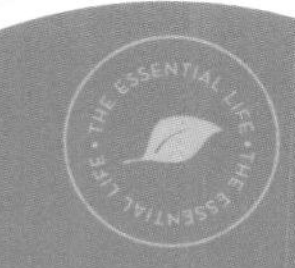

ease • relax • compose

REASSURING

BLEND

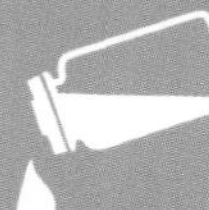

MAIN INGREDIENTS
Vetiver
Lavender
Ylang Ylang
Frankincense
Clary Sage
Marjoram
Spearmint

SAFETY
Safe for NEAT application. Caution for use during early stages of pregnancy.

TOP USES

RESTLESSNESS & CONFUSION
Inhale aromatically and apply to forehead and back of neck.

ADDICTIONS & ANOREXIA
Apply topically to wrist pulse points and inhale aromatically.

ADD, ADHD & FOCUS ISSUES
Inhale aromatically and apply to forehead and back of neck.

MENTAL STRAIN & HYPERACTIVITY
Apply topically to forehead, shoulders, and back.

CHILDBIRTH & RECOVERY
Apply topically to abdomen, as a foot massage, or inhale.

ALLERGIES & OVERREACTION
Apply topically to affected area, bottoms of feet and diffuse.

COLIC & CALMING
Apply topically to bottoms of feet and abdomen.

STRESS
Diffuse aromatically and inhale from hands for relaxation and deep release.

INFERTILITY & FRIGIDITY
Apply topically to bottoms of feet, back, and inhale.

No matter what is happening in life, this blend can bring a sense of reassurance and promote focus on true sources of happiness.

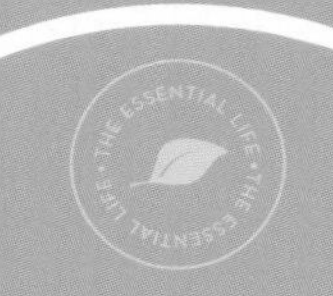

RENEWING

BLEND

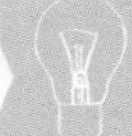

Holding onto things that no longer serve can limit personal growth. This blends invites you to trust the process of life and move forward with confidence.

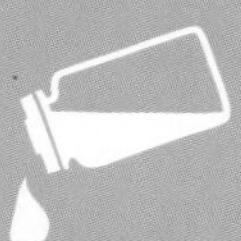

MAIN INGREDIENTS
Spruce
Bergamot
Juniper Berry
Myrrh
Arborvitae
Thyme

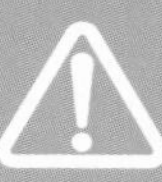

SAFETY
Dilute for skin sensitivity. If pregnant or nursing, consult your physician. Avoid exposure to direct sunlight or UV rays for up to 12 hours after topical use.

relieve • release • liberate

TOP USES

ULCERS & LIVER ISSUES
Apply topically over affected areas with carrier oil.

ANXIETY
Apply topically to bottoms of feet, back of neck, and under nose to soothe and ground.

EMOTIONAL BALANCE
Diffuse aromatically or inhale from cupped hands to get from fear or frigidity to passion or intimacy.

SKIN INFECTION & DAMAGE
Apply topically to affected areas with carrier oil.

ADDICTIONS & IRRITABILITY
Diffuse aromatically and apply topically to wrist pulse points.

CIRCULATION
Apply topically to chest and inhale or diffuse.

ATTACHMENT & HOLDING ON
Apply topically to temples and back of neck or diffuse to promote letting go.

FUNGUS & PARASITES
Apply topically to bottoms of feet.

SPIRITUAL & EMOTIONAL TOXICITY
Diffuse aromatically and apply topically to chest.

HAIR LOSS, PROSTATE ISSUES & LIBIDO
Apply to affected areas or bottoms of feet.

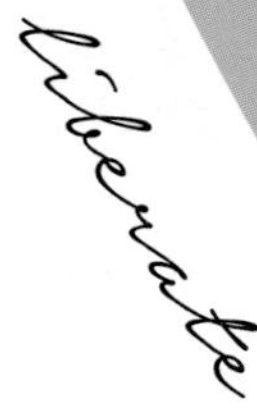

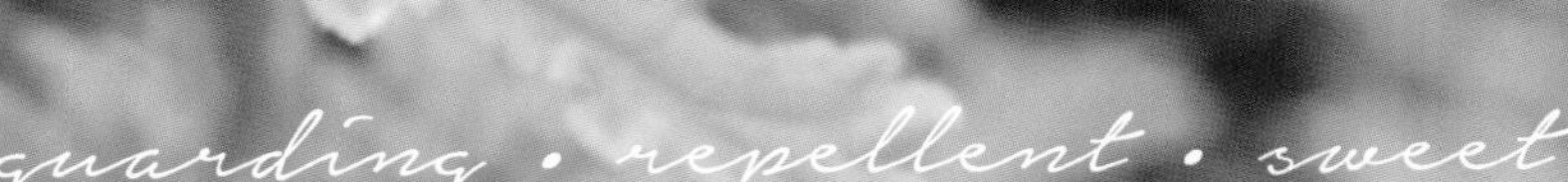

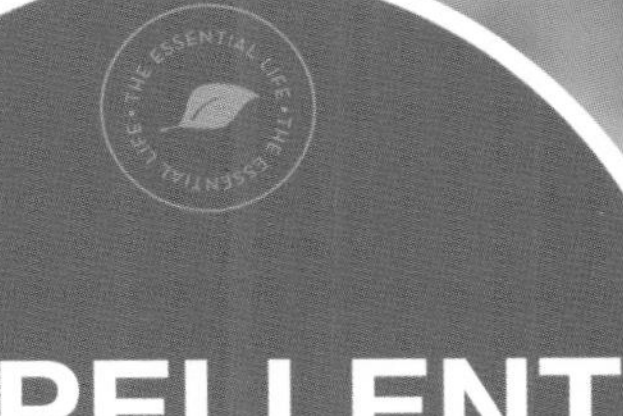

REPELLENT
BLEND

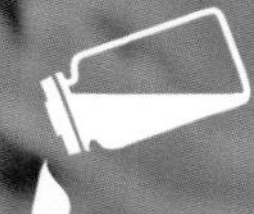

MAIN INGREDIENTS
Skimmia laureola
Catnip
Amyris
African sandalwood
Cabrueva balsam
Wild orange
White fir
Cedarwood
Citronella
Eucalyptus
Hawaiian sandalwood
Genet
Rose

SAFETY
Safe for NEAT application.

OIL BLENDS

TOP USES

REPELLENT
Diffuse, spray on surfaces, or apply topically to repel bugs and insects.

CELLULAR HEALTH
Apply topically to pulse points and bottoms of feet to promote healthy cell function.

SUNSCREEN
Apply topically with helichrysum or lavender to protect against sun exposure.

SKIN COMPLAINTS
Apply topically with lavender to troubled skin.

HEALTHY BOUNDARIES
Diffuse, spray on surfaces or apply topically to repel bugs and insects.

WOOD POLISH
Mix 4 drops with fractionated coconut oil to polish and preserve wood.

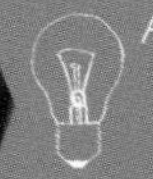

A toxic-free alternative to guard against bugs and pests. Fractionated coconut oil helps the blend stay on the skin longer, prolonging its effect.

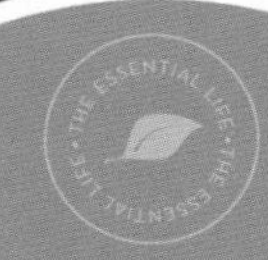

RESPIRATION

BLEND

airy
expanding
supportive

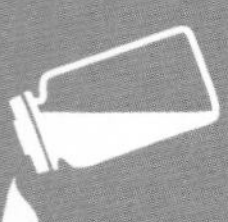

MAIN INGREDIENTS
Laurel
Peppermint
Eucalyptus
Melaleuca
Lemon
Ravensara
Cardamom

TOP USES

PNEUMONIA & ASTHMA
Diffuse aromatically or apply topically under nose and on chest.

ALLERGIES
Inhale aromatically from cupped hands or apply topically on or under nose.

COUGH & CONGESTION
Diffuse aromatically or apply topically to chest.

BRONCHITIS & INFLUENZA
Diffuse aromatically and apply topically to chest.

SINUSITIS & NASAL POLYPS
Apply topically on or under nose.

SLEEP ISSUES
Diffuse aromatically with lavender and apply topically to bottoms of feet.

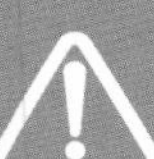

SAFETY
Dilute for young or sensitive skin.

Healthy airflow and oxygen supply bring life and energy with each breath. Enjoy a restful sleep with this blend.

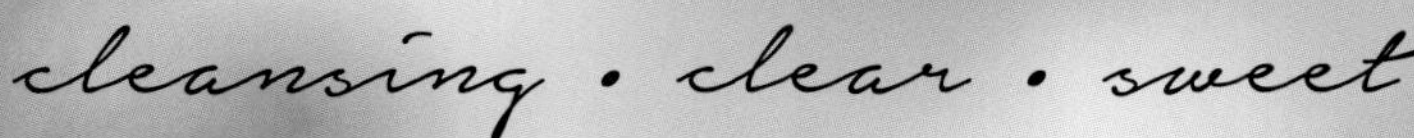

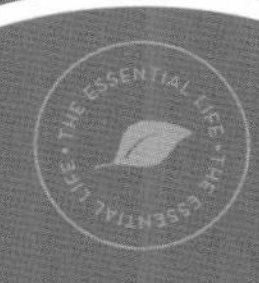

SKIN CLEARING

BLEND

TOP USES

ACNE & PIMPLES
Apply topically to area of concern.

OILY SKIN & OVERACTIVE SEBACEOUS GLANDS
Apply topically to area of concern.

SKIN BLEMISHES & IRRITATIONS
Apply topically to area of concern.

DERMATITIS & ECZEMA
Apply topically to area of concern.

FUNGAL ISSUES
Apply topically to area of concern.

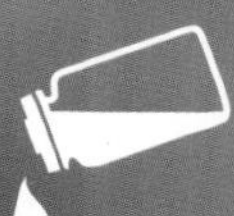

MAIN INGREDIENTS
Black cumin
Ho wood
Melaleuca
Litsea
Eucalyptus
Geranium

SAFETY
Dilute if irritation occurs.

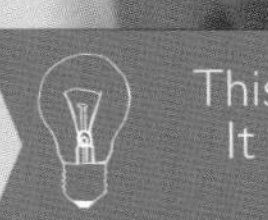

This blend is cleansing and calming to the skin. It reduces two components that encourage acne: bacteria and inflammation.

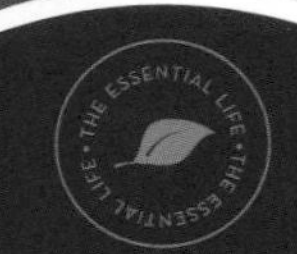

SOOTHING

BLEND

minty
athletic
cooling

TOP USES

MUSCLE, BACK & JOINT PAIN
Apply topically to affected area.

ARTHRITIS & ACHES
Apply topically to affected area.

FIBROMYALGIA & LUPUS
Apply topically to affected area.

WHIPLASH & MUSCLE TENSION
Apply topically to affected area.

PRE- & POST-WORKOUT
Apply topically to affected area.

GROWING PAINS
Apply topically to affected area.

HEADACHE & NECK PAIN
Apply topically to back of neck, shoulders, and temples.

BRUISES & INJURIES
Apply topically to affected area to reduce inflammation and scar tissue.

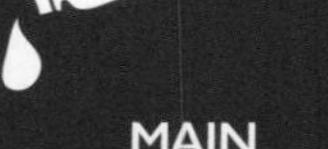

MAIN INGREDIENTS
Wintergreen
Camphor
Peppermint
Blue tansy
Blue chamomile
Helichrysum

SAFETY
Apply diluted for young or sensitive skin.

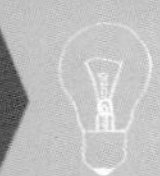

A toxic-free substitute for topical ointments and creams. This blend naturally reduces pain and inflammation.

relieving • renewing • awakening

TENSION

BLEND

TOP USES

HEADACHES & MIGRAINES
Apply topically to temples, forehead, and back of neck.

MUSCLE ACHES, SWELLING & CRAMPING
Apply topically to area of concern.

BRUISES & BURNS
Apply topically to area of concern.

JOINT PAIN
Apply topically to area of concern.

TENSION & STRESS
Apply topically to pulse points and inhale.

NECK & SHOULDER PAIN
Apply topically to area of discomfort.

ARTHRITIS
Apply topically to area of discomfort.

RESTFUL SLEEP
Apply topically to back of neck.

MAIN INGREDIENTS
Wintergreen
Lavender
Peppermint
Frankincense
Cilantro
Marjoram
Roman chamomile
Basil
Rosemary

SAFETY
Dilute if irritation occurs.

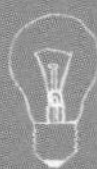

Tension is the cause of many neurological complaints including headaches. This blend relieves tension and increases blood flow.

UPLIFTING
BLEND

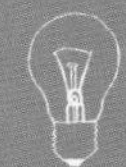

Encourage an optimistic attitude, promote focus on what really matters, and nurture an uplifted state of mind with this blend.

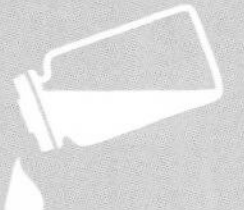

MAIN INGREDIENTS
Wild orange
Clove
Star Anise
Lemon Myrtle
Nutmeg

gladden · illuminate · delight

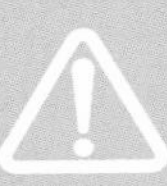

SAFETY
Dilute for skin sensitivity. If pregnant or nursing, consult your physician. Avoid exposure to direct sunlight or UV rays for up to 12 hours after topical use.

TOP USES

DEPRESSION & PMS
Inhale aromatically or apply topically with carrier oil to abdomen or pressure points on inside and outside below ankle bones.

HYSTERIA & ANXIETY
Diffuse aromatically or inhale.

DISCONNECTION
Inhale aromatically in palms of hands or diffuse.

CELLULAR HEALTH
Apply topically to bottoms of feet.

INFLAMMATION & STIFFNESS
Apply topically to affected areas with carrier oil.

INDIGESTION & IRRITABLE BOWELS
Apply topically to abdomen with carrier oil and bottoms of feet.

BLOOD SUGAR & CHOLESTEROL
Apply topically to bottoms of feet and over liver and pancreas areas with carrier oil.

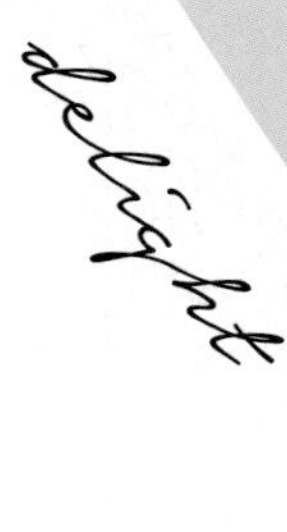

floral • warm • calming

WOMEN'S

MONTHLY BLEND

TOP USES

HORMONE BALANCING
Apply topically to back of neck or bottoms of feet.

HEAVY PERIODS, PMS & CRAMPS
Apply topically to abdomen, back of neck, or bottoms of feet.

PRE & PERIMENOPAUSE
Apply topically to abdomen, back of neck, or bottoms of feet.

HOT FLASHES
Apply topically to abdomen or back of neck.

MOOD SWINGS
Apply topically to abdomen, back of neck, or bottoms of feet.

BLOOD SUGAR ISSUES
Apply topically to back of neck or bottoms of feet.

SKIN ISSUES & WOUNDS
Apply topically to area of concern.

MAIN INGREDIENTS
Clary sage
Lavender
Bergamot
Roman chamomile
Cedarwood
Ylang ylang
Geranium
Fennel
Carrot
Palmarosa
Vitex

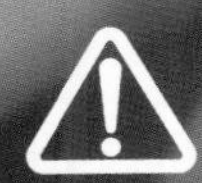

SAFETY
Safe for NEAT application.

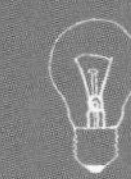

This gentle and safe blend brings harmony by balancing and stabilizing hormones.

WOMEN'S

OR PERFUME BLEND

Each woman's unique body chemistry makes the scent of this blend her own.

MAIN INGREDIENTS
Bergamot
Ylang ylang
Patchouli
Vanilla bean
Jasmine
Cinnamon
Labdanum
Vetiver
Sandalwood
Cocoa bean
Rose

fresh • balancing • cleansing

SAFETY
Safe for NEAT application.

TOP USES

BALANCE HORMONES
Apply topically to pulse points.

PERFUME
Apply topically to pulse points and cleavage.

CALMING
Diffuse aromatically or apply topically to back of neck.

HOT FLASH
Apply topically to back of neck.

LIBIDO & SEX DRIVE
Apply topically to pulse points.

ANGER
Diffuse aromatically or apply topically to pulse points.

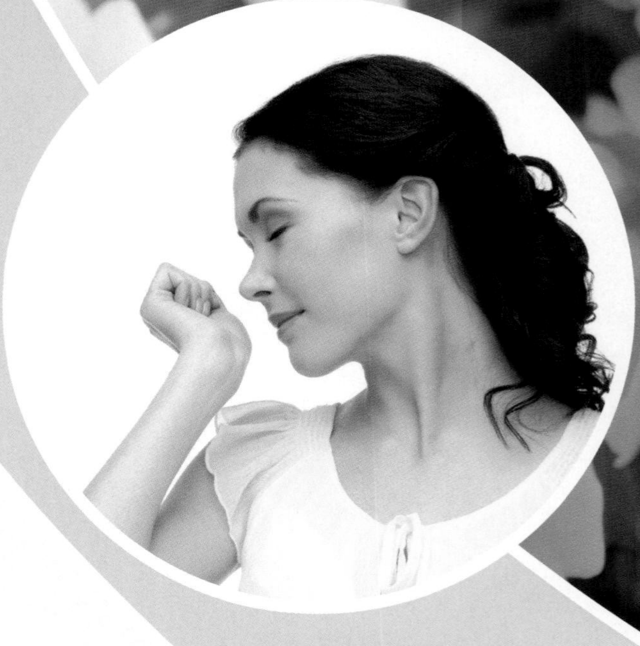

SUPPLEMENTARY PRODUCTS

Is your energy low? Do you experience chronic pain or discomfort in your body? Dealing with challenges in sustaining energy and concentration throughout the day, along with maintaining adequate immune and physical health, are the norm for many. However, virtually any health compromise or issue can be traced to some kind of underlying deficiency or toxicity. Numerous studies have been conducted over decades to determine the optimal nutritional state for the human body. The scientific community agrees that virtually everyone falls short in obtaining the bare minimum of recommended daily nutritional requirements in at least some areas.

These declines can be attributed to two main factors. The first is the increasing level of compromises in farming practices and the rising interest by food growers to genetically modify foods. Even those eating a wholesome, balanced diet find it challenging to consume adequate levels of certain nutrients. The second factor contributing to decline is our consumption of refined, processed, nutrient-void foods loaded with empty calories, which has been on the increase globally for decades. Similarly, adults and children alike are consuming excessive amounts of animal protein while consuming far too few fresh fruits and vegetables.

With these drastic changes in both food supply and consumption, examining one's own nutritional status is a worthy course of action. Consider asking yourself if you have any diet, health, or lifestyle habits or compromises that contribute to a lack in health and vitality and make adjustments accordingly. Whether feeling healthy or not, anyone can benefit from commitment to a daily supplemental program.

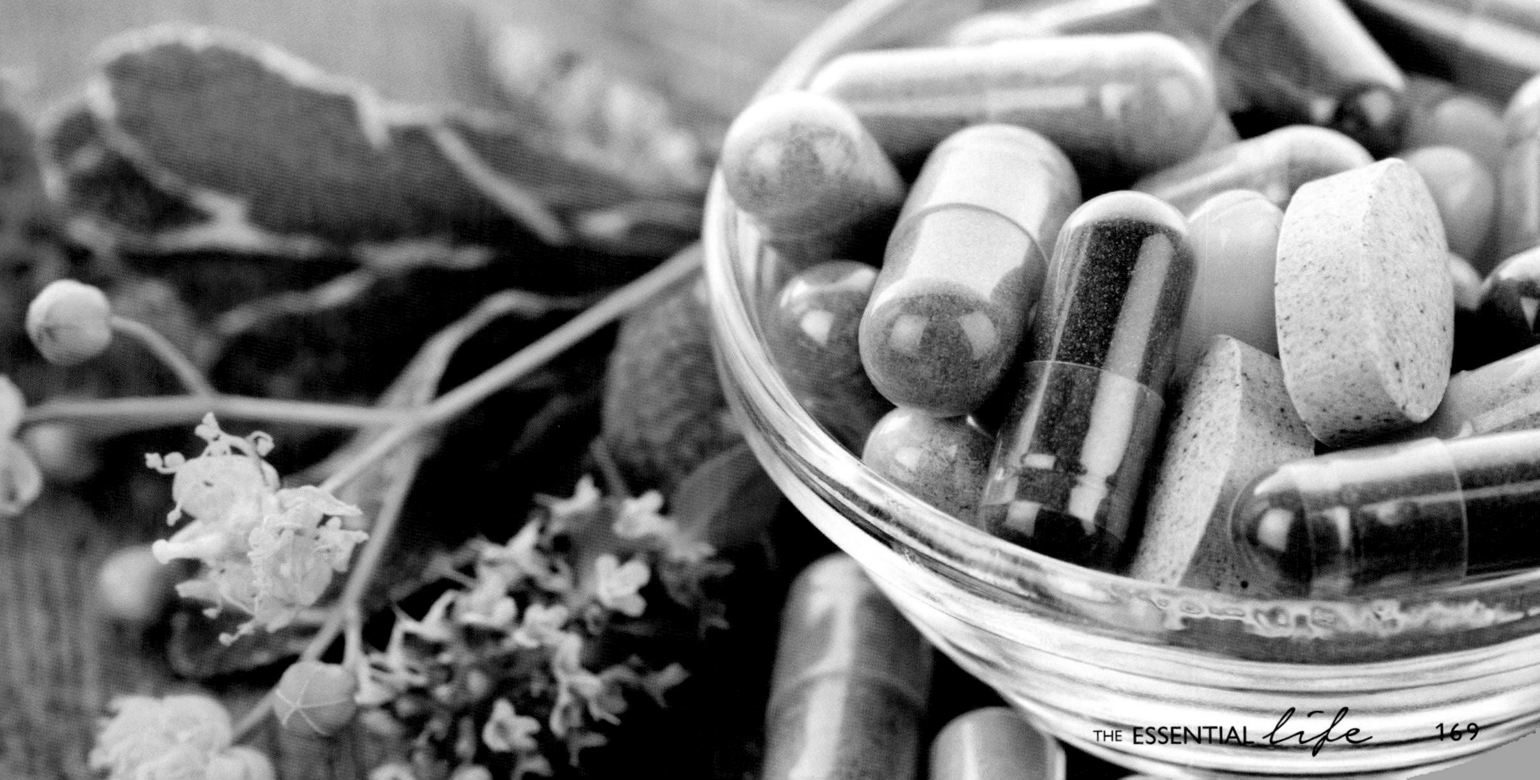

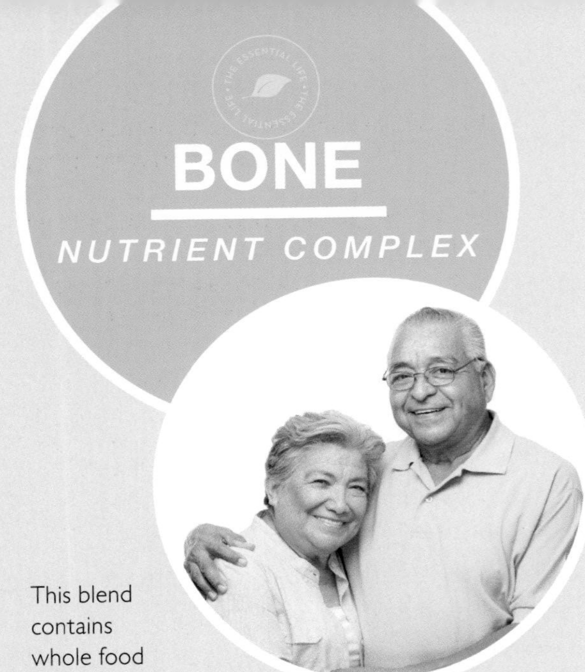

This blend contains whole food created vitamins, minerals and other cofactors necessary for bone integrity, strength and overall health. Not just for women, this complex is bioavailable to the body so the cells not only will recognize, but also utilize the compounds for bone reformation.

TOP USES

Weak or fragile bones, osteopenia and osteoporosis prone individuals, bone fractures, growing individuals, and anyone needing more bone density.

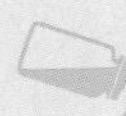

INGREDIENTS

- Vitamin C: Protective role in building strong bones and preventing fractures.
- Vitamin D2 and D3: Increases the absorption of calcium and other minerals by the intestines, increasing utilization of minerals for bone density.
- Biotin: Increase efficiency of bone marrow cell function as well as plays a role in the growth of hair, skin, and nails.
- Calcium, magnesium, zinc, copper, manganese, and boron: Work synergistically to build the foundation of bone tissue and integrity.

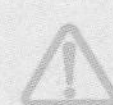

SAFETY

Safe for use by women, teens and men. Pregnant or lactating women should consult a physician or health care provider before use.

Association between serum 25-hydroxyvitamin d levels, bone geometry, and bone mineral density in healthy older adults, Mosele M, Coin A, Manzato E, et al, *The Journals of Gerontology Series A: Biological Sciences and Medical Sciences.* 2013

Nutritional aspects of the prevention and treatment of osteoporosis, Peters BS, Martini LA, *Arquivos Brasileiros de Endocrinologia & Metabologia*, 2010

Minerals and vitamins in bone health: the potential value of dietary enhancement, Bonjour JP, Gueguen L, Palacios C, et al, 2009

Magnesium and osteoporosis: current state of knowledge and future research directions, Castiglioni S, Cazzaniga A, Albisetti W, Maier JA, *Nutrients*, 2013

The physiological effects of dietary boron, Devirian TA, Volpe SL, *Critical Reviews in Food Science and Nutrition*, 2003

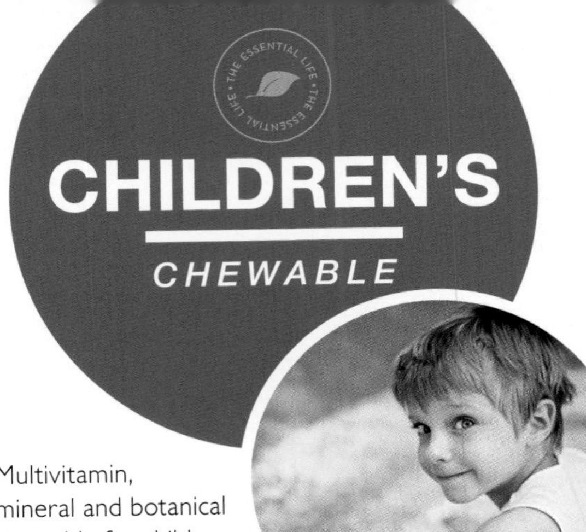

Multivitamin, mineral and botanical chewable for children and adults that have difficulty swallowing. Blended with antioxidants and herbal compounds that increase overall health and wellness.

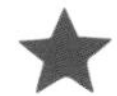

TOP USES

Low energy and fatigue, compromised digestion and immunity, brain fog, oxidative cell damage, malnutrition, and poor health.

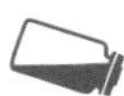

INGREDIENTS

- Vitamins A, C, D3 and full B-complex: Antioxidants and cellular energy, bringing synergy and vital nutrients to the cells of the body and brain. Also supports a healthy immune function.
- Calcium, copper, iron, iodine, magnesium, manganese, potassium and zinc: Bioavailable minerals which lay the foundation for bone health and nerve cell functions. Also supports fluid transportation and utilization by the cells.
- Superfood Blend of pineapple, pomegranate extract, lemon bioflavonoids, spirulina, sunflower oil, rice bran, beet greens, broccoli, brown rice, carrot, mango, cranberry, rose hips, acerola cherry extract: Blend of antioxidants and whole food nutrients to support healthy cell function and increase utilization of other nutrients throughout the body.
- Cellular Vitality Complex of tomato extract, turmeric extract, boswellia serrata extract, grape seed extract, marigold flower extract: Synergistic blend of natural anti-inflammatories, antioxidants and cellular repair compounds.

SAFETY

No gluten, wheat, dairy, soy or nut products. Pregnant or lactating women should consult a physician or health care provider before use.

Selected vitamins and trace elements support immune function by strengthening epithelial barriers and cellular and humoral immune responses, Maggini S, Wintergerst ES, Beveridge S, Hornig DH, *British Journal of Nutrition*, 2007

Contribution of selected vitamins and trace elements to immune function, Wintergerst ES, Maggini S, Hornig DH, *Ann Nutr Met*, 2007

Minerals and vitamins in bone health: The potential value of dietary enhancement, Bonjour JP, Gueguen L, Palacios C, et al, *Bri J Nutr*, 2009

The immunological functions of the vitamin D endocrine system, Hayes CE, Nashold FE, Spach KM & Pedersen LB, *Cell Molec Biol*, 2003

Possible role for dietary lutein and zeaxanthin in visual development, Hammond BR, *Nutr Rev*, 2008

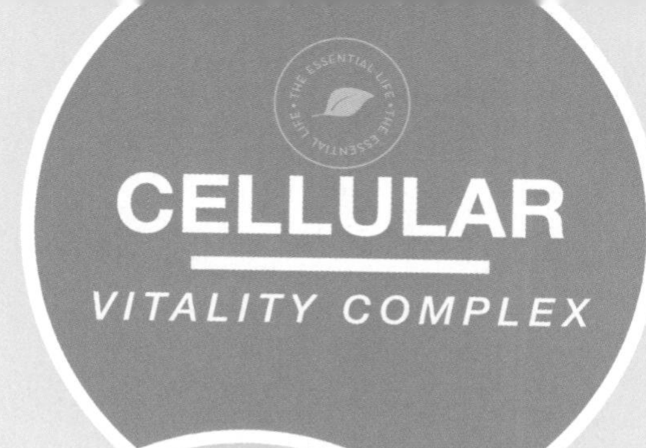

CELLULAR VITALITY COMPLEX

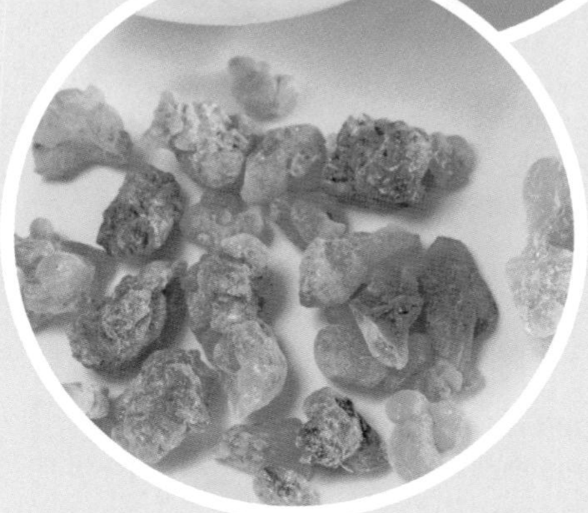

Packed with nature's most potent antioxidants, natural anti-inflammatories, and energy cofactors, this blend of synergistic herbs will give life and energy to the cells and a sense of well being to the body.

TOP USES

Pain and inflammation, arthritis, osteoarthritis, fibromyalgia, foggy brain, cirrhosis, jaundice, cellular repair, fatigue, mood, and cancer prevention.

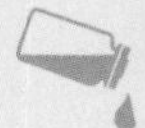

INGREDIENTS

- Boswellia serrata gum resin: Inflammatory modulator (helps regulate and decrease inflammation and pain).
- Scutellaria Root (baicalin): Inflammatory modulator and cellular damage repair, supports liver and kidney health.
- Milk Thistle (silymarin): Powerful liver protectant and free radical scavenger.
- Polygonum cuspidatum (resveratrol): Increases healthy cell proliferation and decreases free radical damage from cells.
- Green Tea Leaf (EGCG): Powerful antioxidant, free radical scavenger, and anticancer properties.
- Pomegranate Fruit extract: Antioxidant shown to lower LDL cholesterol, blood pressure, and increase heart health.
- Pineapple (bromelain): An enzyme shown to decrease pain and inflammation.
- Turmeric extract (curcumin): Powerful anti-inflammatory and anticancer compound.
- Grape Seed extract: Proanthocyanidins shown to decrease free radical damage and increase cellular repair.
- Sesame seed extract: Antioxidant shown to protect liver from oxidative damage.
- Pine Bark extract (pycnogenol): Antioxidant shown to increase vasodilation of the arteries and decrease free radical damage.
- Gingko Biloba Leaf: Increases circulation to the brain and brings mental clarity.
- Acetyl-L-Carnitine: Increases energy production by the mitochondria and increases glutathione (internal antioxidant) levels in the body.
- Alpha-Lipoic Acid: Antioxidant vital for cellular energy and neutralizing free radicals.
- Coenzyme Q10: Plays a significant role in energy production for the heart and muscle cells.
- Quercetin: Potent antioxidant flavonoid known to decrease cell damage and increase recovery.

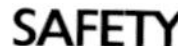

SAFETY

For men, women and teens. Pregnant or lactating women should consult a physician or health care provider before use.

Gene Expression Profiling of Aging in Multiple Mouse Strains: Identification of Aging Biomarkers and Impact of Dietary Antioxidants, Park SK, Kim K, Page GP, Allison DB, Weindruch R, Prolla TA, *Aging Cell*, 2009

Antioxidative and anti-inflammatory activities of polyhydroxyflavonoids of Scutellaria baicalensis GEORGI, Huang WH, Lee AR, Yang CH, *Biosci Biotechnol Biochem*, 2006 Oct

New therapeutic aspects of flavones: the anticancer properties of Scutellaria and its main active constituents Wogonin, Baicalein and Baicalin, Li-Weber M, *Cancer Treat Rev*, 2009 Feb

The SIRT1 activator resveratrol protects SK-N-BE cells from oxidative stress and against toxicity caused by alpha-synuclein or amyloid-beta (1-42) peptide, Albani D, Polito L, Batelli S, De Mauro S, Fracasso C, Martelli G, Colombo L, Manzoni C, Salmona M, Caccia S, Negro A, Forloni G, *J Neurochem*, 2009

Resveratrol induces mitochondrial biogenesis in endothelial cells, Csiszar A, Labinskyy N, Pinto JT, Ballabh P, Zhang H, Losonczy G, Pearson K, de Cabo R, Pacher P, Zhang C, Ungvari Z, *Am J Physiol Heart Circ Physiol*, 2009 Jul

In vitro effects of tea polyphenols on redox metabolism, oxidative stress, and apoptosis in PC12 cells, Raza H, John A, *Ann N Y Acad Sci*, 2008 Sep

Orally administered green tea polyphenols prevent ultraviolet radiation-induced skin cancer in mice through activation of cytotoxic T cells and inhibition of angiogenesis in tumors, Mantena SK, Meeran SM, Elmets CA, Katiyar SK, *J Nutr*, 2005 Dec

Grape seed and red wine polyphenol extracts inhibit cellular cholesterol uptake, cell proliferation, and 5-lipoxygenase activity, Leifert WR, Abeywardena MY, *Nutr Res*, 2008 Dec

Quercetin increases brain and muscle mitochondrial biogenesis and exercise tolerance, Davis JM, Murphy EA, Carmichael MD, Davis B, *Am J Physiol Regul Integr Comp Physiol*, 2009 Apr

Mineral and vitamin deficiencies can accelerate the mitochondrial decay of aging, Ames BN, Atamna H, Killilea DW, *Mol Aspects Med*, 2005 Aug-Oct

Boswellic acid inhibits growth and metastasis of human colorectal cancer in orthotopic mouse model by downregulating inflammatory, proliferative, invasive and angiogenic biomarkers, Yadav, VR, Prasad S, Sung, B, Gelovani, JG, Guha, S, Krishnan, S, Aggarwal, BB *Int. J. Cancer*, 2012

Plant food supplements with anti-inflammatory properties: A systematic review, Di Lorenzo C, Dell'agli M, Badea M, et al, *Critical Reviews in Food Science and Nutrition*, 2013

Polyphenols, inflammation, and cardiovascular disease, Tangney CC, Rasmussen HE, *Curr Atheroscler Rep*, 2013

Bioavailability and activity of phytosome complexes from botanical polyphenols: The silymarin, curcumin, green tea, and grape seed extracts, Kidd PM, *Alternative Medicine Review*, 2009

Open, randomized controlled clinical trial of Boswellia serrata extract as compared to valdecoxib in osteoarthritis of knee, Sontakke S, Thawani V, Pimpalkhute S, Kapra P, Babhulkar S, Hingorani L, *Indian Journal of Pharmacology*. 2007

Baicalin, an emerging multi-therapeutic agent: pharmacodynamics, pharmacokinetics, and considerations from drug development perspectives, Srinivas NR, *Xenobiotica, 2010*

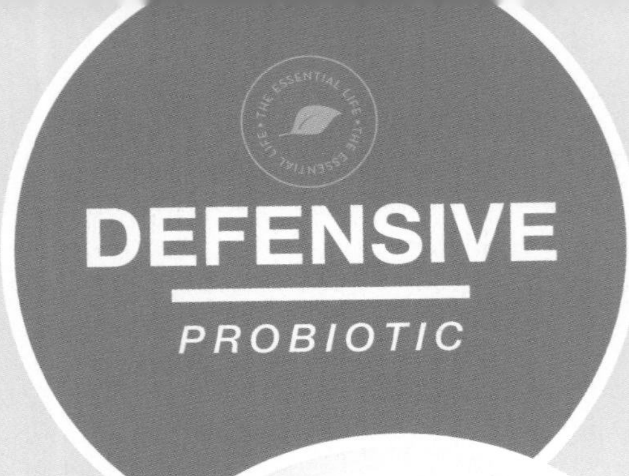

DEFENSIVE

PROBIOTIC

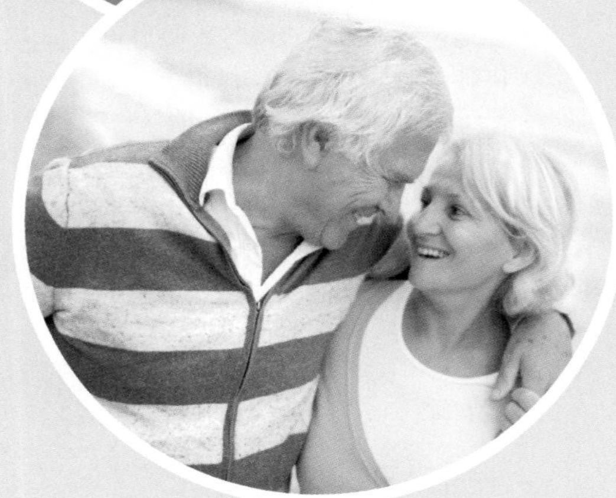

SUPPLEMENTARY PRODUCTS

A double-encapsulated, time-release probiotic made with six different strains of good bacteria and prebiotic fiber for maximum delivery and cultivation of healthy gut flora.

TOP USES

Flatulence, constipation or diarrhea, malabsorption, irritable bowel, compromised immune system, leaky gut, allergies, autoimmune diseases, malabsorption, anxiety and depression, mental disorders, and infections.

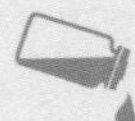

INGREDIENTS

- L. acidophilus, L. salivarius, L. casei: Lactobacillus strains of bacteria which increase the integrity of the villi of the upper intestinal tract to improve the absorption of other nutrients. Also enhancing immunity and the gut-brain connection increasing proper neurotransmitter and brain function.
- B. lactis, B. bifidum, B. longum: Bifidobacterium strains that help digestion and immunity of the large intestines and enhance overall colon health. Also increasing the functions of the brain and improving mood.
- FOS (fructooligosaccharides) prebiotic: Indigestible fibers that enhance the growth and cultivation of good bacteria while decreasing growth of bad bacteria.

SAFETY

For all ages.

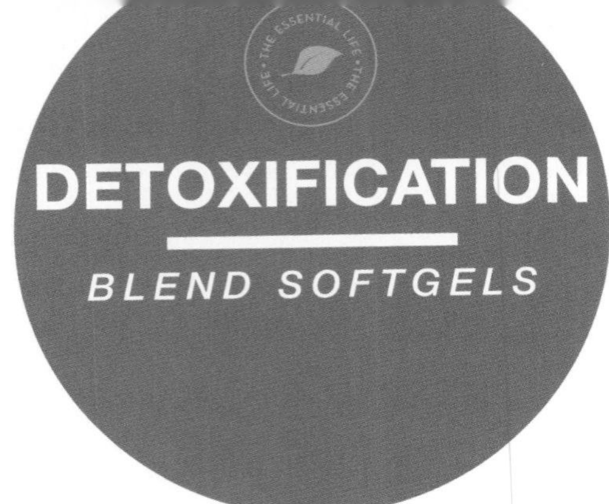

DETOXIFICATION

BLEND SOFTGELS

A blend of essential oils that support natural detoxification of the body to help cleanse it of toxins and free radicals that can slow your systems down, leaving a heavy, weighted feeling.

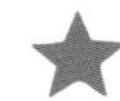

TOP USES

Toxic liver, jaundice, cirrhosis, bloating, toxic gallbladder, pancreatitis, kidney damage, and hormonal imbalances.

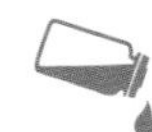

INGREDIENTS

- Tangerine Peel: Antioxidant and cleansing properties of the liver and kidneys.
- Rosemary Leaf: Supports a healthy liver and gallbladder as well as reduces xenoestrogens (foreign estrogens form plastics, growth hormones and environmental toxins).
- Geranium Plant: Cleanses liver, gallbladder and balances hormones and rids the body of unwanted estrogens.
- Juniper Berry: Powerful detoxifier of the kidneys and decreases water retention.
- Cilantro Herb: Powerful cleansing agent that eliminates toxins from the body, including heavy metals.

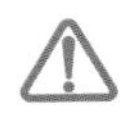

SAFETY

Not for children. Keep out of reach of small children. If pregnant or lactating, women should consult a physician or health care provider before use.

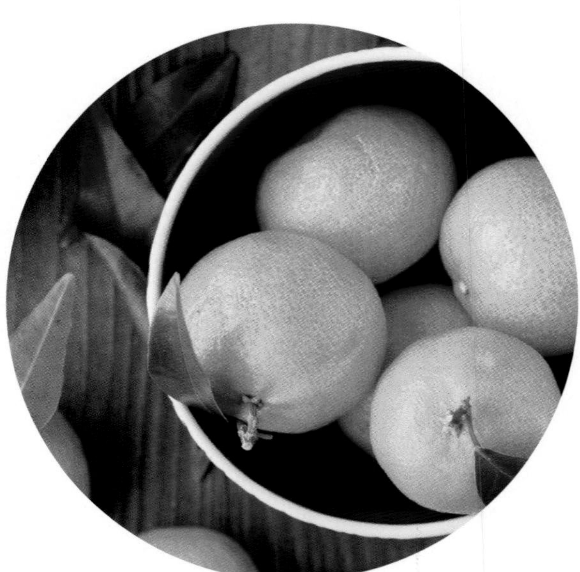

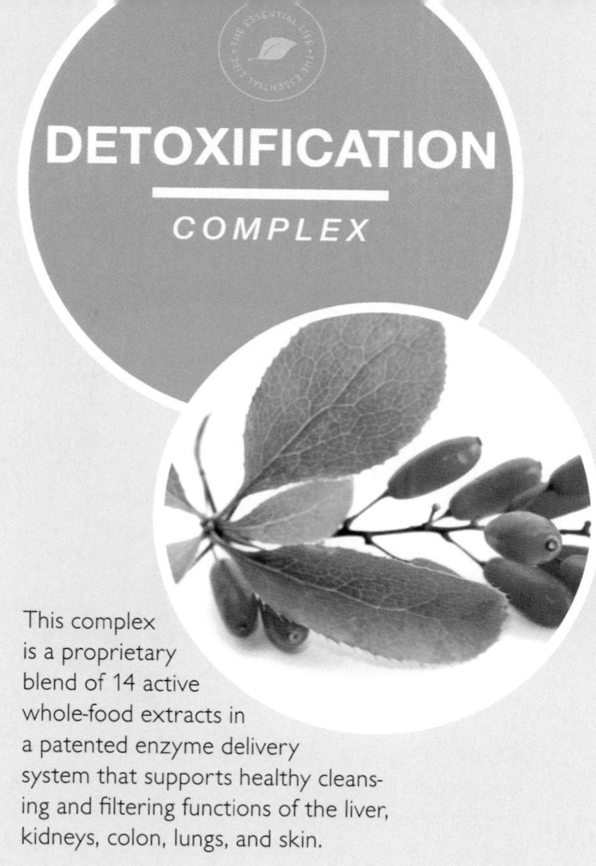

DETOXIFICATION
COMPLEX

This complex is a proprietary blend of 14 active whole-food extracts in a patented enzyme delivery system that supports healthy cleansing and filtering functions of the liver, kidneys, colon, lungs, and skin.

TOP USES

Toxic liver, jaundice, cirrhosis, bloating, toxic gallbladder, pancreatitis, kidney damage, respiratory issues, colon issues and constipation.

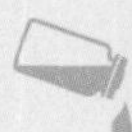

INGREDIENTS

- Barberry leaf, milk thistle seed, burdock root, clove bud, dandelion root, garlic fruit, red clover leaf: Targets the cleansing and support of the liver and helps filter the blood of toxins.
- Turkish rhubarb stem, burdock root, clove bud, dandelion root: Targets the cleansing of the kidneys while bringing strength and integrity to it.
- Psyllium seed husk, turkish rhubarb stem, acacia gum bark, marshmallow root: Helps to strengthen the elimination process of the colon and colon health.
- Osha root, safflower petals: Helps to strengthen and cleanse the lungs from environmental and other toxins.
- Kelp, milk thistle seed, burdock root, clove bud, garlic fruit: Helps support the cleansing of toxins from the skin.
- Enzyme assimilation system of amylase and cellulase their natural mineral cofactors magnesium and manganese: Increases digestion and utilization of the rest of the ingredients.

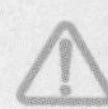

SAFETY

Not for children. Keep out of reach of small children. If pregnant or lactating, women should consult a physician or health care provider before use.

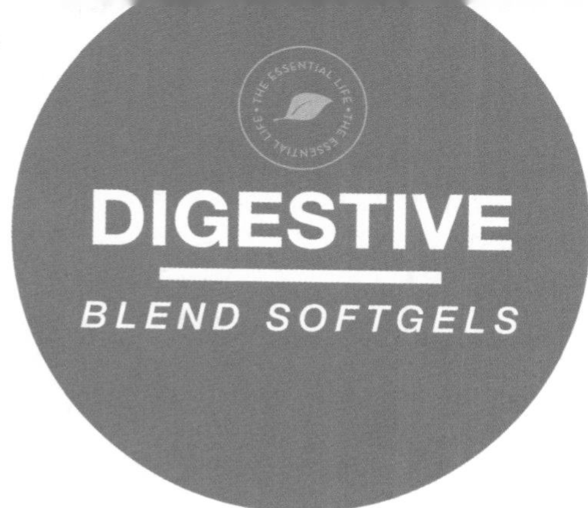

DIGESTIVE
BLEND SOFTGELS

A synergistic blend of essential oils that help ease digestion and increase digestive health.

TOP USES

Upset stomach, constipation, diarrhea, IBS, vomiting, heartburn and acid indigestion/reflux.

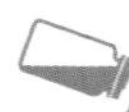

INGREDIENTS

- Ginger: Renowned for its ability to soothe stomach upset and ease indigestion.
- Peppermint: Supports healthy gastrointestinal function and aids in digestion.
- Tarragon: Promotes healthy digestion.
- Fennel: Helps relieve indigestion and a myriad of stomach issues.
- Caraway: Acts as a natural carminative while supporting a healthy gastrointestinal tract.
- Coriander: Eases occasional stomach upset.
- Anise: Promotes healthy digestion.

SAFETY

Can be taken by all ages that can swallow capsules. Keep out of reach of small children.

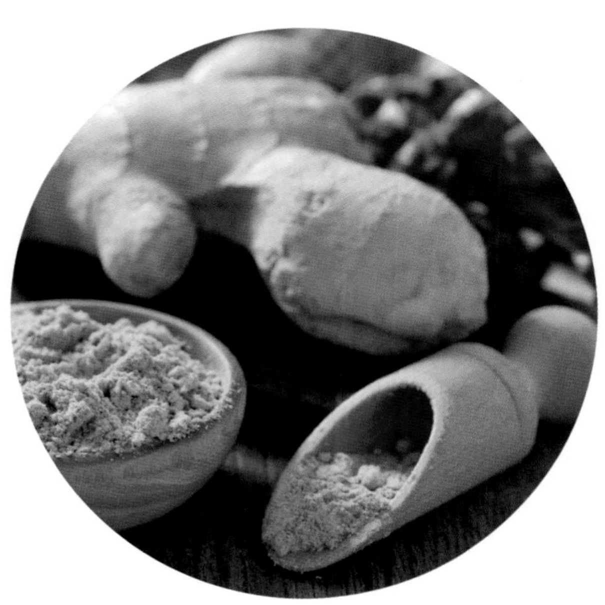

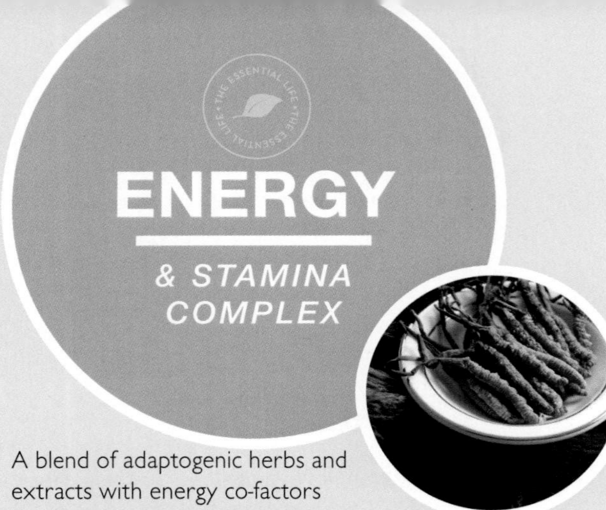

A blend of adaptogenic herbs and extracts with energy co-factors made to increase mitochondrial biogenesis and overall energy while decreasing the stress response due to physical activity and daily life.

TOP USES

Body fatigue and tiredness, adrenal fatigue, hormonal imbalance, libido, physical stress, anxiety, and poor circulation.

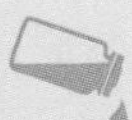

INGREDIENTS

- Acetyl-L-Carnitine HCL: Increases energy production by the mitochondria and increases glutathione (internal antioxidant) levels in the body.
- Alpha-Lipoic Acid: Antioxidant vital for cellular energy and neutralizing free radicals.
- Coenzyme Q10: Plays a significant role in energy production for the heart and muscle cells.
- Lychee Fruit Extract and Green Tea Leaf Polyphenol Extract: Increases circulation, decreases inflammation, and decreases oxidative stress.
- Quercetin dihydrate: Potent antioxidant flavonoid known to decrease cell damage and increase recovery.
- Cordyceps Mycelium: An Adaptogen which enhances respiratory health and physical endurance, hormonal health, increased libido and liver function.
- Ginseng (Panax quinquefolius) root extract: Increases energy and adaption to stress as well stimulates the immune system by increasing the amount of white blood cells in the blood.
- Ashwagandha (withania somnifera) root extract: Powerful Adaptogen that lowers cortisol by decreasing the mental and physical stress response. Also gives energy and vitality to the body.

SAFETY

Not for children. Keep out of reach of small children. If pregnant or lactating, women should consult a physician or health care provider before use.

Ginkgo biloba special extract EGb 761 in generalized anxiety disorder and adjustment disorder with anxious mood: A randomized, double-blind, placebo-controlled trial, Woelk H, Arnoldt KH, Kieser M, Hoerr R, *Journal of Psychiatric Research* 2007

Effects of ginkgo biloba on mental functioning in healthy volunteers, Cieza A, Maier P, Poppel E, *Archives of Medical Research*, 2002

Translating the basic knowledge of mitochondrial functions to metabolic therapy: role of L-carnitine, Marcovina SM, Sirtori C, Peracino A, et al, *Translational Research* 2013

Effects of Ð-lipoic acid on mtDNA damage following isolated muscle contractions, Fogarty MC, Deviot G, Hughes CM, et al, *Med Sci Sports Exerc*, 2013

The effects and mechanisms of mitochondrial nutrient a-lipoic acid on improved age-associated mitochondrial and cognitive dysfunction: An overview, Liu J, *Neurochem Res*, 2008

Effect of Cs-4 (Cordyceps sinensis) on exercise performance in healthy older subjects: A double-blind, placebo controlled trial, Chen S, Li Z, Krochmal R, et al, *The Journal of Alternative and Complementary Medicine*. 2010

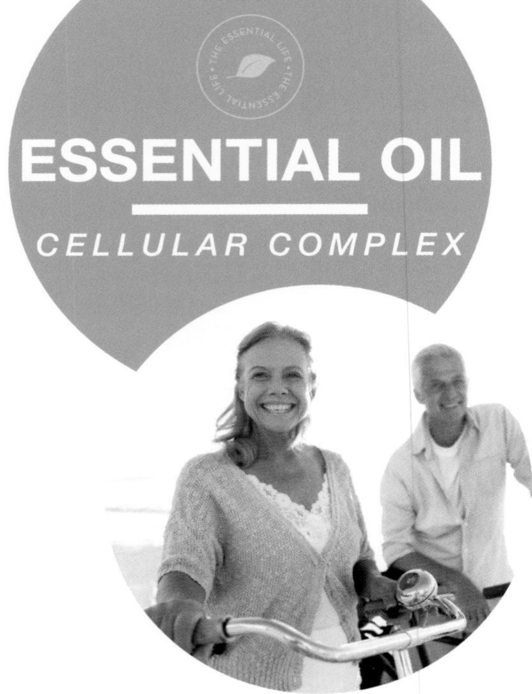

A blend of essential oils that have been shown in clinical studies to help protect cells against free radical damage while supporting cellular function through apoptosis of damaged and mutated cells, and proliferation of healthy cells.

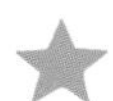

TOP USES

Damaged or mutated cellular diseases, oxidative stress, autoimmune diseases and anything that requires cellular regeneration and healthy cellular function.

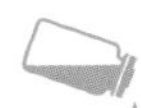

INGREDIENTS

- Frankincense oil: Anti-inflammatory and immune-stimulant properties. Is often used to help support the body's response to cancer and other cellular diseases.
- Wild orange oil: High levels of d-Limonene, which helps inhibit cancer tumor growth and reduction of cholesterol.
- Lemongrass oil: Anti-inflammatory and antiseptic and has the ability to inhibit cancer cell growth and to induce apoptosis (cellular death).
- Thyme oil: Strong antioxidant and antiseptic. Supports the brain as it ages.
- Summer Savory oil: Antifungal and anti-inflammatory properties. Shows ability to reduce DNA damage from oxidative stress.
- Clove Bud oil: Powerful antioxidant and anti-infectious and helps support healthy liver and thyroid function.
- Niaouli oil: Powerful antifungal and anti-inflammatory, helps protect against radiation, and helps to regenerate damaged tissues.

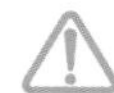

SAFETY

Not for small children. If pregnant or lactating, women should consult a physician or health care provider before use.

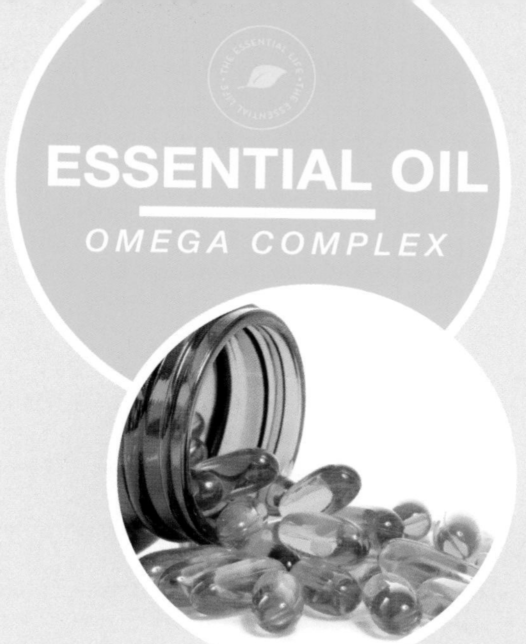

A blend of marine base and land base omega essential fatty acids in a unique assimilation capsule with essential oils and fat-soluble vitamins.

TOP USES

Inflammation and pain, arthritis, anything "itis", compromised immune system, brain fog, concentration, ADD/ADHD, aging skin, PMS, post-partum depression, depression and anxiety, cardiovascular disease, dry skin and skin issues.

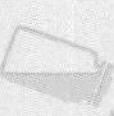

INGREDIENTS

- Fish oil (from Anchovy, Sardine, Mackerel, and Calamari) concentrate: EPA and DHA essential fatty acids that support brain function and increase mood, heart and cardiovascular function, decrease LDL and triglyceride levels, increase attention, memory, concentration, joint health, skin health, immunity and decrease inflammation.
- Echium plantagineum Seed Oil: a blend of ALA, SDA, and GLA essential fatty acids that support the cardiovascular system, decrease LDL and increase HDL triglyceride levels, balances inflammatory markers, enhances mood, brain, and skin health.
- Pomegranate seed oil: Antioxidant oil that increases skin health and decreases inflammation in the skin.
- Vitamin A (as Alpha and Beta carotene): Antioxidants that promote eye health and fight free radicals.
- Vitamin D3 (as natural Cholecalciferol): Supports immune system function, enhances macro-mineral absorption, hormone balance, muscle health, and increases cognitive function.
- Vitamin E: Protects cell membranes against oxidative damage and promotes eye health.
- Astaxanthin: Powerful carotenoid that promotes cellular regeneration, heart and cardiovascular strength, decreases macular degeneration and strengthens the eyes.
- Lutein: Shown to increase strength of the eyes, heart and cells.
- Zeaxanthin: Potent antioxidant good for the eyes and cardiovascular system.
- Essential oil blend of caraway, clove, cumin, frankincense, German chamomile, ginger, peppermint, thyme, and wild orange: Powerful antioxidant properties, immune system properties, promotes healthy digestion, cellular function, and anti-inflammation.

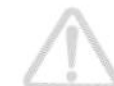

SAFETY

Can be taken by all ages that can swallow capsules.
If pregnant or lactating, women should consult a physician or health care provider before use.

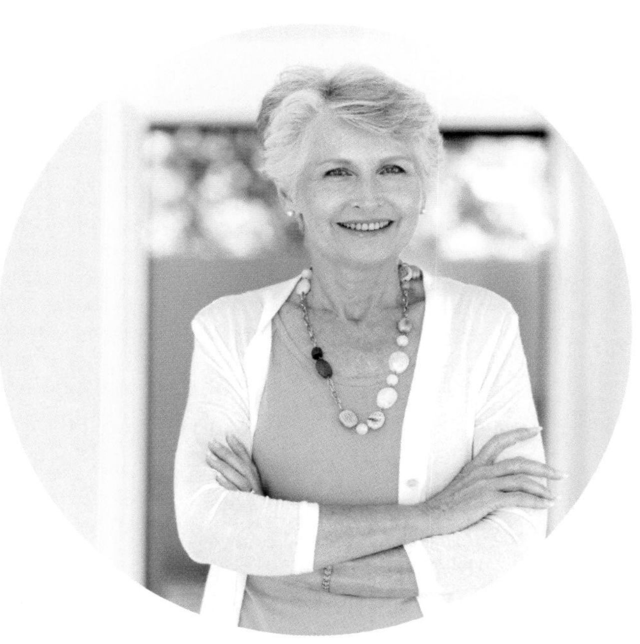

Serum and macular responses to multiple xanthophyll supplements in patients with early age-related macular degeneration, Huang YM, Yan SF, Ma L, et al, *Nutrition*, 2013
a-Linolenic acid and risk of cardiovascular disease: a systematic review and meta-analysis, Pan A, Chen M, Chowdhury R, et al, *The American Journal of Clinical Nutrition*, 2012
Protective effect of borage seed oil and gamma linolenic acid on DNA: In Vivo and In Vitro Studies, Tasset-Cuevas I, Fernandez-Bedmar Z, Lozano-Baena MD, et al, *PLoS ONE*, 2013
Fish oil omega-3 fatty acids and cardio-metabolic health, alone or with statins, Minihane AM, *European Journal of Clinical Nutrition*, 2013
Essential fatty acids as potential anti-inflammatory agents in the treatment of affective disorders, Song C, *Mod Trends Pharmacopsychiatry*, 2013

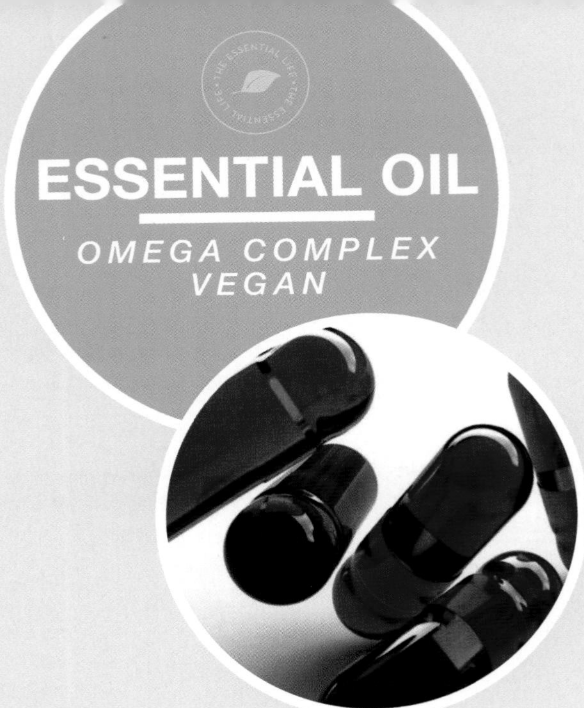

ESSENTIAL OIL

OMEGA COMPLEX VEGAN

A blend of marine base and land base omega essential fatty acids in a unique assimilation capsule with essential oils and fat-soluble vitamins.

TOP USES

Inflammation and pain, arthritis, anything "itis", compromised immune system, brain fog, concentration, ADD/ADHD, aging skin, PMS, postpartum depression, depression and anxiety, cardiovascular disease, dry skin and skin issues.

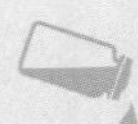

INGREDIENTS

- Flax seed oil: ALA essential fatty acid that support the production of EPA and DHA in the body increasing all the benefits of omega-3 fatty acids.
- Algae oil (DHA): Essential fatty acid that support brain function and increase mood, heart, and cardiovascular function, decreases LDL and triglyceride levels, increased attention, memory, concentration, joint health, skin health, immunity and decreases inflammation.
- Inca Inchi seed oil: Essential fatty acid that promotes inflammatory modulation and decreases oxidative stress.
- Borage seed oil: GLA essential fatty acid that supports inflammatory markers in the body, clears skin, and balances out the mood and hormones.
- Cranberry seed oil: Shown to decrease LDL and triglyceride levels, enhances mood and concentration as well as provides beneficial fats for skin health.
- Pomegranate seed oil: Antioxidant oil that increases skin health and decreases inflammation in the skin.
- Pumpkin seed oil: Helps to increase HDL (good) cholesterol and can promotes energy in the brain.
- Grape seed oil: Promotes a reduction in LDL (bad) cholesterol and triglyceride levels.
- Natural vitamin D: Supports immune system function, enhances macro-mineral absorption, hormone balance, muscle health and increases cognitive function.
- Natural vitamin E: Protects cell membranes against oxidative damage and promotes eye health.
- Astaxanthin: Powerful carotenoid that promotes cellular regeneration, heart and cardiovascular strength, decreases macular degeneration and strengthens the eyes.
- Lutein: Shown to increase strength of the eyes, heart and cells.
- Zeaxanthin: Potent antioxidant good for the eyes and cardiovascular system.
- Lycopene: Fights free radicals and strengthens the integrity of the cell membranes.
- Alpha and Beta carotene: Antioxidants that promote eye health and fight free radicals.
- Essential oil blend of: caraway, clove, cumin, frankincense, German chamomile, ginger, peppermint, thyme, and wild orange: Powerful antioxidant properties, immune system properties, promotes healthy digestion, cellular function, and anti-inflammation.

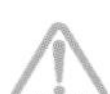

SAFETY

Can be taken by all ages that can swallow capsules. If pregnant or lactating, women should consult a physician or health care provider before use.

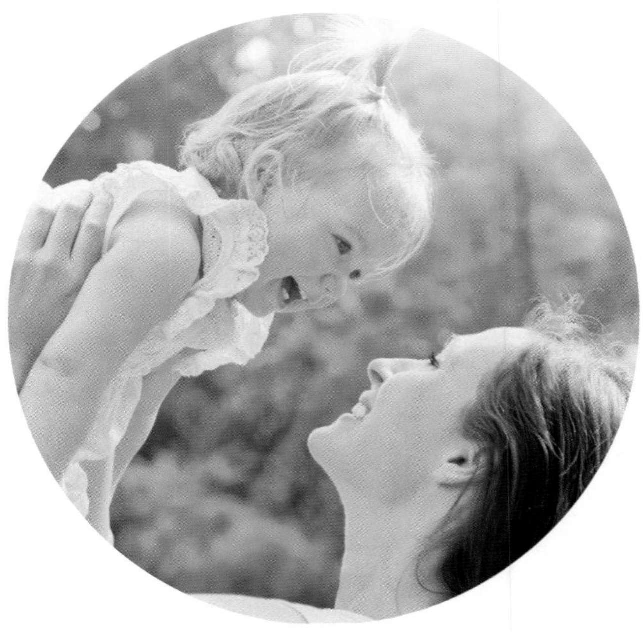

A meta-analysis shows that docosahexaenoic acid from algal oil reduces serum triglycerides and increases HDL-cholesterol and LDL-cholesterol in person without coronary heart disease, Bernstein AM, Ding EL, Willett WC, Rimm EB, *The Journal of Nutrition*, 2012
Astaxanthin, cell membrane nutrient with diverse clinical benefits and anti-aging potential, Kidd P, *Alternative Medicine Review*, 2011
a-Linolenic acid and risk of cardiovascular disease: a systematic review and meta-analysis, Pan A, Chen M, Chowdhury R, et al, *The American Journal of Clinical Nutrition*, 2012
The cardiovascular effects of flaxseed and its omega-3 fatty acid, alpha-linolenic acid, Rodriguez-Leyva D, Bassett CMC, McCullough R, Pierce GN, *Can J Cardiol*, 2010
Macular pigment optical density and eye health, Alexander DE, *Kemin Technical Literature*, 2010

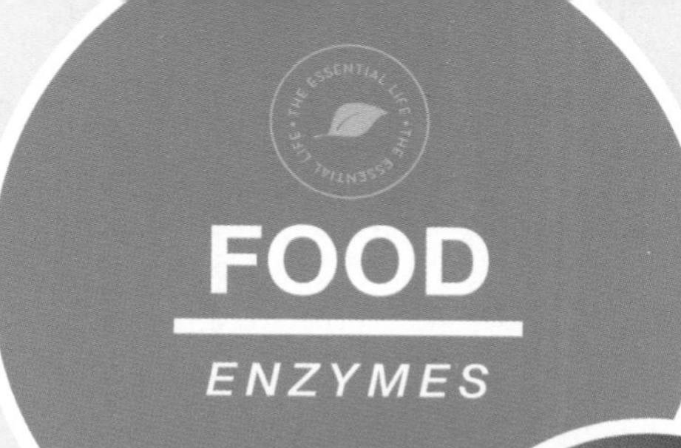

FOOD

ENZYMES

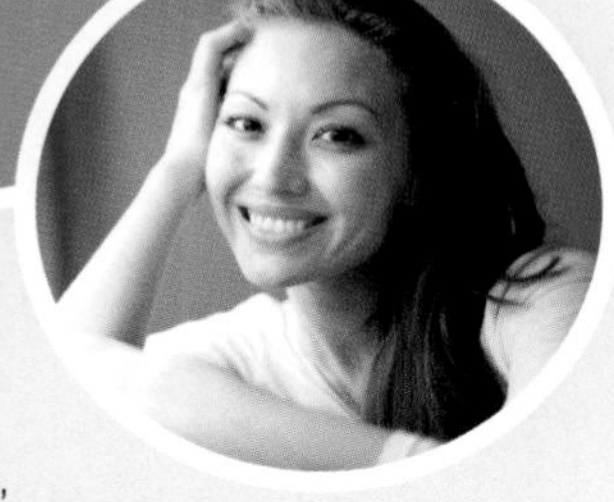

A blend of several, active, whole-food enzymes and mineral cofactors that help the breakdown of proteins, fats, complex carbohydrates, sugars, and fiber, giving the body better digestion nutrients readily available by for absorption and utilization.

TOP USES

Poor nutrition, heartburn or indigestion, slow metabolism, upset stomach, bloating, and flatulence.

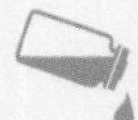

INGREDIENTS

- Protease: Breaks down protein to peptides and amino acids.
- Papain: Breaks down protein.
- Amylase: Breaks down carbohydrates, starches, and sugars.
- Lipase: Breaks down fats and oils to be absorbed in the intestine.
- Lactase: Breaks down lactose in milk sugars.
- Alpha Galactosidase: Breaks down complex polysaccharide sugars in legumes and cruciferous vegetables that can cause bloating and gas.
- Cellulase: Breaks down fiber to help digest fruits and vegetables.
- Sucrase: Breaks down sucrose to fructose and glucose for energy.
- Anti-Gluten Enzyme Blend: Assists in breaking down gluten.
- Glucoamylase: Breaks down starch.
- Betaine HCL: Aids in protein digestion.
- Digestion blend of peppermint leaf, ginger root, caraway seed: Helps soothe the digestive process and tames the stomach.

SAFETY

Can be taken by all ages that can swallow capsules. If pregnant or lactating, women should consult a physician or health care provider before use.

A broader view: Microbial enzymes and their relevance in industries, medicine, and beyond, Gurung N, Ray S, Bose S, Rai V, *Biomed Res Int* 2013

Enzyme replacement therapy for pancreatic insufficiency: Present and future, Fieker A, philpott J, Armand M, *Clinical and Experimental Gastroenterology*, 2011

Randomised clinical trial: A 1-week, double-blind, placebo-controlled study of pancreatin 25000 Ph. Eur. Minimicrospheres for pancreatic exocrine insufficiency after pancreatic surgery, with a 1-year open-label extension, Seiler Cm, Izbicki J, Varga-Szabo L, et al, *Aliment Pharmacol Ther*, 2013

Fate of pancreatic enzymes during small intestinal aboral transit in humans, Layer P, Go VLW, DiMagno EP, *Intraluminal Fate of Pancreatic Enzymes*, 1986

Effects of different levels of supplementary alpha-amylase on digestive enzyme activities and pancreatic amylase mRNA expression of young broilers, Jiang Z, Zhou Y, Lu F, et al, *Asian-Aust J Anim Sci*. 2008

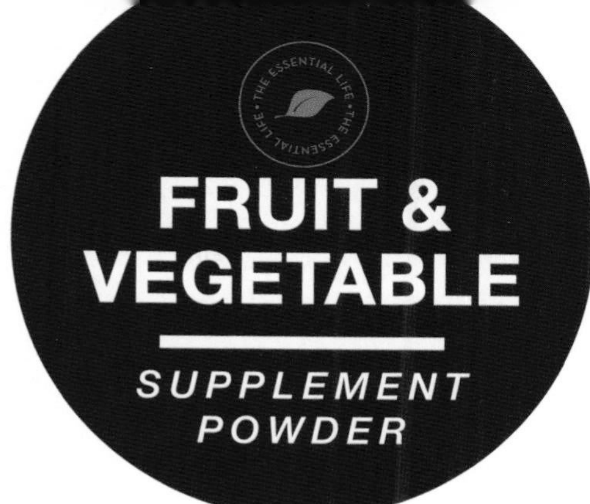

FRUIT & VEGETABLE

SUPPLEMENT POWDER

TOP USES

For people with poor nutrition, busy and stressful lifestyle habits, weight management, compromised digestion and immunity.

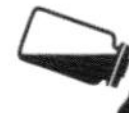

INGREDIENTS

- Green Powder Blend (kale, dandelion greens, spinach, parsley, collard greens leaf, broccoli, cabbage): Phytonutrients, which are cleansing to the body and immune building. Also anticancer and antioxidant properties.
- Grass Powder blend (wheat grass, alfalfa juice, oat grass, barley grass, oat grass juice and barley grass juice): High in chlorophyll and other phytonutrients which have powerful blood-cleansing and -strengthening properties as well as enhancing immune function.
- Fruit Powder blend (pineapple juice, guava fruit, mango juice, goji berry, mangosteen, and acerola cherry): Powerful antioxidant and free radical scavenging properties.
- Lemon Peel and Ginger Root Essential Oils: Aids in digestive and metabolic functions.

SAFETY

For all ages. Gluten-free and non-GMO. Vegan-friendly.

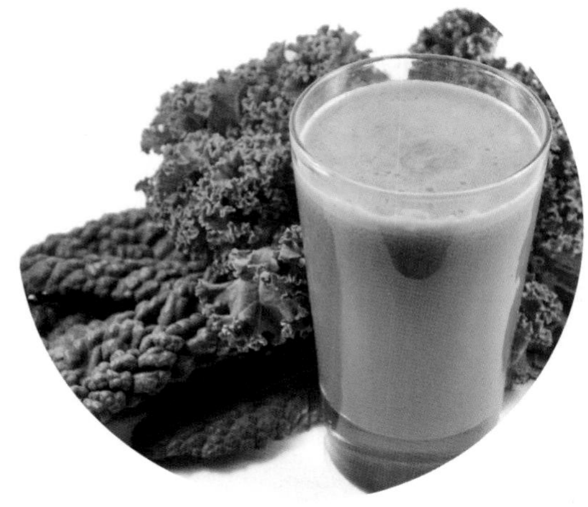

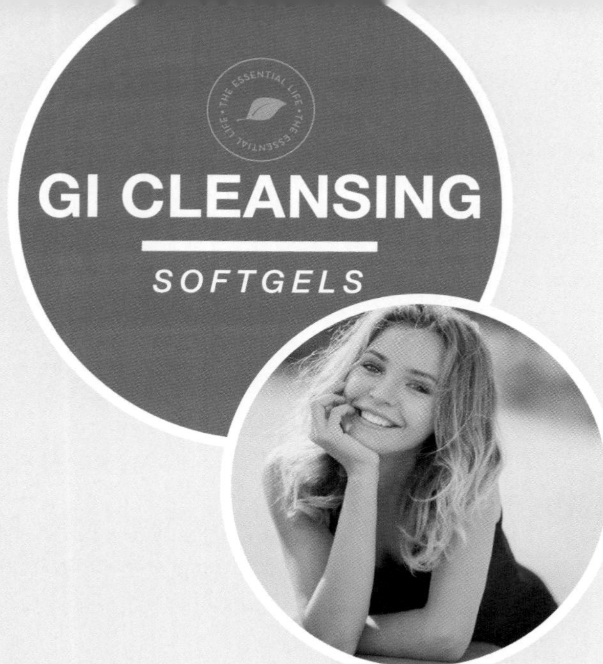

GI CLEANSING

SOFTGELS

A blend of essential oils that support a healthy gastrointestinal (GI) tract by decreasing the overgrowth of pathogens in the gut; thereby increasing gut integrity and creating a healthy environment for new, good bacteria to thrive.

TOP USES

For overgrowth of candida albicans and other negative pathogens, autoimmune diseases, compromised digestive system, brain fog, illness and infections.

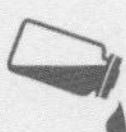

INGREDIENTS

- Oregano: Anti-fungal, anti-bacterial, anti-parasitic, decreases allergies, heartburn and bloating.
- Melaleuca: Fights bad bacteria, fungus, and yeast infections and supports the immune system.
- Lemon: Antioxidant, anti-microbial, increases liver health and glutathione (internal antioxidant) production.
- Lemongrass: Anti-inflammatory, anti-microbial, supports immunity and digestive health.
- Peppermint: Soothes digestion, decreases heartburn and upset stomach.
- Thyme: Decreases inflammation, nausea and fatigue, anti-parasitic and fights bad bacteria.

SAFETY

Keep out of reach of small children. If pregnant or lactating, women should consult a physician or health care provider before use.

Effect of thyme oil on small intestine integrity and antioxidant status, phagocytic activity and gastrointestinal microbiota in rabbits, Placha I, Chrastinova L, Laukova A, et al, Acta Veterinaria Hungarica. 2013

Antimicrobial activity of essential oils against Helicobacter pylori, Ohno T, Kita M, Yamaoka Y, et al, *Helicobacter*, 2003

Inhibition of enteric parasites by emulsified oil of oregano in vivo, Force M, Sparks WS, Ronzio RA, *Phytotherapy Research*, 2000

Antimicrobial activity of five essential oils against origin strains of the Enterobacteriaceae family, Penalver P, Huerta B, Borge C, et al, *APMIS*, 2005

In vitro antibacterial activity of some plant essential oils, Prabuseenivasan S, Jayakumar M, Ignacimuthu S, *BMC Complementary and Alternative Medicine*, 2006

Antimicrobial and antioxidant activities of three Mentha species essential oils, Mimica-Dukic N, Bozin B, Sokovic M, et al, *Planta Med*, 2003

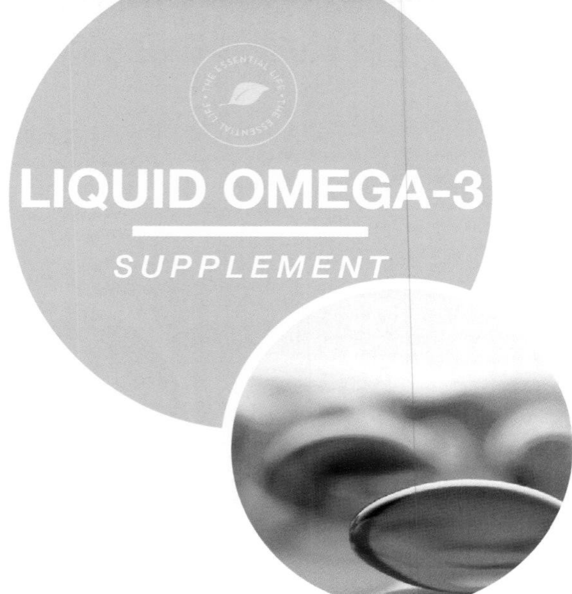

LIQUID OMEGA-3

SUPPLEMENT

This product has both eicosapentaenoic acid (EPA) and docosahexaenoic acid (DHA) which combine to make up a balance of omega 3 essential fatty acids in fish oil form. Blended with essential oils to bring a less fishy flavor and more pleasant one.

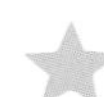

TOP USES

Brain fog, ADD/ADHD, Cardiovascular disease, dry skin, joint pain and arthritis, anything "itis", weak muscles, and compromised immune system.

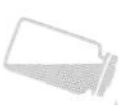

INGREDIENTS

- EPA: Essential fatty acid shown to increase mood, well being, cognitive function, nerve cell function and overall health of joints and inflammation in the body.
- DHA: Essential fatty acid shown to increase brain function, concentration, attention, memory, joint health, cell membrane integrity, nerve cell function, immunity and decrease inflammation.
- Essential oils blend, wild orange: For flavor

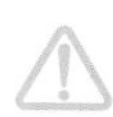

SAFETY

Keep out of reach of small children, keep refrigerated after opening.

Omega-3 fatty acid intakes are inversely related to elevated depressive symptoms among United States women, Beydoun MA, Kuczmarski MTF, Beydoun HA, et a, *J Nutr* 2013

Low blood long chain omega-3 fatty acids in UK children are associated with poor cognitive performance and behavior: A cross-sectional analysis from the DOLAB study, Montgomery P, Burton JR, Sewell RP, et al, *PLoS ONE*. 2013

Omega-3 fatty acids; Their beneficial role in cardiovascular health, Schwalfenberg G, *Can Fam Physician*. 2006

Omega-3 polyunsaturated fatty acids and the treatment of rheumatoid arthritis; a meta-analysis, Lee YH, Bae SC, Song GG, *Arch Med Res*, 2012

Effect of omega-3 fatty acids supplementation on endothelial function: A meta-analysis of randomized controlled trials, Wang Q, Liang X, Wang L, et al, *Atherosclerosis*. 2012

The importance of the ratio of omega-6/omega-3 essential fatty acids, Simopoulos AP, *Biomed Pharmacother*, 2002

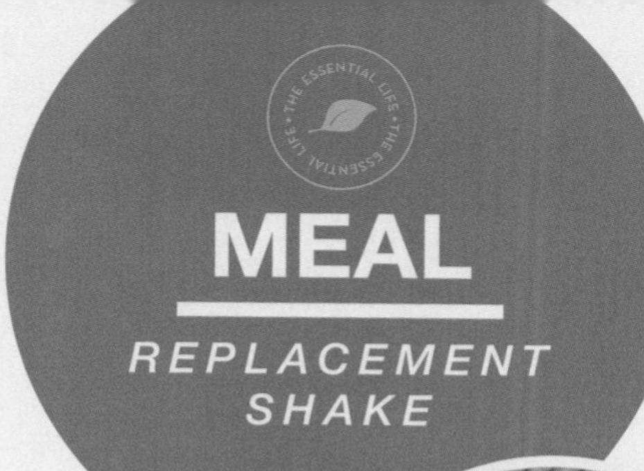

MEAL

REPLACEMENT SHAKE

A convenient and delicious weight management shake mix that provides low-fat, low-calorie, high-protein, high-fiber, nutrients as a lean alternative for individuals trying to lose fat or maintain a lean body composition through calorie reduction and exercise.

TOP USES

Weight management, poor nutrition, slow metabolism, and stressful lifestyle habits.

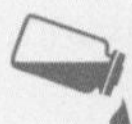

INGREDIENTS

- Protein Blend (Whey protein isolate and egg white protein): Proteins necessary for lean muscle recovery and development while promoting a healthy lifestyle through diet and exercise.
- Fiber Blend (Non-GMO soluble corn fiber, xanthan gum, citrus fiber, tara gum, oligofructose): A mixture of insoluble and prebiotic soluble fiber that promotes beneficial bacterial function and elimination.
- Ashwagandha root/leaf extract: An adaptogen for energy production, helps control the release of the stress hormone cortisol, which is associated with the accumulation of fat, particularly around the stomach, hips, and thighs. Has also been demonstrated to help control stress induced appetite, overeating, and carbohydrate cravings, helps support blood sugar levels, enhances energy, and alleviates fatigue.
- Potato Protein Powder: Supports an increased feeling of satiety, and helps to control snacking between meals, portion control, and feeling full faster and longer.
- Vitamin and mineral blend: Creates a synergy of nutrients similar to whole foods.

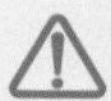

SAFETY

For all ages. Gluten free and non GMO.

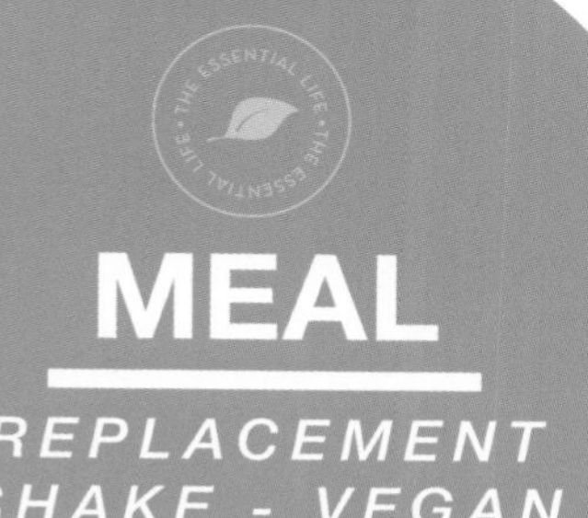

MEAL

REPLACEMENT SHAKE - VEGAN

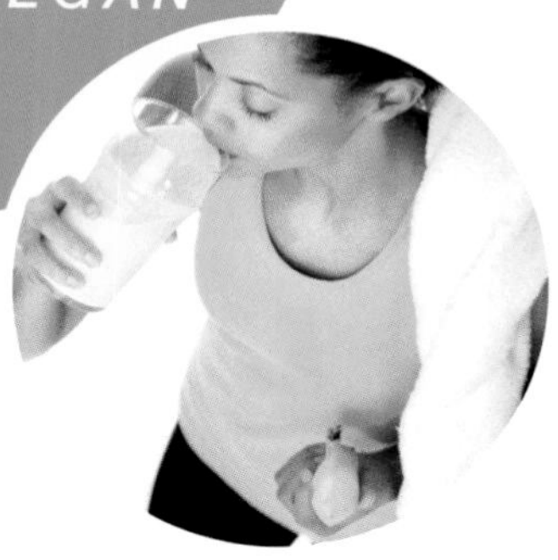

A convenient and delicious weight management vegan shake mix that provides low-fat, low-calorie, high-protein, high-fiber, nutrients as a lean alternative for individuals trying to lose fat or maintain a lean body composition through calorie reduction and exercise.

TOP USES

Weight management, poor nutrition, slow metabolism, stressful lifestyle habits, and vegan alternative.

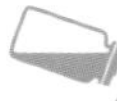

INGREDIENTS

- Protein Blend (Pea protein, quinoa, and amaranth): Proteins necessary for lean muscle recovery and development while promoting a healthy lifestyle through diet and exercise.
- Fiber Blend (Non-GMO soluble corn fiber, xanthan gum, citrus fiber, tara gum, oligofructose): A mixture of insoluble and prebiotic soluble fiber that promotes beneficial bacterial function and elimination.
- Ashwagandha root/leaf extract: An adaptogen for energy production, helps control the release of the stress hormone cortisol, which is associated with the accumulation of fat, particularly around the stomach, hips, and thighs. Has also been demonstrated to help control stress induced appetite, overeating, and carbohydrate cravings, helps support blood sugar levels, enhances energy, and alleviates fatigue.
- Potato Protein Powder: Supports an increased feeling of satiety, and helps to control snacking between meals, portion control, and feeling full faster and longer.
- Vitamin and mineral blend: Creates a synergy of nutrients similar to whole foods.

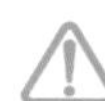

SAFETY

For all ages. Gluten-free, and non-GMO.

Slows gastric emptying, reducing postprandial levels of insulin and glucose Schwartz JG, Guan D, Green GM, Phillips WT, *Diabetes Care*, 1994

Protease inhibitor concentrate derived from potato reduced food intake and weight gain in healthy rats by increasing CCK levels, Komarnytsky S, Cook A, Raskin I, *International Journal of Obesity*, 2011

Taking two capsules a day of 300 mg ashwagandha root extract each for 60 days resulted in a significant reduction in cortisol levels, Chandrasekhar K, Kapoor J, Anishetty S, *Indian Journal of Psychological Medicine*, 2012

A low-fat, high–protein diet seems to enhance weight loss and provide a better long term maintenance of reduced intra-abdominal fat stores, Due A, Toubro S, Skov AR, Astrup A, *International Journal of Obesity*. 2004

An energy-restricted, high-protein, low-fat diet provides nutritional and metabolic benefits that are equal to and sometimes greater than those observed with a high-carbohydrate diet, Noakes M, Keogh JB, Foster PR, Clifton PM, *American Journal of Clinical Nutrition*, 2005

A standardized withania somnifera extract significantly reduces stress-related parameters in chronically stressed humans: A double-blind, randomized, placebo controlled study, Auddy B, Hazra J, Mitra A, et al, *The Journal of the American Nutraceutical Association*, 2008

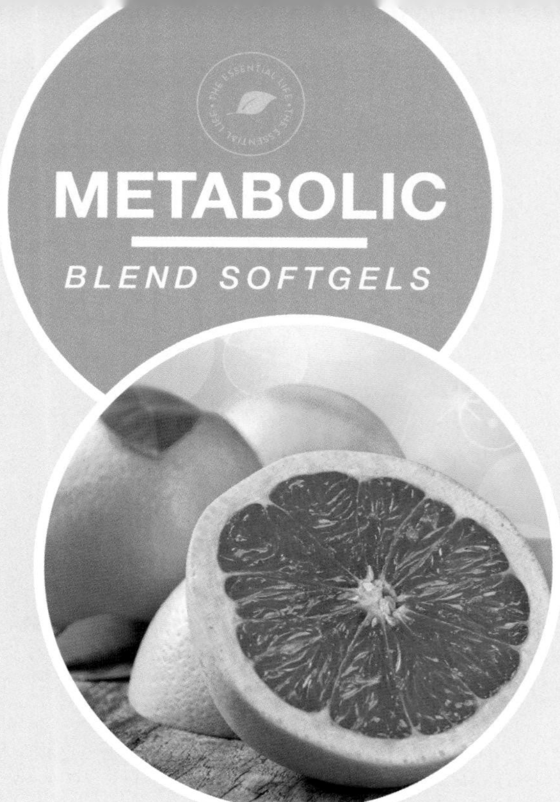

METABOLIC

BLEND SOFTGELS

A blend of essential oils in convenient softgels to help manage hunger throughout the day while boosting metabolism and promoting a positive mood, cleanse the body, aide digestion, curb the appetite, provide a stimulating and positive effect on the endocrine system and to assist with weight loss.

TOP USES

Slow metabolism, overweight or obese individuals, lack of energy (fatigue), diabetes, toxic liver, and compromised endocrine system.

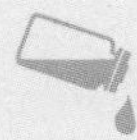

INGREDIENTS

- Grapefruit: Promotes cleansing, detoxifying, decreases appetite, and induces lipolysis (mobilization of fat cells from stored fat).
- Lemon: Cleansing, aids digestion, powerful antioxidant, increases lipolysis, and elevates the mood.
- Peppermint: Helps manage hunger cravings, soothes digestion, and invigorates the mind.
- Ginger: Promotes healthy digestion and enhances metabolism and thermogenesis (increased heat through metabolic stimulation).
- Cinnamon: Has a positive effect on the endocrine system to assist with weight loss, lowers blood sugar, and balances insulin response. Also inhibits adipogenesis (fat storage).

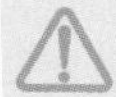

SAFETY

Not for children. Keep out of reach of small children. If pregnant or lactating, women should consult a physician or health care provider before use.

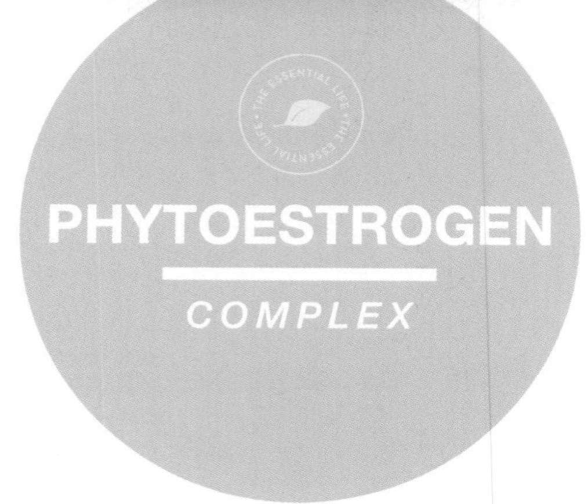

PHYTOESTROGEN

COMPLEX

Blend of standardized extracts of plant (phyto) estrogens and lignans to help create a balance of hormones throughout the body and eliminate unwanted metabolites.

TOP USES

Menopause, perimenopause, andropause, hormonal imbalances and mood swings (PMS).

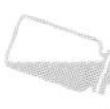

INGREDIENTS

- Genistein (soy extract): An isoflavone antioxidant that promotes healthy breast and uterine tissue and brings balance to hormones in both men and women. Also shown to help prevent prostate cancer in men and ovarian and breast cancer in women.
- Flax seed extract (lignans): Decreases estrogen metabolites for further hormone balance and protection of the sex organ tissues and cells.
- Pomegranate extract: Powerful antioxidant shown to help the reduction of free radical damage to the cells.

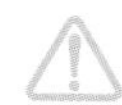

SAFETY

Not for children. Keep out of reach of small children. Okay for men and women. If pregnant or lactating, women should consult a physician or health care provider before use.

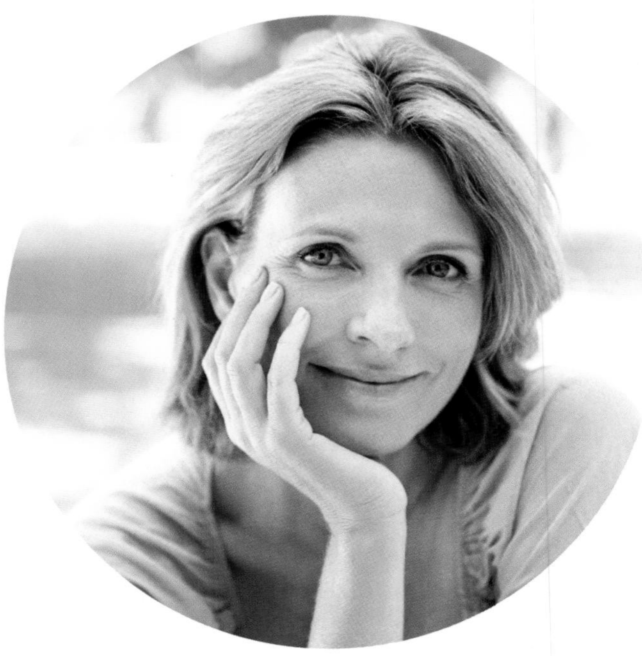

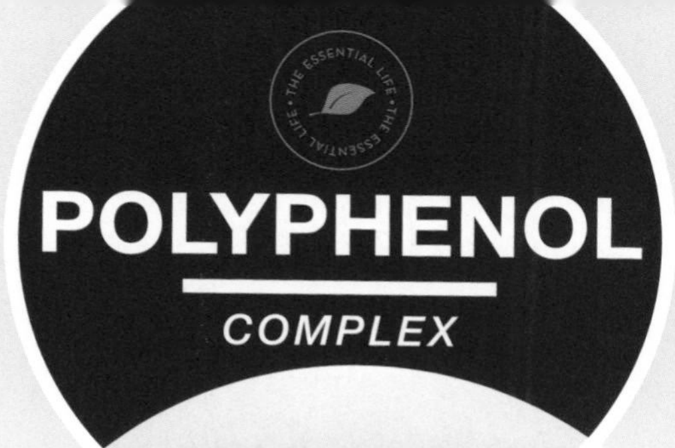

POLYPHENOL
COMPLEX

A blend of powerful polyphenols clinically tested to help soreness and discomfort from physical activities and daily life.

TOP USES

Joint pain, inflammation, arthritis, rheumatoid arthritis and anything "itis", fibromyalgia, sore muscles, Alzheimer's Disease, and cancer prevention.

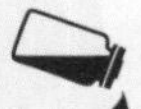

INGREDIENTS

- Frankincense (Boswellia serrata) gum resin extract: Inflammatory modulator which helps regulate and decrease inflammation and pain.
- Curcumin: Extract from turmeric, has been shown to inhibit amyloid beta plaque formation and decrease risk of Alzheimer's Disease. Also shows powerful anti-inflammatory properties.
- Ginger root extract: Reduces pain and inflammation, warming effect and increases circulation.
- Green Tea Leaf extract (caffeine-free): Powerful antioxidant, free radical scavenger, and anticancer properties
- Pomegranate Fruit extract: Antioxidant shown to lower LDL cholesterol, blood pressure, and increase heart health.
- Grape Seed extract: 95% polyphenols shown to decrease free radical damage and increase cellular repair.
- Resveratrol: Increases healthy cell proliferation and inhibits proliferation of damaged and mutated cells.
- Digestion blend of peppermint leaf, ginger root, caraway seed: Helps soothe the digestive process and tames the stomach.

SAFETY

Not for use for children. If pregnant or lactating, women should consult a physician or health care provider before use.

J Biol Chem. 2005 Feb 18;280(7):5892-901. Epub 2004 Dec 7.Curcumin inhibits formation of amyloid beta oligomers and fibrils, binds plaques, and reduces amyloid in vivo.Yang F1, Lim GP, Begum AN, Ubeda OJ, Simmons MR, Ambegaokar SS, Chen PP, Kayed R, Glabe CG, Frautschy SA, Cole GM.

BMC Cancer. 2015;15(1):1119. doi: 10.1186/s12885-015-1119-y. Epub 2015 Mar 5. Resveratrol suppresses epithelial-to-mesenchymal transition in colorectal cancer through TGF-Ð1/Smads signaling pathway mediated Snail/E-cadherin expression. Ji Q1, Liu X, Han Z, Zhou L, Sui H, Yan L, Jiang H, Ren J, Cai J, Li Q.

Yadav, V.R., Prasad S., Sung, B., Gelovani, J. G., Guha, S., Krishnan, S. and Aggarwal, B.B. Boswellic acid inhibits growth and metastasis of human colorectal cancer in orthotopic mouse model by downregulating inflammatory, proliferative, invasive and angiogenic biomarkers. Int. J. Cancer: 2012 130: 2176–2184.

Di Lorenzo C, Dell'agli M, Badea M, et al. Plant food supplements with anti-inflammatory properties: A systematic review. Critical Reviews in Food Science and Nutrition. 2013;53(5):507-516.

Int J Rheum Dis. 2013 Apr;16(2):219-29. doi: 10.1111/1756-185X.12054. Epub 2013 Apr 4. Protective effects of ginger-turmeric rhizomes mixture on joint inflammation, atherogenesis, kidney dysfunction and other complications in a rat model of human rheumatoid arthritis. Ramadan G1, El-Menshawy O.

Tangney CC, Rasmussen HE. Polyphenols, inflammation, and cardiovascular disease. Curr Atheroscler Rep. 2013;15:324-334.

Kidd PM. Bioavailability and activity of phytosome complexes from botanical polyphenols: The silymarin, curcumin, green tea, and grape seed extracts. Alternative Medicine Review. 2009;14(3):226-246

Sontakke S, Thawani V, Pimpalkhute S, Kapra P, Babhulkar S, Hingorani L. Open, randomized controlled clinical trial of Boswellia serrata extract as compared to valdecoxib in osteoarthritis of knee. Indian Journal of Pharmacology. 2007;39:27-29.

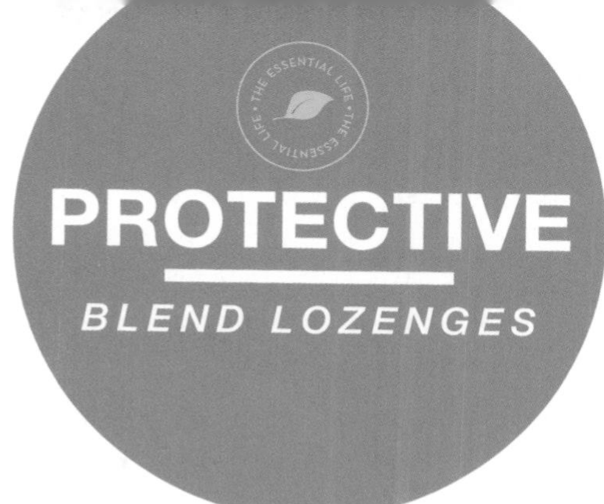

PROTECTIVE
BLEND LOZENGES

A blend of several essential oils in a convenient, organically sweetened throat lozenge that soothe the throat and protect the immune system from foreign invaders. (pathogens).

TOP USES

Sore or dry throat, cough, colds and flu, illness, laryngitis, preventative care, and compromised immunity.

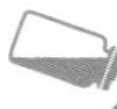

INGREDIENTS

- Wild orange: Antioxidant and anti-inflammatory properties, antimicrobial and promotes healthy digestion.
- Clove: Powerful antioxidant, anti-parasitic and anti-fungal properties, improves blood circulation, decreases pain (numbing agent) and inflammation, and inhibits pathogenic activity.
- Cinnamon: Highly anti-bacterial, anti-fungal, and anti-microbial, promotes healthy blood sugar and insulin balance.
- Eucalyptus: Decreases fevers, congestion and body pains, and has anti-viral effects on the respiratory system.
- Rosemary: Great expectorant/decongestant, increases memory and concentration, inflammation and has a balancing effect on the endocrine system.
- Myrrh: Supports blood flow to gums and teeth, antioxidant properties.
- Organic cane juice: Natural sweetener
- Organic brown rice syrup: Natural sweetener

SAFETY

Be aware of small children that are prone to choking.

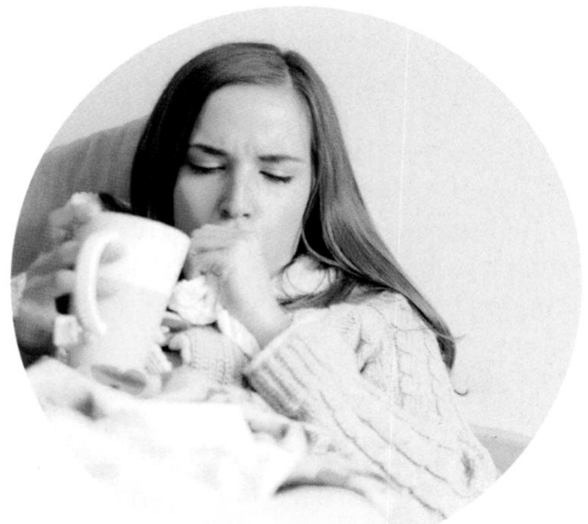

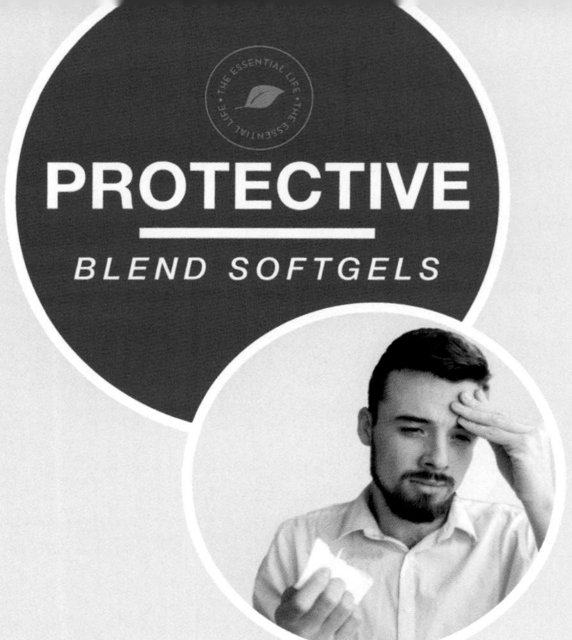

PROTECTIVE

BLEND SOFTGELS

A blend of several essential oils in a convenient softgel that protect the immune system from foreign invaders (pathogens).

TOP USES

Sore or dry throat, cough, colds and flus, illness, laryngitis, preventative care, and compromised immunity.

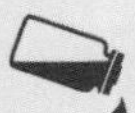

INGREDIENTS

- Wild Orange Peel oil: Antioxidant and anti-inflammatory properties, antimicrobial and promotes healthy digestion.
- Clove Bud oil: Powerful antioxidant, anti-parasitic and anti-fungal properties, improves blood circulation, decreases pain (numbing agent) and inflammation, and inhibits pathogenic activity.
- Black Pepper Seed oil: Antiseptic, anti-catarrhal, and expectorant properties. Helps respiratory system by promoting blood flow and circulation.
- Cinnamon Bark oil: Highly anti-bacterial, anti-fungal, and anti-microbial, promotes healthy blood sugar and insulin balance.
- Eucalyptus Leaf oil: Decreases fevers, congestion and body pains, and has anti-viral effects on the respiratory system.
- Oregano Leaf oil: Powerful antibacterial, antiviral, and antifungal properties. Helps support the immune system against ailments.
- Rosemary Leaf/Flower oil: Great expectorant/decongestant, increases memory and concentration, inflammation and has a balancing effect on the endocrine system.
- Melissa Leaf oil: Antiviral properties and supports against respiratory ailments.

SAFETY

Not for children. Keep out of reach of small children. If pregnant or lactating, women should consult a physician or health care provider before use.

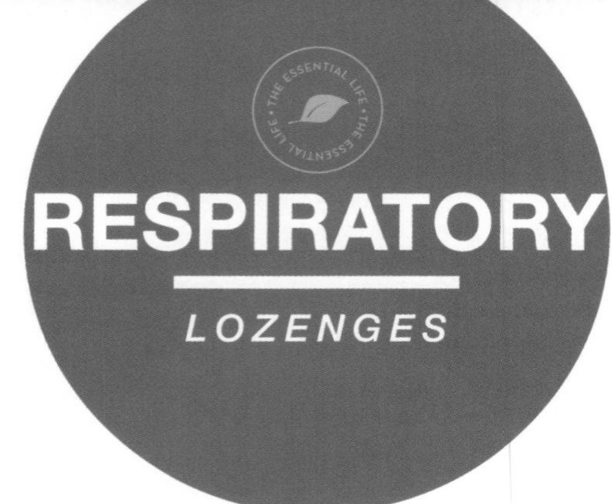

RESPIRATORY

LOZENGES

A blend of essential oils in a convenient, organically sweetened throat lozenge for the use of opening the airways a supporting the respiratory system.

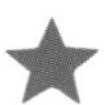

TOP USES

Congestion, head cold, sore throat, bronchitis, asthma, allergies, cough, sinusitis, bad breath, and motion sickness.

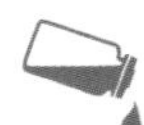

INGREDIENTS

- Laurel Leaf: Shown to decrease symptoms of bronchitis, asthma, and viral infections.
- Cardamom: Clears and opens respiratory system, promotes digestion, decreases nausea and motion sickness.
- Peppermint: Bronchodilator, soothes digestion, anti-inflammatory, stimulates brain.
- Eucalyptus: Decreases fevers, congestion and body pains; and antiviral effects on the respiratory system.
- Melaleuca: Fights bad bacteria and fungus, and supports a healthy immune system.
- Lemon: Antioxidant, antiseptic, promotes physical energy, health and cleansing.
- Ravensara: Powerful antioxidant, antifungal, and anti-infectious, opens and strengthens the respiratory system.

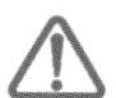

SAFETY

Be aware of small children that are prone to choking.

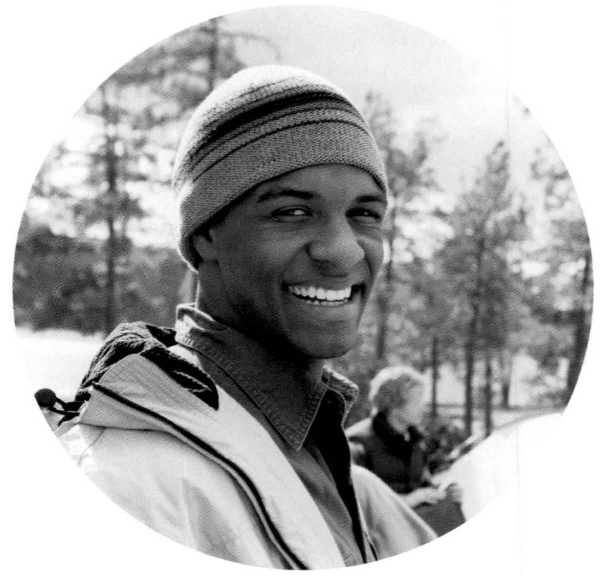

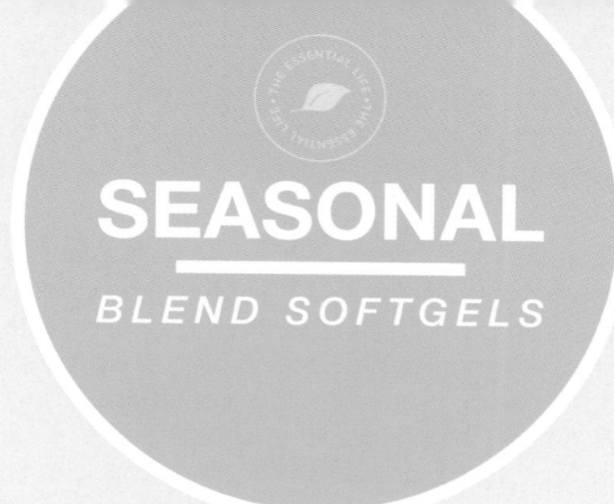

A blend of essential oils in a convenient softgel to be consumed quickly and easily when traveling, attending outdoor events, or when seasonal or environmental elements are particularly high, or on a daily basis during times of seasonal discomfort to promote clear breathing and overall respiratory health.

TOP USES

Seasonal allergies, hay fever, congestion, head colds and headaches, bronchitis, asthma, and sinusitis

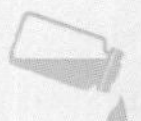

INGREDIENTS

- Lemon: Antioxidant, antiseptic, promotes respiratory health and cleansing.
- Lavender: Renowned for its calming and balancing effects, both internally and externally.
- Peppermint: Bronchodilator, soothes digestion, stimulates brain and helps decrease allergy symptoms.

SAFETY

Be aware of small children that are prone to choking.

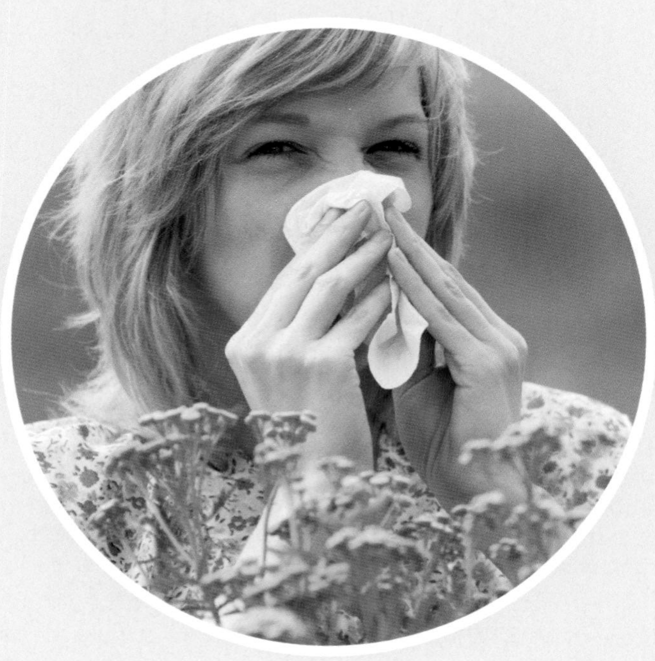

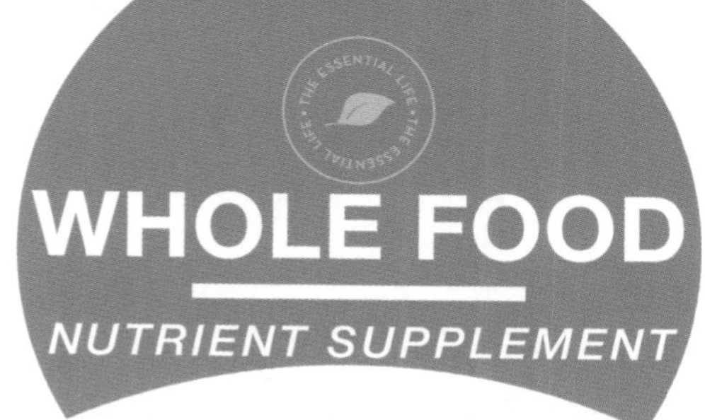

Revolutionary micronutrient supplement providing naturally balanced amounts of all vitamins, minerals, trace elements, phytonutrients and antioxidants that give your body the most beneficial and safe amounts needed for long term health and vitality.

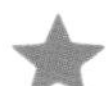

TOP USES

Low energy and fatigue, compromised digestion and immunity, oxidative cell damage, malnutrition, poor health and imbalanced nutrition.

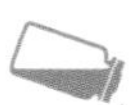

INGREDIENTS

- Water soluble vitamins, B-complex and C: Support energy and enhances macronutrient metabolism, transportation and elimination; enhances immunity and cognitive function, and strengthens the viscosity of the mucosa membranes lining the smooth muscle of the GI tract.
- Fat soluble vitamins A, E and K: Increases free radical scavenging, enhances utilization of macro-minerals and increases immune function.
- Vitamin D3: Immune system regulator. Enhances maro- mineral absorption, hormone balance, muscle health. Increases cognitive function.
- Macro-minerals (calcium, iron, iodine, magnesium, zinc, selenium, copper, manganese and chromium): Supports and enhances bone strength and density, proper bowel health, muscle contraction and release, fluid balance, nervous system health, cell function, immunity, anti-oxidation and hormone health.
- Polyphenol Blend (Grape seed extract, Quercetin, rutin, pomegranate fruit extract, citrus fruit polyphenol extract, resveratrol, Indian kino tree wood extract): enhances free radical scavenging, decreases inflammation, increases proper cellular function and proliferation.
- Whole Foods Blend (Kale leaf extract, dandelion leaf powder, parsley leaf powder, spinach leaf powder, broccoli aerial parts powder, cabbage leaf extract, Brussels sprout immature inflorescences powder): A blend of whole foods and phytonutrients which enhance digestion and absorption of micronutrients and give balanced nutrition.
- Stomach Comfort Blend of ginger root extract, peppermint extract and caraway seed extract: Calms and soothes the digestive process.

SAFETY

Can be taken by all ages that can swallow capsules.

Selected vitamins and trace elements support immune function by strengthening epithelial barriers and cellular and humoral immune responses, Maggini S, Wintergerst ES, Beveridge S, Hornig DH, *British Journal of Nutrition*. 2007
Contribution of selected vitamins and trace elements to immune function, Wintergerst ES, Maggini S, Hornig DH, *Ann Nutr Met*, 2007
Efficacy and tolerability of a fixed combination of peppermint oil and caraway oil in patients suffering from functional dyspepsia, May B, Kohler S, Schneider B, *Aliment Pharmacol Therapy*. 2000
The immunological functions of the vitamin D endocrine system, Hayes CE, Nashold FE, Spach KM & Pedersen LB, *Cell Molec Biol*, 2003
Use of calcium or calcium in combination with vitamin D supplementation to prevent fractures and bone loss in people aged 50 years and older: a meta-analysis, Tang BMP, Eslick GD, Nowson C, et al, *The Lancet*, 2007

Tips for Taking Supplements

- **Partner with quality.** Use supplements with optimal, not exaggerated or deficient, levels of nutrients by buying from a reputable source.
- **Dose diligence.** All products provide dose recommendations. Maximal benefit comes from the consistent use of a variety of specific and complementary supplements. When first starting a program, some individuals may choose to start with a lower dose and work up. The basic recommendations may be adequate or even excessive for a healthy person who has implemented a healthy diet, lifestyle, and regular supplementation program. However, someone with longstanding health issues may require an extensive regimen that may include consumption beyond label recommendations.
- **Start slowly.** Over the course of the first week, start with a few supplements at lower doses and then add from there. This will support awareness of how individual supplements make you feel. Gradually add others and increase doses of each supplement. Synergy between supplements coupled with using the proper therapeutic dose is generally required to achieve optimal benefit. Most supplements can be taken at the same time.
- **Time it right.** Most people do better taking supplements with food while digestive processes are in action. Use on an empty stomach (except at bedtime) can trigger nausea. Just a few bites of food can be enough (e.g. half a banana). Avoid taking with tea, coffee, soda, or even some dairy products as this can interfere with absorption. Dinner and bedtime are also excellent times of day as the body's repair mode and hormone secretions are at their highest capacity while sleeping. Most products recommend dividing doses, say two or three times during the day. Spreading consumption over the course of the day maximizes absorption.
- **Make it a habit.** Consider targeting two set times per day to establish routine or ritual for basic daily nutrition habits. This is what most people can handle and remember. Add additional times for other supplemental needs. In the beginning, or as needed, place reminders in line of sight or set alarms.
- **Be practical.** Keep your supplements in locations that provide easy access. Most do not require refrigeration, so keeping them out on kitchen and bathroom counters creates visibility and supports routine use. Many people find it useful to purchase some kind of pill box or container that allows a week's worth of supplements to be pre-counted and organized for each day. This way, consumption can be accomplished quickly or supplements easily placed in a pocket or small container to consume later. Marking on lids with markers or posting a sheet on the inside of a cupboard door for dose instruction can also be helpful. Use a small cup or glass to put the capsules in before you take them. Keep it close by for reuse.
- **Stay the course.** Most people experience an increased sense of well being when beginning a supplementation program. Some individuals are an exception and feel worse before starting to feel better. A few common causes of discomfort are the elimination of microbes or dealing with chronic illness or disease. In Lyme disease treatment, this phenomenon is referred to as a Herxheimer reaction, but it can occur with any microbial infection. If a new symptom occurs that can be specifically defined as a side effect to a particular supplement (such as nausea after taking a certain supplement), consider first if it was taken with food. If an exacerbation of symptoms occurs, reduce the dose of supplements until symptoms ease and then gradually increase the dose again over time. If adverse reactions occur that seem beyond these parameters, consider discontinuing use until issues can be addressed or a more suitable choice can be made.
- **Make supplements part of your lifestyle.** Supplements to support general health can be continued indefinitely and are an excellent component of a healthy lifestyle. Supplements that support immune function, reduce inflammation, and provide antimicrobial properties should be continued at the higher doses recommended until symptoms subside, when doses may be reduced or supplements discontinued completely. Rotate different supplements over time as needed. Consider intermittent programs to maintain health results. For example, engage in a quarterly detox program for the duration of fourteen to thirty days as a complementary commitment to a basic daily routine.

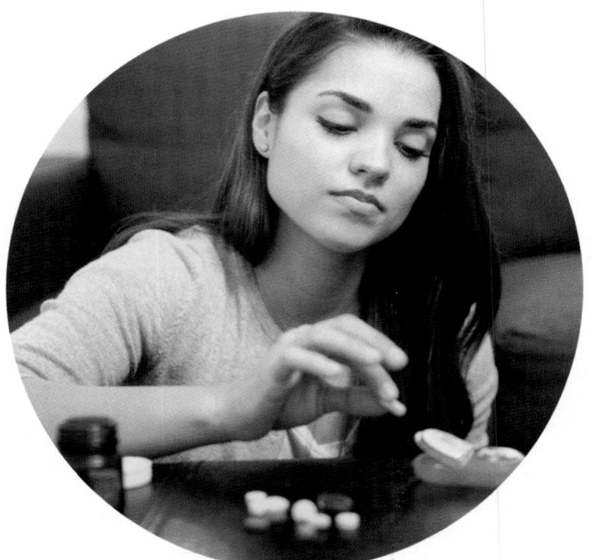

- **Take them along.** When you travel, take your supplements with you. Get a pill box that contains specific, marked sections for different times of the day. Most allow for a week's worth of doses. Plastic baggies can hold capsules for single use or to contain individual products. Use a permanent marker to label the baggies "am" or "pm" or identify the product contained.
- **Store them right.** Keep supplements out of windowsills or away from other sources of bright light. Store in dark or opaque bottles away from microwaves and other electromagnetic sources.

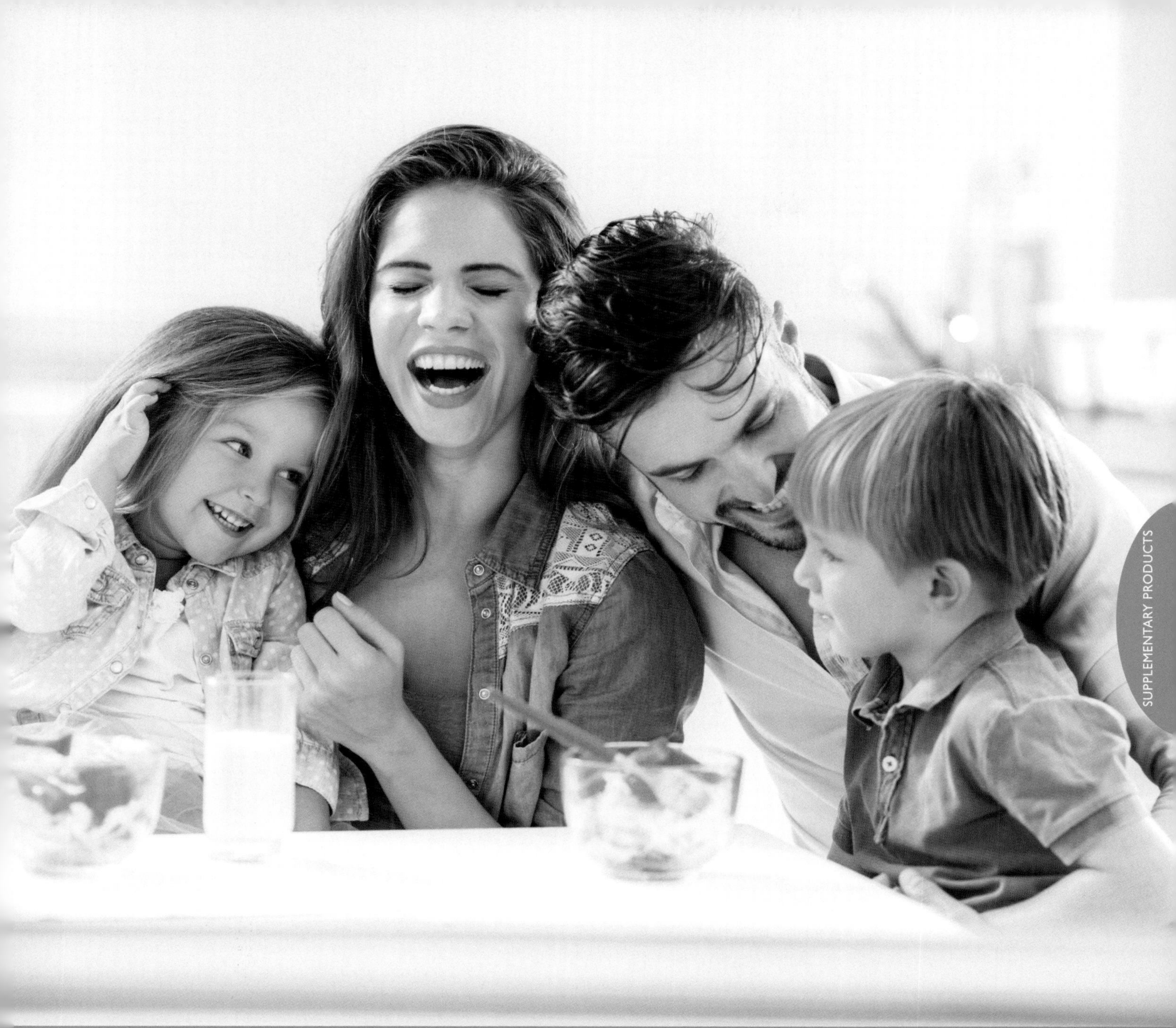

Additional Information

- **Herxheimer reactions.** Die-off of bacteria can intensify symptoms of fatigue, muscle pain, and feeling flu-like. Generally, herxheimer reactions are more common and more intense with conventional antibiotic therapy, but they can still occur with natural supplements. If you feel that you are having herxheimer reactions, back off on dose and then increase gradually and slowly.
- **Excessive stimulation.** One of the greatest benefits of natural supplementation is an increased energy and reserves. Generally this is welcomed during the day but can be a problem at night while trying to sleep. If you notice an effect, take primary supplements in the morning and afternoon.
- **Dealing with adverse effects:** Adverse effects associated with taking natural supplements are uncommon, but possible. Fortunately, most are mild and transient, and you should be able to work around them.
- **Upset stomach.** The most common adverse effects are an upset stomach, indigestion, mild nausea, and discomfort mid-chest or on the left side under the lower rib cage (where the stomach is located). First consider if consumption occurred on an empty or overly full stomach and adjust accordingly. Otherwise, if necessary, take a break from the supplements for a few days to a week. Consider adding an essential oil such as ginger, peppermint, or digestive blend to soothe upset. If chronic digestive issues already existed, additional considerations may need to be made.

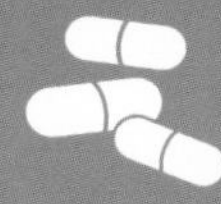

SECTION 4

BODY SYSTEMS & FOCUS AREAS

Take a holistic approach to wellness by learning to address wellness in terms of body systems. Think beyond the disease-symptom model, and instead focus on systems that govern the function of your entire body.

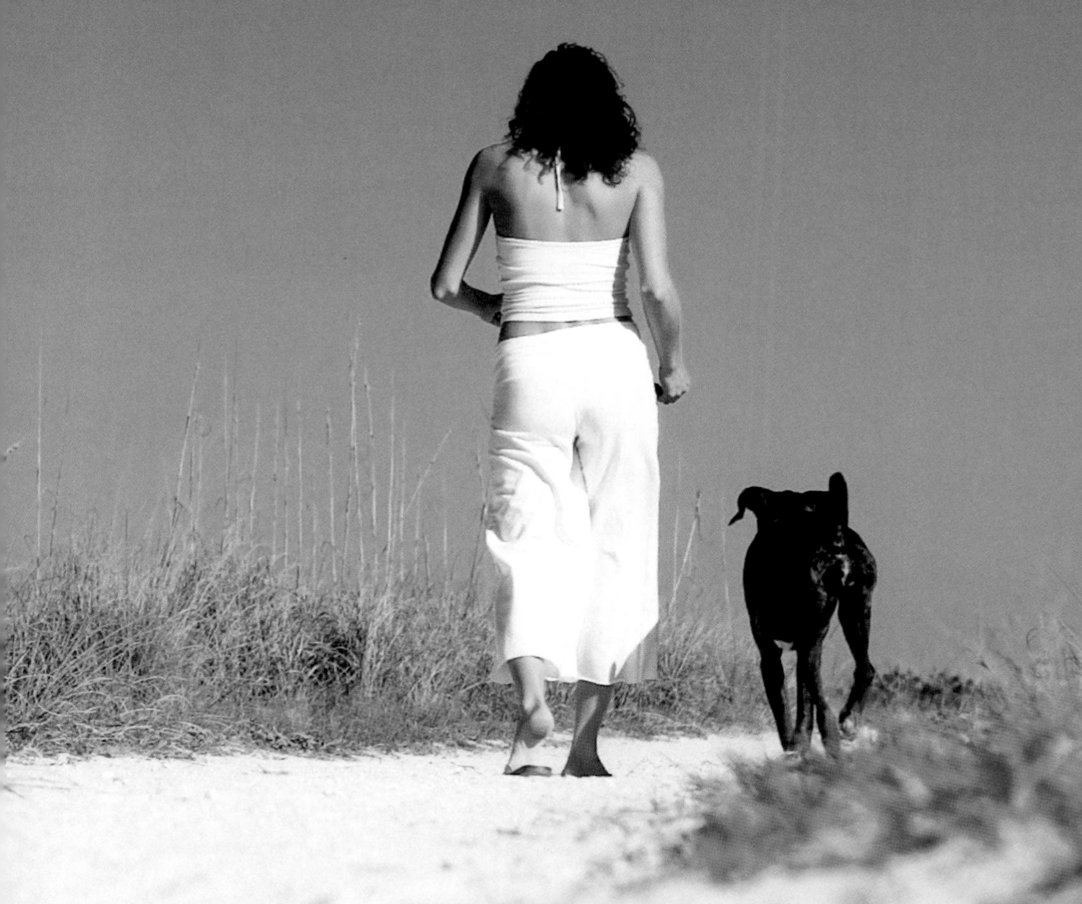

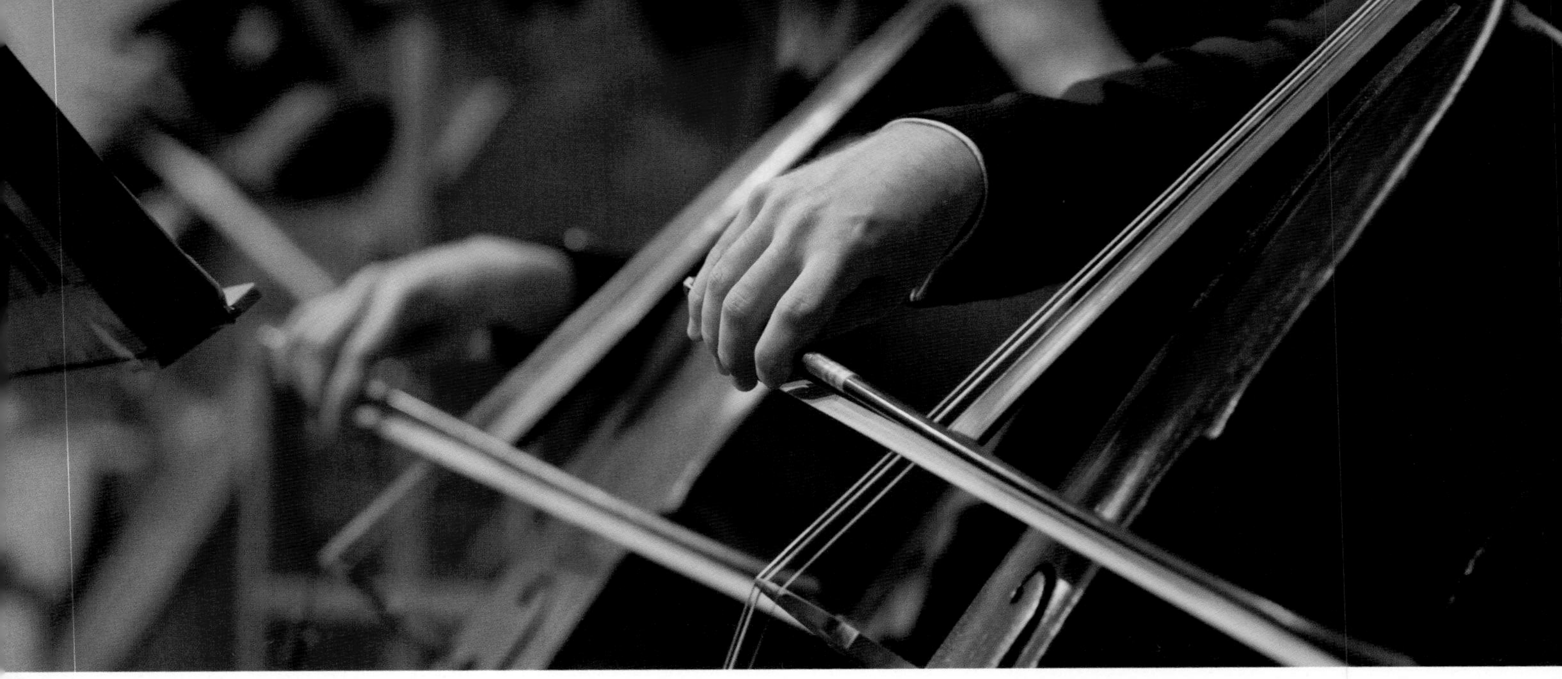

A HEALTHY BODY is like a finely tuned symphony orchestra. An orchestra is divided into sections, and sections are comprised of individual instruments. Similarly, the body is divided into sections called body systems that are comprised of individual organs. During a musical performance when out-of-tune sounds come from a single instrument, it affects not only that section, but the quality of music coming from entire orchestra. The conductor's role is to identify the underlying cause behind the affected sound, tuning and refining where necessary. So, too, is every individual the conductor of their own body's orchestrations and internal harmony in partnership with the body itself.

Take a Holistic Approach

By addressing wellness in terms of body systems, each individual is taking a holistic approach to wellness. Thinking beyond a disease-symptom model and focusing on the systems that govern the function of the entire body allows one to shift away from an ambulance mentality of "if it ain't broke don't fix it" to true whole-body thinking and a prevention mindset.

A holistic approach to wellness promotes living with a prevention mindset and addressing root causes when symptoms arise by providing support to entire body systems.

AMBULANCE APPROACH

ACKNOWLEDGE FEELING BAD → IDENTIFY SYMPTOMS → SEEK REMEDY FOR SYMPTOMS Seek prescribed advice to manage → OUTCOME
- Temporarily address symptoms
- Neglect underlying causes and body systems needs

→ SIDE EFFECTS APPEAR OR SYMPTOMS RETURN → (back to ACKNOWLEDGE FEELING BAD)

HOLISTIC APPROACH

PAY ATTENTION TO BODY → IDENTIFY SYMPTOMS Consider what body system(s) is affected and where symptoms are coming from → SEARCH BODY SYSTEMS Find conditions within system that best relate to what is being experienced → LEARN WHICH OILS ADDRESS CONDITION Address conditions by strengthening body with natural solutions → OUTCOME
- Gain knowledge and understanding of body systems and organ functions
- Consider underlying concerns that contribute (diet, sleep, stress, activity, etc.)
- Prevent issues from occurring and nurture lasting health results

Interconnectivity of All Body Systems

All body systems are interconnected. When one system is hindered or malfunctions other systems are impacted. Likewise, when one system is repaired and strengthened the whole body benefits and functions can be restored. For best success, think in terms of body systems to create true wellness, and learn to use natural healing tools to aid in this process.

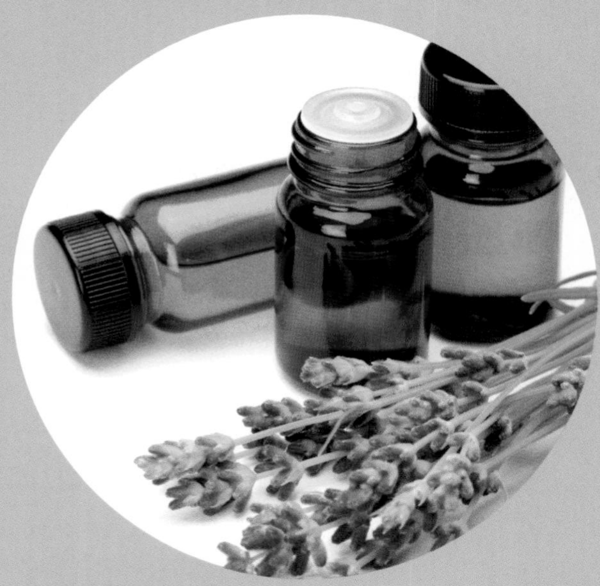

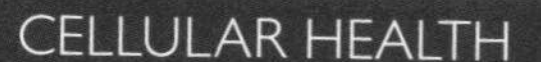

BIOLOGICAL TERRAIN

- Quality nutrients
- Water
- Oxygen
- Waste removal
- Chemical and temperature regulation
- Healthy cells are at the core of wellness.

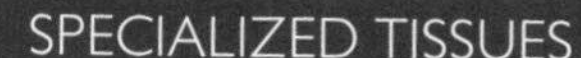

CELLULAR HEALTH

- Unhealthy cells, caused by deficiencies and toxicities, result in ailments or a diseased body.

SPECIALIZED TISSUES

- The needs of healthy cells are met by groups of specialized tissues. These tissues form organs and body systems. They perform functions to support cellular health, and consequently, the health of the whole body.

BODY SYSTEMS

- As body systems operate normally, they function synergistically together to create overall well being. Conditions form as specialized tissues and body systems fail to perform their normal functions. Failure to function eventually gives rise to ailments, the level where most people become conscious of their health.

tips

The Body Talks
Use the *Body Systems* sections to search conditions for solutions. The body uses specific symptoms to communicate it has unmet needs.

The Long and the Short of It
Oils provide support to systems and organs for resolving current conditions and root causes as well as long-term prevention.

The Multitaskers
While essential oil use is supporting one system, their complex chemistry supports other systems and organs simultaneously.

Using the Body Systems Effectively

The Body Systems section of this book is designed to create an opportunity to learn, first, about a body system itself and gain a basic understanding of its purpose or role, its working parts, and what can potentially go wrong. Second, each section contains common ailments that can occur (solutions located in the Quick Reference A-Z), key oils and supplements to be learned as go-to solutions, usage tips, additional solutions to numerous conditions, and user recommended remedies.

One additional component of each section is "By Related Properties." This section allows the user to search for solutions by related properties to certain oils. For example, if one wanted to sleep better, one would search for a properties category such as "Calming" and find an oil of choice such as lavender or roman chamomile. To take this process to a "Power Oil User" (420) level, discover the properties chart in the back of the book and learn numerous properties of each single oil. This is the best way to comprehend and learn the multiplicity of actions an oil is capable of.

In conclusion, the desired outcome from use of *Body Systems* is to become a more experienced oil user, knowing how to "think for yourself," taking attention from symptoms to root causes, solutions, and preventative actions.

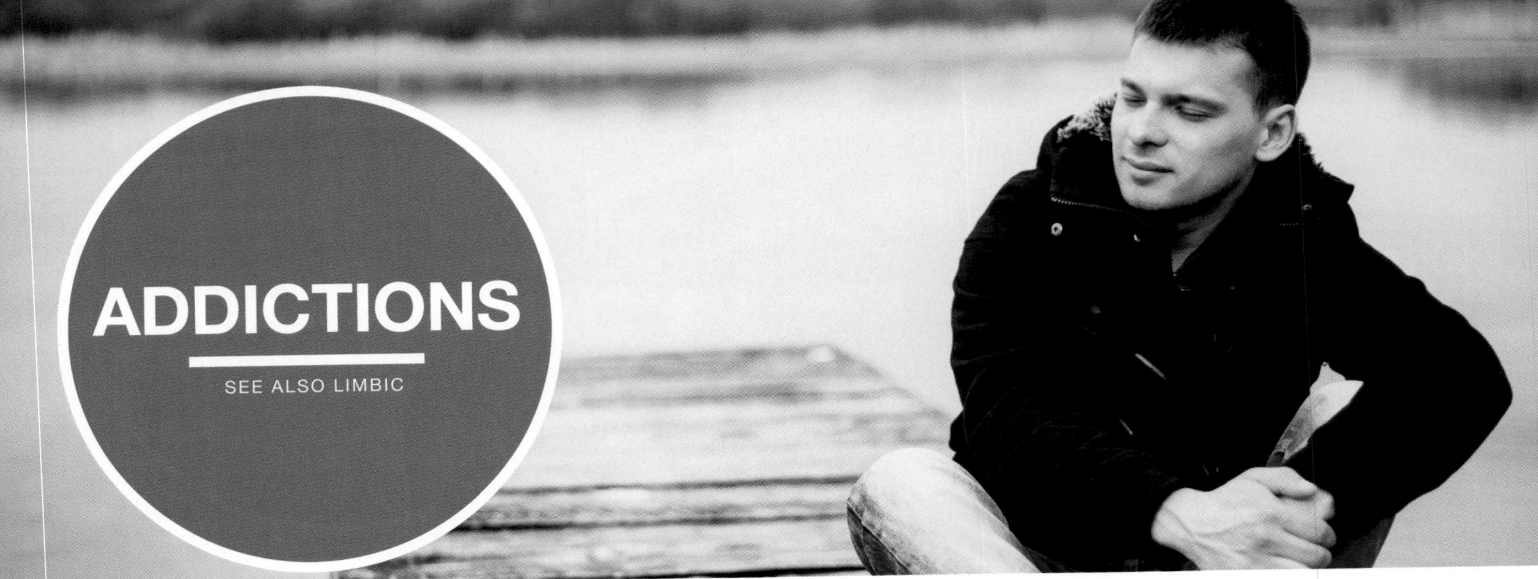

THE WORD "ADDICT" has a negative connotation, leading people to think of base individuals living among the dregs of society. But anyone can develop an addiction. To the brain, all addictions, regardless of the type, have similar damaging effects. The only difference is to the degree to which they occur. Although the substance or the body releases chemicals which enhance a "high," or feeling of euphoria, the pleasure response or relief from pain is only temporary.

Drug addiction is a powerful force that can take control of the lives of users. In the past, addiction was thought to be a weakness of character, but now research is proving that addiction is a matter of brain chemistry.

Dr. Nora Volkow, the director of the National Institute on Drug Abuse, says "the way a brain becomes addicted to a drug is related to how a drug increases levels of the naturally occurring neurotransmitter dopamine, which modulates the brain's ability to perceive reward reinforcement. The pleasure sensation that the brain gets when dopamine levels are elevated creates the motivation for us to proactively perform actions that are indispensable to our survival (like eating or procreation). Dopamine is what conditions us to do the things we need to do.

"Using addictive drugs floods the limbic brain with dopamine—taking it up to as much as five or ten times the normal level. With these levels elevated, the user's brain begins to associate the drug with an outsize neurochemical reward. Over time, by artificially raising the amount of dopamine our brains think is "normal," the drugs create a need that only they can meet." *

When the body starts to expect and incorporate this extra chemical release as part of normal body function, the addict experiences chemical addiction and will suffer from withdrawal symptoms if he or she tries to stop. To make matters worse, most addicts suffer from worsening problems in interpersonal relationships, since their psychological and physical need for relief takes over and replaces all other responsibilities that would enable them to lead a healthy, normal life (such as working, fully participating in family and social relationships, etc.). The results of addiction are typically nothing short of debilitating and eventually devastating.

There are many types of addiction, including but not limited to: alcohol, drugs, food, sugar, exercise, computer (including computer games and social media), pornography (online or other), sex, shopping, gambling, emotional intimacy (including unreasonable expectations and compulsive patterns of romance, sexuality, and relationships), texting, risky behaviors or thrill seeking ("adrenaline junkies"), and more.

Addictions that center on ingested substances (known as exogenous addictions) change body chemistry; addictions to activities or behaviors (known as endogenous addictions) cause the body to produce extra endorphins and other chemicals that make a person feel good temporarily. Either way, changes in body chemistry create a dependency on the activity or substance. The greater the exposure, the more the body becomes desensitized to the excess chemicals.

Individuals who are addicted to substances or activities often feel helpless, frustrated, and ashamed of their situation. Often, most don't realize or admit they are addicted until they try to stop, only to find that they keep regressing to participation in the addictive behavior. Until an addict is ready to be honest and take responsibility for his or her choices, ask for help, and fully participate in successful rehabilitation programs (such as treatment programs, counseling, and twelve step programs), he or she faces a downward spiral that can include marital/family ruin or dissolution, financial devastation, criminal activity, and/or sickness or death.

Because they are chemical in nature, essential oils can assist recovering addicts with emotional and chemical support for the brain as they are seeking to get their lives under control again. To gain additional insight on how they powerfully affect the brain, read the introduction to *Limbic*.

There are essential oils that can help reprogram the body's cravings for specific substances and that can strengthen the resolution to abstain. Essential oils are also able to support and strengthen the very emotional areas of pain that caused the individual to participate in the addictive behavior in the first place, leading the individual to adopt a healthier lifestyle. Loved ones often suffer alongside the addict, as they feel helpless to prevent the collateral damage they see happening right in front of their eyes; essential oils can be a tremendous emotional support for these individuals as well.

TOP SOLUTIONS

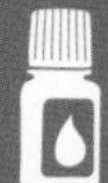

SINGLE OILS

Grapefruit - dissipates cravings; supports detoxification, renewed energy (pg. 104)

Basil - clears negative thought patterns that block change; restores mental energy (pg. 76)

Bergamot - gives sense of empowerment and self-worth (pg. 79)

Peppermint - supports sense of buoyancy and recovery, reprieve from painful emotions (pg. 122)

By Related Properties

For definitions of the properties listed below and more oil options, see Oil Properties Glossary (pg. 435) and Oil Properties (pg. 436).

Anaphrodisiac - arborvitae, marjoram

Analgesic - bergamot, birch, black pepper, clary sage, clove, eucalyptus, fennel, frankincense, helichrysum, juniper berry, lavender, marjoram, melaleuca, oregano, peppermint, ravensara, white fir, wild orange, wintergreen

Antidepressant - bergamot, cinnamon, clary sage, frankincense, geranium, lavender, lemongrass, melissa, oregano, patchouli, ravensara, sandalwood, wild orange

Anti-parasitic - bergamot, cinnamon, clove, frankincense, lavender, melaleuca, oregano, rosemary, thyme

Antitoxic - bergamot, black pepper, cinnamon, coriander, fennel, geranium, grapefruit, juniper berry, lavender, lemon, lemongrass, patchouli, thyme

Calming - bergamot, black pepper, cassia, clary sage, coriander, frankincense, geranium, juniper berry, lavender, oregano, patchouli, roman chamomile, sandalwood, tangerine, vetiver

Regenerative - cedarwood, clove, coriander, geranium, jasmine, lemongrass, myrrh, patchouli, sandalwood, wild orange

Relaxing - basil, cassia, cedarwood, clary sage, cypress, fennel, geranium, jasmine, lime, patchouli, rosemary, sandalwood, spearmint

Restorative - basil, frankincense, lime, patchouli, rosemary, sandalwood, spearmint

Sedative - bergamot, cedarwood, clary sage, frankincense, geranium, juniper berry, lavender, marjoram, melissa, patchouli, roman chamomile, rose, spikenard, ylang ylang

Stimulant - basil, bergamot, black pepper, cardamom, clove, coriander, dill, fennel, grapefruit, juniper berry, lime, melaleuca, patchouli, rosemary, thyme, white fir

Stomachic - cardamom, cinnamon, clary sage, coriander, fennel, ginger, juniper berry, marjoram, melissa, peppermint, rosemary, wild orange, yarrow

Uplifting - cardamom, cedarwood, clary sage, cypress, grapefruit, lemon, lime, melissa, tangerine, wild orange

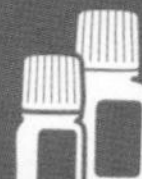

BLENDS

Calming blend - promotes calm, peaceful, tranquil state of being; quiets mind (pg. 142)

Detoxification blend - promotes elimination, detoxification of toxins (pg. 146)

Encouraging blend - promotes self-belief, confidence, trust (pg. 148)

Grounding blend - restores sense of solidity/feeling grounded in life (pg. 150)

Cleansing blend - cleanses and detoxifies (pg. 144)

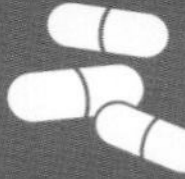

SUPPLEMENTS

Cellular vitality complex, **energy & stamina complex (pg. 174)**, essential oils cellular complex, **essential oil omega complex (pg. 175)**, detoxification complex, food enzymes, **liquid omega-3 supplement (pg. 178)**, metabolic blend softgels, whole food nutrient supplement

Related Ailments: Adrenaline, Alcohol Addiction, Drug Addiction, Food Addiction, Smoking Addiction, Video Game Addiction, Withdrawal Symptoms, Work Addiction

USAGE TIPS: For best support for addiction recovery

- **Aromatic:** Choose an oil(s) to diffuse or inhale from a bottle or hands, or whatever method seems most effective at the time. Wear an oil(s) as perfume/cologne.
- **Topical:** Apply under nose, behind ears, to base of skull (especially in suboccipital triangles) and forehead, and on roof of mouth (closest location to the amygdala; place on pad of thumb, then suck on thumb); place oil that is best match to emotional state over heart area. Use a carrier oil as needed for sensitive skin or "hot" oils. Use to prevent and eliminate urges.
- **Internal:** For immediate impact, in addition to inhalation, place a drop or two of chosen oil under tongue, hold for 30 seconds, swallow; take oils in capsule or in glass of water. Consider detoxification products/oils or a program - see *Detoxification.*

Conditions

Accountability, lack of - fennel, ginger, grounding blend
Anesthetize pain, attempting to - birch, clove, helichrysum, wintergreen, soothing blend
Antisocial - cardamom, cedarwood, marjoram, grounding blend
Anguish - melissa, helichrysum, joyful blend
Anxiety - basil, bergamot, frankincense, juniper berry, lavender, vetiver, ylang ylang, calming blend, encouraging blend, focus blend, grounding blend, joyful blend, reassuring blend
Appetite stimulant - ginger, myrrh, metabolic blend
Appetite, excessive - cassia, cinnamon, ginger, grapefruit, metabolic blend
Checked out - basil, cedarwood, clary sage, frankincense, patchouli, sandalwood, focus blend, grounding blend, inspiring blend
Control, loss of - clove, grounding blend
Cravings - clove, cilantro, cinnamon, grapefruit, peppermint, calming blend, grounding blend, metabolic blend
Deceptive/lying/secretive - clary sage
Despairing/hopeless - bergamot, clary sage, lemongrass, melissa, encouraging blend, joyful blend, renewing blend, reassuring blend
Dishonest - black pepper, clary sage, frankincense, melissa, lavender, calming blend, cleansing blend, women's monthly blend
Dopamine levels, low - basil, bergamot, cedarwood, frankincense, jasmine, lemon, patchouli, roman chamomile, rosemary, sandalwood, wild orange, uplifting blend
Financial issues - wild orange, encouraging blend,
Guilt - bergamot, lemon, peppermint, skin clearing blend, renewing blend
Hangover - cassia, cinnamon, geranium, grapefruit, lemon, detoxification blend, metabolic blend, tension blend
Irrational - cedarwood, lemon, focus blend
Irresponsible - fennel, ginger, grounding blend
Irritable - rose, calming blend, women's blend, women's monthly blend
Obsession/fixation with drug of choice - cypress, patchouli, ylang ylang, grounding blend; see *Limbic "Obsessive/compulsive thoughts/behaviors"*
Relapsing - clove, ginger, lavender blend, melissa, detoxification blend, encouraging blend, focus blend, inspiring blend
Stealing - black pepper, cassia, clary sage, frankincense, geranium, lavender, vetiver, ylang ylang, calming blend, cleansing blend, detoxification blend, women's monthly blend
Stress management, poor - lavender, calming blend; see *Stress*
Thrill seeking, excessive - birch, clove, frankincense, helichrysum, oregano, peppermint, white fir, wintergreen, soothing blend
Urges, intense - cedarwood, patchouli
Withdrawal - cilantro, cinnamon, grapefruit, juniper berry, lavender, marjoram, sandalwood, wild orange, cellular complex blend, encouraging blend, joyful blend, inspiring blend, reassuring blend, and other citrus essential oils

*http://bigthink.com/going-mental/your-brain-on-drugs-dopamine-and-addiction

Remedies

ALCOHOL CRAVINGS
- 1 or 2 drops of cassia on the tongue when cravings hit.
- Consume 2 drops twice per day of helichrysum in a capsule or under tongue.

CHEWING TOBACCO CRAVINGS: Apply coriander outside of lip, thumb to roof of mouth, and a few drops in a cotton ball in snuff container.

TOBACCO/NICOTINE CRAVINGS (top oils: black pepper, clove, protective blend) - Suggestions:
- Aromatically use black pepper to alleviate cravings; diffuse, inhale.
- Clary sage, patchouli, spikenard - use topically, internally, aromatically.
- Put a drop of protective blend or cinnamon oil on toothbrush, brush teeth.
- Combine 2 drops each of clove, frankincense, peppermint oils. Inhale in palms, apply to bottom of feet, or drink one drop of mixture with water.
- Use protective blend on the tongue or in water when the urge strikes; additional considerations: cassia, cinnamon.

PORNOGRAPHY ADDICTION RECOVERY SUPPORT: Use 1-2 drops frankincense under tongue one to two times per day. Apply helichrysum or vetiver over lower abdomen as least once per day. Determine which aromas (basil, cardamom, frankincense, grapefruit, helichrysum, cleansing blend, grounding blend, protective blend) are preferred and utilize both preventatively (e.g. wear as cologne/perfume) and when urges arise.

WORK ADDICTION: Diffuse 5-10 drops oil(s) in work space for a minimum of 2-3 hours per day as needed. Use any of following oils alone or combined as desired: basil, geranium, wild orange, and/or ylang ylang or calming blend to create the 10 drops for diffuser. Experiment with what combination best serves needs. Here are some suggested combinations:
- 3 drops wild orange and 2 drops ylang ylang.
- 2 drops geranium, 2 drops ylang ylang, and 3 drops women's blend.
- 2 drops basil, 3 drops wild orange, and 2 drops ylang ylang.
- 6 drops calming blend and1-2 drops ylang ylang.

VIDEO GAME & INTERNET ADDICTION: Place a few drops of calming blend or vetiver on temples two to three times per day. Inhale aroma from hands after applying. Use 2-3 drops of grounding blend on bottoms of feet each day. If vetiver aroma is too intense, layer with wild orange of invigorating blend.

ENERGY DRINK & CAFFEINE ADDICTION: Place 3 drops basil oil on bottom of each foot and inhale regularly throughout the day. Drink 5 drops of metabolic blend in water or a capsule three to five times daily. Place one drop grapefruit oil under tongue, hold for 30 seconds, swallow anytime experiencing cravings.

DRUG & ALCOHOL ADDICTION: Place 2-3 drops of any one or more oil listed on bottoms of feet, abdomen (specifically over liver area), and forehead. Choose from basil, frankincense, roman chamomile and/or detoxification blend. Dilute with fractionate coconut oil as needed or desired.

OILS TO ADDRESS EMOTIONAL STATES FOR ADDICTION RECOVERY

For emotional states associated with addictions - see *Mood & Behavior*

SINGLES

Basil - overcomes chronic fatigue (creates desire for stimulants); release toxins

Bergamot - encourages self-love, restores sense of self worth

Cardamom - helps overcoming objectifying (common problem with addictions)

Cedarwood - supports healthy GABA (anti-excitatory), serotonin levels

Clary sage - dispels darkness and illusion

Coriander - effective with any addiction

Clove - restores healthy boundaries

Frankincense - connects to divine love/acceptance, purpose, higher brain function

Geranium - assists with love and acceptance

Ginger - supports being fully present, taking full responsibility

Grapefruit - reduces cravings; restores relationship with body's natural energy

Helichrysum - supports healing from deep, intense pain, trauma

Juniper berry - supports accessing, releasing unaccessed/unresolved fears

Lemon - supports restoration of logical thinking; clears generational patterns

Melissa - restores connection to reality, truth, light; instills courage

Patchouli - grounds and stabilizes; get the "guts" to take a leap of faith

Peppermint - promotes sense of recovery

Roman chamomile - helps one live true to one's self

Thyme - releases and resolves toxic emotions

Vetiver - gets to "root" cause and face it head on; supports amygdala

White fir - clears inherited/passed on addictions; tendencies in families

Wild orange - supports creative thoughts, expression; restores playfulness

Ylang ylang - releases trauma; recovers connection to the heart, to feel/trust again

BLENDS

Calming blend - quiets mind; encourages facing issues; helps balance expectations

Cellular complex blend - supports knowing what's worth keeping vs. releasing

Cleansing blend - supports detoxification; provides freedom from past habits/patterns

Detoxification blend - supports detox processes; detoxing old habits, beliefs

Focus blend - normalizes, stabilizes brain activity; invites acceptance of reality

Grounding blend - restores sense of solidity/feeling grounded in life; brings electrical balance to body and focus to mind

Joyful blend - soothes heart, balances emotions; stabilizes mood, supports serotonin

Metabolic blend - supports restoration of a positive relationship to one's body and natural sources of energy

Soothing blend - supports deep emotional healing; restores normal endorphin levels

Tension blend - invites releasing fears, relaxing and enjoying life again

SOLUTIONS FOR SPECIFIC ADDICTIONS:

Adrenaline - basil, bergamot, clary sage, oregano, patchouli, rosemary, calming blend, comforting blend, encouragin blend, focus blend, grounding blend

Alcohol - basil, cassia, eucalyptus, frankincense, ginger, helichrysum, juniper berry, lemon, marjoram, melissa, myrrh, roman chamomile, rosemary, calming blend, grounding blend, cleansing blend, reassuring blend, renewing blend, uplifting blend

Anger - geranium, helichrysum, marjoram, rosemary, thyme, wintergreen, calming blend, cleansing blend, encouraging blend, joyful blend, reassuring blend, renewing blend, uplifting blend, women's blend; see *Mood & Behavior*

Caffeine - basil, grapefruit, patchouli, inspiring blend, metabolic blend, reassuring blend

Controlling, overly/"control freak" - cilantro, cinnamon, cypress, sandalwood, wintergreen, patchouli, inspiring blend, invigorating blend, metabolic blend

Cutting/self harm/self inflicted pain - bergamot, geranium, myrrh, rose, wintergreen, anti-aging blend, joyful blend, protective blend, skin clearing blend, comforting blend, reassuring blend, renewing blend, women's blend, women's monthly blend

Drugs - basil, clary sage, grapefruit, patchouli, roman chamomile, comforting blend, encouraging blend, inspiring blend, reassuring blend, uplifting blend,

Eating Disorders (anorexia, bulimia) - bergamot, cardamom, cinnamon, grapefruit, patchouli, comforting blend, inspiring blend, invigorating blend, reassuring blend, respiration blend, respiration blend lozenges; see *Eating Disorders*

Entertainment - peppermint, vetiver, calming blend, comforting blend, grounding blend, inspiring blend, joyful blend

Fear - cassia, cinnamon, ginger, juniper berry, myrrh, patchouli, reassuring blend; see *Mood & Behavior*

Food - basil, cardamom, ginger, grapefruit, myrrh, comforting blend, encouraging blend, inspiring blend, metabolic blend; see *Eating Disorders*

Gaming - comforting blend, joyful blend, repellent blend, skin clearing blend, soothing blend, uplifting blend, women's blend

Marijuana - basil, patchouli, inspiring blend, reassuring blend

Nicotine - bergamot, black pepper, cinnamon (on tongue), cassia, cinnamon, clove, eucalyptus, ginger, inspiring blend, protective blend, reassuring blend, protective blend lozenges; see "Tobacco" below

Pain meds - birch, clove, eucalyptus, patchouli, wintergreen, comforting blend, inspiring blend, reassuring blend, soothing blend

Pornography - basil, cardamom, frankincense, grapefruit, helichrysum, cleansing blend, comforting blend, grounding blend, protective blend

Sex - arborvitae, basil, cardamom, geranium, marjoram, sandalwood, encouraging blend, inspiring blend, reassuring blend, women's blend

Sugar - cardamom, cassia, cinnamon, clove, dill, grapefruit, helichrysum, encouraging blend, inspiring blend, metabolic blend, uplifting blend, reassuring blend

Technology - patchouli, peppermint, encouraging blend, focus blend, inspiring blend, renewing blend, uplifting blend; see "Entertainment" above

Tobacco/smoking - basil, bergamot, black pepper, cassia, cinnamon, clove, eucalyptus, frankincense, ginger, patchouli, peppermint, spikenard, calming blend, inspiring blend, invigorating blend, protective blend, reassuring blend, renewing blend, respiration blend, uplifting blend, protective blend lozenges, respiration blend lozenges

Tobacco/chewing - bergamot, cassia, cinnamon, clove, coriander, frankincense, inspiring blend, protective blend, reassuring blend, renewing blend, uplifting blend, protective blend lozenges

Work - arborvitae, basil, geranium, lavender, marjoram, wild orange, ylang ylang, uplifting blend, reassuring blend, renewing blend

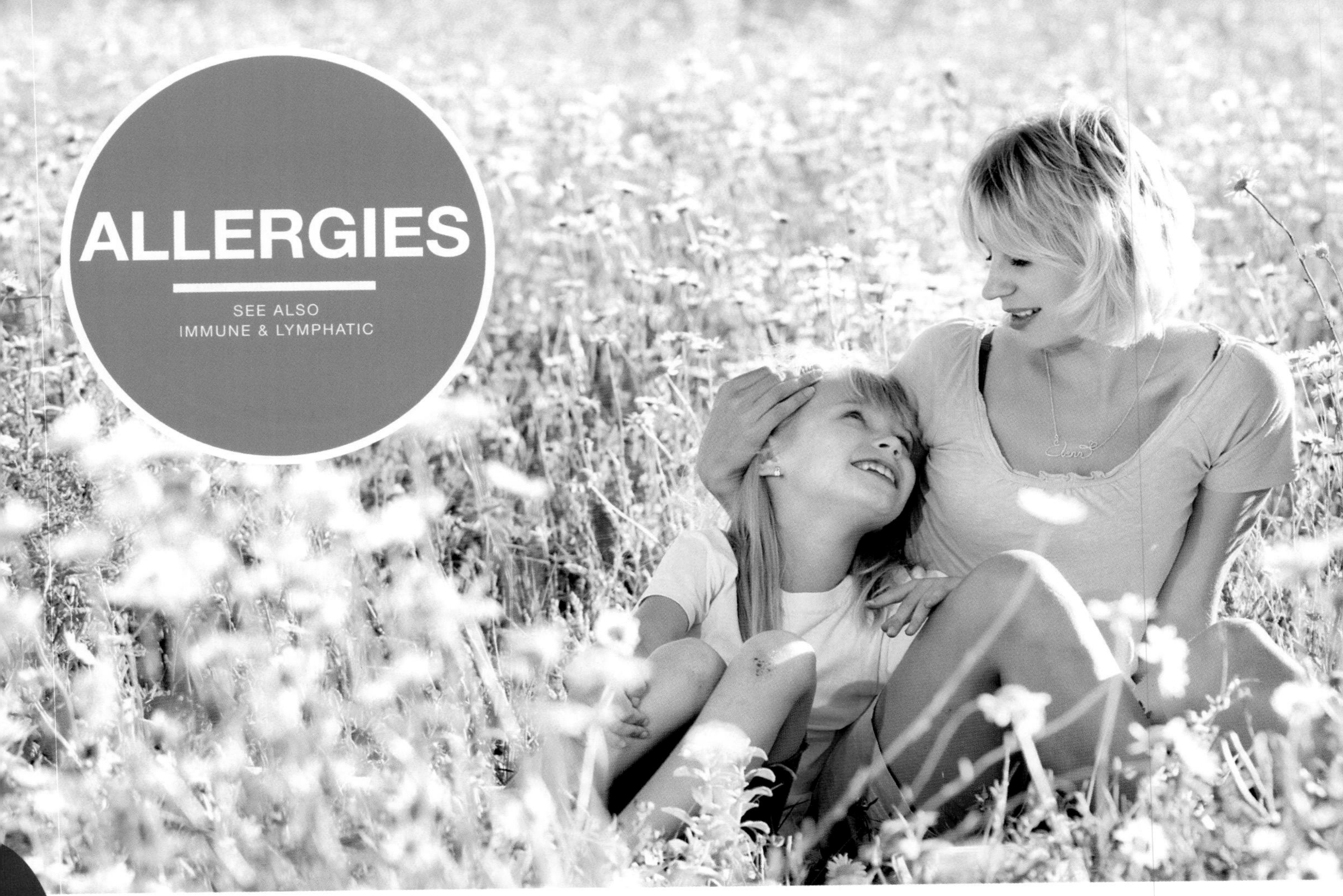

ALLERGIC REACTIONS occur when the immune system reacts to foreign substances in the environment that are normally harmless to most people, such as pollen, bee venom, or pet dander. A substance that causes a reaction is called an allergen. These reactions are generally considered to be acquired. A true allergic reaction is an immediate form of hypersensitivity and is distinctive because the immune response over-activates specific white blood cells that are triggered by antibodies.

When allergies occur, the immune system identifies a particular allergen as harmful—even if it isn't—and creates antibodies to fight it. When contact is made with the allergen, the immune system's reaction will typically inflame skin, sinuses, airways or digestive system. This reaction is known as an inflammatory response.

The severity of allergies varies from person to person and can range from minor irritation to anaphylaxis, which is a severe reaction to an allergen that can be a life-threatening emergency. Common triggers for severe reactions include insect bites or stings (wasps, bees) and certain food allergies (i.e. peanuts, shellfish). It is important to note that not all reactions or intolerances are forms of allergic responses.

Allergy symptoms depend on the allergens/substances involved and can impact the airways, sinuses and nasal passages, skin, the digestive system, and other parts of the body. Allergies are typically categorized as either respiratory or systemic (involving multiple organs - esp. digestive, respiratory, circulatory).

Common allergens include airborne particles (i.e. animal hair, car exhaust, cigarette smoke, dust, dust mites, fragrances, fungi, herbicides, mold, paint fumes, perfume, pesticides, pet dander, pollens, weeds); chemicals, latex, petroleum and automotive products; foods (i.e. peanuts, genetically modified soy products); insect stings and bites; insect or reptile venom; medications (i.e. aspirin, antibiotics such as penicillin or sulfa drugs).

Traditional treatments for allergies include avoiding known allergens or administering steroids that modify the immune system in general and medications such as antihistamines and decongestants to reduce symptoms. Essential oils have the ability to chemically support the body in its capacity to reduce and overcome acute or chronic hypersensitivity. For allergy support specifically, it is especially important to be familiar with three properties of oils and the particular oils associated with the related actions: anti-allergenic (e.g. geranium, helichrysum), antihistamine (e.g. lavender, melissa, roman chamomile), and steroidal (e.g. basil, rosemary). See "By Related Properties" for more information. Additional, for numerous related respiratory needs refer to *Respiratory* section of this book.

TOP SOLUTIONS

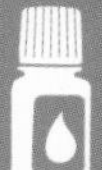

SINGLE OILS

Basil, rosemary - reduces inflammatory response and supports adrenal glands (pgs. 76 & 127)

Lavender - acts as an antihistamine and calms irritation (pg. 108)

Lemon - decongests and reduces mucus (pg. 110)

Peppermint - discharges phlegm and reduces inflammation (pg. 122)

By Related Properties

For definitions of the properties listed below and more oil options, see Oil Properties Glossary (pg. 435) and Oil Properties (pg. 436).

Anti-allergenic - geranium, helichrysum
Antihistamine - lavender, melissa, roman chamomile
Anti-inflammatory - arborvitae, basil, bergamot, birch, black pepper, cardamom, cassia, cedarwood, cinnamon, coriander, cypress, dill, eucalyptus, fennel, frankincense, geranium, ginger, helichrysum, lavender, lemongrass, lime, melaleuca, myrrh, oregano, patchouli, peppermint, roman chamomile, rosemary, sandalwood
Antitoxic - bergamot, black pepper, coriander, grapefruit, juniper berry, lavender, lemon, lemongrass, thyme
Calming - basil, bergamot, black pepper, cassia, clary sage, coriander, fennel, frankincense, geranium, jasmine, juniper berry, lavender, patchouli, roman chamomile, sandalwood, tangerine, vetiver, yarrow
Cleanser - arborvitae, cilantro, eucalyptus, grapefruit, juniper berry, lemon, thyme, wild orange
Detoxifier - cilantro, juniper berry, lime, patchouli, wild orange
Steroidal - basil, bergamot, birch, cedarwood, clove, fennel, patchouli, rosemary, thyme

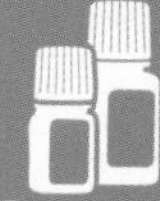

BLENDS

Respiration blend - supports reduction and recovery from allergic responses (pg. 162)

Detoxification blend - supports permanent reduction of reactivity (pg. 146)

Cleansing blend - alleviates allergic responses to bites and stings (pg. 144)

Digestion blend - supports digestion to calm food allergy responses (pg. 147)

Protective blend - supports immune system (pg. 158)

Calming blend - acts as an antihistamine (pg. 142)

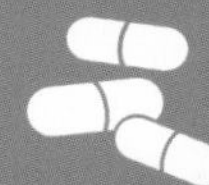

SUPPLEMENTS

Cellular vitality complex, detoxification complex, detoxification blend softgels, energy & stamina complex, **food enzymes (pg. 177)**, phytoestrogen multiplex, **respiration blend lozenges (pg. 182)**, **seasonal blend softgels (pg. 183)**, whole food nutrient supplement

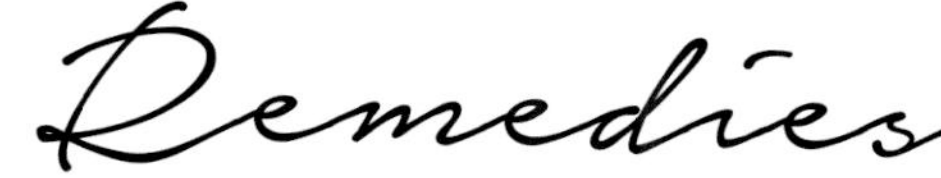

Remedies

EYE ALLERGIES: Layer 2 drops lavender and melaleuca under the pads of the index toe and middle toe and then rub in. Use a few drops of lavender at the temples and gently rubbed in. Take care to stay close to the hairline to avoid eye contact.

ALLERGY POWER TRIO: Take 2 drops lavender, 2 drops lemon, 2 drops peppermint one of three ways:

- Under the tongue, wait thirty seconds, swallow; repeat as necessary.
- Mix in 1/8 to ½ cup water, drink; repeat as necessary until symptoms subside.
- Consume blend in a capsule; repeat as necessary.
- OR Take seasonal blend softgels

SKIN RASH/HIVES: Dilute lavender or melaleuca with carrier oil and rub into skin. A toxic, burdened, sluggish liver is a major culprit of allergic response. Layering oils over the liver area supports its ability to flush toxins that burden other organs, including skin and kidneys. The skin is a secondary pathway of elimination for the liver, and rashes can be indicative of its toxicity.

THE ALLERGY BOMB: Take 2-3 drops each of cilantro, melaleuca and lavender in a capsule.

ALLERGY RELIEF COMBINATION: Lemon, lavender, eucalyptus, and roman chamomile - use in equal parts in a capsule (for example, 1 drop of each). This blend of essential oils has been effective for relieving hay fever and other airborne, allergy-type symptoms that result in sneezing, runny nose, watery eyes, and so on.

ALLERGIES
6 drops lavender
6 drops roman chamomile
2 drops myrrh
1 drop peppermint
Blend and apply one drop behind ears, temples, and thymus.

Related Ailments: Chemical Sensitivity Reaction [Detoxification, Immune & Lymphatic], Hay Fever [Immune & Lymphatic, Respiratory], Hives [Integumentary], Lactose Intolerance, Loss of Smell, Multiple Chemical Sensitivity Reaction, Olfactory Loss, Pet Dander

Conditions

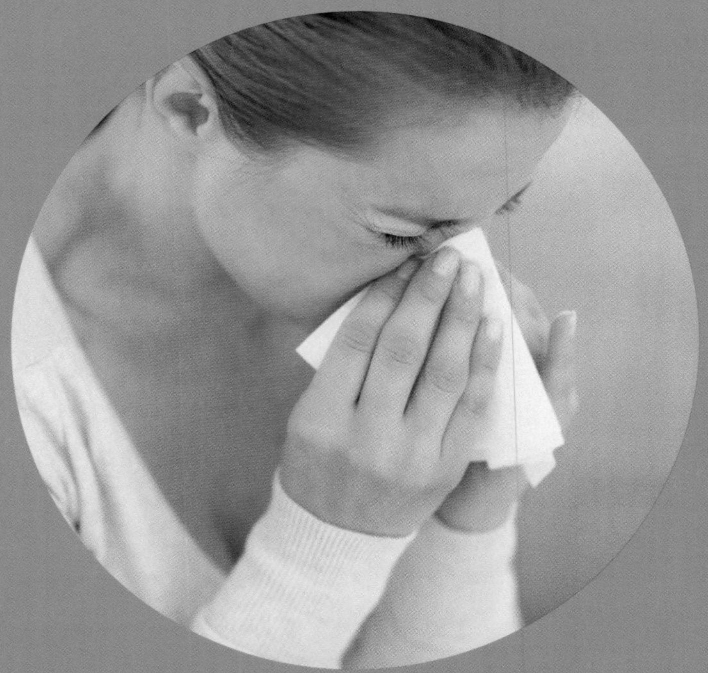

Adrenal fatigue - See *Endocrine*
Abdominal cramping/spasms - See *Digestive & Intestinal*
Airways, narrowing/constriction - birch, cinnamon, douglas fir, eucalyptus, frankincense, helichrysum, lavender, lemon, marjoram, myrrh, peppermint, rosemary, thyme, white fir, wintergreen, calming blend, cellular complex blend, encouraging blend, respiration blend, respiration blend lozenges
Allergies, chronic - basil, ginger, lemon, lemongrass, thyme
Allergies, general - cilantro, frankincense, lavender, melaleuca, peppermint, comforting blend, detoxification blend, reassuring blend
Anxiety - See *Mood & Behavior*
Blood pressure, high or low - See *Cardiovascular*
Chemical sensitivity - arborvitae, cilantro, coriander, eucalyptus, lemon, peppermint, sandalwood, wild orange, cellular complex blend, cleansing blend, detoxification blend, women's blend
Congestion - See *Respiratory*
Cough - See *Respiratory*
Energy, loss of/fatigue, chronic - See *Energy & Vitality*
Facial pressure and pain - helichrysum, myrrh, cellular complex blend, digestion blend
Glands, enlarged/swollen - arborvitae, cilantro, lemon, lime, oregano, roman chamomile, wintergreen, protective blend
Hay fever - cilantro, lavender, lemon, melaleuca, yarrow, cleansing blend, encouraging blend, respiration blend
Headache - see *Pain & Inflammation*
Hives - basil, cilantro, frankincense, lavender, lemongrass, melaleuca, peppermint, roman chamomile, rosemary, cellular complex blend
Inflammation, joints - See *Skeletal*
Inflammation, skin - See *Integumentary*
Immune system, overactive - peppermint, rosemary, joyful blend
Insect bite - See *First Aid*
Itching/urge to scratch, burning - See *Integumentary*
Itchy eyes/mouth/throat - cilantro, lavender, lemon, melaleuca, peppermint, cleansing blend, detoxification blend, encouraging blend, metabolic blend, seasonal blend
Joint pain - See *Skeletal*
Liver - See *Digestive & Intestinal*
Liver, toxic load - See *Digestive & Intestinal*; see "Anti-allergenic" property
Mold sensitivity - arborvitae, melaleuca, oregano, thyme, cleansing blend, detoxification blend
Nasal congestion/drip - See *Respiratory*
Nausea - See *Digestive & Intestinal*
Poison oak - See *First Aid*
Pollen sensitivity - cilantro, juniper berry, lavender, cleansing blend, detoxification blend
Rapid pulse - cardamom, cedarwood, frankincense, rosemary, ylang ylang, calming blend, cleansing blend, encouraging blend, joyful blend; see *Cardiovascular*
Rash - arborvitae, cedarwood, frankincense, lavender, lemon, melaleuca, roman chamomile, sandalwood, anti-aging blend, calming blend, cleansing blend, detoxification blend, metabolic blend, women's monthly blend
Reaction - roman chamomile
Runny nose - grapefruit, lavender, lemon, myrrh, peppermint, detoxification blend, digestion blend, encouraging blend
Shock - See *First Aid*
Skin bumps - See *Integumentary*
Skin cracking/peeling/scaling - See *Integumentary*
Skin flushed - See *Integumentary*
Skin irritation - melaleuca, peppermint, calming blend, cleansing blend, digestion blend, metabolic blend, corrective ointment
Skin reddening - See *Integumentary*
Smoke sensitivity - black pepper, lavender, peppermint, calming blend, detoxification blend
Sneezing - lavender, douglas fir, lemon, peppermint, cleansing blend, encouraging blend, respiration blend
Swallowing, difficulty - lavender, detoxification blend, encouraging blend
Swelling of lips, face, tongue, throat, etc. - lavender, wintergreen, cleansing blend, detoxification blend
Throat, dry - See *Respiratory*
Throat, sore - See *Respiratory*
Voice, loss of/raspy/hoarseness - See *Respiratory*
Vomiting - See *Digestive & Intestinal*
Watery/itchy/red eyes - eucalyptus, lavender, lemon, melaleuca, roman chamomile, cleansing blend, detoxification blend
Welts - arborvitae, myrrh, vetiver, cleansing blend
Wheezing - birch, lavender, wintergreen, respiration blend

USAGE TIPS: For best support in overcoming allergies:

- **Internal:** Take drops of oils in water and drink, take oil(s) in a capsule, or place a drop on or under tongue.
- **Aromatic:** Diffuse chosen oils; apply to chest, clothing, bedding, or other to inhale.
- **Topical:** Apply oils topically to forehead, cheeks (avoid eyes), chest, bottoms of feet.

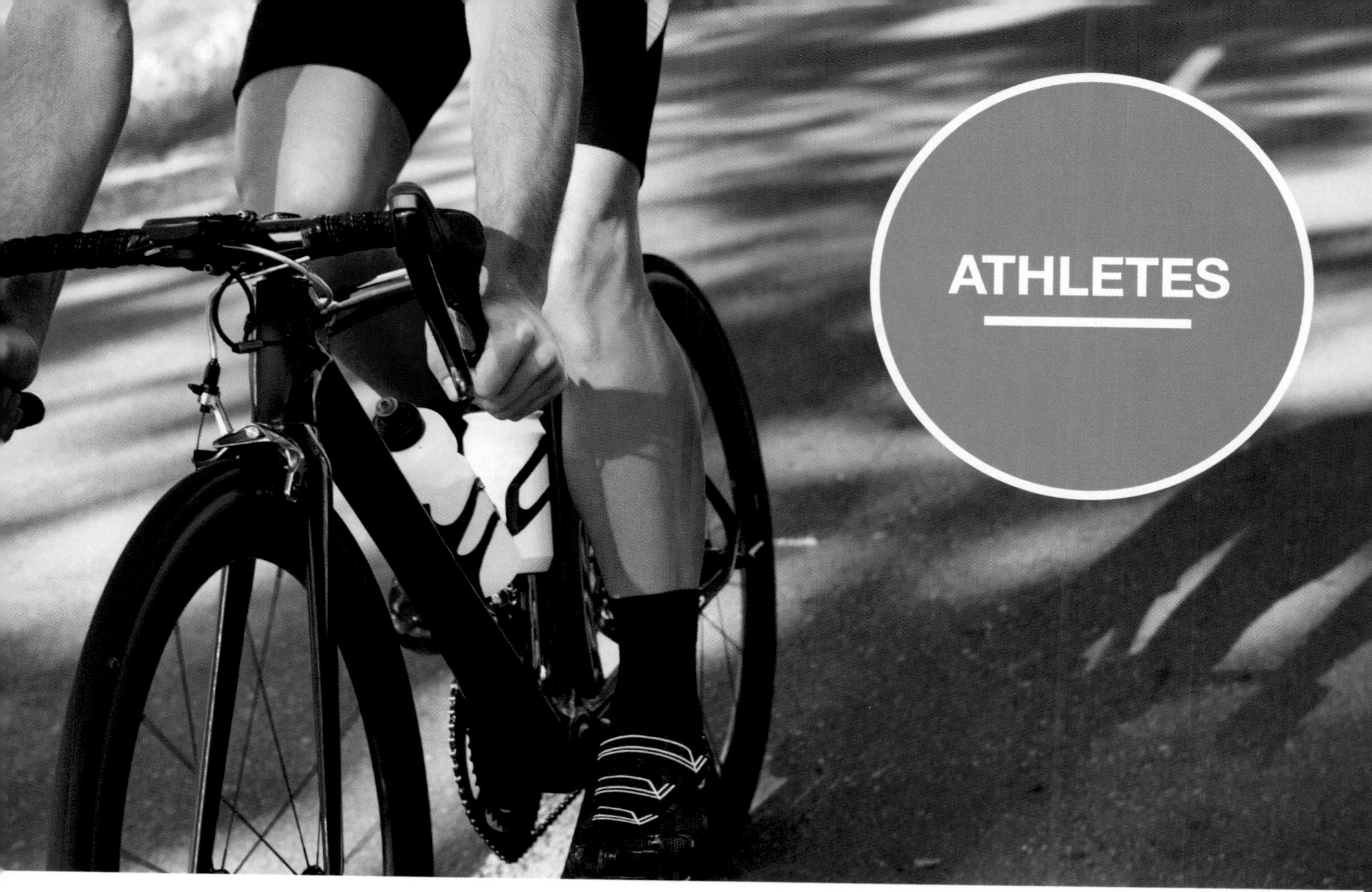

AS THEY PREPARE for their sport of preference, many athletes participate in one or more training programs that can include (but is not limited to): circuit training (develops a broad range of skills by providing stations with various exercises); interval training (short periods of vigorous activity interspersed with shorter resting periods; helps build speed endurance); Plyometrics (bounding exercises to help improve strength and speed); tempo training (the athlete maintains a faster pace than is comfortable to increase endurance ability); strength training (the use of various pieces of equipment increases muscle resistance and inspires faster conditioning); resisted and/or assisted training (helps develop faster speed as the athlete uses resistance equipment, such as bands, or participates in assistance-based exercise, such as running downhill).

As athletes push their bodies for greater conditioning and/or endurance in fitness training or sports, the potential for injury is present. Often these injuries are a result of inadequate recovery (rest) time for muscles/body tissues to adequately rebuild or repair.

Some of these injuries include:

- Muscle pain and soreness
- Overusing tendons
- "Runner's Knee" – a generic term to describe anterior knee pain
- IT Band (iliotibial band) stress/injury – affects approximately 12 percent of runners
- Shin splints
- Pain in Achilles tendon
- Stress fracture

Other common conditions athletes may experience during training/sports:

- Exercise-induced asthma
- Exercise-associated collapse
- Effects resulting from overtraining - concentration, lack of; depression, heart rate (resting) changes, injuries (increased), insomnia/restless sleep, insatiable thirst, motivation and/or self esteem diminished, muscle soreness lasting more than 72 hours, personality changes, progress hindered, sick more often

Athletes can combine sound principles of sports medicine (icing, heating, resting, etc., as appropriate) with natural remedies to increase the body's recovery time. There are oils known specifically for their ability to support connective tissue (involved in all sports injuries), to reduce inflammation, to support cellular regeneration for faster recovery time, and/or to help warm up/cool down muscle groups for better overall performance.

Adding whole-food, bio-available supplements gives cells the support they need to enhance restorative and repairing activities. Supplementation can also increase energy levels during a workout to reduce fatigue. An easily digestible protein drink consumed just after a cardio workout gives the body readily accessible protein so it doesn't have to break down proteins in the body. All these good practices help to minimize breakdown and overuse injuries in the first place, help provide energy, and increase the body's capacity to restore tissues to good health quickly.

TOP SOLUTIONS

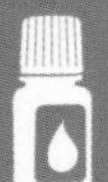

SINGLE OILS

Peppermint - pre-exercise support (pg. 122)
Lemongrass - connective tissue support (pg. 112)
Marjoram - muscle support (pg. 114)

By Related Properties

For definitions of the properties listed below and more oil options, see Oil Properties Glossary (pg. 435) and Oil Properties (pg. 436).

Analgesic - basil, bergamot, birch, black pepper, clove, eucalyptus, ginger, helichrysum, juniper berry, lavender, lemongrass, melaleuca, oregano, peppermint, rosemary, white fir, wintergreen
Anti-inflammatory - arborvitae, basil, birch, black pepper, cardamom, cassia, cedarwood, cinnamon, cypress, eucalyptus, fennel, frankincense, geranium, ginger, helichrysum, lavender, lemongrass, lime, melaleuca, oregano, patchouli, peppermint, rosemary, sandalwood, spearmint, spikenard, wild orange, wintergreen, yarrow
Energizing - basil, cypress, ginger, grapefruit, lemongrass, lime, rosemary, white fir, wild orange
Relaxing - basil, cedarwood, cypress, geranium, helichrysum, lavender, marjoram, roman chamomile, white fir, wild orange, ylang ylang
Regenerative - basil, clove, frankincense, geranium, helichrysum, lavender, helichrysum, lemongrass, melaleuca, myrrh, patchouli, wild orange, ylang ylang
Steroidal - basil, bergamot, birch, cedarwood, clove, fennel, patchouli, rosemary, thyme
Vasodilator - lemongrass, marjoram, peppermint, rosemary, thyme
Warming - birch, black pepper, cassia, cinnamon, clary sage, ginger, marjoram, peppermint, wintergreen

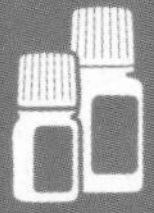

BLENDS

Massage blend - post-exercise recovery (pg. 155)
Soothing blend, soothing blend rub - post-exercise recovery (pg. 164)

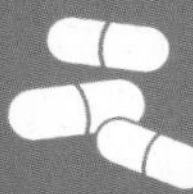

SUPPLEMENTS

Bone support complex (pg. 170), cellular vitality complex, detoxification complex, digestion blend softgels, essential oil cellular complex, essential oil omega complex, **energy & stamina complex (pg. 174)**, food enzymes, **polyphenol complex (pg. 181)**, whole food nutrient supplement, **meal replacement shake (pg. 142)**, **metabolic blend softgels (pg. 180)**

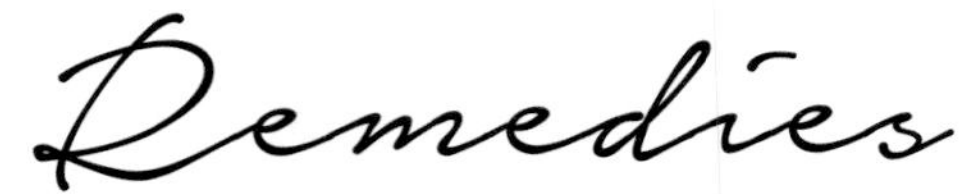

PRE/POST-WORKOUT TIPS

- Sniff peppermint or an invigorating blend before your workout to give you a boost to get you going, better your mood, and reduce fatigue.
- Add 2 drops of lemon or metabolic blend to your water to keep you hydrated.
- Apply peppermint alone or with cypress, lemongrass, and/or marjoram, or peppermint before your workout routine to increase circulation, warm muscles (reduce possibility of injury), and oxygenate muscles.
- After your workout, apply soothing blend rub.
- For a more intense post-workout treatment, layer fractionated coconut oil, lemongrass, and/or marjoram, and then top off with soothing rub blend to aching muscles to reduce inflammation, improve recovery, and support injury repair.

FOR OVERHEATED/HEAT STROKE/HEAT EXHAUSTION: Place peppermint in a spritzer bottle with water and spray back of neck; massage a drop of peppermint on back of neck for cooling.

FOR OXYGEN UPTAKE: Place a few drops of peppermint or metabolic blend in water and sip/drink; swipe a drop of frankincense under nose.

FOR NAUSEA: Place a few drops of peppermint in water, or use peppermint beadlets.

FOR INFLAMMATION/PAIN/STIFFNESS: Mix together 30 drops of soothing blend and 25 drops of frankincense in a 10ml roller bottle; fill the rest with fractionated coconut oil and shake to blend; rub onto affected area as needed.

AFTER-SPORTS BATH: 3 drops lavender, 2 drops roman chamomile, 2 drops marjoram, 1 drop helichrysum, 2 cups Epsom salts; stir oils with salts before dissolving mixture in bathwater to help oils disperse; soak for twelve to twenty minutes.

SHIN SPLINTS AND RUNNER'S KNEE REMEDIES

- Step One: In a 10ml roller bottle, combine one of following recipes. Add fractionated coconut oil to fill remainder of bottle after essential oils are added. Shake to blend. Apply frequently. Massage oil into both the front and the back of the leg in area(s) of concern.
  - Recipe #1: 45 drops each lemongrass and rosemary oils
  - Recipe #2: 50 drops lemongrass oil, 30 drops marjoram oil, 35 drops wintergreen oil
- Optional - Step 2: Layer soothing blend or rub on top of either recipe and massage into tissue.

Conditions

Appetite, excessive - bergamot, cassia, cinnamon, ginger, grapefruit, lemon, metabolic blend; see *Weight*

Appetite, loss of - bergamot, black pepper, ginger, lemon, metabolic blend; see *Weight*

Appetite, imbalanced - wild orange, metabolic blend; see *Weight*

Athlete's foot - arborvitae, cardamom, clove, lavender, lemongrass, melaleuca, myrrh, oregano, massage blend; see *Candida*

Blood pressure, low - See *Cardiovascular*

Body temperature, too cool - cinnamon, ginger, oregano, wintergreen

Body temperature, too high - bergamot, black pepper, lemon, peppermint, soothing blend, tension blend; see "Warming" property

Bone, pain - birch, eucalyptus, helichrysum, white fir, wintergreen, soothing blend; see *Skeletal*

Breathing, constricted - douglas fir, massage blend, respiration blend, soothing blend; see *Respiratory*

Breathing, labored - ravensara, respiration blend; see *Respiratory*

Cartilage injury - basil, birch, helichrysum, wintergreen, marjoram, lemongrass, white fir, peppermint, soothing blend; see *Skeletal*

Circulation, poor - basil, cypress, douglas fir, ginger, marjoram, massage blend; see *Cardiovascular*

Concussion - bergamot, cypress, frankincense, sandalwood, focus blend, grounding blend; see *Brain*

Consciousness, loss of - basil, frankincense, peppermint, rosemary; see *Brain*

Dehydration - lemon, peppermint, metabolic blend

Dizziness - See *Brain*

Fatigue/Exhaustion - basil, bergamot, cinnamon, cypress, douglas fir, eucalyptus, frankincense, lavender, lemon, peppermint, ravensara, rosemary, sandalwood, wild orange, ylang ylang, cellular complex blend, detoxification blend, invigorating blend, joyful blend, metabolic blend; see *Energy & Vitality*

Feet, sore - lemongrass, marjoram, massage blend

Headache - See *Pain & Inflammation*

Heat exhaustion/stroke - bergamot, black pepper, dill, lemon, peppermint, detoxification blend, tension blend

Inflammation - birch, cypress, frankincense, lavender, peppermint, rosemary, wintergreen, cellular complex blend, cellular vitality complex, essential oil cellular complex, soothing blend; see "Anti-inflammatory" property

Injury - birch, helichrysum, lemongrass, white fir, wintergreen, massage blend; see the area of injury - muscles, bones, connective tissue, bruising/skin, etc.; see *Skeletal, Muscular*

Involuntary muscle contractions - clary sage, geranium, lavender, marjoram; see *Nervous*

Jock itch - See *Candida*

Joint, inflammation/stiffness - arborvitae, basil, birch, cinnamon, clove, cypress, douglas fir, eucalyptus, frankincense, ginger, lavender, lemon, marjoram, peppermint, ravensara, rosemary, thyme, vetiver, white fir, wild orange, wintergreen, cellular complex blend, detoxification blend, soothing blend, soothing blend rub; see *Skeletal*

Lactic acid buildup - dill, juniper berry, lemon, lemongrass

Ligaments/tendons/connective tissue - basil, clove (dilute for topical use), eucalyptus, helichrysum, lemongrass, white fir, see "Tendonitis" below see *Skeletal*

Lower back pain - birch, eucalyptus, frankincense, lavender, lemongrass, ginger, marjoram, peppermint, white fir, wintergreen, cellular complex blend, massage blend, soothing blend, soothing blend rub, tension blend; see *Skeletal*

Lymphatic, congestion - ginger, grapefruit, lavender, lemon, lemongrass, sandalwood, cleansing blend, massage blend; see *Immune & Lymphatic*

Mental strength/clarity - basil, patchouli, peppermint, vetiver, focus blend, grounding blend; see *Focus & Concentration*

Muscle, cramps/charley horse - basil, cypress, lemongrass, marjoram, peppermint, spikenard, white fir, wintergreen, massage blend, soothing blend, tension blend; see *Muscular*

Muscle, fatigue/overworked - basil, black pepper, cypress, douglas fir, eucalyptus, marjoram, rosemary, white fir, massage blend; see *Muscular*

Muscle, pain/sprain/strain/injury - clove (dilute for topical use), douglas fir, eucalyptus, ginger, lavender, lemongrass, marjoram, peppermint, rosemary, thyme, vetiver, white fir, wintergreen, massage blend, soothing blend; see *Muscular*

Muscle spasms - arborvitae, basil, birch, black pepper, cardamom, coriander, cypress, eucalyptus, frankincense, ginger, lavender, lemongrass, marjoram, myrrh, oregano, patchouli, peppermint, roman chamomile, rosemary, spearmint, wild orange, wintergreen, yarrow; see *Muscular*

Muscle, stiffness/tension - basil, douglas fir, ginger, grapefruit, rosemary, white fir, massage blend, soothing blend, soothing blend rub, tension blend; see *Muscular*

Muscle, weak - basil, bergamot, birch, black pepper, clary sage, clove, coriander, cypress, frankincense, ginger, helichrysum, lavender, lemongrass, jasmine, marjoram, patchouli, rosemary, wintergreen; see *Muscular*

Nausea/Vomiting - See *Digestive & Intestinal*

Nerve damage - bergamot, frankincense, helichrysum, peppermint, calming blend; see *Nervous*

Nerve pain - basil, birch, ginger, helichrysum, wintergreen, soothing blend; see *Nervous*

Pain - birch, cypress, eucalyptus, helichrysum, lemongrass, peppermint, wintergreen, soothing blend; see *Pain & Inflammation*

Perspiration, lack of - black pepper, cilantro, coriander, cypress, ginger, yarrow; see *Detoxification*

Perspiration, excess - cypress, lemongrass, peppermint; see *Detoxification*

Pulse, weak - cinnamon, coriander, ginger; see *Cardiovascular*

Pulse, rapid - cedarwood, lavender, rosemary, ylang ylang, calming blend; see *Cardiovascular*

Sciatica, issues with - basil, birch, cardamom, cypress, frankincense, helichrysum, lavender, peppermint, sandalwood, thyme, wintergreen, calming blend, soothing blend, soothing blend rub; see *Skeletal*

Stamina, lack of - cinnamon, peppermint, rosemary; see *Energy & Vitality*

Stress, performance - bergamot, clary sage, sandalwood, calming blend, grounding blend; see *Stress*

Tendonitis - basil, birch, cardamom, cypress, eucalyptus, helichrysum, lavender, lemon, lemongrass, marjoram, oregano, peppermint, rosemary, wintergreen, massage blend, soothing blend; see *Skeletal*

USAGE TIPS: For best methods of use for athletes:

- **Topical:** Use oils topically is for muscle/joint pain and injuries.
- **Aromatic:** Inhaling certain oils before and during workouts can invigorate, energize, and improve respiration.

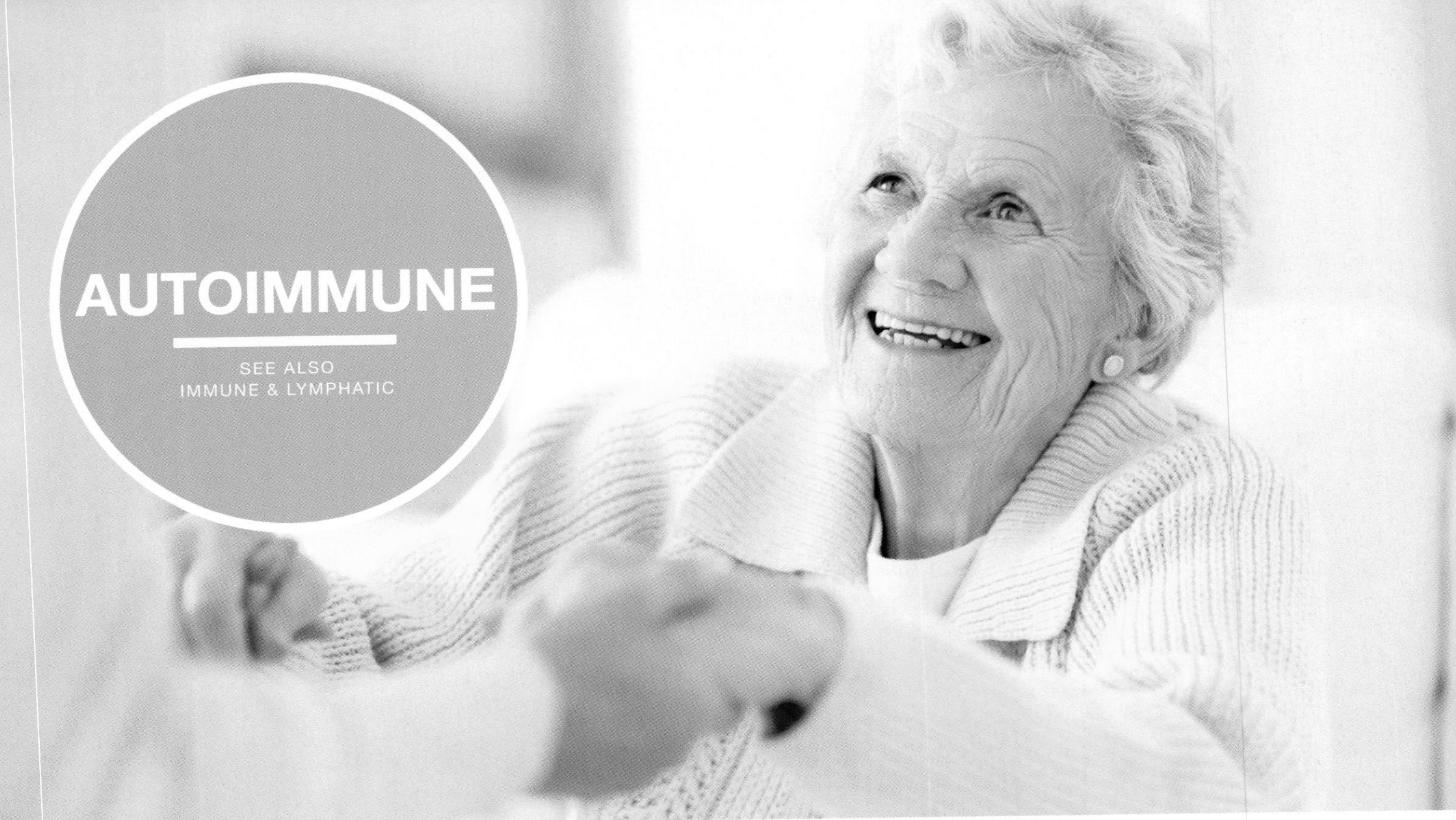

AUTOIMMUNE DISEASES occur when the body has either an abnormally low immune response to pathogens, or when the body's immune system fails to distinguish the difference between pathogens and healthy body tissues. When normal body tissue is identified as a pathogen, or invader, the adaptive immune system creates antibodies that target the destruction of these tissues.

Because they attack the body's organs in a similar manner, many autoimmune disorders tend to have similar symptoms, making it difficult to diagnose them. It is possible for individuals to have multiple conditions simultaneously. There are no known medical cures for autoimmune conditions, so treatment focuses on using medications to suppress the immune response, leaving the individual vulnerable to sickness and disease, and to manage symptoms.

Approximately 75 percent of those suffering from autoimmune disorders are women. Autoimmune disorders are among the top ten causes of death in women. A number of factors contribute to conditions leading to an autoimmune disorder. These factors include genetics, toxins from heavy metals, candida, Epstein-Barr, herpes simplex virus, nerve damage due to excessive exposure to neurotoxins, and chronic inflammation related to food sensitivities, particularly gluten intolerance.

Some of the symptoms characteristic of autoimmune conditions include: joint and/or muscle pain, weakness, tremors, weight loss, insomnia, heat intolerance, rapid heartbeat, recurrent rashes or hives, sun sensitivity, difficulty concentrating or focusing, glandular imbalances such as hypothyroidism or hyperthyroidism, fatigue, weight gain, cold intolerance, hair loss, white patches on skin or inside mouth, abdominal pain, blood or mucus in stool, diarrhea, mouth ulcers, dry eyes/mouth/skin, numbness or tingling in the extremities, blood clots, and multiple miscarriages.

Eighty percent of the immune system is directly connected to gut health, making it a vital area of focus to restore health. Using natural remedies together with a healthy diet can be an effective, non-invasive way to improve gut health. By using a consist program such as a whole food nutrient supplement, essential oil omega complex, and cellular vitality complex in a consistent program, along with food enzymes, a detoxification complex, lemon oil, GI cleansing softgels, and a defensive probiotic, an individual can nourish and support the body in an effort to reclaim health.

Repeating a healthy cleanse the first three to four months in a row can also help the body improve its capacity to take care of itself. Targeted support using natural remedies for certain conditions individualizes a program and targets symptoms of discomfort and disease. It is empowering to exercise options for natural solutions to target root causes, since most modern medical approaches to autoimmune conditions seek to only manage symptoms.

Additionally, a great way to help the immune system function optimally and to reduce environmental stress on the body is to perform the Oil Touch technique as it is explained in the introduction to this book. The technique is a systematic application of eight different essential oils that serves to strengthen the immune system, eliminate pathogens, reduce stress, and bring the body into homeostasis, enabling the body to function more optimally. A weekly application for three to four months is ideal. See Oil Touch technique, page 14.

TOP SOLUTIONS

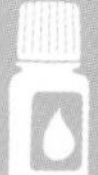

SINGLE OILS

Lemongrass - stimulates nerves and supports digestion (pg. 112)
Juniper berry - antioxidant and supports digestion (pg. 107)
Ginger - invigorates nerves and cleanses (pg. 103)
Clary sage - invigorates nerves and supports endocrine system (pg. 88)

By Related Properties

For definitions of the properties listed below and more oil options, see Oil Properties Glossary (pg. 435) and Oil Properties (pg. 436).

Analgesic - basil, birch, cassia, cinnamon, clary sage, clove, coriander, eucalyptus, fennel, frankincense, helichrysum, lavender, melaleuca, peppermint, white fir, wintergreen
Antiarthritic - arborvitae, basil, birch, cassia, cypress, ginger, white fir, wintergreen
Antidepressant - bergamot, clary sage, frankincense, geranium, jasmine, lavender, lemon, melissa, ravensara, rose, ylang ylang
Anti-infectious - basil, bergamot, cedarwood, cinnamon, clove, cypress, frankincense, geranium, lavender, marjoram, melaleuca, patchouli, rosemary
Anti-inflammatory - basil, birch, cardamom, cassia, cedarwood, cinnamon, coriander, cypress, eucalyptus, frankincense, geranium, helichrysum, lemongrass, lime, melissa, myrrh, peppermint, rosemary, sandalwood, spikenard, wintergreen
Antioxidant - basil, black pepper, cassia, cilantro, cinnamon, clove, frankincense, ginger, grapefruit, helichrysum, juniper berry, lemongrass, lime, melaleuca, oregano, thyme, vetiver, wild orange
Anti-parasitic - cinnamon, clove, frankincense, juniper berry, lavender, melaleuca, oregano, rosemary, thyme
Regenerative - cedarwood, clove, coriander, frankincense, geranium, helichrysum, jasmine, myrrh, patchouli, sandalwood, wild orange
Stomachic - cardamom, cinnamon, clary sage, coriander, fennel, ginger, juniper berry, marjoram, melissa, peppermint, rose, rosemary, tangerine, wild orange, yarrow
Tonic - arborvitae, basil, birch, cardamom, cedarwood, clary sage, coriander, cypress, fennel, frankincense, geranium, ginger, grapefruit, lavender, lemon, lime, marjoram, melissa, myrrh, patchouli, roman chamomile, rose, rosemary, sandalwood, tangerine, thyme, vetiver, white fir, wild orange, ylang ylang
Uplifting - bergamot, cardamom, cedarwood, clary sage, cypress, grapefruit, lime, melissa, sandalwood, tangerine, wild orange, ylang ylang

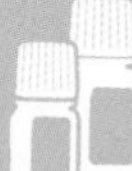

BLENDS

Cellular complex blend - supports nerves and glands (pg. 143)
Detoxification blend - detoxifies and supports proper digestive function (pg. 146)
Metabolic blend - antioxidant and improves digestion (pg. 157)

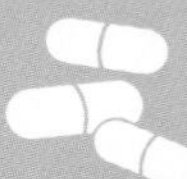

SUPPLEMENTS

Bone support complex, **cellular vitality complex (pg. 171), defensive probiotic (pg. 172)**, digestion blend softgels, energy & stamina complex, **essential oil cellular complex (pg. 174), essential oil omega complex (pg. 175), food enzymes (pg. 177)**, liquid omega-3 supplement, **polyphenol complex (pg. 181)**, protective blend lozenges, protective blend softgels (use with grounding blend), whole food supplement

CRITICAL AUTOIMMUNE SUPPLEMENTATION PROGRAM

- **Cellular vitality complex** with antioxidants, flavonoids, additional cellular support
- **Essential oil omega complex** with land and sea omega sources, astaxanthin (use a liquid omega-3 supplement for children and elderly who can't swallow pills)
- **Food enzymes** for proper digestion; add digestion blend softgels as needed
- **Whole food supplement** as a high potency multivitamin/mineral

Add as needed for desired target support:

- **Bone support complex** necessary for numerous cellular, structural functions
- **Defensive probiotic** to establish and maintain healthy gut flora, eliminate harmful microorganisms
- **Detoxification complex** and **detoxification blend** to promote detoxification, proper elimination
- **Energy & stamina complex** with CoQ10 for energy, improve circulation
- **Essential oil cellular complex** to establish and maintain healthy cell vitality and apoptosis
- **Polyphenol complex** to reduce or eliminate pain/inflammation, inflammatory responses

Remedies

For ALL autoimmune diseases consider the following:

- Critical Supplemental Program - see above
- See *Digestive & Intestinal* for digestive/intestinal issues, leaky gut
- See *Immune & Lymphatic* to manage/eliminate/prevent microorganisms
- See *Candida* to manage/eliminate/prevent candida
- Oil Touch technique or other massage techniques and heat treatments - see page 14

For the following specific autoimmune conditions, all suggestions below are recommended in addition to using the suggested critical supplements daily program and the Oil Touch technique weekly.

CELIAC DISEASE PROTOCOL

Combine in a capsule or in 12 ounces water:
2 drops lemon (tonic for the liver)
2 drops grapefruit (dissolves toxins stored in fat cells)
2 drops ginger (digestive support)
1 drop cinnamon (regulates blood sugar levels)
OR
6-7 drops of metabolic blend (Includes lemon, grapefruit, ginger, cinnamon)
Take two times daily for ongoing support.

Additional Support

- Rub digestion blend on stomach **OR** take 2-4 drops in capsule **OR** use 1-2 digestion blend softgels during digestive discomfort or upset stomach.
- Diffuse frankincense, joyful blend, or invigorating blend to combat depression or irritability.
- Take 2-3 food enzyme capsules daily.

CROHN'S DISEASE

In addition to a whole food nutrient supplement and essential oil omega complex Critical Autoimmune Supplemental Program (see above), additional specific targeted support suggestions are:

- Defensive probiotic three times daily for six months
- Take 2-3 food enzyme capsules daily (at least one per meal)
- Rub digestion blend on abdomen two times daily for 2 months
- Rub digestion blend and ginger on bottoms of feet daily for six months
- Place 2 drops digestion blend, 2 drops frankincense, and fractionated coconut oil (if desired) in a capsule. Take twice a day for two weeks. Then change formula to 5 drops ginger, 5 drops peppermint or marjoram, and 4 drops frankincense for two weeks.
- Topically apply cassia (dilute with a carrier oil), digestion blend, or peppermint for abdominal pain
- Topically apply or diffuse lavender or calming blend to manage stress

Consider a candida cleanse. See *Candida* section for details.

SJOGREN'S

In addition to Critical Autoimmune Supplementation Program (including the cellular vitality complex) twice per day, take 2 -3 drops of frankincense two to four times daily under the tongue or in a capsule. Use additional oils as symptoms occur; soothing blend for painful joints, digestion blend for digestive problems, lavender or geranium for skin problems, etc.

Additional suggestions:

Candida cleanse and other detoxing programs - see *Candida; Detoxification*

Chronic Dry Eye

Gently dab lavender (frankincense, myrrh, sandalwood are additional options) on the facial bones surrounding the eye, being careful to avoid the eye itself. Within minutes the dry, irritated eyes will soothe and feel better. Should you accidentally get too close to eye with any essential oil, dilute with carrier oil, never water!

Chronic Dry Mouth

Try oil pulling (see *Detoxification - Oil Pulling*) for a week and see if it helps the salivary glands to kick in.
Here is one oil pulling recipe:
1 tablespoon fractionated coconut oil
2 drop clove
2 drops oregano
Put mixture in mouth, swish in mouth for twenty minutes, then spit into the sink; repeat daily.

HASHIMOTO'S

Choose from the following protocols or use progressively over time.

- **Protocol 1:**
  40 drops each grounding blend and geranium placed in 10ml roller bottle with carrier oil.
  34 drops lemongrass and 40 myrrh placed in a different 10ml roller bottle with carrier oil.
  Shake each blend after adding to roller bottle. Alternate the above two combinations weekly. Apply them directly to thyroid area and reflex points on big toe, thumb multiple times per day.

- **Protocol 2:**
  25 drops lemongrass
  25 drops clove
  10 drops frankincense
  4 drops peppermint
  Prepare the above blend in a 10ml roller bottle, fill with fractionated coconut oil, and apply topically to thyroid and reflexology points three times daily.

- **Protocol 3:**
  Apply 2-3 drops of frankincense and 1 drop peppermint topically to thyroid and reflexology points three times daily to reduce goiter size.

AUTOIMMUNE

Conditions

Abdominal pain - marjoram, massage blend; see *Digestive & Intestinal, Muscles*

Blood clots - encouraging blend, protective blend, soothing blend, tension blend; see *Cardiovascular*

Blood in stool - birch (ulcer), geranium (bleeding), helichrysum (bleeding), wintergreen (ulcer); see *Digestive & Intestinal (Ulcers)*

Blood pressure changes - clary sage, ylang ylang (if too high); rosemary, thyme (if too low); see *Cardiovascular*

Cold intolerance - black pepper, cinnamon, eucalyptus, cellular complex blend; see *Endocrine (Thyroid), Cardiovascular (Poor circulation; Warming property)*

Diarrhea or constipation - black pepper, cardamom, douglas fir, ginger, digestion blend, encouraging blend; see *Digestive & Intestinal*

Dry eyes, mouth, or skin - See *Respiratory, Oral Health, Integumentary*

Hair loss - clary sage, eucalyptus, rosemary, encouraging blend; see *Integumentary*

Heat intolerance - eucalyptus, peppermint; see *Endocrine (Thyroid)*

Inflammation - birch, cypress, peppermint, wintergreen, encouraging blend; see *Pain & Inflammation*

Insomnia - lavender, frankincense, vetiver, calming blend, focus blend; see *Sleep*

Joint pain - lemongrass, massage blend, soothing blend; see *Skeletal, Pain & Inflammation*

Lack of concentration or focus - basil, rosemary, encouraging blend, focus blend; see *Focus & Concentration*

Mucus in stool - cardamom, ginger, digestion blend, encouraging blend; see *Digestive & Intestinal*

Muscle pain, weakness, tremor, or cramps - marjoram, inspiring blend, massage blend, soothing blend; see *Muscular, Pain & Inflammation*

Mouth ulcers - clove, myrrh, wild orange; see *Oral Health*

Multiple miscarriages - clary sage, grapefruit, thyme, encouraging blend; see *Women's Health*

Numbness or tingling in the hands or feet - cypress, peppermint, massage blend, soothing blend; see *Nervous*

Overactive immune system - basil, frankincense, helichrysum, lavender, grounding blend

Paralysis, facial - helichrysum, patchouli, peppermint, encouraging blend; see *Nervous*

Rapid heartbeat - frankincense, sandalwood, ylang ylang; see *Cardiovascular*

Rashes or hives - lavender, roman chamomile; see *Allergies*

Salt cravings - see "Critical Autoimmune Supplementation Program" above"

Skin pigmentation - cedarwood, sandalwood, anti-aging blend; see *Integumentary*

Sore throat, chronic - basil, cassia, cinnamon, eucalyptus, fennel, ginger, lemon, oregano, thyme, respiration blend, protective blend

Sun sensitivity - lavender, myrrh, essential oil omega complex with astaxanthin; see *Integumentary*

Tiredness or fatigue - cinnamon, cypress, douglas fir, peppermint, encouraging blend, uplifting blend; see *Energy & Vitality*

Weight gain or loss - cinnamon, ginger, metabolic blend; see *Weight*

White patches on skin, inside mouth - myrrh, sandalwood; see

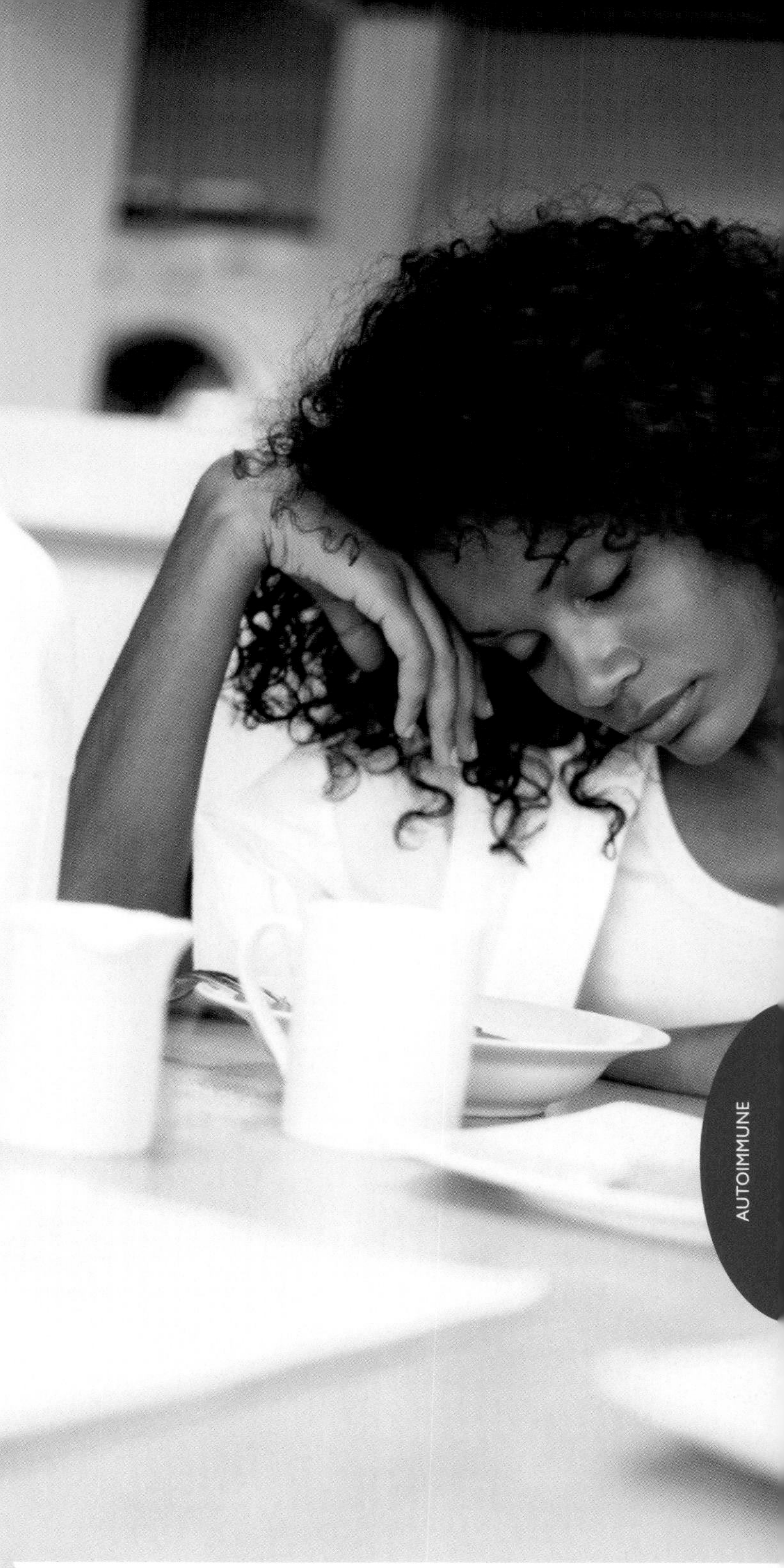

USAGE TIPS: For best support in resolving autoimmune conditions:

- **Internal:** Take oils in a capsule, drop under tongue (hold 30 seconds; swallow).
- **Topical:** Use Oil Touch technique at least one to two times monthly; weekly if possible; apply oils on bottoms of feet, rub oils down spine and on any specific area of concern.
- **Aromatic:** Diffuse chosen oils

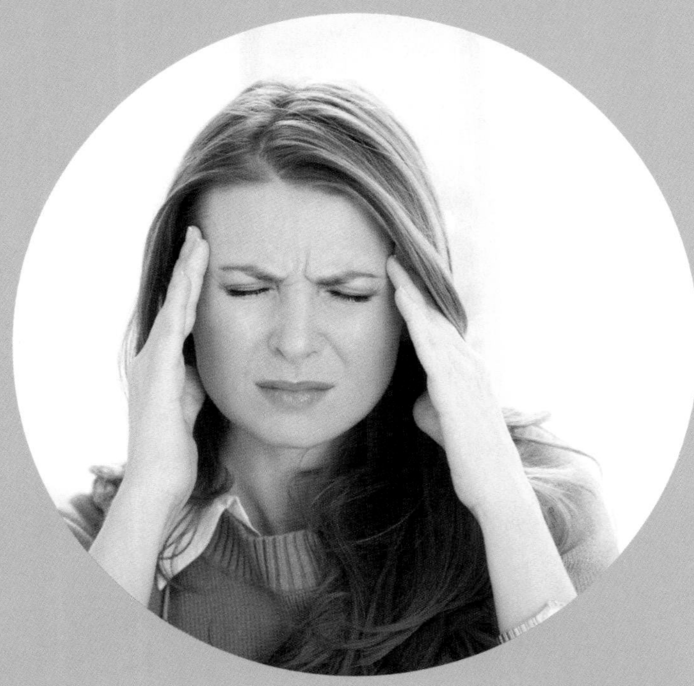

LUPUS

Cleanse (in addition to basic critical supplementation):
Do a candida cleanse. See *Immune & Lymphatic - Candida* section for details.

Address Inflammation
- Ingest citrus oils as a daily priority. Use your favorite 3-5 drops three times per day in water or veggie capsule.
- For liver and anti-inflammatory support:
  - Place 4 drops each geranium, helichrysum or lemongrass, rosemary oils in a capsule and take daily.
  - Use detoxification blend

For localized pain, use soothing blend, wintergreen, or birch topically.

For systemic pain, combine (in capsule), consume every four hours or as needed:
- 2-4 drops lavender
- 2-4 drops helichrysum
- 2-4 drops clove or thyme

  Additionally, for a soothing bath, add above oils to: 1-2 cups Epsom salt (4 drops of oil per cup Epsom salt). Mix oils in salt prior to placing in tub water as hot as is tolerated. Dissolve the salt mixture in the water and soak for twenty minutes. Other oils to consider: cinnamon, clove, coriander, frankincense, geranium, ginger, lavender, lemongrass, myrrh, roman chamomile, wintergreen. Change oil choices/combinations as needed and desired.

SCLERODERMA

Initial Cleanse
- The Critical Supplementation Program is a must.
- Do a candida cleanse. See *Candida* section for details. Repeat the cleanse twice; take a 10 day break in between the first and second; then repeat every other month as needed. Be sure to follow up each round with five days of increased amounts of defensive probiotic.
- Drop 2-3 drops of frankincense under the tongue four times a day for two weeks.
- Pain Relief blend - use at least two times per day:
  - 3 drops each lavender, soothing blend, and birch OR wintergreen
  - 4 drops each myrrh and sandalwood
  - Apply topically to bottoms of feet, along spine, and outside of ears, alternating daily between blends.

Ongoing Support
Continue supplementation program.
- Daily - apply soothing blend to areas of concern morning, midday, evening, and anytime intense pain occurs.
- Morning:
  - Topically apply peppermint to the bottoms of feet.
  - Take 3-4 drops of peppermint, digestion blend, frankincense, basil in capsule.
- During the day:
  - Add 1-3 drops of lemon to each glass of water. Drink lots of water. Glass containers only.
- Evening:
  - Take 3-4 drops each of peppermint, lemongrass, marjoram in capsule.
- Topically apply 2-3 drops of frankincense to bottoms of feet. Layer 2-4 drops geranium oil, massage blend.

Specific Issues:
- Breathing issues - rub 2-4 drops of peppermint and/or respiration blend on chest, on/in nasal passages.
- Digestive issues - rub 3-4 drops of digestion blend over abdomen.

Related Ailments: Addison's Disease (adrenals) [Endocrine], Autoimmune Hepatitis (liver) [Digestive & Intestinal], Celiac Sprue Disease (GI tract) [Digestive & Intestinal], Crohn's Disease [Digestive & Intestinal], Diabetes Type 1 [Blood Sugar], Glomerulonephritis (kidneys) [Urinary], Grave Disease (thyroid) [Endocrine], Gout (joints, big toe) [Skeletal], Hashimoto's (thyroid) [Endocrine], Huntington Disease (nerve cells in brain) [Brain, Nervous], Inflammatory myopathies [Muscles], Lou Gehrig's/ALS (nerve cells in brain, spinal cord) [Brain, Nervous], Lupus (any part of the body such as skin, joints, and/or organs), Multiple Sclerosis (myelin sheath) [Nervous], Pernicious Anemia (failure to produce red blood cells [Cardiovascular] and failure to absorb vitamin B12 - liver) [Digestive & Intestinal], Rheumatoid Arthritis (joints in hands, feet) [Skeletal], Sarcoidosis/sarcoid (primarily lungs, lymph nodes) [Respiratory, Immune & Lymphatic; Digestive & Intestinal (leaky gut)], Schmidt's Syndrome (Scleroderma (connective tissue) [Muscles, Skeletal], Sjogrens (salivary, tear duct glands) [Oral Health, Respiratory], Vitiligo (skin pigment cells) [Integumentary, Endocrine (thyroid), Women's Health, Stress]

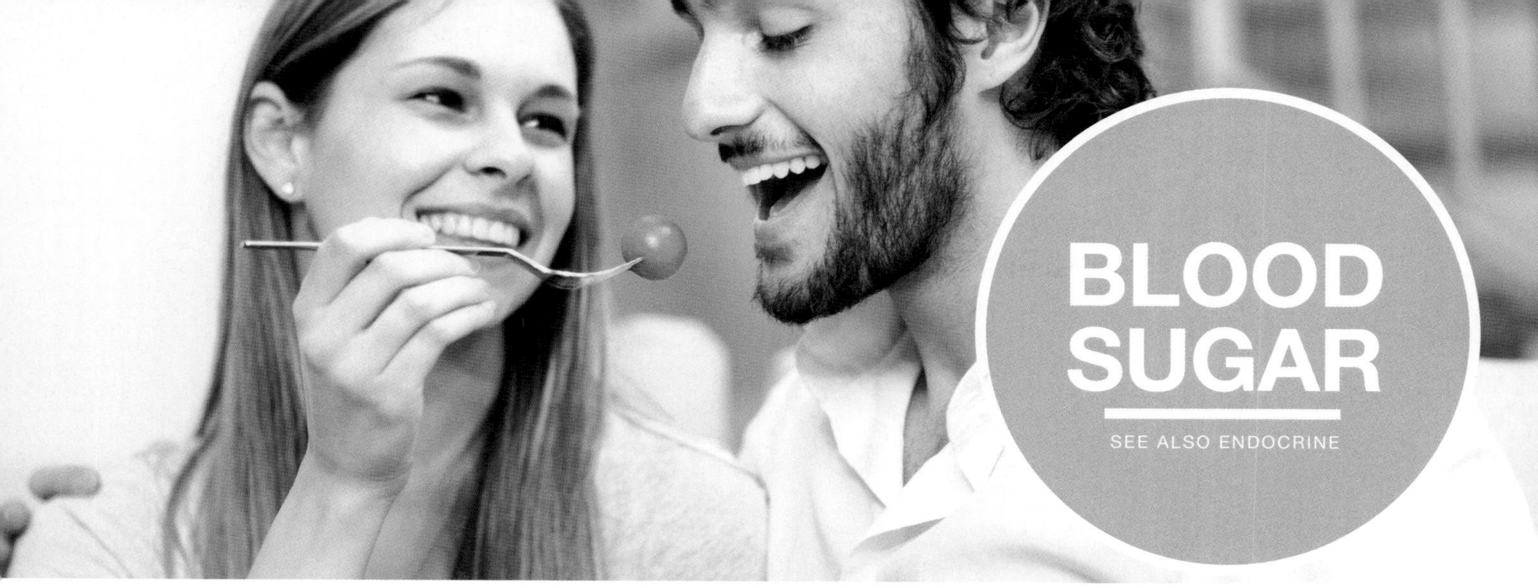

BLOOD SUGAR

SEE ALSO ENDOCRINE

INSULIN is a hormone that regulates blood sugar levels, shuttling the right amount of glucose into the cells where it is used for energy. When the body doesn't have enough insulin, blood-sugar levels become too high and cells don't have enough energy to function properly.

Diabetes is the most common endocrine disorder; it occurs when pancreas doesn't produce enough insulin (type 1 - typical onset is before age 20), or if the body is unable to use insulin (type 2 - typically over age 40). The onset age for type 2 is decreasing with an increasingly younger population suffering from what is a preventable disease. A third type, gestational diabetes, can occur during pregnancy and create potential long-term issues for both mother and child.

Hypoglycemia is a condition characterized by too little glucose in the blood. When severe, is also called "insulin reaction" or "insulin shock" and can lead to accidents, injuries, even coma and death.

When we consume healthy sources of carbohydrates with plenty of good fats and protein, the glucose from the meal enters the blood slowly and the pancreas responds by secreting a measured amount of insulin. Keeping blood sugar balanced throughout the day is the best way to avoid "sugar highs" and "sugar lows." A healthy individual can easily go three hours or more between meals without experiencing sugar cravings or feeling shaky, irritable, or tired.

Eating habits can influence the likelihood of developing blood sugar issues. When individuals consume foods too high in sugar or refined carbohydrates, these simple carbs enter the bloodstream almost immediately through the intestines, resulting in higher-than-normal blood sugar levels. The body then needs to produce more insulin to process the excess glucose. As the presence of elevated insulin levels becomes chronic, the body's sensitivity to insulin decreases (known as insulin resistance), forcing blood glucose levels to rise. Insulin is also an inflammatory agent.

Additionally, blood sugar imbalances and elevated insulin levels affect a number of functions, from hormones to heart to mood to cellular health to fertility... as well as perpetuate inflammation, which is considered to be a prime contributor to disease. One lesser known fact is that high blood pressure is another common symptom which is caused by high circulating levels of insulin in the blood. Common conditions resulting from blood sugar issues can be found in *Endocrine* and *Cardiovascular*.

Insulin and glucose levels are easily improved by positive changes in lifestyle, exercise, and diet. One of the benefits of stable blood sugar is the natural reduction of inflammation and the resulting balance of hormones. Healthy dietary changes (elimination of harmful sugars and refined carbohydrates), commitments, and consistencies are therefore significant. A study reported in the Journal of the American Medical Association (JAMA) stated, "Duration and degree of sugar exposure correlated significantly with diabetes prevalence while declines in sugar exposure correlated with significant subsequent declines in diabetes rates." *

Natural solutions can be incredibly effective in supporting the body to generate a healthy insulin response and blood-sugar regulation. Because stable blood sugar levels diminish or eliminate sugar and carb cravings, even stubborn weight can melt away and longevity may be extended.

In addition to necessary dietary and lifestyle commitments, essential oils are powerful allies in achieving and maintaining healthy blood sugar and insulin levels, improving insulin receptivity, and resolving a surprising number of related health concerns. Additionally, essential oils support bringing other body systems into balance, which is particularly helpful given the number of diabetes-related disorders. Essential oils positively impact blood sugar management. For example, coriander oil lowers glucose levels by normalizing insulin levels and supporting pancreatic function. Cinnamon oil aids in managing blood glucose levels and strengthens the circulatory and immune systems.

NOTE: Every condition listed below is considered potentially related to or associated with imbalanced blood sugar and/or insulin levels. Addressing both blood sugar and insulin levels through diet, supplementation, and the use of essential oils is critical to success. The use of suggestions below to manage symptoms is intended to be paired with these critical diet and lifestyle changes.

TOP SOLUTIONS

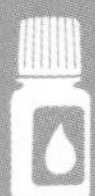

SINGLE OILS

Coriander - promotes a healthy insulin response (pg. 92)
Cinnamon - balances blood sugar levels (pg. 86)
Cassia - balances blood sugar levels (pg. 83)

By Related Properties

For definitions of the properties listed below and more oil options, see Oil Properties Glossary (pg. 435) and Oil Properties (pg. 436).

Antifungal - bergamot, cinnamon, clove, coriander, fennel, helichrysum, lemongrass, melaleuca, oregano, ravensara, thyme
Anti-inflammatory - birch, cardamom, cassia, cinnamon, clove, coriander, frankincense, ginger, lavender, lemongrass, myrrh, oregano, patchouli, rosemary, spikenard, yarrow
Antioxidant - black pepper, cinnamon, coriander, frankincense, ginger, helichrysum, juniper berry, lemon, lemongrass, oregano, vetiver, wild orange
Detoxifier - arborvitae, cassia, cilantro, geranium, juniper berry, lemon, lime, patchouli
Invigorating - grapefruit, lemon, peppermint, wild orange
Stomachic - cardamom, cinnamon, clary sage, coriander, eucalyptus, juniper berry, marjoram, melissa, peppermint, rosemary, wild orange, yarrow
Stimulant - basil, cedarwood, cinnamon, coriander, thyme, wintergreen
Vasodilator - lemongrass, marjoram, rosemary, thyme

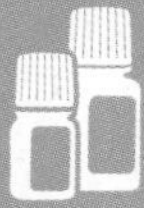

BLENDS

Protective blend - balances blood sugar levels (pg. 158)
Cellular complex blend - improves insulin receptivity (pg. 143)
Cleansing blend - improves insulin receptivity (pg. 144)

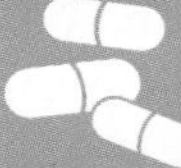

SUPPLEMENTS

Cellular vitality complex (pg. 171), digestion blend softgels, essential oil omega complex, **metabolic blend softgels (pg. 180)**, whole food nutrient supplement

Related Ailments: Blood Sugar Headaches, Blood Sugar Imbalance, Diabetes, Diabetic Sores, Hypoglycemia, Insulin, Insulin Imbalances, Insulin Resistance, Low Blood Sugar, Sugar Headache

BLOOD SUGAR

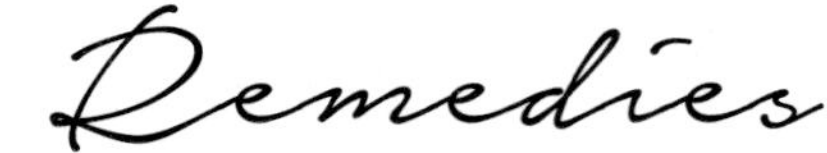

Remedies

HIGH BLOOD SUGAR REDUCER
3 drops coriander or basil
3 drops metabolic blend
1 drop oregano
Taken two to three times per day in capsule.

LOW BLOOD SUGAR (use to improve)
2 drops rosemary
1 drop geranium
1 drop cypress
Apply to chest and reflexology points on feet and hands (dilute if needed), or diffuse.

BLOOD SUGAR BALANCE BLEND
- Recipe #1: 2 drops cinnamon, 2 drops clove, 4 drops rosemary, 3 drops thyme oils;
  Combine in 10ml roller bottle; fill remainder with carrier oil; apply to bottoms of feet, massage; focus on arch of foot to target pancreas reflex point(s).
- Recipe #2: 2 drops cinnamon + 5 drops cypress
  Combine in palm of one hand then distribute across bottoms of feet, center of abdomen just below the ribs (over the pancreas).

DAILY ROUTINE FOR SUPPORTING HEALTHY BLOOD SUGAR
- Rub 1-2 drops of grounding blend on bottoms of feet in morning
- Use "High Blood Sugar" remedy three times daily
- Rub 1-2 drops of lavender on feet at night prior to sleep

CDF BLEND (coriander, dill, fennel)
- Apply 2-3 drops coriander, dill, fennel in equal parts on feet first thing in morning. At night apply same oils on pancreas area of body with a warm compress (warm, damp cloth). Dilute if desired to lessen sensation of heat.
- Place 2 drops each of coriander, dill, fennel in capsule, fill with carrier oil, and take one time per day. Can also be placed on a spoon and swallowed.

NEUROPATHY NEUTRALIZER
Apply 3-4 drops of cypress, coriander, and/or soothing blend to legs below knees all the way to bottoms of feet; massage. Use at least morning and night.

BLOOD SUGAR BALANCING CINNAMON TEA
Place 1-2 drops of cinnamon bark in ½ cup warm water, sweeten with 1 teaspoon raw honey or agave nectar if needed.

GRAPEFRUIT DETOX DELIGHT
1-2 drops cassia or cinnamon + 3 drops grapefruit in a 24-ounce water bottle. Shake, do not stir. Drink throughout day.

EMOTIONAL RELIEF AND PANCREAS SUPPORT
Apply 1-2 drops of geranium to bottoms of feet.

Conditions

Anxiety - cilantro, coriander, melaleuca, peppermint, calming blend, detoxification blend, grounding blend, tension blend; see *Mood & Behavior*

Apple-shaped body/abdominal excess weight - See "Insulin resistance...", "Insulin, excessive," "Glucose levels, high...", See *Weight*

Blurred/compromised vision - cilantro, coriander, helichrysum, lemongrass, melissa, rose, thyme, anti-aging blend, cellular complex blend, detoxification blend, joyful blend

Circulation issues/foot issues/gangrene - See *Cardiovascular*

Cravings for sweets - cassia, cinnamon, grapefruit, metabolic blend; see *Eating Disorders, Weight*

Concentration, poor/Brain fog - See *Focus & Concentration*

Depression - bergamot, geranium, wild orange, ylang ylang, joyful blend; see *Mood & Behavior*

Digestive issues/chronic constipation or diarrhea - See *Digestion & Intestinal*

Dizziness - dill, helichrysum, cellular complex blend, detoxification blend; see "Glucose levels, low (Hypoglycemia)" below

Energy dips/fatigue/drowsiness - basil, cinnamon, ginger, lemon, lime, peppermint, rosemary, wild orange, wintergreen, metabolic blend, uplifting blend; see *Energy & Vitality*

Feeling frequent urination - detoxification blend; see *Urinary*

Glucose levels, high (hyperglycemia) - basil, cinnamon, coriander, dill, eucalyptus, fennel, ginger, lemon, oregano, rosemary, ylang ylang, detoxification blend, metabolic blend

Glucose levels, low (hypoglycemia) - cassia, cypress, eucalyptus, geranium, juniper berry, lavender, lemongrass, detoxification blend, metabolic blend

Headache - frankincense, lavender, peppermint, wintergreen, metabolic blend, tension blend; see *Pain & Inflammation*

Heart palpitations/irregular/rapid heartbeat - See *Cardiovascular*

High blood pressure (due to the circulation of excessive insulin) - See "Glucose levels, high (Hyperglycemia)"

Hunger/excessive hunger - See *Weight*

Infections, skin/vaginal - melaleuca, protective blend

Insulin, excessive - coriander, lemongrass

Insulin, insufficient - dill, wild orange

Insulin resistance or poor response to - cassia, coriander, cypress, juniper berry, lavender, lemongrass, oregano, rosemary, ylang ylang, cellular complex blend, cleansing blend, detoxification blend, metabolic blend, protective blend

Irritability - See *Mood & Behavior*

Kidney/urinary issues - See *Urinary*

Mood swings/sudden changes - geranium, patchouli, calming blend, focus blend, grounding blend, joyful blend; see *Mood & Behavior*

Nausea - basil, bergamot, ginger, juniper berry,digestion blend; see *Digestion & Intestinal*

Nerve damage (i.e. painful cold or insensitive feet, loss of hair on the lower extremities, or erectile dysfunction, tingling skin) - basil; see *Nervous*

Nervousness, sudden - cedarwood, frankincense, calming blend, grounding blend; see *Mood & Behavior*

Shaky/weak - black pepper, frankincense, vetiver, calming blend, joyful blend, tension blend

Skin, pale - cypress, wild orange, massage blend

Sleep, want excessive amount - geranium, wild orange

Sleep, difficulty - geranium, lavender, marjoram, patchouli, roman chamomile, ylang ylang; see *Sleep*

Sweating/hot flashes (due to blood sugar imbalance) - eucalyptus, peppermint

Thirst, excessive/increased - grapefruit, lemon, metabolic blend

Urination, frequent - basil, cinnamon, cypress, detoxification blend, massage blend, protective blend; see *Urinary*

Weight loss, sudden/excessive - cinnamon, metabolic blend; see *Weight*

Wound healing, poor/slow - cypress, frankincense, helichrysum, lavender, myrrh, white fir, anti-aging blend; see *First Aid*

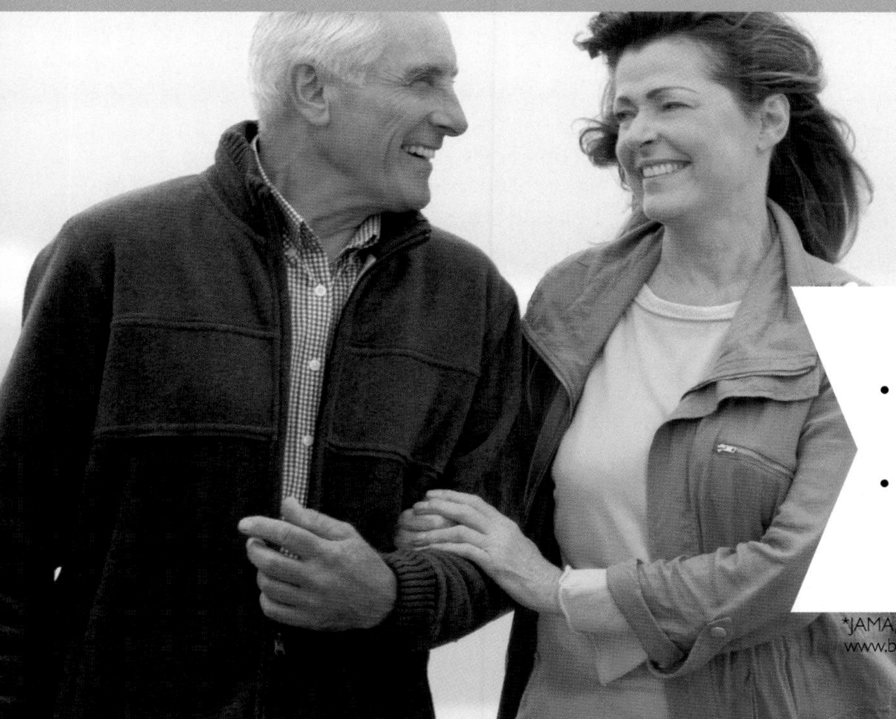

USAGE TIPS: For best success at targeting blood sugar and insulin levels:

- **Internal:** Place 1-5 drops in water to drink, take oil(s) in a capsule, place a drop(s) on or under tongue, or lick them off back of hand.
- **Topical:** Apply oils topically on bottoms of feet targeting reflex points for pancreas and other endocrine partners such as adrenal and thyroid locations; see Reflexology.

*JAMA, 2004; Diabetes Care, 2010; PLOS ONE, 2013. Reported by Business Insider: www.businessinsider.com/effects-of-eating-too-much-sugar-2014-3#ixzz3UKTXOpuy

BRAIN

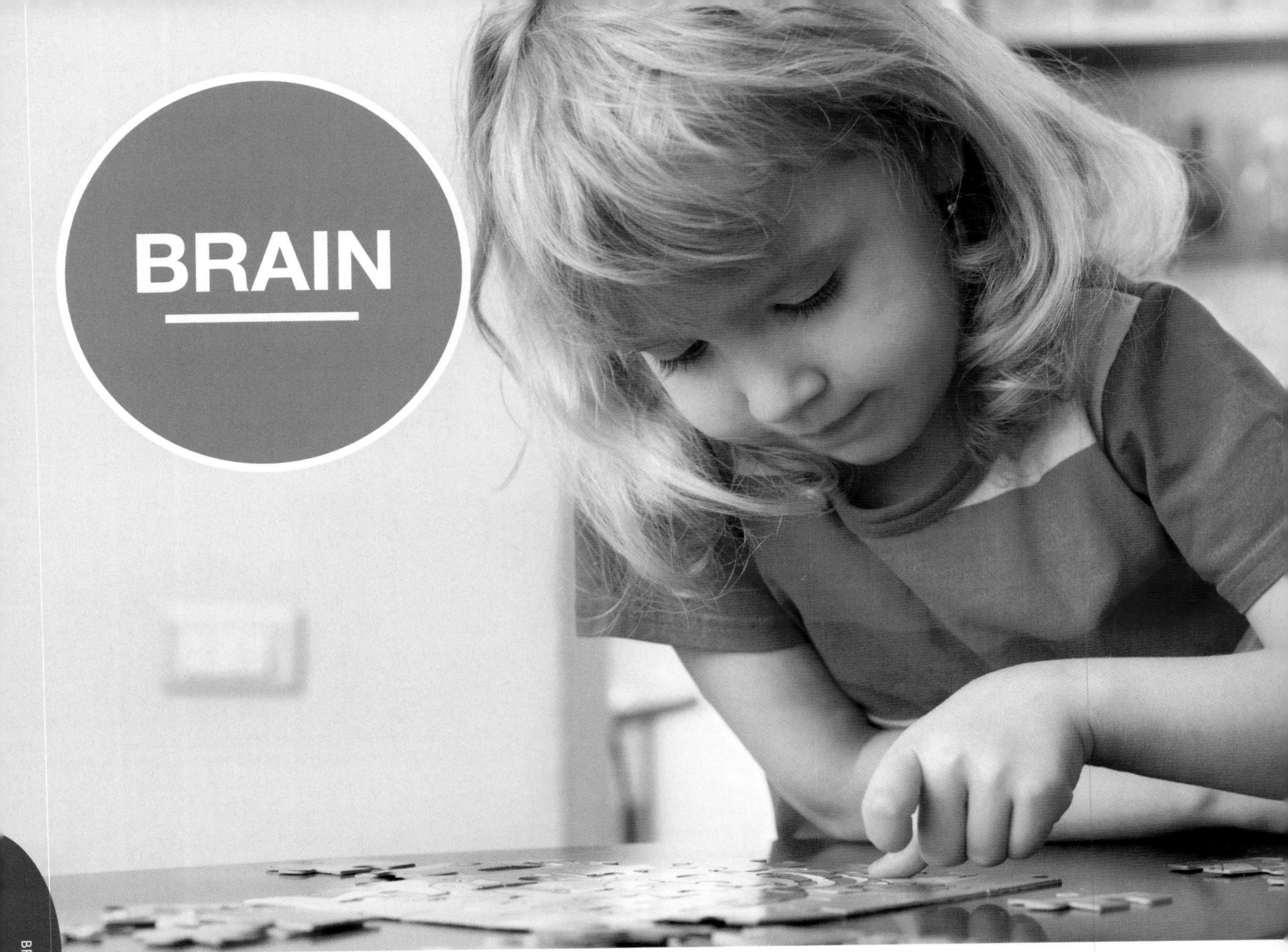

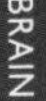

THE BRAIN, an organ the size of a small head of cauliflower, resides in the skull and is the control center of the body. The brain is the most vital organ to everyday life functioning and, together with the spinal cord and peripheral nerves, makes up the central nervous system, which directs, coordinates, and regulates voluntary (conscious) and involuntary (unconscious) processes. Sensory nerves throughout the body constantly gather information from the environment and send it to the brain via the spinal cord. The brain rapidly interprets the data and responds by sending messages with motor neurons to the rest of the body.

Scientists have found that certain parts of the brain perform certain functions. The frontal lobe, where the limbic system is located, helps regulate emotions and trauma, assists with reasoning, planning, and problem solving, and is involved with some language skills. The parietal lobe aids with recognition and interpreting data, orientation, and movement. The occipital lobe is connected to visual processing, and the temporal lobe supports perception, auditory processing, memory, and speech.

Due to its important role in managing and directing all organs, systems, and body processes, the brain has several layers of protection including the skull, the meninges (thin membranes), and cerebrospinal fluid. The brain also has what has come to be called the "blood-brain barrier," which keeps cells of the nervous system separate from cells throughout the vascular system (the rest of the body).

Essential oils powerfully benefit brain function and processes. When used aromatically, such as diffusing oils into the air or inhaling oils directly from bottle or palms of the hands, essential oils directly access the brain through the olfactory bulb and are able to initiate almost immediate physical and emotional responses in the brain.

Due to their unique chemical constituents and the fact that they are carbon based, essential oils are able to permeate the protective blood-brain barrier and provide support for such things as headaches, migraines, vertigo, emotions, and mood. Certain essential oils that are comprised of specific chemical constituents like sesquiterpenes, such as frankincense and sandalwood, have a particular affinity for supporting the brain. Essential oils with antioxidant and anti-inflammatory properties are also particularly important for maintaining a healthy brain.

TOP SOLUTIONS

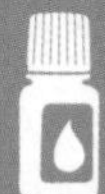

SINGLE OILS

Sandalwood - promotes optimal brain function, repair; crosses blood-brain barrier (pg. 128)
Frankincense - crosses blood-brain barrier; anti-aging brain support (pg. 100)
Cedarwood - calms, stimulates, and protects brain (pg. 84)
Rosemary - enhances brain, cognitive performance; relieves mental fatigue (pg. 127)
Clove and thyme - provides brain protective antioxidants (pgs. 90 & 133)

By Related Properties

For definitions of the properties listed below and more oil options, see Oil Properties Glossary (pg. 435) and Oil Properties (pg. 436).

Anticonvulsant - clary sage, fennel, geranium, lavender
Anti-inflammatory - basil, bergamot, birch, black pepper, cardamom, cedarwood, cinnamon, clove, coriander, dill, eucalyptus, fennel, frankincense, geranium, helichrysum, jasmine, lavender, lemongrass, lime, melaleuca, melissa, myrrh, oregano, patchouli, peppermint, roman chamomile, rosemary, sandalwood, spearmint, wild orange, wintergreen
Antioxidant - arborvitae, basil, black pepper, cassia, cilantro, cinnamon, clove, coriander, eucalyptus, frankincense, ginger, grapefruit, helichrysum, juniper berry, lemon, lemongrass, lime, melaleuca, oregano, rosemary, thyme, vetiver, wild orange
Anti-parasitic - bergamot, cinnamon, clove, fennel, frankincense, juniper berry, lavender, melaleuca, oregano, roman chamomile, rosemary, thyme
Nervine - basil, clary sage, clove, helichrysum, juniper berry, lavender, lemongrass, melissa, patchouli, peppermint, rosemary, thyme
Neuroprotective - frankincense, lavender, roman chamomile, thyme, vetiver
Neurotonic - arborvitae, basil, bergamot, black pepper, clary sage, cypress, ginger, melaleuca
Regenerative - frankincense, geranium, helichrysum, melaleuca, patchouli, rose, sandalwood, wild orange
Stimulant - arborvitae, basil, bergamot, birch, black pepper, cardamom, cedarwood, cinnamon, clove, coriander, cypress, dill, eucalyptus, fennel, ginger, grapefruit, juniper berry, lime, melaleuca, patchouli, rosemary, spearmint, thyme, vetiver, white fir, wintergreen, ylang ylang

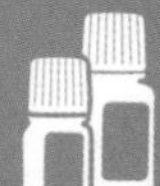

BLENDS

Cellular complex blend - provides antioxidants and brain protection (pg. 143)
Detoxification blend - supports relief from mental fatigue and toxins (pg. 146)
Focus blend - supports oxygen and blood flow to brain, blood brain barrier (pg. 149)

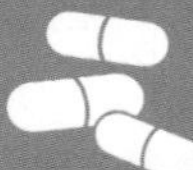

SUPPLEMENTS

Cellular vitality complex (pg. 171), essential oil cellular complex, **essential oil omega complex (pg. 175)**, detoxification complex capsules, **liquid omega-3 supplement (pg. 178)**, whole food nutrient complex

USAGE TIPS: Some best ways to apply oils for brain health are where there's more direct access to the brain:

- **Topically:** Apply to forehead, back of skull (especially in occipital triangles), under nose, roof of mouth (place oil on pad of thumb, place on roof, "suck")
  Use reflex points on foot for brain, namely big toe, underside pad.
- **Aromatically:** Diffuse oils of choice to stimulate brain allowing entry through nose to olfactory system.

Related Ailments: Absentmindedness, Alertness, Alzheimer's Disease, Amnesia, Ataxia, Autism [Focus & Concentration], Bipolar Disorder [Mood & Behavior], Body Dysmorphic Disorder, Brain Fog, Brain Injury, Chemical Imbalance [Endocrine], Coma, Concussion, Creutzfeldt-Jakob Disease [Immune & Lymphatic], Dementia, Down Syndrome, Epilepsy, Huntington's Disease [Nervous], Hydrocephalus, Learning Difficulties, Lou Gehrig's Disease, Meniere's Disease, Mental Fatigue, Narcolepsy, Obsessive-Compulsive Disorder, Parkinson's Disease, Schizophrenia, Seizures, Social Anxiety Disorder [Mood & Behavior], Stroke, Transverse Myelitis

Remedies

ALZHEIMER'S PROTOCOL

Internal:

- Take 4-5 drops each frankincense, thyme, patchouli in a capsule daily.
- Take 4-5 drops each clove, melissa, vetiver in a capsule weekly.
- Eat 1 teaspoon of virgin coconut oil a day. Work up to 3 tablespoons a day. Great on toast.
- Take energy & stamina complex and cellular vitality complex daily.
- Blood sugar support: Drop metabolic blend under the tongue three to five times per day.

Topical:

Rub frankincense on base of skull and neck twice daily.

Brain support: Rub anti-aging blend on spine and suboccipital triangle area at the base of the skull at least twice daily, occasionally rotate with focus blend and patchouli. Diffuse these oils as well.

BRAIN-FOG BUSTER: (good for overall brain support): Layer 1 drop of each cedarwood, frankincense, patchouli, sandalwood, and vetiver on back of neck with a few drops of carrier oil to enhance circulation to the brain. Note: A carrier oil can be applied before, mixed with, or after essential oils are applied. If carrier oil is applied before or mixed with the essential oil, it slows the absorption. If the carrier oil is applied after, it enhances accelerates absorption.

COGNITIVE IMPROVEMENT: Place 1-2 drops melissa, frankincense, patchouli on suboccipital triangle area at the base of the skull, the bottoms of the feet, and under tongue twice daily to support improvement of cognitive impairment and help dispel agitation and depression.

BRAIN

AUTISM SUPPORT PROTOCOL

- **Overall detox**
  - › Layer 1 drop of rosemary and wild orange on each foot at bedtime
  - › Apply 2 drops detoxification blend on each foot on top of the single oils at bedtime
- **Cleanse gut**
  - › Take 2 children's chewable vitamins daily
  - › Take 1 GI cleansing softgels daily if child can swallow capsules, if not, use a good quality powder or liquid GI cleansing supplement
  - › Follow up with defensive probiotics as recommended, or if not able to swallow capsules, then use a good quality powder or liquid probiotic supplement
- **Brain repair**
  Take liquid omega-3 supplements twice daily
  Apply 1 drop cellular complex blend on the base of the skull at least morning and evening, up to five times daily
- **Emotional support** - use the following aromatically in hands or in a diffuser unless otherwise directed, apply to spine or bottoms of feet if the aroma is not tolerated.
  - › Use cypress, oregano (with a carrier oil), or wintergreen as needed for inflexibility
  - › Use juniper berry or wintergreen morning and night to lift mood and instill courage
  - › Use lime as needed for overstimulation or feelings of being overwhelmed
  - › Use patchouli as needed when agitated
  - › Use roman chamomile morning and night to soothe nerves and excessive reactions
  - › Use 1 drop protective blend or repellent blend every morning on bottom of each foot to increase sense of security

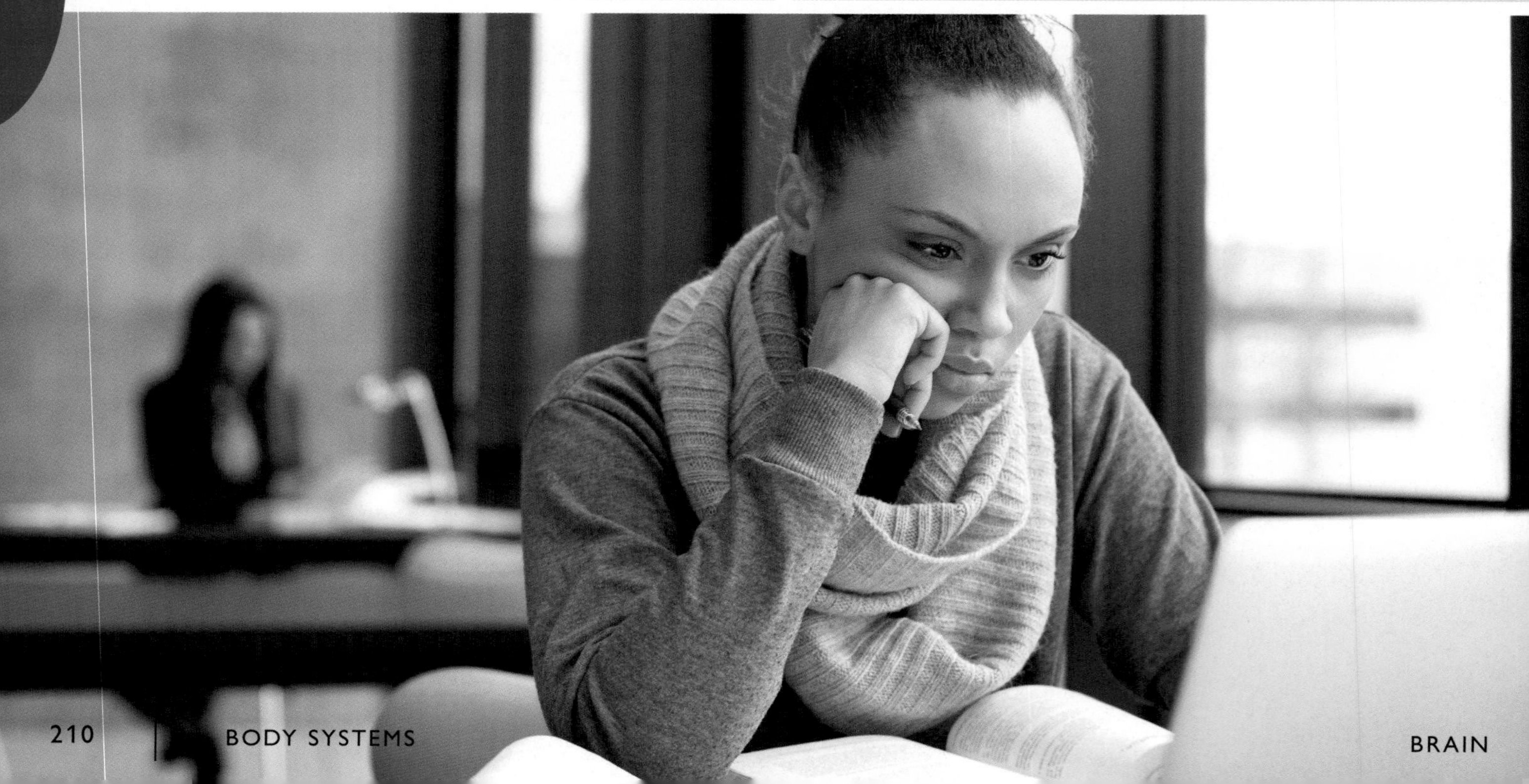

Conditions

Alzheimer's - clove, coriander, frankincense, lemon, melissa, sandalwood, thyme, vetiver, cellular complex blend, comforting blend, focus blend, grounding blend, renewing blend; see *Focus & Concentration*

Autism - basil, bergamot, clary sage, frankincense, geranium, peppermint, rosemary, vetiver, calming blend, cellular complex blend, focus blend, grounding blend, soothing blend

Balance/equilibrium - See "Dizziness" and "Vertigo" below

Blood-brain barrier - cedarwood, frankincense, ginger, myrrh, sandalwood, patchouli, vetiver, ylang ylang, cellular complex blend, focus blend, grounding blend, women's blend

Brain - arborvitae, cedarwood, clove, eucalyptus, frankincense, ginger, patchouli, rosemary, sandalwood, thyme, vetiver, cellular complex blend, detoxification blend, encouraging blend, focus blend, grounding blend, protective blend, women's blend

Brain, aging - clove, douglas fir, frankincense, oregano, thyme, cellular vitality complex, comforting blend, focus blend, grounding blend, protective blend, reassuring blend; see "Brain" above

Brain, aneurysm - bergamot, frankincense, helichrysum, myrrh, cellular complex blend

Brain, blood flow - basil, cedarwood, cypress, eucalyptus, ginger, lemongrass, oregano, patchouli, peppermint, rosemary, sandalwood, tangerine, thyme, cellular complex blending, energy & stamina complex, massage blend, women's blend

Brain, injury - arborvitae, bergamot, douglas fir, frankincense, helichrysum, lemon, myrrh, peppermint, cellular complex blend, comforting blend

Brain, lesions - frankincense, peppermint, rosemary, sandalwood, cellular complex blend, grounding blend

Central nervous system - bergamot, black pepper, myrrh, patchouli, rosemary, sandalwood

Chemical imbalance - cilantro, cinnamon, geranium, frankincense, patchouli, cellular complex blend, detoxification blend, focus blend, joyful blend

Coma - cedarwood, helichrysum, frankincense, myrrh, sandalwood, cellular complex, encouraging blend, grounding blend

Concussion - bergamot, cypress, frankincense, sandalwood, focus blend, grounding blend

Dizziness - arborvitae, cedarwood, douglas fir, ginger, frankincense, lavender, spearmint, rosemary, cellular complex blend, comforting blend, detoxification blend, focus blend, grounding blend, invigorating blend

Free radicals, neutralization of - cilantro, cinnamon, coriander, clove, ginger, lemongrass, rosemary, any citrus oil; see oils with "Antioxidant" properties

GABA, lack of - basil, cedarwood, rosemary, thyme, ylang ylang, calming blend, citrus blend, encouraging blend, focus blend, grounding blend; see *Endocrine (adrenals)*

Heat stroke - bergamot, black pepper, dill, lemon, peppermint, detoxification blend, soothing blend, tension blend

Heavy metal toxicity - cilantro; see *Detoxification*

Memory, poor - clove, douglas fir, frankincense, ginger, rosemary, peppermint, sandalwood, focus blend

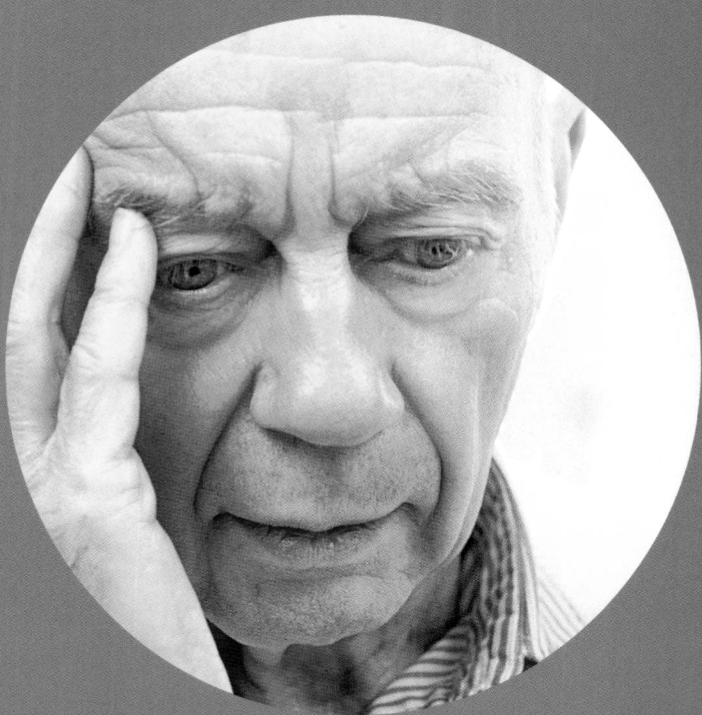

Mental fatigue - basil, bergamot, cardamom, frankincense, lemon, lavender, lemongrass, peppermint, ravensara, rose, rosemary, sandalwood, spearmint, white fir, ylang ylang, comforting blend, encouraging blend, invigorating blend, renewing blend, reassuring blend, respiration blend

Oxygen, lack of - cedarwood, cypress, eucalyptus, frankincense, ginger, patchouli, sandalwood, vetiver; see oils with "Antioxidant" properties

Parasites - See oils with "Anti-parasitic" properties; see *Parasites*

Parkinson's - basil, bergamot, clary sage, clove, cypress, frankincense, geranium, helichrysum, jasmine, juniper berry, lavender, lemon, marjoram, peppermint, rosemary, sandalwood, thyme, vetiver, wild orange, calming blend, cellular complex blend, comforting blend, detoxification blend, grounding blend; see *Addictions (oils to support dopamine levels)*

Seizures/convulsions, involuntary - basil, cardamom, cedarwood, clary sage, douglas fir, fennel, frankincense, geranium, lavender, myrrh, peppermint, rose (delay onset), sandalwood, uplifting blend; see oils with "Anticonvulsant" properties

Senility - frankincense, sandalwood; see oils with "Stimulant" properties

Sensory systems, closed/blocked - birch, wintergreen

Speech, slurred words/trouble speaking/difficulty understanding speech - arborvitae, patchouli, detoxification blend, women's blend

Stroke - basil, bergamot, cedarwood, cypress, fennel, frankincense, helichrysum, wintergreen, cleansing blend, protective blend; see oils with "Anti-inflammatory" and "Antioxidant" properties

Vertigo - cedarwood, frankincense, geranium, ginger, helichrysum, lavender, melissa, rosemary, cellular complex blend, focus blend, grounding blend, invigorating blend, reassuring blend

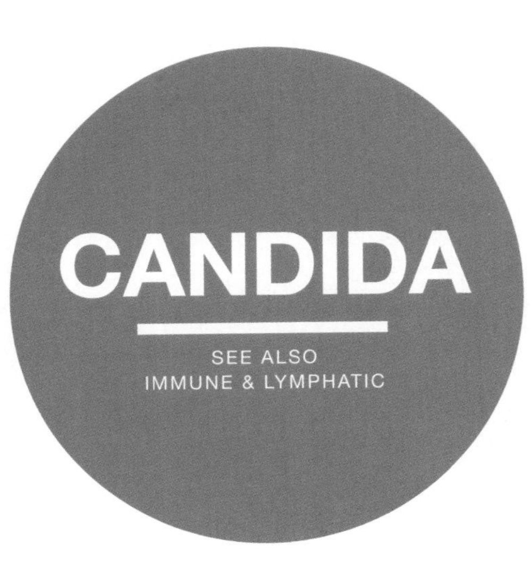

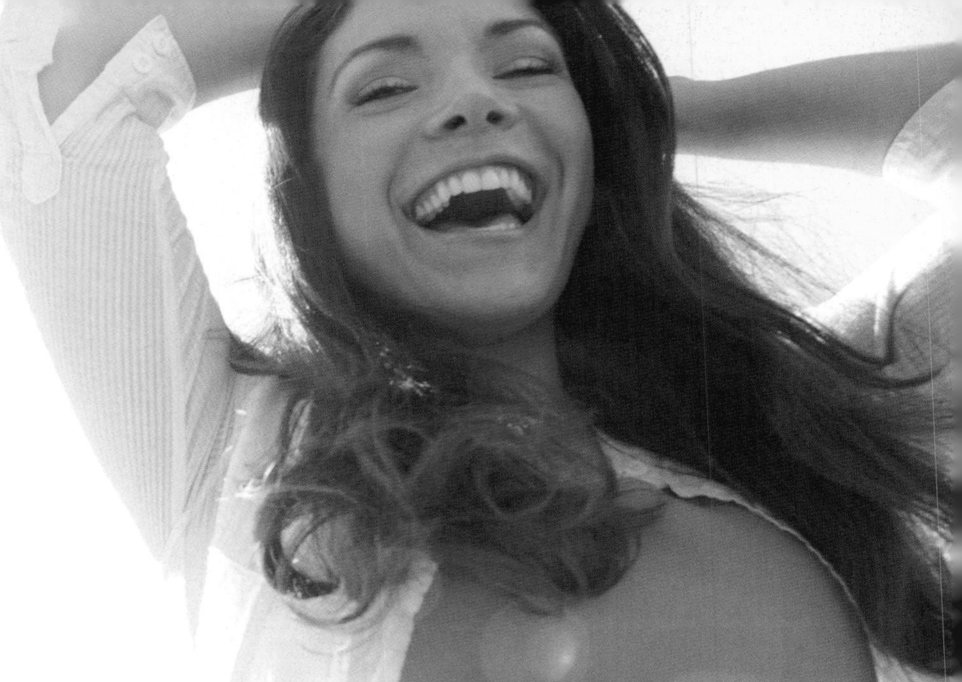

CANDIDA

CANDIDA ALBICANS is a type of yeast that grows on the warm interior membranes of the body such as the digestive, respiratory, gastrointestinal, and female and uro-genital tracts. Candidiasis, the overgrowth of candida, can cause detrimental effects throughout the body and occurs when the balance between candida organisms and helpful bacteria in the gastrointestinal tract is disrupted. Candida mutates and grows rapidly in such situations and can cause frustrating and/or dangerous conditions in the body as it flourishes out of control.

Conditions that can result from candidiasis include headaches, autoimmune diseases, allergies, fatigue, digestive disorders (including IBS), yeast infections, infertility, skin and nail conditions/infections (such as toenail fungus or psoriasis), and strong sugar cravings or addiction.

Certain factors increase the risk of candidiasis. When these are acknowledged, awareness increases, and it becomes easier to remedy and avoid such situations:

- Candida and other microorganisms thrive when there is a lack of competing healthy organisms; a lack of friendly bacteria predisposes one to candidiasis.
- Diets high in sugar, high-fructose corn syrup, processed foods, yeast, or alcohol can depress the immune system and/or offset the delicate bacterial balance in the gut, allowing opportunity for candida to multiply.
- A single round of antibiotics is enough to kill both good and bad bacteria, leaving opportunity for harmful candida organisms to encroach. Prolonged or repeated use of antibiotics or other medications (i.e. contraceptive pills, steroidal drugs) increases risk dramatically.

Use of probiotic supplements is one of the most effective ways to restore gut flora when compromised.

- Poorly digested food particles, especially proteins, are known irritants that often stimulate mucus production as a defense or coping mechanism from the body; these affected areas can become feasting ground for microorganisms like candida albicans.

A diet rich in raw, live food as well supplementing with digestive enzymes assists in restoring proper digestion. Utilizing these enzymes as well as essential oils like a digestion blend helps to clear both unwanted food particles and mucus accumulation.

- Stress can lead to candida in one of two ways: first, the body can respond to stressful situations by releasing cortisol, a hormone that elicits the same responses as does excess sugar. Second, stress can weaken the immune system and adrenal glands leading to exhaustion or lack of energy. Individuals in this weakened state typically don't eat well, further decreasing the body's ability to respond to pathogens such as candida.

Use of immune boosting essential oil blends such as a protective blend as well as caring for adrenal gland health with proper rest, nutrition, and essential oils such as rosemary or basil helps preserve the body's defense system.

- One of candida albicans' toxic byproducts is estrogenic-like, and its presence "tricks" the body, influencing delicate hormonal states in both men and women. This toxic state undermines important functions such as fertility, negatively affects weight, and impacts prostate inflammation. This kind of activity can go undetected for years and is a culprit of many other health issues.

Use of essential oils such as clary sage and thyme combined supports the body's ability to correct exaggerated estrogen and deficient progesterone levels. Grapefruit, oregano, and thyme essential oils have demonstrated positive effects on healthy progesterone levels.

While it is important to work with expert medical professionals, especially when candidiasis has caused extensive system upset in the body, restoring the body's bio terrain to a balanced state can be done very effectively with natural remedies. Essential oils help clear toxins and harmful microorganisms gently and effectively from the gastrointestinal tract, address improved insulin response, and support digestion. Probiotics help restore balance and immune support.

TOP SOLUTIONS

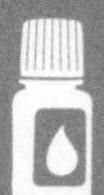

SINGLE OILS

Melaleuca - eliminates candida yeast and prevents mutation (pg. 116)
Oregano - eliminates and prevents candida yeast and fungus (pg. 120)
Thyme - eliminates and prevents candida yeast and fungus (pg. 133)

By Related Properties

For definitions of the properties listed below and more oil options, see Oil Properties Glossary (pg. 435) and Oil Properties (pg. 436).

Anti-carcinogeniz - arborvitae, clove, frankincense, lemongrass, myrrh, tangerine, wild orange; see *Cellular Health*
Antifungal - arborvitae, cardamom, cassia, cedarwood, cilantro, cinnamon, clary sage, clove, coriander, ginger, helichrysum, lemongrass, marjoram, melaleuca, melissa, myrrh, oregano, patchouli, ravensara, rosemary, spearmint, thyme
Antimicrobial - arborvitae, cassia, cilantro, cinnamon, dill, fennel, lemongrass, myrrh, oregano, spearmint; see *Immune & Lymphatic*
Antimutagenic - ginger, lavender, lemongrass; see *Cellular Health*
Antioxidant - basil, cinnamon, clove, cassia, coriander, lemongrass, melaleuca, thyme, juniper berry
Vermifuge - arborvitae, black pepper, fennel, frankincense, geranium, lavender, lemon, roman chamomile - see *Parasites*

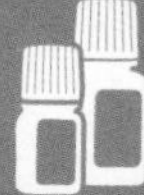

BLENDS

Cellular complex blend - restores health of cells (pg. 143)
Detoxification blend - detoxifies and eliminates free radicals (pg. 146)
Skin clearing blend - cleanses skin (pg. 163)
Protective blend - helps eliminate candida/fungus (pg. 158)

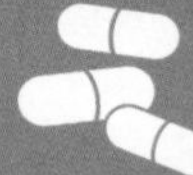

SUPPLEMENTS

Defensive probiotic, detoxification complex capsules, essential oil omega complex, **food enzymes (pg. 177)**, whole food nutrient supplement, **GI cleansing softgels (pg. 178)**

Related Ailments: Athlete's foot, Candidiasis, Fungal Skin Infection, Fungus, Yeast

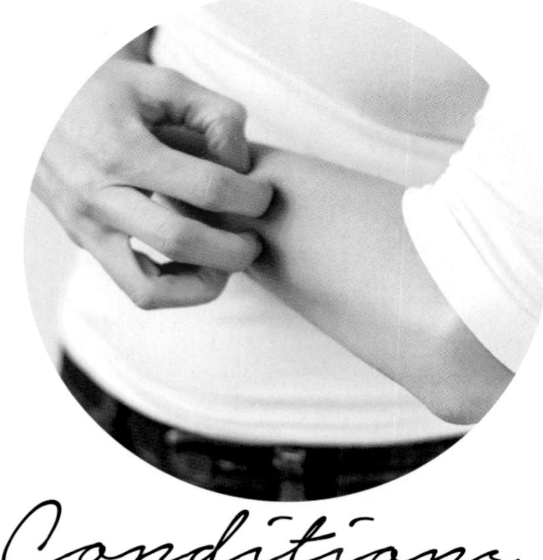

Conditions

Athlete's foot - arborvitae, cardamom, clove, lavender, lemongrass, melaleuca, myrrh, oregano, massage blend; see "Antifungal" property
Autoimmune disease - See *Autoimmune*
Brain fog - See *Focus & Concentration*
Concentration, poor - See *Focus & Concentration*
Cravings, sugar/refined carbohydrate - See *Weight*
Fatigue - See *Energy & Vitality*
Focus, lack of - See *Focus & Concentration*
Memory, poor - See *Focus & Concentration*
Mood swings, depression/anxiety/irritability - See *Mood & Behavior*
Severe seasonal allergies - See *Allergies*
Sinus infection, chronic - arborvitae, cardamom, melissa, myrrh, oregano, rosemary; consider a chronic fungal condition; see "Antifungal" property
Skin/nail infection - melaleuca, myrrh, cedarwood, protective blend
Skin, eczema/psoriasis - arborvitae, birch, bergamot, cedarwood, geranium, helichrysum, juniper berry, melissa, myrrh, oregano, patchouli, peppermint, roman chamomile, rosemary, spearmint, thyme, wintergreen
Thrush - arborvitae, clary sage, dill, fennel, lemon, bergamot, clove (diluted), lavender, dill, melaleuca, oregano (diluted), wild orange, metabolic blend, protective blend (diluted)
Urinary infection/fungal - basil, cypress, eucalyptus, juniper berry, lemon, lemongrass, melaleuca, thyme, cleansing blend, detoxification blend, protective blend, renewing blend; consider a chronic fungal condition; see "Antifungal" property
Vagina, mild discharge - bergamot, women's monthly blend
Vaginal inflammation/infection - cinnamon (internal or diluted on bottoms of feet only), spearmint, protective blend (internal or diluted on bottoms of feet only), women's blend
Vaginal itching - bergamot, women's blend
Vaginal thrush - frankincense (topical, internal), oregano (internal or diluted on bottoms of feet only), melaleuca (topical - diluted, internal), women's blend
Weak immune system - cinnamon, protective blend; see *Immune & Lymphatic*
Weakness, chronic - frankincense, rosemary, encouraging blend, protective blend; see *Energy & Vitality*

Remedies

CANDIDA SIMPLE TREATMENT
Combine basil and melaleuca and massage onto bottoms of feet.

CANDIDA MONTHLY PROTOCOL
- Step 1: 1 GI cleansing softgel three times per day with meals for ten days.
- Step 2: 1 capsule defensive probiotic each meal daily for at least next ten days.
- Step 3: Continue defensive probiotic if desired; rest for ten days.
- Step 4: Repeat steps one and two monthly as needed.
- For the entire 30 days consume:
  - 1-3 capsules food enzymes with meals and/or on an empty stomach
  - 1-2 detoxification complex capsules with AM and PM meals
  - 2 drops detoxification blend in capsule two times per day with meals
  - 2 drops lemon three times per day in a capsule or in drinking water

CANDIDA QUARTERLY MAINTENANCE CLEANSE
- Step One: Place 5 drops each melaleuca, lemon, and choose from lemongrass, thyme or oregano in a capsule; take two capsules per day for two weeks. If oregano was utilized, after two weeks of usage, take a break for two weeks and replace in capsule with thyme or lemongrass.
- Step Two: After two weeks of usage, reduce consumption to one capsule of above combination per day for two weeks.
- Step Three: Take 2-4 defensive probiotic per day for at least one week.
- Step Four: Repeat cleanse every three months or more frequently as needed.

CANDIDA SUPPOSITORY
1 drop melaleuca
1 drop oregano
1 drop thyme
Combine essential oil(s) with virgin coconut oil and roll into the shape of a large pill. Refrigerate or freeze until solid; insert into the vagina.

CANDIDA FACIAL & SKIN OIL
3 drops clary sage
2 drops frankincense
2 drops geranium
2 drops myrrh
1 drop patchouli
Combine oils in 30ml glass bottle; fill remainder of bottle with fractionated coconut oil. Apply to affected areas to soothe, relieve irritated skin and until symptoms subside.

CANDIDA SKIN RELIEF
Create a paste with ½ cup of aluminum-free baking soda and a few tablespoons of fractionated coconut oil. Then add the following essential oils:
4 drops lavender
3 drops melaleuca
3 drops rosemary
Use paste in shower as cleanser and exfoliator. Apply all over body; gently scrub for a few minutes. Repeat at least twice a week to kill the candida living on the skin.

CANDIDA RELIEF TOPICAL BLEND
9 drops cassia
8 drops clove
6 drops cinnamon
4 drops oregano
Blend oils into a 10ml roller bottle; fill remainder with carrier oil. Use topically as needed.

CANDIDA RELIEF INTERNAL BLEND
2 drops cinnamon
2 drops clove
Place oil drops in an empty capsule; ingest three times per day.

ECZEMA AND PSORIASIS
4 drops bergamot
3 drops roman chamomile
3 drops geranium
2 drops rosemary
1-2 teaspoons carrier oil
Apply to skin twice per day; massage in as tolerated. Additionally, use food enzymes.

VAGINAL THRUSH/YEAST TREATMENT
Apply a few drops of frankincense, myrrh, and/or melaleuca to tip of tampon. Insert.

CANDIDA RASH
12 drops white fir
6 drops geranium
6 drops patchouli
6 drops thyme
5 drops frankincense
Blend oils; add carrier oil. Store in a 10ml glass bottle and distribute from there. Apply to areas where candida rash is expressing. Consider some kind of candida detox.

CANDIDA TAMPON VAGINAL SUPPOSITORY
2 tablespoons of carrier oil (fractionated coconut oil or extra-virgin olive oil)
10 drops clove OR 9 drops lemongrass for a more intense treatment.
OR 15 drops frankincense, melaleuca or myrrh for a more mild treatment.
Dip tampon in oil mixture about halfway up from the insertion tip. Squeeze out excess. Insert. Wear a panty liner. Up to four fresh applications daily are appropriate. Alternate oils: four days of one, then four days of the other. This keeps pathogens from adapting. With the stronger oils it may sting intensely, especially during initial treatments, for about 15 minutes. Quantity of essential oil used can be reduced so as to reduce intensity. Response should calm over time. Use a probiotic simultaneously. Replace lid. Store for future use. Repeat nightly.

CANDIDA BOMB
3 drops cassia
2 drops oregano
Place oils in a capsule; take with meals twice a day for up to ten days. Add 1 drop of melissa or 4 drops of protective blend as needed for more chronic cases where conditions have lasted for long periods of time or are stubborn to resolve.

CANDIDA DOUCHE
1 drop lavender
1 drop melaleuca
1 teaspoon vinegar
1 cup warm water
Combine into squeeze bottle. Douche daily for three days a week.

Candida program

Daily Program to support a balanced system and optimal capacity to experience a successful detox program

STEP ONE

Take daily:

- **Whole Food nutrient supplement** (basic core nutrition for body's daily needs)
- **Defensive probiotic** - use for the first two weeks (to populate the gut with friendly bacteria)
- **Food enzymes** (digestion of food and elimination of waste)
- **Essential oil omega complex** (vital essential fatty acids)
- **Lemon essential oil in drinking water** (to balance and maintain healthy pH; antioxidant and detox support)
- **Optional as needed:** digestion blend (take if experiencing unresolved digestive upset)

STEP TWO

Add detox supplement - day 14:

(to support optimal function and detoxification of eliminative pathways). Length of use of detoxification supplements can vary from one person to another. Some individuals may benefit from brief use, such as two weeks; others will require longer usage, such as 90 days, to obtain desired long-term results.

- **Detoxification complex capsules** (add to program sooner if bowels tend to be sluggish and food enzymes are inadequate to resolve)
- **Detoxification blend softgels**

STEP THREE

Choose one: (core antifungal supplement) - day 14 (for 7-10 days)

- Essential oil cellular complex
- GI cleansing softgels

STEP FOUR

Choose optional additional antifungal target support - day 21 or later

Consider an additional antifungal oil or two to target a specific area(s) of concern. This support can be added at week three or later as determined by tolerance and desired results. Although specific oils are sited for specific areas or organs of the body, all oils listed in this section are antifungal and assist the body in restoring and balancing the bio terrain. It is important for each individual to choose whatever oil feel is best for them. Intuition is a tremendous asset in decision making.

- **Adrenals** - rosemary, ginger, geranium, detoxification blend
- **Brain** - cedarwood, clary sage, frankincense, rosemary, sandalwood
- **Heavy Metals** - cilantro, frankincense, cleansing blend (topical only), detoxification blend
- **Intestinal** - marjoram, melaleuca, oregano, thyme, detoxification blend, protective blend
- **Liver** - helichrysum, lemon, lemongrass, geranium, detoxification blend
- **Mouth** - bergamot, lavender, melaleuca, oregano, metabolic blend, protective blend
- **Mucous membrane** (i.e. stomach, intestines, uro-genital) - melaleuca, lemon, fennel
- **Pancreas** - cassia, cinnamon, coriander, dill, metabolic blend
- **Reproductive** - female/infertility - clary sage, fennel, geranium, oregano, rose, thyme, frankincense, rosemary
- **Reproductive** - male/infertility/prostate - clary sage, cypress, frankincense, geranium, thyme, ginger
- **Respiratory** - arborvitae, cardamom, myrrh, oregano, rosemary, melissa, eucalyptus
- **Skin** (i.e. eczema, psoriasis) - arborvitae, birch, bergamot, cedarwood, geranium, helichrysum, juniper berry, lavender, melissa, myrrh, oregano, patchouli, peppermint, roman chamomile, rosemary, spearmint, thyme, wintergreen
- **Thyroid** - clove, lemongrass, myrrh, rosemary, frankincense, cellular complex blend, protective blend
- **Urinary** - cypress, eucalyptus, juniper berry, lemon, lemongrass, basil, cinnamon, cleansing blend, detoxification blend
- **Vaginal** - cinnamon, thyme, melaleuca, basil, marjoram, spearmint
- **Weight, excessive** - oregano, ginger, grapefruit, metabolic blend

STEP FIVE

Probiotic

After using detoxing supplements for the length of time that is appropriate, a probiotic will further assist in populating the gut with healthy bacteria.

BONUS option: Choose oils by emotional state
Another method of selecting target oils is to search for oils that most closely relate to both the physical and emotional states that are being experienced and choose from there. There are resources available to discover what oils are related to what emotions. Below are a few suggestions that relate candida specifically.

Oils that support empowerment such as ginger are excellent for candida overgrowth. The body is being invaded and overpowered by microorganisms and fungi, promoting an emotional state of feeling powerless along with other states such as anger, blame, defensiveness, feeling out of control, resentment, unprotected.
The following oils may address candida-related emotions:

Bitterness, resentment	thyme, geranium
Blame/victim mentality/defensive	melaleuca
Deprived	myrrh
Used, betrayed	coriander, rose
Feeling out of control/invaded	oregano
Parasitical/co-dependent relationships	clove
Powerless/unprotected	cassia/cinnamon, frankincense

CANDIDA

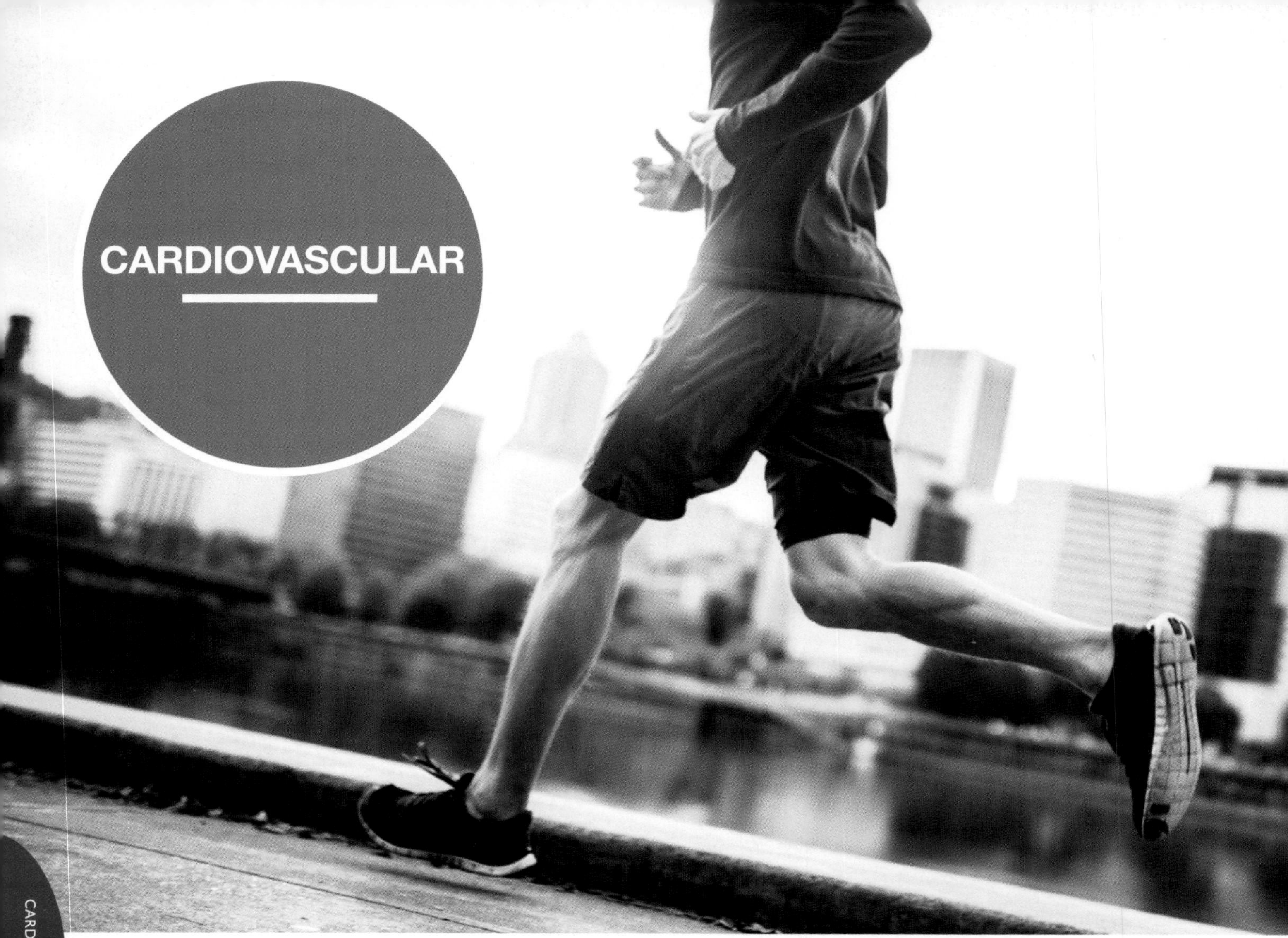

THE HEART and circulatory system make up the cardiovascular system. The heart works as a pump that pushes blood to the organs, tissues, and cells of the body. Blood delivers oxygen and nutrients to every cell and removes carbon dioxide and waste products made by those cells. Blood is carried from the heart to the rest of the body through a complex network of arteries, arterioles, and capillaries. Blood is returned to the heart through venules and veins. Many of vessels are smaller than a hair and only allow one blood cell at a time to circulate. If all the vessels of this network were laid end to end, they would extend for about 60,000 miles (more than 96,500 kilometers), which is far enough to circle the planet more than twice.

In pulmonary circulation, the roles are reversed. The pulmonary artery brings oxygen-poor blood into the lungs, and the pulmonary vein sends oxygen-rich blood back to the heart.

The oxygen and nutrient-rich blood that bring life and health to all the cells and tissues of the body, also transport essential oils. When applied topically, essential oils are absorbed through the skin. They move through the circulatory system within thirty seconds, and are then able to permeate cells and tissues throughout the body for targeted support within fourteen to twenty minutes.

Cardiovascular diseases comprise the leading cause of death globally and can refer to any disease involving the heart or blood vessels. The most common cardiovascular disease is related to arteriosclerosis/atherosclerosis, a process by which plaque causes the blood vessels to harden, stiffen, suffer a loss of elasticity, and narrow. The narrower vessels make blood flow more difficult, and blood clots can more easily block blood flow and cause serious conditions, including death. The good news is that 90% of cardiovascular disease is preventable with good lifestyle choices, including adequate rest, exercise, and nutrition. Risk factors are vast and include stress, excessive use of alcohol or caffeine, high blood pressure, smoking, diabetes, poor diet, obesity, and certain medications.

Any serious issue involving the cardiovascular system should immediately be seen by a qualified medical professional. It should be noted that natural solutions can support heart health, both preventatively and restoratively. Using certain essential oils has been shown to reduce blood pressure and heart rate. As heart disease, one of the leading causes of death, is almost entirely preventable, solutions offered with essential oils and the shifting from an ambulance mentality to a prevention mindset is most prudent.

TOP SOLUTIONS

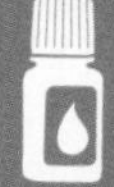

SINGLE OILS

Cypress - promotes proper circulation and blood flow throughout body (pg. 93)
Ylang ylang - balances heart rate and reduces high blood pressure (pg. 139)
Helichrysum - repairs damaged blood vessels; stops bleeding; resolves low blood pressure (pg. 105)
Black pepper - warms and tones blood vessels; decongests circulatory/lymphatic (pg. 81)
Geranium - supports heart, blood, and blood vessel integrity (pg. 102)

By Related Properties

For definitions of the properties listed below and more oil options, see Oil Properties Glossary (pg. 435) and Oil Properties (pg. 436).

Anticoagulant - clary sage, helichrysum, lavender
Antihemorrhagic - geranium, helichrysum, lavender, lemon, lemongrass, melaleuca, myrrh, oregano, patchouli, rosemary, sandalwood, spearmint, thyme
Anti-inflammatory - arborvitae, basil, bergamot, black pepper, cinnamon, clary sage, coriander, cypress, dill, eucalyptus, frankincense, geranium, helichrysum, lavender, lemongrass, lime, melissa, patchouli, peppermint, spikenard, wintergreen
Antitoxic - bergamot, black pepper, cinnamon, coriander, fennel, geranium, grapefruit, juniper berry, lavender, lemon, lemongrass, patchouli, thyme
Calming - basil, clary sage, coriander, frankincense, jasmine, lavender, oregano, patchouli, roman chamomile, sandalwood, vetiver
Cardiotonic - cassia, cypress, ginger lavender, marjoram
Decongestant - basil, black pepper, cardamom, cypress, eucalyptus, ginger, grapefruit, lemon, lemongrass, melaleuca, patchouli, white fir
Detoxifier - arborvitae, cassia, cilantro, cypress, geranium, juniper berry, lemon, lime, patchouli
Hypertensive - melissa, rosemary, thyme
Hypotensive - clary sage, dill, eucalyptus, lavender, lemon, marjoram, white fir, ylang ylang
Regenerative - basil, cedarwood, clove, frankincense, geranium, helichrysum, jasmine, lavender, lemongrass, melaleuca, myrrh, patchouli, wild orange
Relaxing - basil, cypress, geranium, lavender, marjoram, roman chamomile, ylang ylang
Tonic - basil, bergamot, cypress, fennel, frankincense, geranium, lavender, lemon, lemongrass, melissa, patchouli, rose, sandalwood, thyme, vetiver, wild orange
Vasoconstrictor - cypress, helichrysum, peppermint, white fir, ylang ylang
Vasodilator - lemongrass, marjoram, rosemary, thyme
Warming - birch, black pepper, cassia, cinnamon, clary sage, clove, eucalyptus, ginger, lemongrass, marjoram, oregano, peppermint, thyme, wintergreen

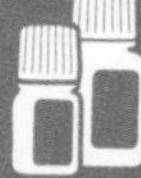

BLENDS

Cleansing blend - decongests circulatory/lymphatic congestion (pg. 144)
Inspiring blend - promotes healthy blood flow (pg. 152)
Massage blend - stimulates circulation and blood flow, especially to extremities (pg. 155)

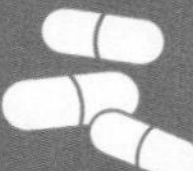

SUPPLEMENTS

Cellular vitality complex (pg. 171), energy & stamina complex (pg. 174), essential oil cellular complex, phytoestrogen complex, polyphenol complex, defensive probiotic, whole food nutrient supplement whole food nutrient supplement

USAGE TIPS: For best methods of use for cardiovascular and circulatory support consider:

- **Topical:** Apply oils directly to chest, bottoms of feet, down spine, and/or on specific areas of concern for direct affect as needed.
- **Aromatic:** Diffuse 5-10 drops of oils of choice, inhale from product bottle or self-made blend, apply a few drops to clothing, or any other method that supports inhalation for oils especially for supporting reducing stress
- **Internal:** Place 1-5 drops in water to drink, take drops in capsule, or place drop(s) under tongue to affect internal activities that impact circulation and heart activity.

Related Ailments: Anemia (iron deficiency), Aneurysm, Angina, Arrhythmia, Arteriosclerosis, Atherosclerosis, Balance Problems, Bleeding, Blood Clot, Broken Capillaries, Broken Heart Syndrome [Mood & Behavior], Bruise [Integumentary], Cardiomyopathy, Cardiovascular Disease, Cholesterol, Cold [Endocrine (Thyroid)], Cold Hands/Feet/Nose, Congenital Heart Disease, Deep Vein Thrombosis (blood clot in vein), Dizziness, Edema (water retention), Fainting [First Aid], Fibrillation (atrial), Fibrillation (ventricular), Gangrene [Immune & Lymphatic], Hardening of Arteries, Hematoma, Hemophilia, Hemorrhage, Hemorrhoids, Hypertension (high blood pressure), Hypotension (low blood pressure), Long QT Syndrome, Marfan Syndrome (connective tissue disorder), Mitral Valve Prolapse, Palpitations, Pericardial Disease, Phlebitis (inflammation of the vein), Pulmonary Embolism, Raynaud's Disease, Renal Artery Stenosis, Sickle Cell, Tachycardia, Thrombosis, Varicose Veins [Integumentary], Vertigo

Conditions

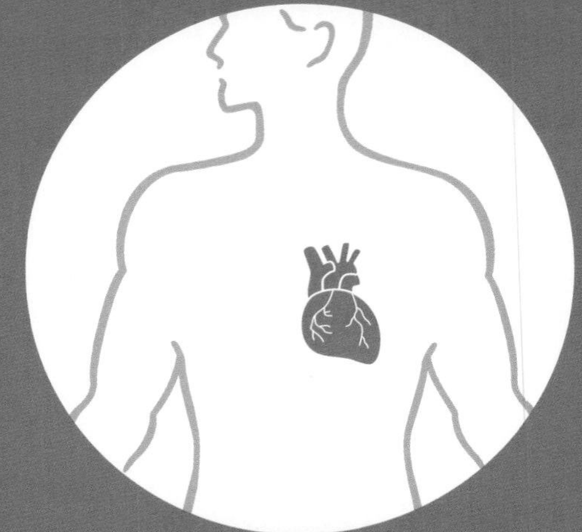

Anemia (iron deficiency) - basil, cinnamon, helichrysum, lemon, rosemary, cellular complex blend, protective blend, whole food nutrient supplement

Aneurysm - cypress, frankincense, helichrysum, marjoram, cellular complex blend

Bleeding/hemorrhaging - arborvitae, cypress, frankincense, geranium, helichrysum, lavender, wild orange, yarrow, cellular complex blend, cleansing blend, detoxification blend

Blood clot - clary sage, coriander, fennel, frankincense, helichrysum, marjoram, melaleuca, myrrh, patchouli, peppermint, thyme, wintergreen, cellular complex blend, cleansing blend, encouraging blend, massage blend, soothing blend

- **Pain** - ylang ylang, massage blend, soothing blend
- **Significant swelling** - clary sage, cleansing blend, cellular complex blend, protective blend
- **Redness** - melaleuca, melissa, ylang ylang, detoxification blend, protective blend
- **Warmth** - fennel, melissa, ylang ylang, detoxification blend, massage blend, tension blend, women's blend

Blood, dirty/toxic - grapefruit, lime, roman chamomile, geranium, helichrysum, white fir, detoxification blend

Blood flow, blocked - cypress, fennel, lavender (arteries), lemon (arteries), ylang ylang, cleansing blend, cellular complex blend, detoxification blend, encouraging blend, massage blend, energy & stamina complex

Blood pressure, high (hypertension) - birch, cypress, dill, eucalyptus, lavender, lemon, lime, marjoram, melissa, patchouli, roman chamomile, spearmint, thyme, wintergreen, ylang ylang, invigorating blend, respiration blend, uplifting blend

Blood pressure, low (hypotension) - helichrysum, lime, rosemary, thyme, cleansing blend, detoxification blend

Blood vessels, blocked/obstructed - cinnamon, lavender, lemongrass, marjoram, cleansing blend, encouraging blend, protective blend

Blood vessels/capillaries, broken - cypress, frankincense, geranium, helichrysum, lemon, lime, cleansing blend, detoxification blend

Blood vessel integrity, lack of - black pepper, helichrysum, lemongrass, marjoram, detoxification blend

Breathing problems - See *Respiratory*

Bruising - arborvitae, cypress, fennel, geranium, helichrysum, oregano, roman chamomile, ylang ylang, cellular complex blend, cleansing blend, detoxification blend

Chest pain/pressure (angina) - basil, cinnamon, douglas fir, ginger, rosemary, thyme, wild orange (for false angina), cellular complex blend, cleansing blend, protective blend

Cholesterol/triglycerides, elevated or imbalanced - basil, coriander, cypress, dill, helichrysum, lavender, lemongrass, marjoram, rosemary, thyme, wild orange, digestion blend, metabolic blend, protective blend, reassuring blend, uplifting blend

Circulatory system tonic - basil, cypress, fennel, lemon, melaleuca, rosemary, wild orange, anti-aging blend, massage blend, renewing blend, soothing blend, tension blend

Circulation, poor/cold extremities - basil, black pepper, cassia, cedarwood, cinnamon, coriander, cypress, eucalyptus, fennel, geranium, ginger, oregano, patchouli, peppermint, rose, rosemary, sandalwood, tangerine, thyme, wintergreen, cellular complex blend, cleansing blend, comforting blend, encouraging blend, inspiring blend, massage blend, protective blend, reassuring blend, uplifting blend, women's blend, energy & stamina complex

Cold, need overall or systemic warming - birch, cassia, cinnamon, eucalyptus, ginger, lemongrass, wintergreen, comforting blend, massage blend, renewing blend

Cold, need localized warming - birch, black pepper, cinnamon, eucalyptus, massage blend

Confusion or trouble walking - cedarwood, frankincense, jasmine, myrrh, peppermint, wild orange, cleansing blend, focus blend; see *Brain*

Dizziness/loss of balance/unsteady - black pepper, marjoram, rosemary, tangerine, ylang ylang, cellular blend, detoxification blend, respiration blend, tension blend, women's blend

Edema (water retention, swelling in hands/ankles/feet) - basil, cypress, ginger, lemon, lemongrass, rosemary, repellent blend, tension blend; see *Urinary, Detoxification*

Fainting/near fainting - basil, bergamot, cinnamon, cypress, frankincense, lavender, patchouli, peppermint, sandalwood, wintergreen, cleansing blend

Fibrillation/atrial fibrillation - arborvitae, black pepper, douglas fir, ginger, lime, marjoram, ylang ylang, cellular complex blend, cleansing blend, massage blend, respiration blend

Gangrene - arborvitae, cypress, lavender, melaleuca, melissa, myrrh, patchouli, cellular complex blend, detoxification blend, metabolic blend, protective blend

Hardening of the arteries (arteriosclerosis) - arborvitae, basil, cardamom, cinnamon, cypress, juniper berry, lavender, marjoram, rosemary, sandalwood, wild orange, protective blend, renewing blend

Heart - cinnamon, geranium, frankincense, lime, patchouli, sandalwood, ylang ylang, massage blend, cleansing blend, detoxification blend

Heart attack, prevention - cassia

Heart, broken - geranium, lime, rose, ylang ylang, joyful blend

Heart infection - oregano; see *Immune & Lymphatic*

Heart murmur - douglas fir, patchouli, peppermint, thyme, white fir, cleansing blend, massage blend, women's blend

Heart muscle, thickening (cardiomyopathy) - basil, marjoram, rosemary, ylang ylang, cleansing blend

Heart muscle, lack of tone - cassia, helichrysum, rose, renewing blend

Heart, weak - cinnamon, coriander, ginger, rosemary, massage blend

Heartbeat, irregular (arrhythmia) - basil, lavender, lemon, melissa, rosemary, ylang ylang, cellular complex blend, protective blend, reassuring blend

Heartbeat, rapid/racing (tachycardia) - arborvitae, cardamom, cedarwood, lavender, melissa, oregano, rosemary, wild orange, ylang ylang, calming blend, detoxification blend

Heartbeat, slow (bradycardia) - douglas fir, patchouli, detoxification blend, encouraging blend, massage blend

Hematoma - basil, cypress, frankincense, helichrysum, marjoram, myrrh, lemongrass, anti-aging blend, massage blend, renewing blend

Hemorrhoids - cypress, frankincense, geranium, helichrysum, juniper berry, myrrh, patchouli, roman chamomile, rosemary, detoxification blend, digestion blend, renewing blend

Lightheaded - douglas fir, grapefruit, melaleuca, oregano, patchouli, detoxification blend, protective blend

Numbness/tingling/paralysis in arm, face, leg - arborvitae, basil, cardamom, cypress, frankincense, geranium, ginger, patchouli, cellular complex blend, cleansing blend, detoxification blend, massage blend

Palpitations - cardamom, cedarwood, frankincense, lavender, oregano, rose, rosemary, thyme, ylang ylang, detoxification blend, massage blend, protective blend

Phlebitis - basil, cypress, helichrysum, lavender, lemon, lemongrass, marjoram, detoxification blend

Plaque, clogged arteries (atherosclerosis) - basil, clove, ginger, lavender, lemon, lemongrass, marjoram, patchouli, rosemary, thyme, wintergreen, cellular complex blend, cleansing blend, detoxification blend, encouraging blend, massage blend, protective blend

Prolapsed mitral valve - marjoram, helichrysum, myrrh

Red blood cells, poor production - lemon

Redness on tip of tongue - arborvitae, ylang ylang, cleansing blend, women's blend

Redness on tip of nose - patchouli, ylang ylang, repellent blend

Restless leg syndrome - arborvitae, basil, cardamom, cypress, wintergreen, massage blend, soothing blend, tension blend

Ringing in ears (see tinnitus) - arborvitae, cypress, detoxification blend, repellent blend

Stenosis (vessel narrowing) - arborvitae, oregano, patchouli, cellular complex blend, cleansing blend

Stroke - See *Brain*

Skin, cold/clammy/cold sweats - patchouli, ylang ylang, massage blend

Skin, color changes to skin on face, feet, hands (bluish cyanosis, grayish, pale/white) - cypress, douglas fir, lemon, patchouli, ylang ylang, cleansing blend

Thrombosis, deep vein:

- **narrowing (stenosis)** - patchouli, detoxification blend
- **leaking (regurgitation or insufficiency)** - grapefruit, ylang ylang, cleansing blend, protective blend
- **improper closing (prolapse)** - melissa, detoxification blend

Tongue, inflamed/red/sore - See *Heart*

Ulcers, leg/varicose - frankincense, geranium, helichrysum, lavender, marjoram, cellular complex blend, detoxification blend, massage blend, metabolic blend

Varicose veins - bergamot, cardamom, coriander, cypress, geranium, helichrysum, lemon, lemongrass, marjoram, melaleuca, patchouli, peppermint, rosemary, detoxification blend, reassuring blend

Vein inflammation (phlebitis) - cypress, frankincense, marjoram, myrrh, cellular complex blend, detoxification blend, tension blend

Vertigo/sense room is spinning/sense of falling/loss of equilibrium (disequilibrium) - melissa, peppermint, rosemary, cellular blend, grounding blend, invigorating blend, reassuring blend

Vision, blurred - arborvitae, douglas fir, juniper berry, lemongrass, peppermint, cellular complex blend, cleansing blend, detoxification blend

Vision, abnormal or jerking eye movements (nystagmus) - cellular complex blend

Vision, trouble with seeing in one or both eyes - arborvitae, cypress, douglas fir, lemongrass, cellular complex blend

Vision, see spots (consider low blood pressure) - arborvitae, rosemary, thyme; see Nervous

Weakness in arms/muscles; reduced ability to exercise - coriander, ginger, helichrysum, lemongrass, rosemary

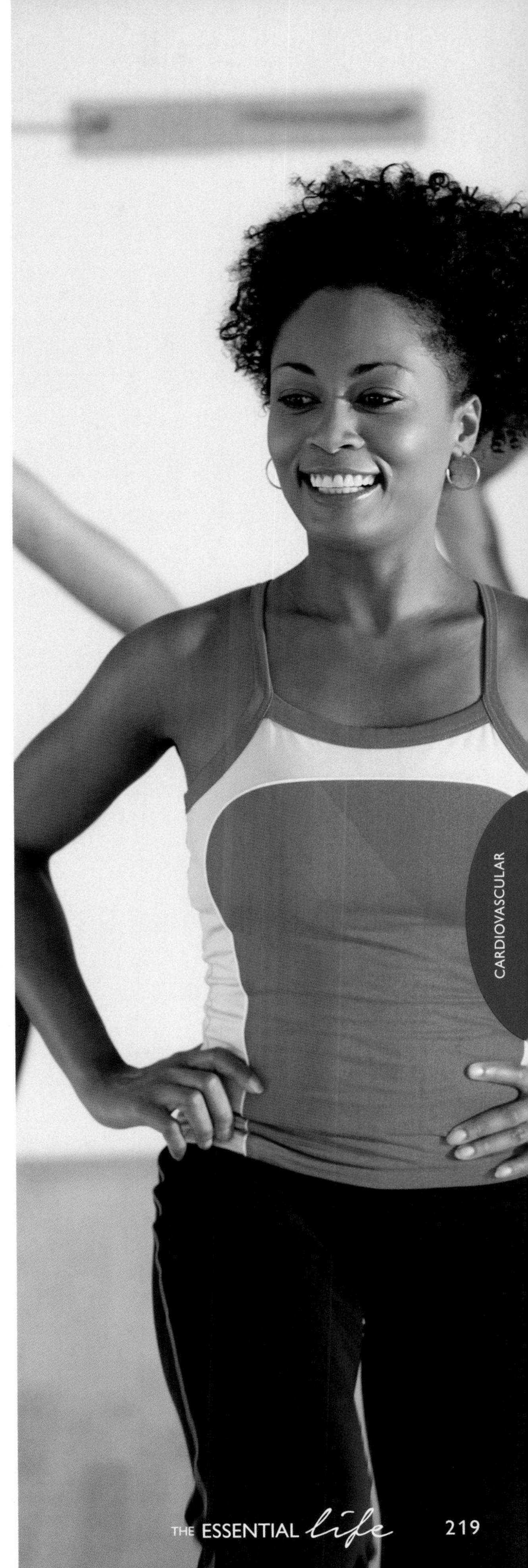

Remedies

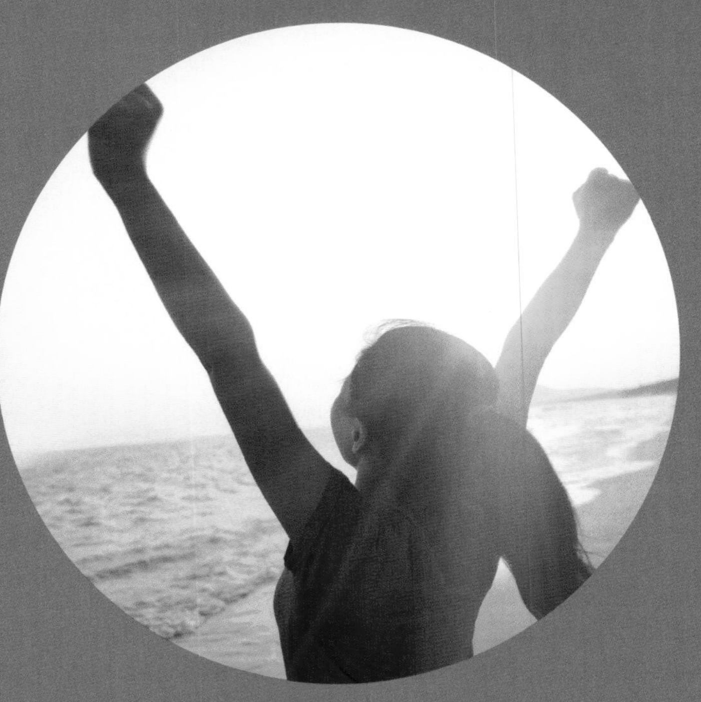

CHOLESTEROL FIGHTER: Combine and ingest frankincense and lemongrass in a capsule two times per day.

CIRCULATION MOVER: Apply essential oils of choice; cover with a warm, moist towel to help drive oils into area and increase circulation.

PROMOTE CIRCULATION AND OXYGENATION
Use massage blend twice per day on legs and feet.

VARICOSE VEIN SOOTHER: Use a warm compress with 3 drops cypress on affected areas at least once per day.

VARICOSE VEIN REPAIR: Apply cypress and helichrysum to veins to encourage supporting tissue to "show up."

ANEMIA RESOLVE
6 drops lavender
4 drops lemon
Combine with 1 teaspoon carrier oil and apply to bottoms of feet and stomach.

ANEURYSM SUPPORT & PREVENTION
5 drops frankincense
1 drop helichrysum
1 drop peppermint
Combine and apply to temples, heart, and feet. Dilute as needed.

BLOOD CLOT SUPPORT
4 drops grapefruit
3 drops clove
3 drops lemon
2 drops helichrysum
Combine and ingest in capsule or apply NEAT to bottoms of feet to support blood flow. Dilute if desired.

HEMORRHOID SUPPORT
10 drops cypress
10 drops helichrysum
10 drops lavender
5 drops basil
5 drops geranium
2 drops peppermint
Place oils in 2 ounce bottle with orifice reducer seal, mix; fill remainder with fractionated coconut oil. Apply 10 drops of mixture to affected areas at least twice per day and/or following bowel movement. Additionally, keep a witch hazel bottle with 5 drops of lavender in it beside toilet area; spray on affected area and use with last wipe when using bathroom. A spritzer may also be made and sprayed to affected area as needed.

CHOLESTEROL BUILD UP BUSTER
2 drops lemongrass
2 drops marjoram
Place in capsule; take two times per day.

HIGH BLOOD PRESSURE RELIEVER
12 drops helichrysum
12 drops ylang ylang
8 drops cassia
8 drops frankincense
8 drops marjoram
Combine in 10ml roller bottle; fill remainder with fractionated coconut oil. Apply blend to the bottoms of feet, wrists, along breastbone, massage over heart, carotid arteries, and/or back of neck as needed at least two times per day.

RAYNAUD'S DISEASE REMEDY
11 drops cypress
5 drops lavender
2 tablespoons carrier oil
Combine in a glass bottle with a dropper top. Drop 6-8 drops of blend into bath. Bathe twice daily (morning and evening). Water is best hot, yet comfortable. While in the bath, massage fingers and toes. After bath, apply blend over whole body except face. If possible, have blend massaged onto back.

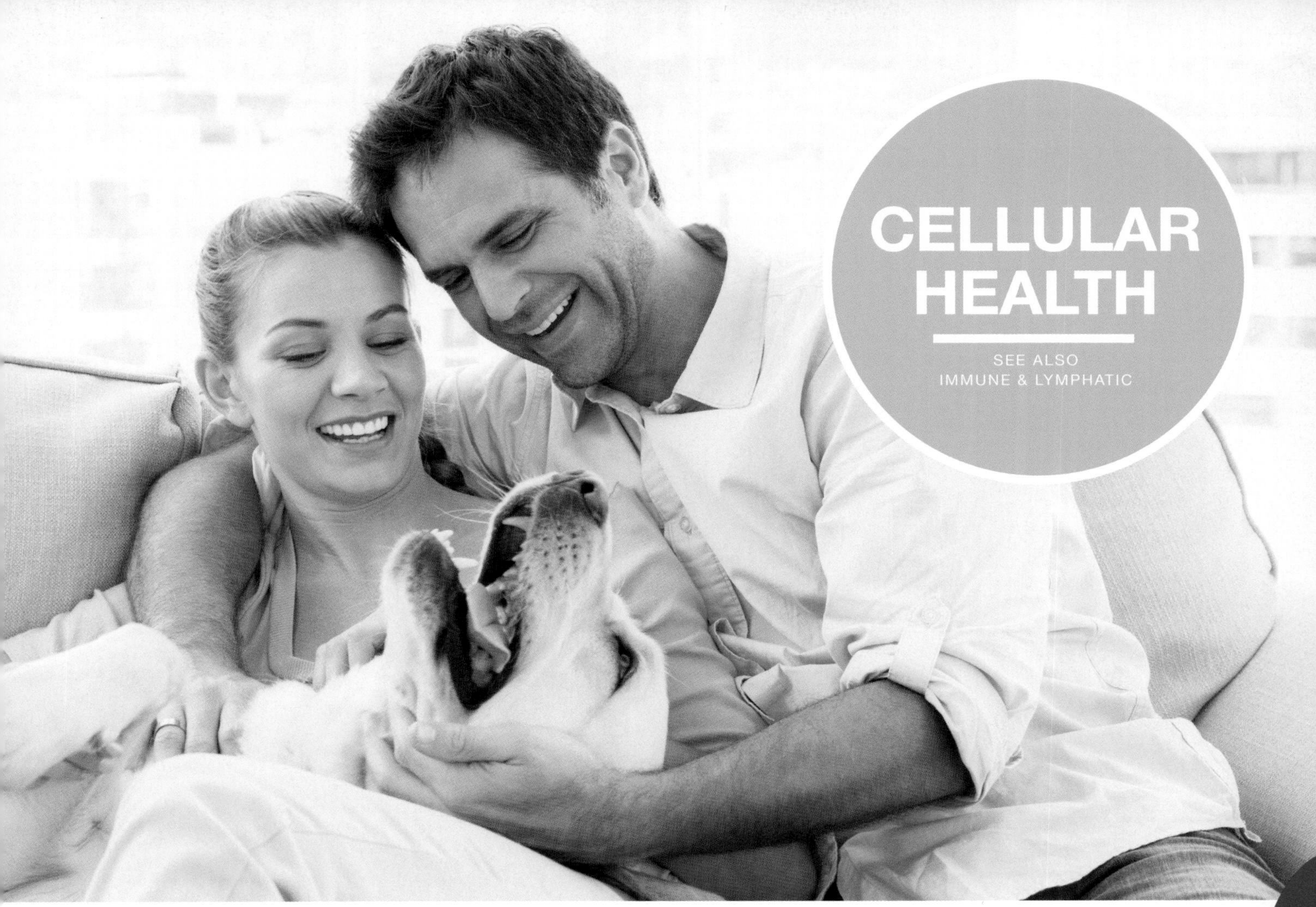

CELLS are the smallest units of life for all living organisms, and they have a lifespan consisting of three primary functions. They replicate themselves through a process called mitosis. They perform different specialized functions , such as epithelial, sensory, blood, hormone secreting, etc. Apoptosis, their final function, is a pre-programmed, healthy, cellular death. To achieve optimal health, it is important to nourish and support the cells throughout each stage.

In his book, Never Be Sick Again, Dr. Raymond Francis teaches that there's only one disease–a malfunctioning cell; there are two causes of disease–deficiency and toxicity; and there are six pathways to health and disease–nutrition, toxins, psychological/emotional state, physical, genetic, and medical. These ideas certainly simplify, and highlight, the most important areas on which to focus to achieve a healthy body. When cells do not operate efficiently, tissue and organ function is compromised, which in turn can diminish physical well being and invite a host of health conditions and diseases. By nourishing the cells, the entire body system is supported.

Safeguarding the DNA (located in the cell's nucleus) and providing energy for all body processes are two of the most critical cellular activities. Research has shown that a diet low in antioxidants and other important phytonutrients, and environmental exposure to toxins such as pesticides, can damage DNA. This damage, called mutation, can affect the cells' ability to produce energy. It can cause cells to die early, resulting in weakened tissue or inflammation, or even worse. And it can also cause cells to replicate themselves in their mutated form.

When using essential oils to support cellular function, it is important to remember that essential oils operate chemically within the body; they do not provide nutrition. When essential oils enter the body, they bring powerful instructions to help "remind" and support cells of their healthy function – but unless the cells are properly nourished, they won't have the energy necessary to perform their desired functions. Eating nutrient-dense raw foods is always a top priority, but many individuals have difficulty eating the quantities and types of quality food that assist cellular health. If this is the case, it's a good idea to find high-quality, bioavailable supplements, such as a whole-food nutrient supplement and essential oil omega complex, to assist with keeping cells well-nourished and safeguarded.

Essential oils are a powerful addition to any regimen targeting cellular health, because they are actually able to permeate the cell membrane and provide powerful support to the structures found within the cell, including safeguarding against inside threats such as viruses. Synthetic or adulterated essential oils are not able to bypass the cell membrane, and therefore are unable to assist on a cellular level in the body.

TOP SOLUTIONS

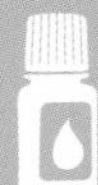

SINGLE OILS

Sandalwood - promotes healthy apoptosis and cellular health (pg. 128)

Frankincense - promotes healthy apoptosis and cellular health (pg. 100)

Lemongrass - cellular detoxifier (pg. 112)

Wild orange - encourages healthy DNA and optimal glutathione levels (pg. 136)

Cinnamon - promotes healthy cellular response to glucose and inflammation (pg. 86)

Patchouli - supports the cell in eliminating harmful toxins (pg. 121)

Clove - powerful antioxidant; supports cellular repair (pg. 90)

Thyme - cellular health and DNA repair (pg. 133)

Arborvitae - stimulates immune support and cellular repair (pg. 75)

By Related Properties

For definitions of the properties listed below and more oil options, see Oil Properties Glossary (pg. 435) and Oil Properties (pg. 436).

Anticarcinogenic - arborvitae, frankincense, myrrh, peppermint

Anti-carcinoma - arborvitae, frankincense, grapefruit, lemon, lemongrass, myrrh, rosemary, sandalwood, wild orange

Anti-inflammatory - basil, bergamot, black pepper, cassia, cinnamon, clove, coriander, cypress, eucalyptus, frankincense, geranium, ginger, lavender, lemongrass, melissa, oregano, patchouli, peppermint, roman chamomile, spearmint, white fir, yarrow

Antimutagenic - cinnamon, ginger, lavender, lemongrass

Antioxidant - arborvitae, basil, black pepper, cassia, cilantro, cinnamon, clove, coriander, eucalyptus, frankincense, ginger, grapefruit, helichrysum, juniper berry, lemon, lemongrass, lime, melaleuca, oregano, patchouli, peppermint, rosemary, thyme, vetiver, wild orange

Antitoxic - black pepper, cinnamon, coriander, fennel, geranium, grapefruit, lemongrass, patchouli, thyme

Anti-tumoral - arborvitae, clove, frankincense, lavender, myrrh, sandalwood

Cleanser - cilantro, grapefruit, lemon, thyme, wild orange

Cytophylactic - arborvitae, frankincense, geranium, lavender, rosemary, tangerine

Detoxifier - cassia, cilantro, geranium, juniper berry, patchouli

Purifier - cinnamon, eucalyptus, grapefruit, lime, marjoram, melaleuca, wild orange

Regenerative - basil, cedarwood, clove, coriander, frankincense, geranium, helichrysum, jasmine, lavender, lemongrass, melaleuca, myrrh, patchouli, sandalwood, wild orange

Tonic - arborvitae, basil, birch, cardamom, coriander, frankincense, geranium, lemon, lemongrass, melissa, Roman chamomile, sandalwood, ylang ylang

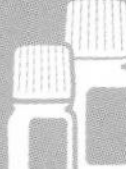

BLENDS

Cellular complex blend - promotes cellular health and DNA repair (pg. 143)

Detoxification blend - helps eliminate free radicals and heavy metals (pg. 146)

Uplifting blend - antioxidant; neutralizes free radicals and supports cells (pg. 166)

Cleansing blend - detoxifies cells and lymphatic system (pg. 144)

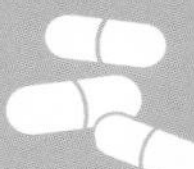

SUPPLEMENTS

Cellular vitality complex (pg. 171), defensive probiotic, digestion blend softgels, energy & stamina supplement, **essential oil cellular complex (pg. 174)**, essential oil omega complex, GI cleansing softgels, polyphenol complex, whole food nutrient supplement

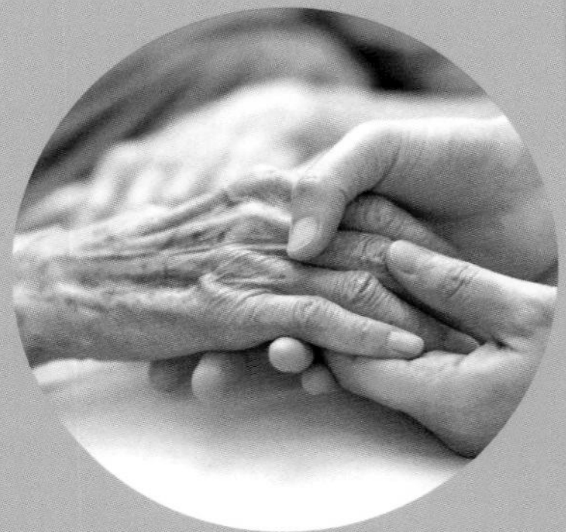

Related Ailments: Basal Cell Carcinoma, Benign Prostatic Hyperplasia, Bone Cancer, Brain Cancer, Breast Cancer, Cells [Integumentary], Cervical Cancer, Colon Cancer, Endometrial Cancer, Hodgkin's Disease, Leukemia, Lipoma, Liver Cancer, Lung Cancer, Lymphoma (Non-Hodgkin's), Melanoma, Mesothelioma, Mouth Cancer, Ovarian Cancer, Pancreatic Cancer, Polyps, Prostate Cancer, Radiation Damage [Immune & Lymphatic], Skin Cancer, Throat Cancer, Tongue Cancer, Tumor, Uterine Cancer

USAGE TIPS: For best success at supporting cellular health:

- **Topical:** Apply oils on bottoms of feet, spine, and/or on any specific area of concern. Use Oil Touch technique regularly as desired or able.
- **Internal:** Consume oils in capsules, drop under tongue, or sip in water.

Conditions

CELLULAR HEALTH:

Acidic, overly - arborvitae, dill, fennel, frankincense, lemon, lime, rosemary, wild orange, cellular complex blend, detoxification blend, grounding blend, metabolic blend

Activity, poor - cinnamon, clove, frankincense, geranium, ginger, rosemary, anti-aging blend, cellular complex blend, detoxification blend, digestion blend, protective blend

Cellular malfunction - arborvitae, black pepper, cedarwood, clove, frankincense, geranium, lavender, lemongrass, rosemary, tangerine, thyme, wild orange, anti-aging blend, cellular complex blend, protective blend, renewing blend

Cellular health, poor/premature aging - anti-aging blend, cellular comforting blend, complex blend, reassuring blend; see "Antioxidant" property

Free radicals, excess damage - arborvitae, basil, cassia, cardamom, cilantro, cinnamon, clove, frankincense, ginger, grapefruit, lemon, lemongrass, lime, melaleuca, rosemary, thyme, anti-aging blend, cellular complex blend, invigorating blend, protective blend, renewing blend; see "Antioxidant" property

Hardening of cell membrane - arborvitae, cinnamon, clove, frankincense, rosemary, sandalwood, thyme, vetiver, anti-aging blend, cellular complex blend, grounding blend, respiration blend; see "Antioxidant" property

Inflammation - basil, bergamot, birch, black pepper, cinnamon, clove, coriander, cypress, douglas fir, eucalyptus, frankincense, geranium, lavender, melissa, patchouli, peppermint, roman chamomile, rosemary, thyme, white fir, wintergreen, yarrow, cellular complex, comforting blend, soothing blend; see "Anti-inflammatory" property, Pain & Inflammation

Nutrient absorption, poor/cellular starvation - cinnamon, ginger, metabolic blend

Oxygen flow to cell, poor - black pepper, cilantro, cypress, frankincense, peppermint, sandalwood, metabolic blend, respiration blend

Radiation damage - cilantro, clove, geranium, patchouli, peppermint, detoxification blend

Toxic/autointoxication - arborvitae, bergamot, douglas fir, frankincense, grapefruit, lemon, lime, sandalwood, wild orange, anti-aging blend, cellular complex blend, cleansing blend, detoxification blend, focus blend, metabolic blend

Vitality, lack of - bergamot, cedarwood, douglas fir, wild orange, ylang ylang, cellular complex blend, cleansing blend, detoxification blend, invigorating blend

CELLULAR HEALTH SUPPORT BY BODY PARTS OR AREAS:

Bladder - basil, cinnamon, cypress, frankincense, juniper berry, lemongrass, rosemary, cellular complex blend, massage blend, metabolic blend

Blood - basil, clary sage, clove, frankincense, geranium, lavender, lemongrass, myrrh, rosemary, thyme, cellular complex blend, cleansing blend, detoxification blend, protective blend

Bone - clary sage, clove, frankincense, helichrysum, lemon, lemongrass, sandalwood, thyme, white fir, cellular complex blend

Brain - arborvitae, cedarwood, clove, frankincense, grapefruit, helichrysum, melissa, myrrh, patchouli, rosemary, sandalwood, thyme, wild orange, anti-aging blend, cellular complex blend

Breast - arborvitae, cinnamon, clary sage, frankincense, lavender, lemongrass, marjoram, oregano, rosemary, sandalwood, thyme, anti-aging blend, cellular complex blend, women's blend

Cervix - clary sage, cypress, frankincense, geranium, lemon, patchouli, sandalwood, thyme, vetiver, white fir, anti-aging blend, detoxification blend, protective blend, women's blend

Fatty tissue - frankincense, grapefruit, helichrysum, lemon, lemongrass, metabolic blend

General - arborvitae, basil, clary sage, clove, eucalyptus, frankincense, geranium, grapefruit, lavender, lemongrass, myrrh, rose, rosemary, sandalwood, tangerine, wild orange, anti-aging blend, cellular complex blend, cleansing blend, detoxification blend, protective blend, women's blend

Large intestines/colon/rectum - arborvitae, basil, cardamom, clove, frankincense, geranium, ginger, lavender, lemongrass, oregano, rosemary, sandalwood, thyme, wild orange, anti-aging, cellular complex blend, cleansing blend, detoxification, women's blend

Liver - clove, frankincense, geranium, grapefruit, lavender, lemon, lemongrass, rosemary, tangerine, thyme, wild orange, cellular complex blend, detoxification blend

Lung - cinnamon, eucalyptus, frankincense, lavender, lemon, melissa, ravensara, rosemary, sandalwood, thyme, wild orange, cellular complex blend, cleansing blend, detoxification blend, protective blend, respiration blend, women's blend

Lymphatic system/lymph/nodes - basil, bergamot, cardamom, cilantro, cinnamon, clary sage, clove, frankincense, lavender, lemon, lemongrass, melaleuca, myrrh, rosemary, sandalwood, thyme, cellular complex blend, cleansing blend, detoxification blend, joyful blend, protective blend, women's blend

Mouth - bergamot, black pepper, frankincense, geranium, lavender, melaleuca, myrrh, peppermint, thyme, cellular complex blend

Mucus membrane - arborvitae, frankincense, geranium, lavender, lemongrass, peppermint

Ovaries - clary sage, frankincense, lemon, geranium, myrrh, rosemary, sandalwood, vetiver, wild orange, anti-aging blend, cellular complex blend, detoxification blend, grounding blend, metabolic blend, women's blend

Pancreas - cinnamon, coriander, frankincense, rosemary, cellular complex blend, cleansing blend, detoxification blend, metabolic blend, protective blend

Prostate - arborvitae, basil, cardamom, cassia, cinnamon, cypress, dill, frankincense, oregano, sandalwood, thyme, anti-aging blend, cellular complex blend, cleansing blend, detoxification blend, massage blend, metabolic blend, protective blend, women's blend

Skin - arborvitae, clove, douglas fir, frankincense, geranium, grapefruit, lavender, lemon, lemongrass, melaleuca, melissa, rosemary, sandalwood, tangerine, thyme, wild orange, anti-aging blend, detoxification blend, protective blend, women's blend

Throat - cinnamon, frankincense, lavender, lemon, rosemary, thyme, anti-aging blend, detoxification blend, protective blend, women's blend

Tongue - cassia, clove, bergamot, frankincense, geranium, ginger, lavender, melaleuca, myrrh, peppermint, thyme, cellular complex blend, detoxification blend, digestion blend

Tissue - clove, frankincense, geranium, grapefruit, melissa, myrrh, patchouli, sandalwood, wild orange, anti-aging blend, cellular complex blend, cleansing blend, detoxification blend, protective blend, women's blend

Uterus - clary sage, cypress, frankincense, geranium, ginger, grapefruit, lemon, lemongrass, rosemary, sandalwood, anti-aging blend, cellular complex blend, cleansing blend, detoxification blend, protective blend, women's blend

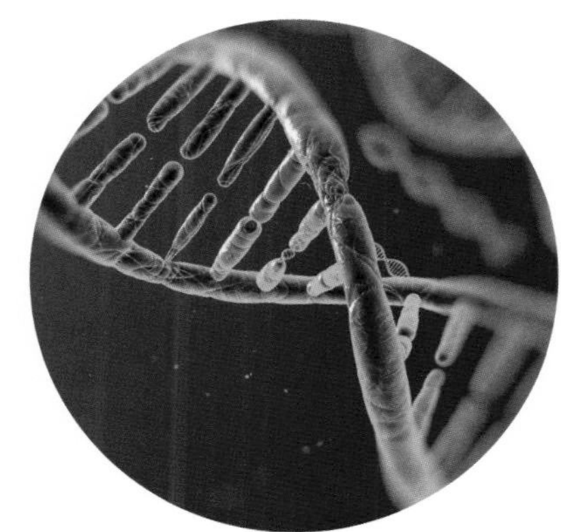

Remedies

NOTE: Diet, exercise, stress, emotional and spiritual issues all contribute to the development of any degenerative disease including cancer. They must all be dealt with in order to truly heal this condition. Any efforts are best conducted with the support and care of a professional health care provider.

CELLULAR HEALTH PROGRAM - choose from the following:

- **Dietary changes** are imperative - research best options
  - › Optional: add fruit & vegetable supplement powder to smoothies or in water
- **Use nutritional supplements** for basic and vital nutrient needs
  - › whole food nutrient supplement - take 2 capsules am and pm with food
  - › cellular vitality complex - take 2 capsules am and pm with food; add as needed
  - › essential oil omega complex - take 2 capsules am and pm with food
- **Support healthy digestion & elimination** - consider the following basics
  - › food enzymes - take 1-2 capsules with meals
  - › defensive probiotic - take 2 capsules at bedtime; add as needed
  - › digestion blend if needed for digestive/intestinal upset or sluggishness
- **Use a citrus oil(s) daily** to raise glutathione levels in body
  Choose citrus oil according to needs; add to drinking water or take in capsule
  - › 2-3 drops grapefruit, lemon, tangerine, and/or wild orange two times per day
- **Engage in detoxification & natural chelation**
  - › **Remove toxins** from diet/lifestyle; reduce exposure to chemicals and toxins
  - › **Open channels of elimination:**
    - Use detoxification complex - take 1-2 capsules am and pm with food
    - See *Detoxification* section in this book for further ideas
  - › **Support liver and rid body of heavy metal toxicity**
    Choose one of following based on what is best match for condition(s):
    - Recipe #1: Use detoxification blend, take 4 drops two times per day
    - Recipe #2: Use 2-3 drops each cilantro, geranium, grapefruit, rosemary oil in a capsule once or twice per day
    - Recipe #3: Use 2 drops helichrysum and 2 drops detoxification blend in capsule two times per day
- **Focus on cellular health, DNA repair, & promoting healthy apoptosis**
  Choose one or two of following:
  - › Use cellular complex blend on bottoms of feet - 4 drops per foot two times per day
  - › Use essential oil cellular complex as a supplement - 2 softgels with meals two to three times per day
  - › 2 drops frankincense under tongue two times daily; hold thirty seconds; swallow
  - › 2 drops clove in capsule each day with meals
  - › 2-3 drops each clove, grapefruit, lavender oil, cellular complex blend in capsule two to three times per day
  - › Research and create own blend using oils that are specific to condition(s)
- **Heal and maintain a healthy emotional state**
  See *Mood & Behavior* section
- **Support a healthy immune system** - consider:
  - › Use protective blend or see *Immune & Lymphatic* section
  - › Consider candida detox program - see Candida section
- **Manage pain** - choose from:
  - › Use polyphenol complex
  - › See *Pain & Inflammation, Muscular, Nervous, Skeletal* sections
- **Maintain energy levels**
  - › Use energy & stamina complex
  - › See *Energy & Vitality* section
- **Use a specified topical application** once or more per day
  Choose from the following:
  - › Conduct the Basic Application Technique once daily - see below
  - › Choose a topical application recipe or create one - see below

OPTIONAL TOPICAL APPLICATION RECIPES

Apply blends below to affected area(s) one to two times daily. Also apply to spine one time per day and bottoms of feet two times per day. Blends may be multiplied and stored in a glass bottle with lid to create reserves for future applications. Mix in a glass bowl or container.

- **Breast**
  2 drops frankincense + 3 drops white fir + 3 drops wild orange + 2 drops grapefruit blended into 10 drops skin clearing oil; IF lymph gland involvement, add 2 drops lemongrass; place oils in 1 ounce glass bottle; fill remainder with high quality aloe vera gel. Mix thoroughly. Apply blend to entire breast area, and underarms (if area is affected). Use twice per day.
- **Lung**
  6 drops respiration blend + 4 drops clove + 4 drops myrrh + 5 drops frankincense, 2 drops sage + 1 tablespoon carrier oil
- **Lymph**
  15 drops frankincense + 6 drops clove + 1 tablespoon carrier oil
- **Ovaries**
  15 drops frankincense + 5 drops myrrh + 6 drops geranium + 1 tablespoon carrier oil
- **Skin**
  3 drops lavender + 4 drops frankincense + 1 tablespoon carrier oil

BREAST DETOX SALVE

Melt 2 tablespoons shea butter over low heat; removed from heat as soon as butter has liquified. Cool to room temperature, then add essential oils listed below. When salve begins to solidify, stir well. Cover and use within about two weeks.

4 drops cinnamon
4 drops roman chamomile
3 drops thyme
2 drops frankincense
2 drops jasmine or ylang ylang

CELLULAR HEALTH LAYERING APPLICATION TECHNIQUE

1. Apply a base coat using 1-2 teaspoons fractionated coconut oil
2. Once daily, layer following oils, one at a time, on back. First drip 5-6 drops of one oil up spine; distribute across back; massage lightly. Repeat until all oils are applied:
   - clove or thyme - frankincense - lemongrass - rosemary - sandalwood
3. Alter recipe according to needs and conditions. Choose oils from particular cancer lists.

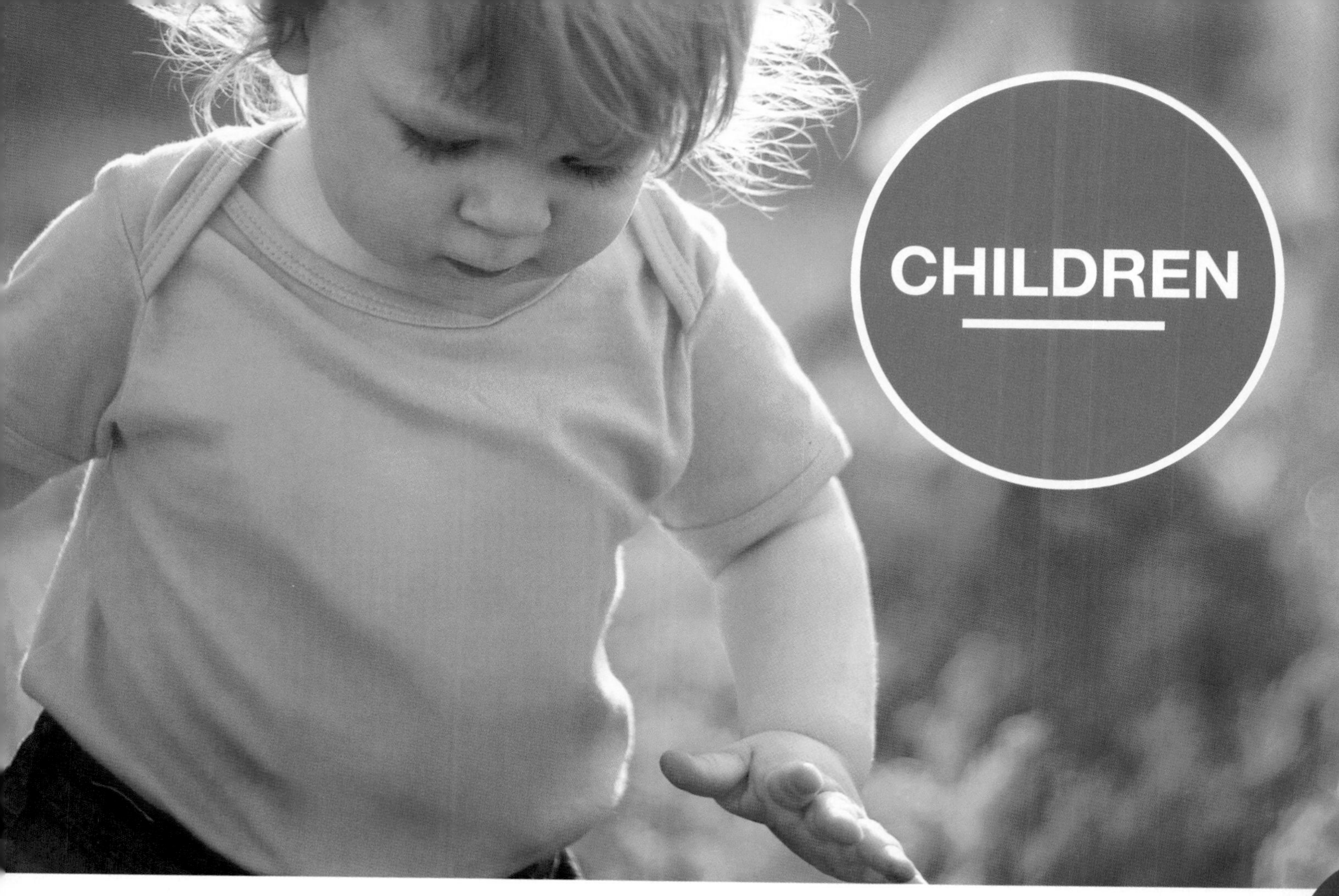

CHILDREN'S HEALTH involves both physical and mental well being. Physical health concerns range from irritating (i.e. diaper rash, crying, colic) to concerns that can quickly become serious if not addressed (i.e. scarlet fever, strep throat). Once a child begins socializing outside the home, exposure to bacterial and viral infections becomes commonplace. Since their immune systems are immature, children can more easily succumb to infectious diseases. They are also exposed to a number of compromising situations that increase risk for injury. See the First Aid section for tips on addressing issues resulting while engaged in typical childhood play.

Just like adults, children have mental health needs and are affected by perceived stress and trauma, responding with typical emotions such as fear, sadness, and anger. Parents and caregivers often feel poorly equipped with the knowledge and tools they need to properly care for their children. It is difficult and frustrating to have limited resources when trying to help a child resolve emotional upset, stress, hyperactivity, sadness, illness, injury, and any other potential concern.

Children are particularly responsive to aromas and healthy touch. Simply smelling or experiencing the application of an essential oil followed by a simple massage technique is very comforting to a child and can support rapid changes in behavior and responsiveness to trauma or difficult situations. Many real life situations have demonstrated that a room full of children under a variety of circumstances have a nearly universal positive response in mood, outlook, and behavior through the diffusing or dispersing of essential oils into the air.

Most children naturally love essential oils, and many seem to know what they need and when to use them. They respond particularly well to opportunities to discover their favorite oils and make their own personalized roller-bottle blend (see Blending and Layering for further information). For further ideas for mood support, see *Mood & Behavior*.

While proper medical care is always advised when needed, there are many situations in the home and family when natural solutions can be used as a first line of defense. Parents and caregivers are more intimately acquainted with their children than anyone else, and typically have excellent insight into the nature or causes of many issues their children encounter. It is empowering to know a few natural remedy basics that may help prevent potential issues and that will support health and wellness.

Teaching children self care at an early age creates an empowering environment in which they may grow and advance as confident and balanced individuals. Essential oils offer an excellent opportunity to participate in this self-care process. When partnered with children's nutritional supplements and a healthy diet, a foundation of health is laid that positively affects a young person's health status for decades to come.

TOP SOLUTIONS

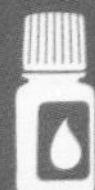

SINGLE OILS

Lavender - most used essential oil for children; all things calming (pg. 108)

Wild orange - gentle/powerful calming/uplifting; digestive support; boost immune/anti-infectious; promotes sense of abundance "there is enough for me!" (pg. 136)

Frankincense - supports brain, mood, wound healing, feeling grounded and safe/secure (pg. 100)

Roman chamomile - supports sense of calm/relaxation; sedative effect; diffuses agitated negative thoughts/moods; detoxifying (pg. 125)

By Related Properties

For definitions of the properties listed below and more oil options, see Oil Properties Glossary (pg. 435) and Oil Properties (pg. 436).

Antibacterial - arborvitae, bergamot, black pepper, cardamom, cedarwood, cinnamon, eucalyptus, ginger, lemongrass, marjoram, melaleuca, myrrh, oregano, patchouli, rosemary, tangerine, thyme

Anticatarrhal - black pepper, frankincense, helichrysum, myrrh, rosemary, spearmint, white fir

Antidepressant - basil, bergamot, clary sage, coriander, frankincense, geranium, lemon, lemongrass, rose, sandalwood, wild orange

Anti-inflammatory - arborvitae, basil, bergamot, cedarwood, coriander, cypress, eucalyptus, frankincense, geranium, ginger, helichrysum, lavender, lemongrass, lime, marjoram, melaleuca, myrrh, peppermint, roman chamomile, rosemary, sandalwood, wintergreen

Antiseptic - basil, bergamot, black pepper, cardamom, cedarwood, clary sage, cypress, geranium, helichrysum, jasmine, lavender, lemon, lime, marjoram, melaleuca, melissa, oregano, patchouli, ravensara, rosemary, sandalwood, tangerine, thyme, white fir, wild orange, yarrow, ylang ylang

Antiviral - arborvitae, cassia, cinnamon, clove, eucalyptus, lime, melaleuca, melissa, oregano, thyme, white fir

Calming - basil, lavender, patchouli, roman chamomile, tangerine, vetiver

Decongestant - cypress, eucalyptus, lemon, melissa, rosemary, white fir

Expectorant - cardamom, dill, eucalyptus, fennel, helichrysum, jasmine, lemongrass, marjoram, melaleuca, oregano, rosemary, sandalwood, thyme, white fir

Immunostimulant - arborvitae, cassia, cinnamon, clove, eucalyptus, frankincense, lime, melissa, rosemary, white fir, wild orange

Invigorating - grapefruit, lemon, peppermint, spearmint, wild orange, wintergreen

Mucolytic - basil, cedarwood, clary sage, cypress, fennel, helichrysum, lemon, myrrh

Regenerative - basil, cedarwood, clove, cypress, frankincense, geranium, helichrysum, lavender, lemongrass, melaleuca, patchouli, sandalwood

Relaxing - basil, cassia, cedarwood, geranium, jasmine, lavender, marjoram, myrrh, ravensara, roman chamomile, ylang ylang

Sedative - basil, bergamot, cedarwood, coriander, frankincense, juniper berry, lavender, patchouli, roman chamomile, sandalwood, vetiver, ylang ylang

Stomachic - basil, cardamom, fennel, ginger, juniper berry, peppermint, rosemary, yarrow

Uplifting - bergamot, cardamom, cedarwood, clary sage, cypress, grapefruit, sandalwood, tangerine, wild orange

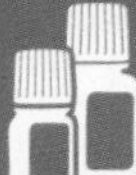

BLENDS

Calming blend - supports sense of peace and calm (pg. 142)

Grounding blend - supports feeling grounded and stable (pg. 150)

Digestion blend - supports digestion and elimination (pg. 147)

Protective blend - boosts immune system (pg. 158)

Focus blend - supports optimal focus and concentration (pg. 149)

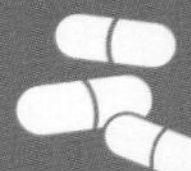

SUPPLEMENTS

Children's chewable (pg. 170), defensive probiotic, **liquid omega-3 supplement (pg. 178)**, meal replacement shake, respiration blend lozenges

Related Ailments: Colic, Crying Baby, Diaper Rash, Fifth's Disease (human parvovirus B19), Gastroenteritis (stomach flu) [Digestive & Intestinal; Immune & Lymphatic], Hand, Foot and Mouth Disease [Immune & Lymphatic - Viral], Infant Reflux, Legg-Calve-Perthes Disease [Skeletal], Roseola, RSV, Scarlet Fever, Thrush [Candida]

USAGE TIPS: Children are wonderfully responsive to the use of essential oils, love to learn about them and what they do, and be involved in the process of selecting what oils are used on their behalf. They love to nurture others with the oils as well and participate in making their own personalized roller bottle blend. Allowing a child to smell an oil prior to use creates a sense of safety.

- **Aromatic:** Use of oils at bedtime with a diffuser or smelling oils from some kind of sealed container during school can bring both peace and calming, also mental focus and concentration support. Oils supply a vast variety of emotional support.
- **Topical:** Use of oils with children is most effective when oils are combined with a carrier oil and are massaged on back, abdomen or feet (NEAT - undiluted - application on feet with 1-2 drops depending on body weight is acceptable in older children; for infants and toddlers, dilute oils with a carrier oil prior to application in most cases).

Conditions

EMOTIONAL/MENTAL STATES

Children naturally experience any number of emotional states, as do adults. Common expressions can be anxious or stressed, defiant, excessive crying, willful, grumpy or irritable, overly reactive or over-sensitive, shy, sad, whiny or pouty, and excessively wound up or hyperactive. See *Mood & Behavior* for suggested solutions. For attention deficits or issues with focus and concentration, see *Focus & Concentration.*

PHYSICAL STATES

Acne, baby - melaleuca, skin clearing blend (dilute); see *Integumentary*

Allergies - cilantro, lemon, lavender, melaleuca, peppermint, detoxification; see *Allergies*

Antibiotic recovery - cilantro, detoxification blend, defensive probiotic; see *Candida*

Bed-wetting - black pepper, cilantro, cypress, rosemary, spearmint, thyme, grounding blend, massage blend

Birth - arborvitae, clary sage, frankincense, melaleuca, melissa, myrrh, sandalwood, patchouli, wild orange, calming blend, encouraging blend, grounding blend; see *Pregnancy, Labor & Nursing*

Bronchitis - cardamom, clary sage, eucalyptus, encouraging blend,protective blend, respiration blend; see *Respiratory*

Bug bites/stings - lavender and cleansing blend; see *First Aid*

Bumps/bruises - fennel, geranium, helichrysum, lavender, soothing blend; see *First Aid*

Colic - bergamot, black pepper, cardamom, cilantro, clove, coriander, cypress, dill, fennel, ginger, lavender, marjoram, roman chamomile, rosemary, spearmint, wild orange, ylang ylang, calming blend, digestion blend; see *Digestive & Intestinal*

Common cold/flu - cardamom, cedarwood, lemon, melaleuca, melissa, rose, rosemary, sandalwood, thyme, protective blend, respiration blend; see *Immune & Lymphatic*

Constipation - cardamom, cilantro, douglas fir, ginger, lemongrass, rosemary, wild orange, detoxification blend, digestion blend; see *Digestive & Intestinal*

Cradle cap - arborvitae, cedarwood, clary sage, geranium, lavender, lemon, sandalwood, anti-aging blend, corrective ointment; see *Integumentary*

Croup - arborvitae, douglas fir, eucalyptus, lemon, marjoram, ravensara, patchouli, sandalwood, thyme, wild orange, protective blend, respiration blend; see *Respiratory*

Cuts - frankincense, lavender, melaleuca, myrrh, sandalwood, corrective ointment; see *First Aid*

Diaper rash - dilute: frankincense, lavender, melaleuca, patchouli, roman chamomile, ylang ylang; see *Integumentary*

Dry lips/above lips - cedarwood, jasmine, myrrh, sandalwood, corrective ointment, fractionated coconut oil; see *Integumentary*

Dry skin - arborvitae, lavender, lemon (skin cleansing), melaleuca, myrrh, sandalwood, anti-aging blend, diluted; see *Integumentary*

Earache - basil, clary sage, cypress, fennel, ginger, helichrysum, lavender, melaleuca, roman chamomile, thyme, wild orange, soothing blend; see *Respiratory*

Eczema/Psoriasis - arborvitae, cedarwood, douglas fir, geranium, helichrysum, myrrh, patchouli, roman chamomile, sandalwood, ylang ylang, corrective ointment, fractionated coconut oil; see *Integumentary*

Fever - cardamom, eucalyptus, frankincense, lavender, lime, peppermint, roman chamomile, tension blend; see *Immune & Lymphatic*

Foot fungus (Athlete's foot) - basil, clove, melaleuca, protective blend; see *Candida*

Hand, foot and mouth - arborvitae, cassia, cinnamon, clove, helichrysum, lemongrass, melaleuca, melissa, oregano, rosemary, thyme, wild orange, wintergreen, protective blend; see *Immune & Lymphatic*

Headache - lavender, peppermint, frankincense, wintergreen, tension blend; see *Pain & Inflammation*

Hiccups - arborvitae, clary sage, fennel, helichrysum, lemon, sandalwood, wild orange, calming blend, detoxification blend; see *Digestive & Intestinal*

Hives - basil, cilantro, frankincense, lavender, melaleuca, peppermint, roman chamomile, rosemary; see *Allergies*

Immune system boost - protective blend; see *Immune & Lymphatic*

Infant reflux - dill, lavender, peppermint, roman chamomile; see *Digestive & Intestinal*

Jaundice - geranium, helichrysum, juniper berry, lemon, lemongrass, lime, rosemary, wild orange, detoxification blend; see *Digestive & Intestinal*

Leg aches/growing pains - arborvitae, birch, cypress, ginger, lavender, lemongrass, marjoram, melissa, rosemary, white fir, wintergreen, massage blend, soothing blend; see *Pain & Inflammation*

Pinkeye (conjunctivitis) - clary sage, melaleuca, frankincense, corrective ointment; see *Immune & Lymphatic*

Rash - arborvitae, cedarwood, lavender, lemon, melaleuca, roman chamomile, rose, sandalwood, detoxification blend; see *Integumentary*

Respiratory support - eucalyptus, rosemary, respiration blend; see *Respiratory*

Runny nose - basil, cedarwood, lemon/lavender/peppermint (use together), respiration blend; see *Allergies, Immune & Lymphatic, Respiratory*

Seizures - cedarwood, frankincense, lavender, myrrh, peppermint, rose (will delay onset), sandalwood; see *Brain*

Sleep, disturbed/irregular/nighttime waking - lavender, vetiver, calming blend, grounding blend; see *Sleep*

Sleep, trouble getting to - lavender, roman chamomile; see *Sleep*

Stomach flu - bergamot, basil, cardamom, clove, dill, ginger, thyme, digestion blend; see *Digestive & Intestinal*

Stuffy nose - douglas fir, lemon, sandalwood, digestion blend, respiration blend; see *Allergies, Immune & Lymphatic, Respiratory*

Sunburn - frankincense, helichrysum, lavender, peppermint, sandalwood, anti-aging blend; see *Integumentary*

Teeth grinding - frankincense, geranium, marjoram, lavender, roman chamomile, wild orange, calming blend; see *Parasites*

Teething pain - clove, frankincense, helichrysum, lavender, roman chamomile, sandalwood; dilute and apply directly to gums

Thumb sucking - clove (diluted) or any other internally safe, unpleasant-tasting oil (diluted)

Thrush - bergamot, clary sage, clove, dill, geranium, fennel, lavender, lemon, melaleuca, oregano, thyme, wild orange, metabolic blend, protective blend; see *Candida*

Tired, overly - lavender, roman chamomile, calming blend, renewing blend; see *Sleep*

Tooth decay - clove, helichrysum, melaleuca; see *Oral Health*

Tooth infection - clove, helichrysum, melaleuca; see *Oral Health*

Tummyache - cardamom, fennel, ginger, peppermint, digestion blend; see *Digestive & Intestinal*

Vomiting - bergamot, cardamom, clove, dill, ginger, cellular complex blend, cleansing blend, detoxification blend, digestion blend, protective blend, dilute; see *Digestive & Intestinal*

Warts - arborvitae, cinnamon, clove, frankincense, lemon, lemongrass, lime, melissa, oregano, thyme, protective blend; see *Integumentary*

Whooping Cough, spastic/persistent cough - cardamom, clary sage, cypress, douglas fir, eucalyptus, frankincense, lavender, roman chamomile, rosemary, calming blend, cleansing blend, respiration blend; see *Respiratory*

Remedies

AID KIDS IN GOING TO SLEEP AND STAYING ASLEEP
Diffuse eight drops lavender or calming blend and three drops wild orange

ANGER MANAGEMENT FOR LITTLE ONES
Use invigorating blend and grounding blend; place a drop of each on palms of hands, rub together, cup over face (without making contact with skin) and inhale; then rub oils on back of neck.

BED-WETTING (for older children who can swallow capsules)
1-2 drops cilantro oil in a capsule one time per day
Increase number of times per day as needed for results.
Apply cypress as needed.
For younger children, apply 1-2 drops cypress to bottoms of feet (dilute with a carrier oil).

CHILL OUT
14 drops cypress
10 drops frankincense
25 drops lavender
12 drops vetiver
18 drops roman chamomile
5 drops ylang ylang
5 drops cedarwood
Mix in a 50/50 ratio of essential oils to carrier oil for children and a 75/25 ratio for adults. Apply to back of neck, inside of wrists, base of skull, along spinal cord.

COLIC BLEND
Combine 2 tablespoons almond oil with 1 drop roman chamomile, 1 drop lavender, and 1 drop geranium or dill. Mix and apply to stomach and back. Note: Burping the baby and keeping the abdomen warm with a warm (not hot) water bottle will often bring relief.

COMMON COLD BLEND
Combine 2 tablespoons of a carrier oil with 2 drops melaleuca, 1 drop lemon, and 1 drop protective blend. Massage a little of the blend on neck and chest.

CRADLE CAP
Combine 2 tablespoons almond oil with 1 drop of melaleuca or lemon oil with 1 drop geranium, OR or 1 drop cedarwood and 1 drop sandalwood. Mix and apply a small amount on scalp.

CURE FOR POUTY KIDS
- Step 1: Take 1-2 drops of joyful blend - a natural anti-neurotic
- Step 2: Massage oil on back of neck of pouty child
- Step 3: Tickle pouty child
- Step 4: If child is still pouty, continue to tickle until poutyness ceases

TIP: Diaper rash may be caused by irritation from stool/urine, reaction to introduction of new foods or products, bacterial or yeast/fungal infection, sensitive skin, chafing or rubbing, or use of antibiotics resulting in a lack of friendly bacteria.

DIAPER RASH BLEND
Combine 1 drop roman chamomile and 1 drop lavender with fractionated coconut oil and apply.

EARACHE BLEND
Basil, helichrysum, lavender, melaleuca, roman chamomile, or thyme.
Put 1 drop of oil diluted in a carrier oil on a cotton ball and place on the surface of the ear, avoiding the ear canal; rub a little bit of diluted oil behind the ear.

FEVER
Dilute 1 drop lavender in carrier oil and massage baby or child (back of neck, feet, behind ear, etc.). Dilute 1 drop peppermint in a carrier oil and rub into bottoms of feet.

FLU
Place 2 drops of cypress, lemon, and melaleuca in a diffuser and diffuse. OR dilute 1 drop of each in 1 tablespoon bath gel base or mix into ½ cup Epsom salts for a bath treatment.

JAUNDICE
Dilute geranium and frankincense in a carrier oil and apply on the liver area and to the liver reflex points on feet.

LIGHTS OUT! (nighty night in minutes)
2 vetiver
2 cedarwood
2 patchouli
2 calming blend
3 ylang ylang
Blend in a 10 ml roller bottle; fill remainder of bottle with a carrier oil. Roll on feet at bedtime.

THRUSH BLEND
8 drops lemon
8 drops melaleuca
2 tablespoons garlic oil
1 ml Vitamin E oil
Combine. Apply a small amount of the mixture to nipples just before nursing, or with a clean finger into baby's mouth and on tongue.

TRANSITION BLEND (Helpful for children facing stressful social environment changes, like going to daycare or school)
Apply 2-3 drops of grounding blend and vetiver on back of neck. (Focus on occipital triangle area and bottoms of feet, especially the big toes.). Apply the night before and the morning of any significant event.

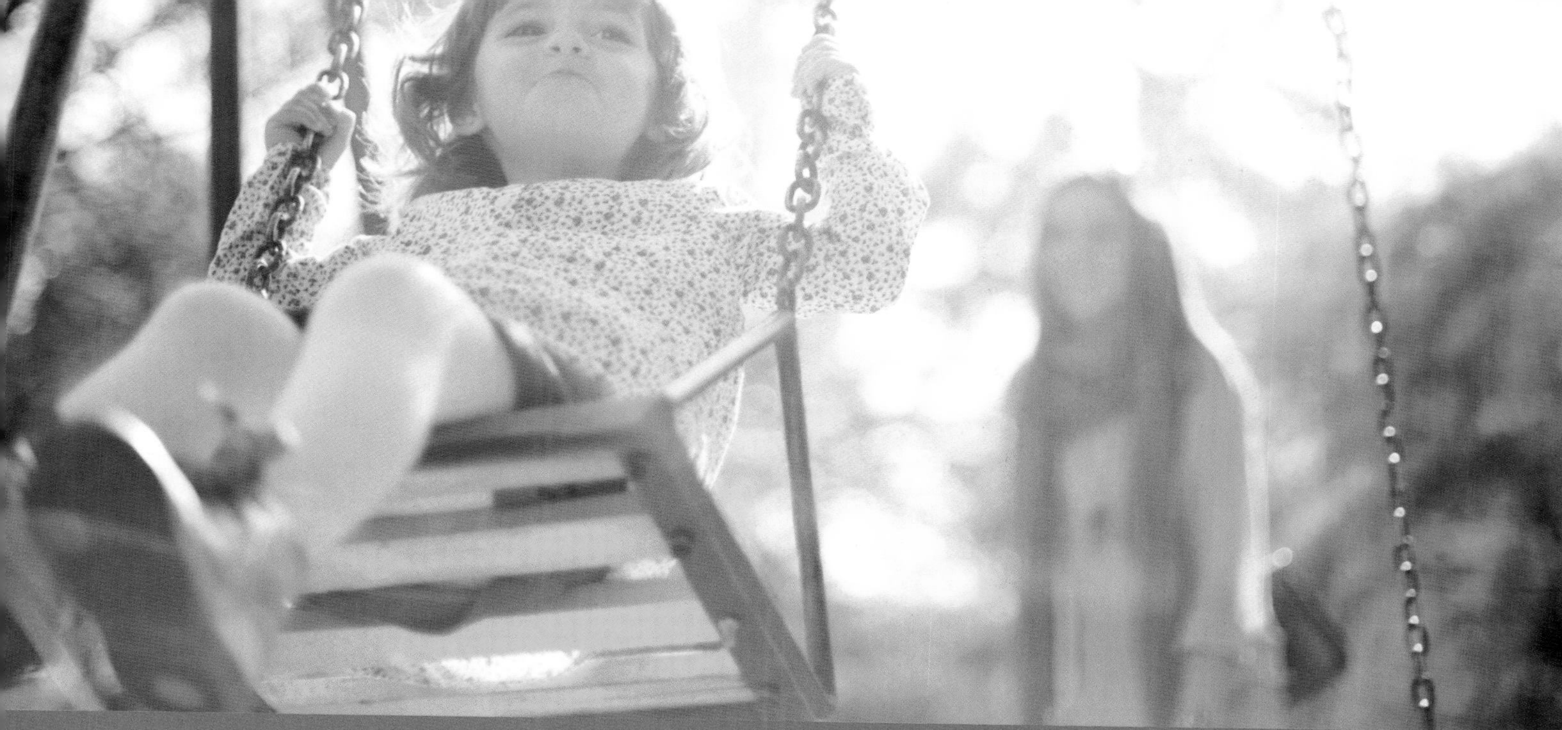

USAGE INFORMATION & NOTE TO PARENTS

Parents and caretakers bear a profound stewardship for the child's health that deserves to be taken seriously and managed responsibly. This involves educating oneself about nutrition, supplementation, preventative care options, and treatment of illnesses and injuries.

Doctors bring a wealth of medical skills and deep knowledge of disease to their work. Few have more than a cursory understanding of health maintenance essentials like supplements and nutrition. Most have no knowledge whatsoever about effective natural health care solutions like essential oils.

A parent who educates herself appropriately can choose a health care provider for her family who is open to natural solutions. Together, they can partner intelligently to provide the child an effective health maintenance program and powerful natural remedies when needed, particularly the implementation of essential oils.

Caution must be taken when researching solutions online. Most information available about aromatherapy reflects the assumption that the product used will contain synthetic ingredients. In the case of these adulterated products, warnings should be heeded as legitimate.

But when pure, unadulterated, genuine essential oils are selected, a parent can treat the family with confidence. In fact, when quality oils are used, parents can experiment much like experimenting with healthy options in the kitchen. One child might thrive on a particular grain; another might find it upsets the tummy and prefer a different selection. But no harm is done. That is what this section is designed to provide: appropriate information to encourage confidence and educated experimentation to have a healthy family.

The invitation to parents and caretakers is to know it isn't about being perfect. It is about being present. Give up the idea of doing it perfectly for the idea of being flexible and teachable. If something isn't generating the desired results, change it up, try something different, diversify efforts. Obtain fearless confidence by freely playing with the oils until you (and your children) figure them out and discover what is right for you.

Some safety rules for essential oil use with children

Generally speaking, use prudence when applying essential oils to children. Keep oils away from eyes and out of reach of children. Generally, dilution of oils with a carrier oil is recommended. When using an oil NEAT (undiluted), it is best applied on the bottoms of a child's feet.

To determine quantities, consider the child's body weight and apply a fraction of the adult recommended dosage. For example, if an adult were to apply 1-2 drops topically of an oil directly to the skin, those same number of drops could be placed in a roller bottle, highly diluted with a carrier oil, and applied repeatedly on an infant. Any oil that contains 1,8 cineole such as cardamom, eucalyptus, rosemary, myrtle, laurel leaf, or niaouli should be diluted with a carrier oil, used in small amounts, or used in a blend (which changes the nature of an oil) especially with children under the age of two.

Avoid putting undiluted peppermint oil on the chest, face, or throat area of a young child (under 30 months), as the sensation and effect can startle the infant and cause them to hold their breath or stop breathing momentarily. Use peppermint diluted on the bottoms of the feet or in a blend, such as in a respiration blend.

As indicated in the safety section of this book, birch, cassia, cinnamon, clove, eucalyptus, ginger, lemongrass, oregano, peppermint, thyme, and wintergreen are all considered to be "hot" essential oils that deserve more caution and care when used in the presence of or on children. Dilution and proper storage (away from children) are essential. Avoid contact with eyes and other sensitive parts of the body.

Premature babies: Since premature babies have very thin and sensitive skin, a very conservative and highly diluted use of essential oils is recommended.

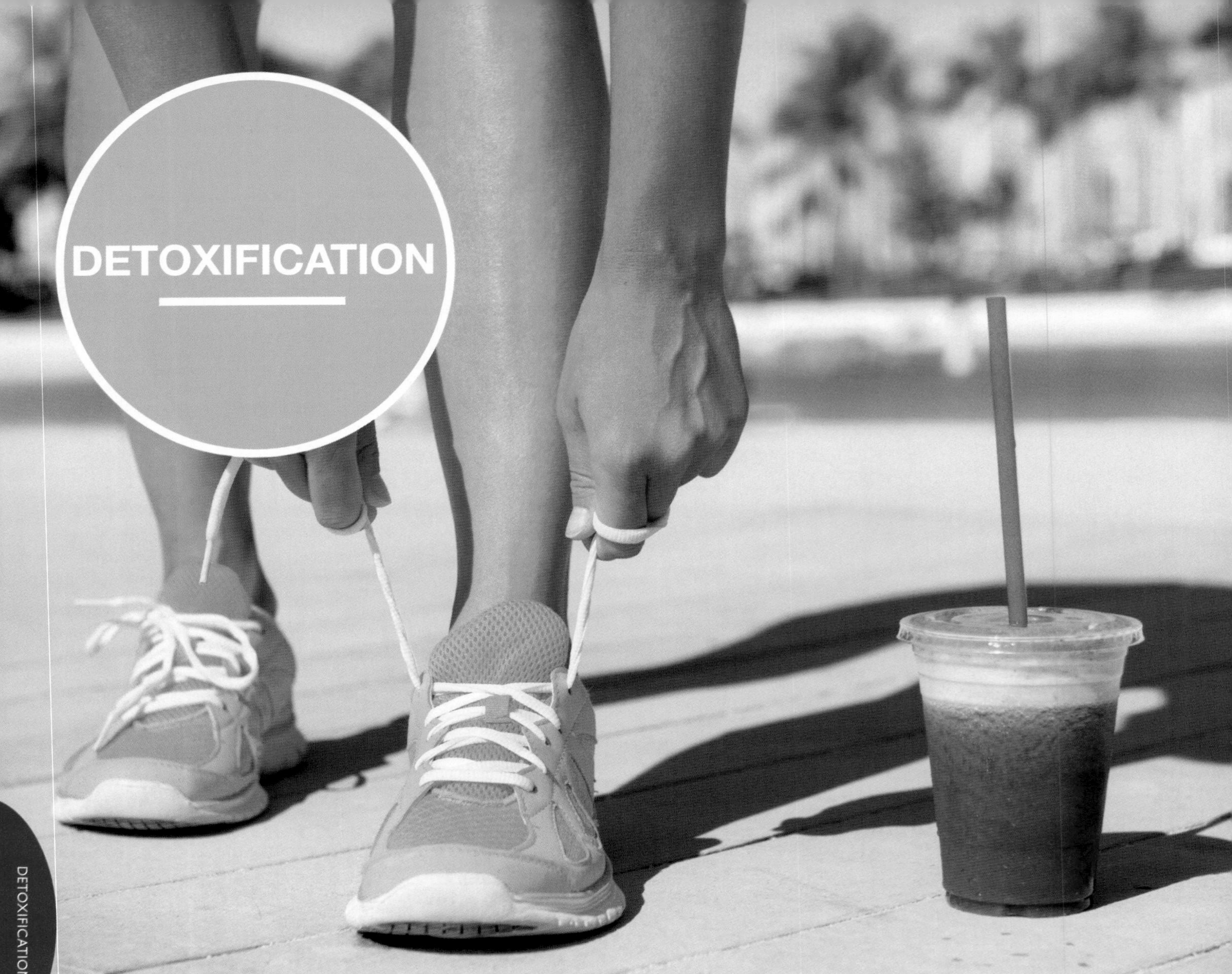

DETOXIFICATION (detoxing or cleansing) is the term used to describe the deliberate use of programs, products, dietary, and lifestyle changes to support the body in the elimination of unwanted substances and circumstances. Releasing toxins allows the body, heart, and mind to dedicate greater amounts of energy to thriving rather than just coping and surviving.

We live, eat, and breathe toxic substances every day. Consider the paint on the walls, the carpet, laundry and cleaning products, pesticides, extermination products, preservatives and chemicals in foods, the "stuff" that goes in and out of cars; personal care products and makeup also contribute to higher toxicity levels in the body. Toxicity must be dealt with even when trying to limit exposure to toxins, since contact with chemicals and other toxic agents occurs every day by eating, breathing, living, and sleeping.

When overwhelmed by toxins, the body cannot properly perform its many functions with full efficiency. Metabolism, immunity, elimination of waste, absorption of nutrients, production of important brain chemicals, reproduction, circulation, respiration, etc., are affected. Even hydration can be compromised. Toxic overload may reveal itself as fevers, headaches, acne, fatigue or lack of energy, sneezing, coughing, vomiting, diarrhea, rashes, allergies, excess weight, cellulite, brain fog or lack of mental clarity, decreased immunity, chronic pain, poor moods, and much more. Sometimes these symptoms are interpreted as sickness, when in reality the body may be trying to eliminate toxins through different systems—and the symptoms are mere side effects. Avoiding toxins and detoxifying are necessary to be healthy, happy, and free of disease.

Essential oils have unique properties that support health on a cellular level, including detoxing. When the body is overwhelmed by excess toxins, the liver will safeguard vital organs by insulating toxins in fat cells; there are oils that help release toxins from fat cells, break them down, and flush them out of the body with good hydration. Other oils stimulate cell receptor sites to greater, more efficient activity. And there are oils that are helpful in clearing the gut of harmful bacteria and restoring balance for healthy digestion and immunity. Consider what actions can reduce the intake of toxins, and how to consistently detox to maintain optimal health.

TOP SOLUTIONS

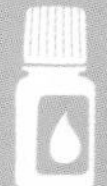

SINGLE OILS

Grapefruit - antioxidant; superb detoxifier of fat, liver, gallbladder (pg. 104)

Lemon - antioxidant; superb detoxifier of fat, chemicals, urinary, liver, lymph (pg. 110)

Lemongrass - powerhouse decongestant for any system of the body (pg. 112)

Clove - powerful antioxidant, blood and cellular cleanser (pg. 90)

By Related Properties

For definitions of the properties listed below and more oil options, see Oil Properties Glossary (pg. 435) and Oil Properties (pg. 436).

Antitoxic - bergamot, black pepper, cinnamon, coriander, fennel, geranium, grapefruit, juniper berry, lavender, lemon, lemongrass, patchouli, thyme

Detoxifier - arborvitae, cassia, cilantro, cypress, geranium, juniper berry, lemon, lime, patchouli, rosemary, wild orange

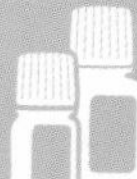

BLENDS

Detoxification blend - detox liver, gallbladder, gut, kidneys, lungs, skin (pg. 146)

Cleansing blend - detox lymph, blood, kidneys, skin (pg. 144)

Cellular complex blend - detox lymph, cells, gut, brain (pg. 143)

Metabolic blend - detox fat, liver, gallbladder (pg. 157)

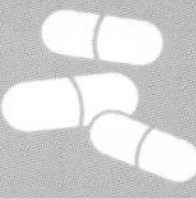

SUPPLEMENTS

Cellular vitality complex, **detoxification blend softgels (pg. 173), detoxification complex (pg. 173)**, energy & stamina complex, essential oil cellular complex, essential oil omega complex, food enzymes, GI cleansing softgels, whole food nutrient supplement

Related Ailments: Acidosis, Alkalosis, Blood Detoxification, Body Odor, Hangover, Lead Poisoning, Metal Toxicity, Xenoestrogens

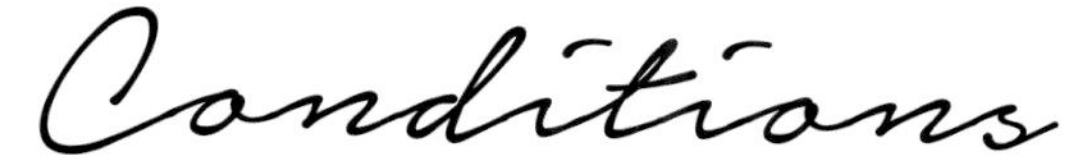

Conditions

Blood toxicity - basil, cassia, clove, frankincense, geranium, grapefruit, lime, roman chamomile, helichrysum, white fir, thyme, cellular complex blend, detoxification blend; see *Cardiovascular*

Brain - arborvitae, basil, bergamot, cedarwood, clove, frankincense, melissa, rosemary, sandalwood, thyme, cellular complex blend

Candida toxicity - arborvitae, basil, lemongrass, melaleuca, oregano, thyme; see *Candida*

Cellular toxicity - arborvitae, clove, frankincense, helichrysum, lemongrass, tangerine, wild orange, cellular complex blend, comforting blend, skin clearing blend; see *Cellular Health*

Cellulite - cypress, douglas fir, eucalyptus, ginger, grapefruit, lemon, thyme, wild orange, metabolic blend; see *Weight*

Gallbladder toxicity - geranium, grapefruit, lemongrass, lime, tangerine, cellular complex blend, detoxification blend, metabolic blend; see *Digestive & Intestinal*

Gut toxicity - bergamot, black pepper, cardamom, cinnamon, fennel, ginger, roman chamomile, wild orange, detoxification blend, digestion blend; see *Digestive & Intestinal*

Heavy metal toxicity - arborvitae, cilantro, frankincense, geranium, helichrysum, juniper berry, rosemary, thyme, cleansing blend, detoxification blend

Kidney/urinary toxicity - bergamot, cardamom, cassia, cilantro, coriander, eucalyptus, fennel, geranium, juniper berry, lemon, lemongrass, rosemary, encouraging blend, invigorating blend; see *Urinary*

Liver toxicity - basil, bergamot, clove, cypress, dill, geranium, grapefruit, helichrysum, juniper berry, lemon, lemongrass, marjoram, peppermint, roman chamomile, rose, rosemary, detoxification blend, metabolic blend; see *Digestive & Intestinal*

Lymphatic toxicity - arborvitae, cypress, lemon, lemongrass, melaleuca, myrrh, rosemary, cleansing blend, encouraging blend, massage blend; see *Immune & Lymphatic*

Lung/respiratory toxicity - arborvitae, cardamom, cedarwood, cinnamon, douglas fir, eucalyptus, lemon, lemongrass, lime, detoxification blend, encouraging blend, protective blend, respiration blend, skin clearing blend; see *Respiratory*

Nerve toxicity - arborvitae, basil, bergamot, black pepper, cypress, frankincense, ginger, helichrysum, lemongrass, myrrh, patchouli, peppermint, grounding blend; see *Nervous*

Pancreas toxicity - cilantro, cinnamon, coriander, lemongrass, rosemary

Parasite, intestinal toxicity - clove, fennel, thyme, oregano, roman chamomile, protective blend; see *Parasites*

Skin toxicity - cedarwood, douglas fir, frankincense, geranium, lavender, lemon, myrrh, sandalwood, vetiver, ylang ylang, anti-aging blend, skin clearing blend; see *Integumentary*

Xenoestrogen toxicity - grapefruit, clary sage, lemon, oregano, thyme, women's monthly blend; see *Men's or Women's Health*

Why Detox?

The body stores toxins in fat to keep harmful substances away from critical organs and functions whenever possible. During a detox program, when nutrients are provided and proper dietary parameters are observed, the body releases toxins and excess fat. Long-lasting results can be achieved when diet and lifestyle habits are supportive.

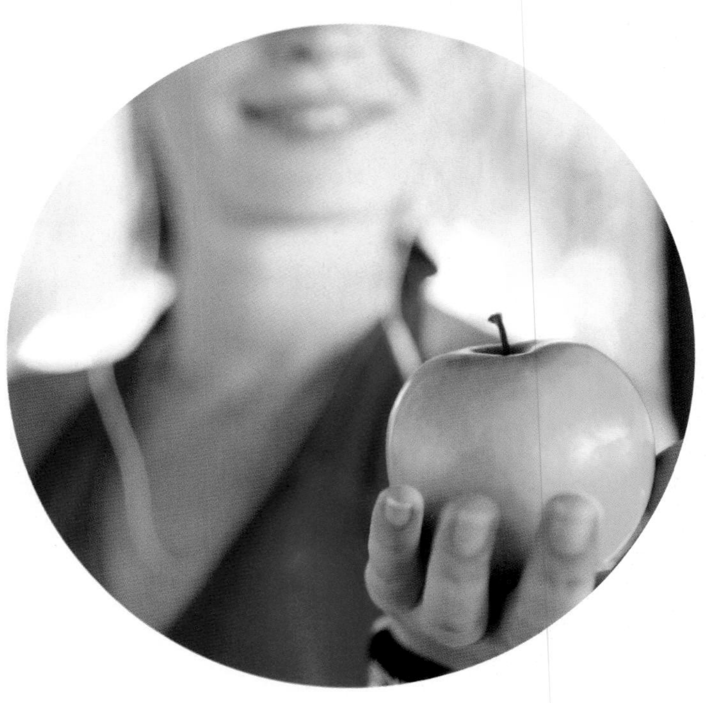

Detox Response Too Intense?

The most common detox discomfort is diarrhea, which often indicates a lack of probiotics and fiber or simply pushing the body too fast. Solutions may include increased consumption of dietary or supplemental fiber and/or probiotics, and if necessary, cut back on detox products. For example, to ease diarrhea, cut back on detoxification blend or essential oil cellular complex; if constipation is an issue, increase the same products along with food enzymes. If additional adverse symptoms occur - congestion, skin eruptions, etc., see the correlating section of this book for suggested solutions - Respiratory, Integumentary, etc.

Basic Detox Program

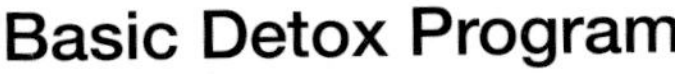

TWO-WEEK PROGRAM	
CLEAN UP DIET	
Make necessary dietary adjustments to achieve results. If desired detox results are not being achieved, make additional dietary adjustments. Eliminate refined sugars, junk foods, and dairy. Increase consumption of fruits and vegetables. Eat a high-fiber diet.	
PROVIDE IMPORTANT NUTRIENTS AND SUPPORT GUT HEALTH	
Whole food nutrient supplement	1-2 capsules AM and PM
Essential oil omega complex	1-2 capsules AM and PM
Cellular vitality complex	1-2 capsules AM and PM
Food enzymes	1-2 capsules with meals BONUS: 1-2 capsules on empty stomach in AM
Defensive probiotic	2 at bedtime
USE DETOX TOOLS	
Lemon oil	3 drops in 24 ounces water three times a day
Detoxification complex	1-2 capsules AM and PM
Detoxification blend	5-8 drops in capsule with dinner or 1-2 softgels

BONUS	
SUPERCHARGE CLEANSE	
Essential oil cellular complex	5-10 drops in capsule or 1-2 softgels twice daily
DAILY ENERGY SUPPORT	
Energy & stamina	1-2 capsules AM and afternoon as needed
TISSUE RELEASE	
Oil Touch technique	Weekly
TARGET EMOTIONS	
When negative emotions are retained, so are toxins. They are inextricably and chemically connected. Consider targeting toxic emotional states during a program. Use grounding blend or choose your own. See Mood & Behavior to select emotion(s) and oil(s) for program.	

Dosage levels are determined by body weight, tolerance, and results. Adjust accordingly.

* To take a detox commitment to the next level, see *Weight* or *Candida* for additional detox, weight management, and candida clearing programs.

Remedies

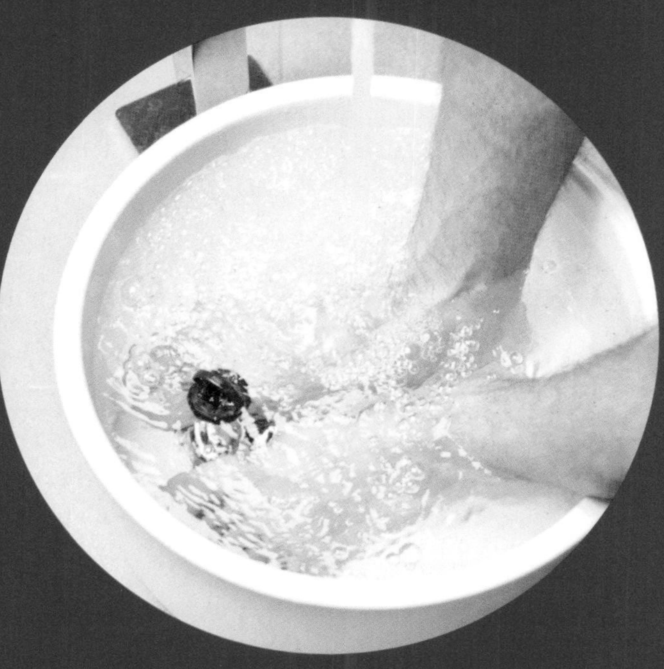

HEAVY METAL DETOX
2 drops geranium
4 drops helichrysum
2 drops lavender
3 drops cilantro
2 drops cypress
2 drops frankincense
Combine oils in a roller bottle. Fill with fractionated coconut oil. Apply to eustachian tubes and neck in downward motion.

FOOT SOAK DETOX
1 cup Epsom salt
1 cup baking soda
⅓ cup sea salt
⅓ cup Redmond Clay powder
Selected essential oil(s)

- Mix the dry ingredients only in a mason jar and store with a lid. When a foot soak is desired, put ¼ cup of dry ingredients in foot bath tub, then mix in oils.
- Add enough warm-to-hot (100-115 degrees F) water to cover feet completely.
- Choose 3-4 drops of one or more of selected oils to direct detox to a specific areas of focus. See Conditions list above for suggestions.

DETOX BODY SCRUB
2 cups salt or sugar (i.e. sea salt, mineral salts, organic sugar)
1 cup almond oil
4 drop wild orange
4 drops basil
4 drops lemongrass
4 drops lime
4 drops thyme
4 drops rosemary
4 drops grapefruit
4 drops lavender
Combine ingredients and store in a glass jar. Apply desired amount and gently massage into skin for exfoliation; rinse.

EVERYDAY MORNING DETOX
1 tablespoon organic apple cider vinegar
1 teaspoon honey
2 drops lemon
2 drops ginger
1 drop cinnamon
10 ounces warm water
Combine in a glass and drink.

SKIN DETOX
½ cup of aluminum-free baking soda
A few tablespoons of fractionated coconut oil
4 drops lavender
3 drops rosemary
3 drops melaleuca
Create a paste; add more or less coconut oil to achieve desired consistency. Use in shower as cleanser and exfoliator. Apply all over the body and gently scrub for a few minutes; then rinse. Repeat at least twice a week. The skin naturally serves as a pathway for detoxification. Keeping the skin clean and open will aid the body in the detoxification process.

USAGE TIPS: For detoxification, various methods will contribute to success. Here are a few to focus on:

- **Internal:** Taking essential oils and supplements internally is one of the most effective ways to deliver detox "instructions" to specific organs and tissues. Consume oils in a capsule, place under tongue, or in water to drink to accomplish these targeted efforts.
- **Topical:** Invite tissue and organs to release fat and toxins by directly applying oils to specific areas of focus. Massage after application to ensure absorption. Applying oils to the bottoms of the feet will have a direct impact on blood and lymphatic fluids of the body, which is vital to detoxification. Additionally, use the Oil Touch technique to increase the success of a detox program.
- **Aromatic:** Consider addressing toxic emotional states during a program, as mood directly impacts health. Negative emotions and toxins are inextricably and chemically connected. Aromatic application immediately and directly impacts the amygdala, the center of emotions in the brain. See *Mood & Behavior* to select emotion(s) and oils that will best support a detox program.

Oil pulling

Oil pulling is an ancient practice and cleansing technique that involves the simple swishing of a specific oil in the mouth for a few minutes each day. One of the main purposes for the habit is "pulling" a variety of toxins from the bloodstream. Some of the benefits include improved gum health, whiter teeth, clear skin, elimination of bad breath, and a healthy complexion. A wide range of additional benefits have been reported that include positive changes in cellular health, immunity, and the ridding of unwanted toxins such as heavy metals and microorganisms, resulting in more energy, and much more. To increase benefits, add an essential oil that targets an area of interest. For example, add frankincense or lemon to support blood cleansing or detoxification respectively; or clove for teeth health.

INSTRUCTIONS

- Oil pulling is to be done first thing in the morning on an empty stomach prior to consumption of any liquids (including water) or foods. It is not recommended to be done at any other time of day.
- Choose a "swishing" oil. Some of the top choices include: sesame, sunflower, olive (cold-pressed, extra virgin), coconut, cod liver, cedar nut, avocado, walnut, castor, black cumin, safflower. Each oil has particular properties that bring specific results. There is a lot of information available on oil pulling and the various oils both online and in written resources.
- Choose an essential oil that supports your particular health concern. Use suggestions in "By Related Properties" or "Conditions" sections of any body system for ideas.

STEP ONE

Pour one tablespoon of selected "swishing" oil in mouth. Add 1-2 drops of chosen essential oil(s) - up to 5 if desired. Older children can also do pulling with less quantity of oil provided they have the ability to not swallow it.

STEP TWO

Swish oil around in mouth. DO NOT swallow it. Move it around in mouth and through teeth, using the tongue to create the movement. Do not tilt head back. The oil will begin to get watery as it mixes with saliva. Keep swishing. If jaw muscles get sore while swishing, relax jaw and use tongue more to help move liquid. This is a gentle and relaxed process that lasts for about twenty minutes. When done correctly, it feels comfortable, especially with repeated practice.

As the oil/saliva mixture is saturated with toxins, it may become more whitish or milk-like in consistency, depending on oil used. Each session varies in results and timing for such an effect. Again, twenty minutes is the general rule.

STEP THREE

As the end of the oil pulling session approaches, spit the oil out in a trash can - not down the drain (can clog the drain). Rinse mouth with warm water. Adding salt to the water (use a good quality sea salt or such) adds antimicrobial action, can soothe any inflammation or irritation, and is effective in rinsing out any residual mouth toxins.

TIP: If experiencing an urge to swallow during pulling session prior to the twenty minute mark (for example, its become too unpleasant), spit the oil out and begin again and resume the session until the above described change in the liquid has occurred to indicate completion. With practice, these urges, if present, diminish over time.

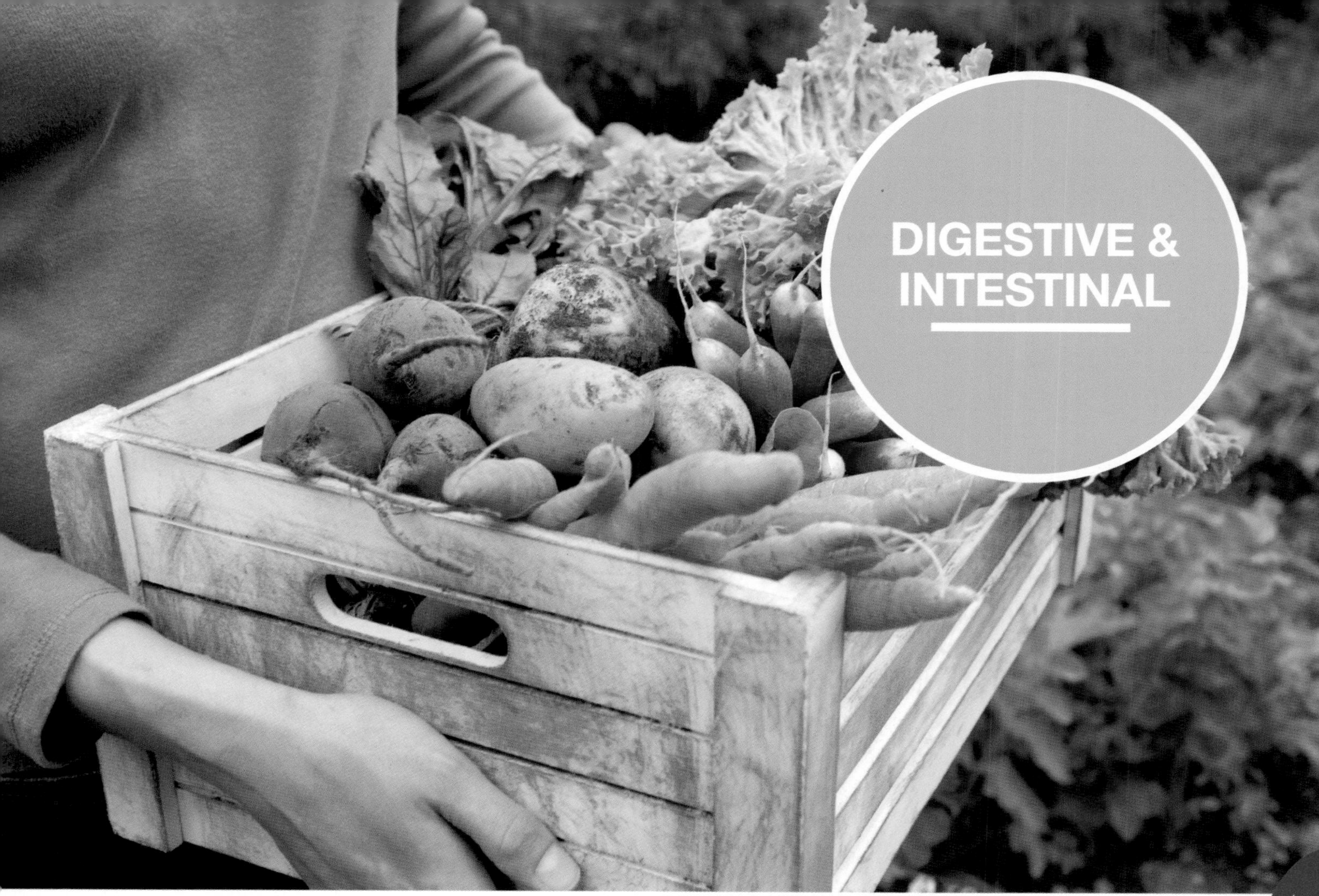

THE DIGESTIVE SYSTEM is comprised of the gastrointestinal (GI) tract and is a series of connected organs along a thirty-foot pathway responsible for chewing food, digesting and absorbing nutrients, and expelling waste. The organs involved in the digestive process are the mouth (chewing), the esophagus (swallowing), the stomach (mixing food with digestive juices), small intestine (mixing food with digestive juices of the pancreas, liver/gallbladder, and intestine, and pushing food forward for further digestion), large intestine (absorbing water and nutrients, changing remaining waste into stool), and the rectum (storing and expelling stool from the body).

The digestive tract works closely with the immune system to protect the body from pathogens and invaders. The GI tract is exposed to high quantities of outside substances including bacteria and viruses and can almost be considered to be an exterior body surface. Without the immune system (lymphoid tissue in the GI produces about 60 percent of the total immunoglobulin produced daily), the long, dark, moist GI tract would be ideal for pathogenic colonization. In return, the digestive system assists the immune system in protecting the rest of the body by breaking down bacteria and pathogens at various stages, starting with lysozyme in the saliva.

There are over one hundred million neurons embedded in the gut, which is more than exist in the spinal column or peripheral nervous system.This mesh-like network of neurons, known as the enteric nervous system (sometimes called the second brain) works together with the central nervous system to oversee every aspect of digestion. It follows then, that brain-gut interactions are highly connected to emotional health; there is a proven correlation between stress, anxiety, and gut disorders such as Crohn's disease and irritable bowel syndrome.

Digestive and eliminative problems are becoming increasingly more prevalent. They create pain, gas, bloating, excessive diarrhea, inability to absorb nutrients, and more. Mood management and emotional health issues are also on the rise. How can the neurons embedded in the gut influence healthy emotions when inflammation, blockages, candida, and other harmful bacteria are overpopulated and system imbalances are standard? They can't.

When digestive system problems are present, natural remedies offer ample opportunity for balance and restoration (see Candida section for additional understanding of GI tract imbalances). Start with good nutrition, clear the primary pathways of elimination so waste and toxins can be eliminated, use essential oils specifically targeted to help remove harmful bacteria, take a good prebiotic to encourage growth of good bacteria, and ingest a probiotic to repopulate the gut with live strains of helpful bacteria. Re-establishing health and balance in the gut can literally be a life-changing experience.

TOP SOLUTIONS

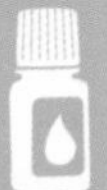

SINGLE OILS

(sorted by ailment)

Stomach - black pepper, fennel, ginger, wild orange
Stomach/intestinal lining - grapefruit, peppermint
Intestines - basil, cardamom, ginger, marjoram, peppermint
Liver - basil, cilantro, geranium, grapefruit, helichrysum, lemon, rosemary
Gallbladder - geranium, grapefruit
Pancreas - dill, fennel, geranium, ginger, thyme

By Related Properties

For definitions of the properties listed below and more oil options, see Oil Properties Glossary (pg. 435) and Oil Properties (pg. 436).

Calming - basil, coriander, jasmine, oregano, roman chamomile, sandalwood, vetiver
Carminative - basil, bergamot, cardamom, cassia, cilantro, cinnamon, clary sage, clove, coriander, cypress, dill, fennel, ginger, jasmine, juniper berry, lavender, lemon, lemongrass, melissa, myrrh, oregano, patchouli, peppermint, roman chamomile, rose, rosemary, sandalwood, spearmint, thyme, vetiver, wild orange, wintergreen, yarrow
Detoxifier - arborvitae, cassia, cilantro, cypress, dill, geranium, lavender, lime, patchouli
Digestive stimulant - basil, bergamot, black pepper, cardamom, cinnamon, clary sage, coriander, dill, fennel, frankincense, grapefruit, helichrysum, juniper berry, lemongrass, marjoram, melaleuca, myrrh, oregano, patchouli, spearmint, wild orange, yarrow
Laxative - bergamot, black pepper, cilantro, fennel, ginger, lemongrass
Regenerative - basil, frankincense, geranium, helichrysum, lavender, myrrh, wild orange
Stimulant - arborvitae, basil, birch, black pepper, cardamom, cedarwood, cinnamon, dill, fennel, ginger, grapefruit, juniper berry, spearmint, thyme, vetiver, white fir, wintergreen
Stomachic - basil, cardamom, cinnamon, clary sage, coriander, fennel, ginger, juniper berry, marjoram, melissa, peppermint, rose, rosemary, tangerine, wild orange, yarrow

USAGE TIPS: for best effect on digestive and intestinal activity:

- **Internal:** Place 1-5 drops in water and drink, take in capsule, lick off back of hand, or place drop(s) on or under tongue to allow impact directly in stomach and intestines.
- **Topical:** Apply oils topically on abdomen and/or bottoms of feet for relief.

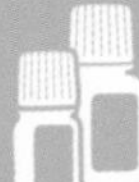

BLENDS

Digestion blend - supports digestion and elimination (pg. 147)
Metabolic blend - supports stomach, intestines, pancreas, liver, gallbladder, fat digestion and satiation (pg. 157)
Massage blend - supports peristalsis and bowel tone (pg. 155)
Detoxification blend - supports gallbladder, liver, and pancreas (pg. 146)

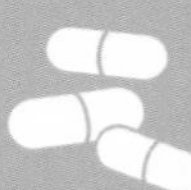

SUPPLEMENTS

Bone support complex, **defensive probiotic (pg. 172)**, detoxification blend softgels, detoxification complex, **digestive blend softgels (pg. 173)**, essential oil cellular complex, essential oil omega complex, **food enzymes (pg. 177)**, **GI cleansing softgels (pg. 178)**, liquid omega-3 supplement, whole food nutrient supplement

Related Ailments:

- **Digestive:** Abdominal Cramps, Acid Reflux, Bloating, Esophagitis, Flatulence, Food Poisoning [Immune & Lymphatic], Gastritis, GERD, Heartburn, Hemochromatosis, Hernia(Hiatal), Indigestion, Metabolism, Motion Sickness, Nausea, Ulcers - Duodenal and Gastric and Peptic, Stomach ache, Vomiting [Detoxification]
- **Intestinal:** Appendicitis, Celiac, Colitis, Constipation, Crohn's Disease, Diarrhea, Dumping Syndrome, Diverticulitis, Dysentery, Giardia [Immune & Lymphatic], Irritable Bowel Syndrome, Leaky Gut Syndrome, Malabsorption Syndrome
- **Liver And Gallbladder:** Cirrhosis, Liver Disease, Gallbladder Infection, Gallbladder Stones, Jaundice [Candida]

Remedies

DIGEST-EASE: Combine digestion blend, detoxification blend, and oregano in a capsule; consume to ease digestive discomfort, stomach pain, and bloating.

HOT BATH: Add 10-15 drops of favorite digestive/intestinal soothing oil(s) to bath salts (i.e. Epsom); stir oils into salts; place salts in hot (as is tolerable) bathwater and soak for 20 minutes.

HOT COMPRESS: Apply digestive/intestinal soothing oil(s) with carrier oil to abdomen. Place warm, moist cloth over top to create soothing compress. Repeat as needed.

INTERNALIZE: Consume favorite digestive/intestinal soothing oil(s) internally: drop 1-2 drops under tongue and hold for thirty seconds before swallowing; sip a few drops of oil(s) in a glass of water; take a few drops in a capsule and consume every twenty to thirty minutes until symptoms subside, then reduce exposure to every two to six hours as needed.

MASSAGE MAGIC FOR RELIEF
- Apply oil(s) to abdomen, over stomach or intestinal area depending on location of discomfort.
- Apply oil(s) to bottoms of feet using the reflexology points provided on charts in *Reflexology*.

NAVEL DROP: Drop a single drop of a selected oil into navel for digestive/intestinal relief.

NO MORE NAUSEA: Aromatic use of an oil can reduce influence of nausea-triggering smells:
- Diffuse essential oil(s) of choice to dispel offensive smells or toxic fumes
- Swipe an oil under nose so unpleasant odors are overridden by the essential oil aroma
- Apply a few drops to a cotton handkerchief or such and inhale as needed

TUMMYACHE SOOTHER: Place 1 drop arborvitae in bellybutton to eliminate gas and pain or other digestive discomfort.

CIRRHOSIS OF THE LIVER
4 drops roman chamomile
2 drops frankincense
2 drops geranium
2 drops lavender
1 drop myrrh
1 drop rosemary
1 drop rose
Place oils in 10ml roller bottle; fill remainder with fractionated coconut oil. Apply to liver area twice per day.

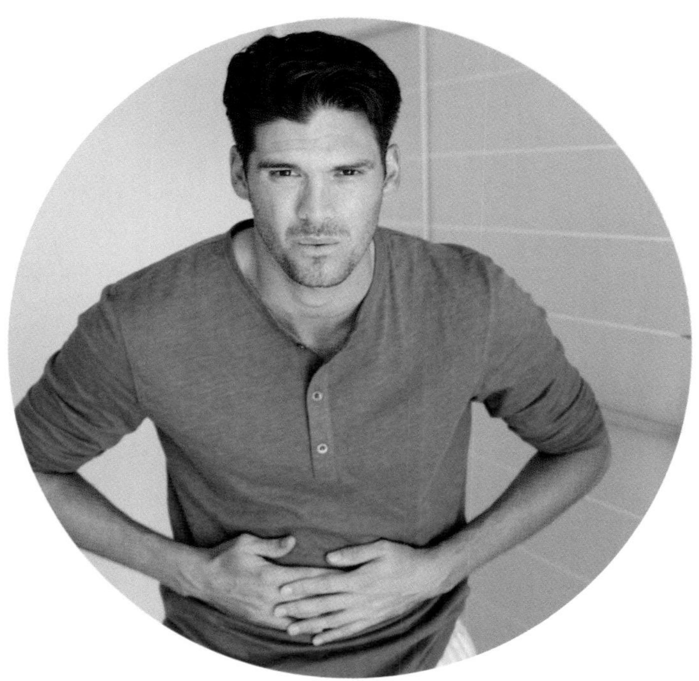

IBS RELIEF
4 drops frankincense
2 drops peppermint
2 drops fennel
2 drops ginger
Combine oils in a capsule; consume three times a day with meals. Also add GI cleansing softgels, defensive probiotic, and a whole food nutrient complex to cleanse and rebuild the gut and to build nutritional strength.

TRAVELER'S DIARRHEA: 3-4 drops digestion blend in a capsule or in water three times a day.
OR
1 drop each melaleuca and digestion blend dropped under tongue every thirty minutes until symptoms subside; usually takes about four doses.
OR
3 drops oregano
3 drops thyme
2 drops cinnamon
2 drops wild orange
1 drop rosemary
Combine and ingest in a capsule three times per day.

CONSTIPATION REMEDY
7 drops wild orange
5 drops coriander
4 drops lemon
4 drops digestion blend
2 drops ginger
Combine in 2-ounce spray bottle; fill about 1/ 2 full of carrier oil. Spray on belly and rub in clockwise motion for three to five minutes.

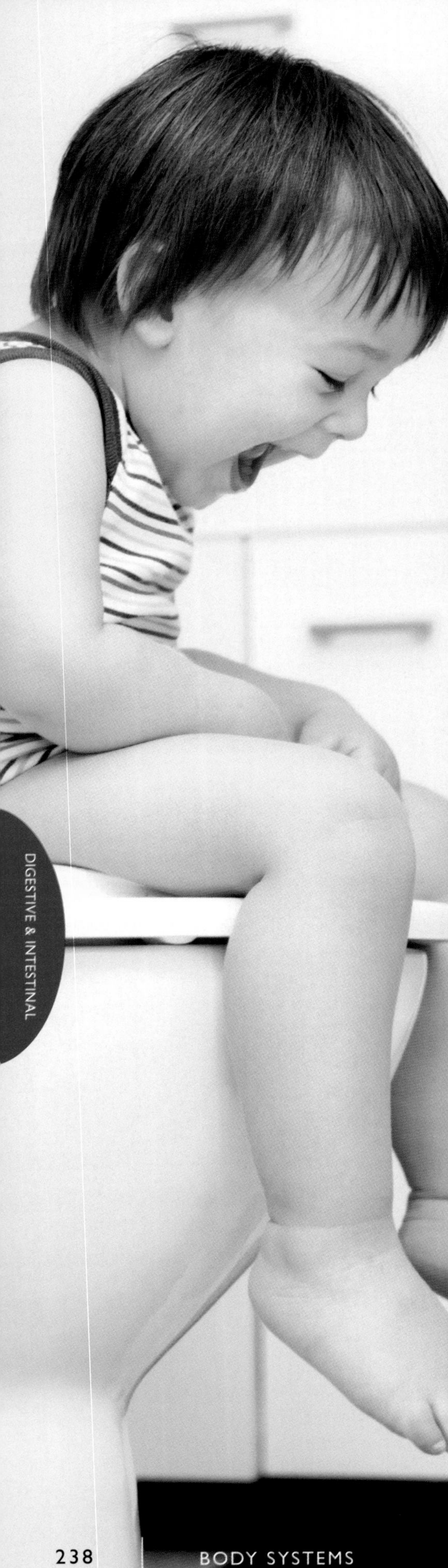

Conditions

Abdominal cramps/pain - basil, birch, cardamom, cinnamon, clove, dill, fennel, ginger, lavender, lemongrass, marjoram, melissa, patchouli, peppermint, detoxification blend, digestion blend, inspiring blend, massage blend, renewing blend

Acid reflux/regurgitation (of food/sour liquid) - cardamom, dill, fennel, ginger, lemon, peppermint, thyme, digestion blend

Alcohol-related conditions - See *Addictions*

Anus, prolapsed - thyme, wild orange

Anus, itching - cypress, geranium, helichrysum, lavender, oregano (internal), anti-aging blend, cellular complex blend

Appendix - basil, ginger, detoxification blend, digestion blend

Appetite, exaggerated - cassia, cinnamon, fennel, ginger, grapefruit, metabolic blend

Appetite, reduced/loss of - ginger, grapefruit, lavender, lemon, wild orange, encouraging blend, metabolic blend, tension blend

Belching/burping - cardamom, fennel, ginger, lavender, thyme, vetiver, detoxification blend, digestion blend

Bloating/swollen belly - cedarwood, cilantro, dill, ginger, melissa, peppermint, myrrh, digestion blend

Bowel constrictions/obstructions - basil, marjoram, rosemary, thyme, detoxification blend, encouraging blend, inspiring blend

Bowel inflammation - basil, ginger, peppermint, thyme, cellular complex blend, detoxification blend

Bowel, lack of tone - cardamom, ginger, lemongrass, marjoram

Bowel, lining (hyperpermeability/ulcerations) - basil, frankincense, geranium, helichrysum, lavender, lemongrass, myrrh, wild orange, cellular complex blend

Bowel, pockets (diverticula) - arborvitae (topical), black pepper, cedarwood (topical), geranium, tangerine, wild orange, detoxification blend

Breath, bad (halitosis) - bergamot, cardamom, lavender, patchouli, peppermint, spearmint, cellular complex blend, detoxification blend, digestion blend, metabolic blend, uplifting blend

Burp, need to - dill, ginger, peppermint

Colic - bergamot, black pepper, cardamom, cilantro, clove (dilute), coriander, cypress (topical only), dill, fennel, ginger, lavender, marjoram, roman chamomile, rosemary, spearmint, wild orange, ylang ylang, calming blend, comforting blend, digestion blend, uplifting blend

Colon polyps - coriander, ginger, lemongrass, peppermint, digestion blend

Constipation/sluggish bowels/inability to defecate despite urgency - arborvitae, black pepper, cardamom, cilantro, dill, douglas fir, fennel, ginger, lemon, lemongrass, marjoram, patchouli, peppermint, rosemary, spearmint, tangerine, vetiver, ylang ylang, comforting blend, digestion blend, detoxing blend, encouraging blend, renewing blend

Dehydration - lemon, wild orange, metabolic blend

Diarrhea/urgency to pass stool - arborvitae, black pepper, cardamom, cinnamon, clove, coriander, cypress, frankincense, geranium, ginger, jasmine, lemon, lemongrass, melissa, myrrh, patchouli, peppermint, roman chamomile, spearmint, tangerine, vetiver, wild orange, comforting blend, detoxing blend, digestion blend, renewing blend, uplifting blend

Digestive disorders - coriander, fennel, ginger, peppermint, tangerine, detoxification blend, digestion blend

Digestion, poor/sluggish - cassia, cinnamon, coriander, geranium, lemon, spearmint, encouraging blend

Distended abdomen (many possible contributors) - cardamom, fennel, ginger, detoxification blend, digestion blend

Diverticulitis - arborvitae, basil, cedarwood, cilantro, cinnamon, ginger, lavender, cellular complex blend, detoxification blend, digestion blend, metabolic blend

Failure to thrive - patchouli, cellular complex blend

Fat digestion - grapefruit, lemon, tangerine, metabolic blend

Flatulence - black pepper, cilantro, coriander, dill, fennel, ginger, lavender, melissa, myrrh, roman chamomile, rosemary, sandalwood, spearmint, tangerine, detoxification blend, digestion blend, metabolic blend

Food poisoning - black pepper, cinnamon, clove, coriander, juniper berry, lemon, melaleuca, peppermint, oregano, rosemary, thyme, cellular complex blend, detoxification blend, digestion blend, renewing blend

Fullness, early (during a meal) - cleansing blend

Fullness, uncomfortable (lasts longer than it should) - arborvitae, digestion blend
Gallbladder, disease - juniper berry, grapefruit, helichrysum, lemongrass
Gallbladder - basil, cypress, geranium, grapefruit, helichrysum, lime, rosemary, tangerine, cellular complex blend, detoxification blend, metabolic blend
Gallstones - bergamot, birch, cilantro, clove, geranium, grapefruit, juniper berry, lavender, lemon, lime, patchouli, rosemary, wild orange, wintergreen, cellular complex blend, detoxification blend, reassuring blend
Gaseousness/bloating - black pepper, cardamom, cinnamon, clove, dill, fennel, frankincense, geranium, ginger, lavender, lemongrass, lime, melissa, peppermint, digestion blend, reassuring blend
Gastric juices, poor production of - cinnamon
Heartburn - black pepper, cardamom, cedarwood (topical), dill, fennel, ginger, lemon, peppermint, wild orange, cellular complex blend, detoxification blend, digestion blend, metabolic blend
Hemorrhoids - cypress, geranium, helichrysum, myrrh, patchouli, roman chamomile, cellular complex blend, detoxification blend, digestion blend
Hiatal hernia - arborvitae, basil, cypress, helichrysum, juniper berry, melissa, patchouli, peppermint, detoxification blend
Hunger pains - fennel, lavender, metabolic blend
Indigestion - arborvitae, black pepper, dill, ginger, lavender, lemon, lemongrass, melissa, peppermint, spearmint, thyme, ylang ylang, digestion blend, inspiring blend, metabolic blend
Indigestion, nervous - cardamom
Inflammation, gut/intestinal - fennel, lemongrass, peppermint, roman chamomile, spearmint, thyme, inspiring blend
Intestinal parasites - clove, fennel, oregano, thyme
Intestinal peristalsis, lack of/spastic - marjoram, digestion blend, massage blend
Jaundice/excess bilirubin - basil, frankincense, geranium, helichrysum, juniper berry, lemon, lemongrass, lime, rosemary, wild orange, cleansing blend, detoxification blend, metabolic blend
Lactose issues - cardamom, coriander, dill, lemongrass, cellular complex blend, detoxification blend, digestion blend, food enzyme
Leaky gut/gut permeability/weak intestinal lining/malabsorption - arborvitae, cardamom, dill, ginger, grapefruit, patchouli, cellular complex blend, digestion blend
Liver - basil, cilantro, clove, cypress, frankincense, geranium, ginger, grapefruit, helichrysum, jasmine, juniper berry, lemon, rosemary, cellular complex blend, comforting blend, detoxification blend, renewing blend, uplifting blend
Liver, low bile production - geranium, helichrysum, lavender, peppermint, roman chamomile, rosemary, detoxification blend
Liver, blocked bile duct/obstruction - cypress, geranium, marjoram, patchouli, detoxification blend
Liver congestion - geranium, helichrysum, peppermint, rose, rosemary, encouraging blend
Liver, fatty - rosemary, metabolic blend, grapefruit
Liver headaches/migraines - grapefruit, helichrysum
Liver, hepatitis - frankincense, jasmine, melaleuca
Liver, overloaded/sluggish/toxic- cilantro, clove, helichrysum, lemon, detoxification blend, encouraging blend
Liver, scarring - helichrysum, myrrh
Liver, weak - dill, geranium, lemon, lime, roman chamomile, rose
Nausea/motion sickness - basil, bergamot, black pepper, cardamom, cassia, clove, coriander, fennel, ginger, lavender, juniper berry, melissa, patchouli, peppermint, roman chamomile, rosemary, sandalwood, spearmint, cellular complex blend, cleansing blend, detoxification blend, digestion blend, reassuring blend, renewing blend
Pancreas - basil, cinnamon, coriander, dill, fennel, frankincense, geranium, ginger, cellular complex blend, metabolic blend, protective blend
Pancreatic, duct blocked - cardamom, helichrysum
Rectal bleeding - geranium, helichrysum, cellular complex blend
Rectal, fissures - geranium, helichrysum, detoxification blend
Rectal pain - frankincense, geranium, helichrysum, detoxification blend
Saliva, lack of - cardamom
Spasms, digestive - cardamom, cassia, cinnamon, clove, coriander, dill, fennel, spearmint, tangerine, wild orange, inspiring blend, renewing blend
Spasms, esophageal - wild orange
Stomach, ache/cramp/pain/inflammation - basil, cardamom, cinnamon, coriander, ginger, helichrysum, peppermint, roman chamomile, sandalwood, ylang ylang, cellular complex blend, comforting blend, detoxification blend, digestion blend, encouraging blend, invigorating blend (topical)
Stomach flu (viral gastroenteritis) - arborvitae, thyme, oregano, cellular complex blend, detoxification blend, invigorating blend (topical), protective blend
Stomach, nervous (due to worry/anxiety/stress) - cardamom, calming blend, wild orange
Stomach, lack of tone - black pepper, rose, tangerine
Stomach, upset (indigestion) - cardamom, cinnamon, clove, dill, fennel, ginger, grapefruit, frankincense, jasmine, lavender, thyme, wild orange, invigorating blend (topical), renewing blend
Stools, bloody - birch (ulcer), geranium (bleeding), frankincense, helichrysum (bleeding), wild orange, wintergreen (ulcer)
Stools, mucus - black pepper, detoxification blend, massage blend, protective blend
Stools, pale in color/clay-like - detoxification blend
Swallowing, difficulty (dysphagia) - arborvitae, frankincense, lavender, wild orange, calming blend, cellular complex blend
Swallowing, painful/tight throat - cardamom, wild orange, detoxification blend, protective blend
Ulcer, duodenal (located in duodenum/upper intestines) - birch, bergamot, ginger, fennel, frankincense, geranium, myrrh, wintergreen, cellular complex blend, cleansing blend, detoxification blend, digestion blend, soothing blend
Ulcer, gastric (located in stomach) - birch, bergamot, frankincense, geranium, myrrh, peppermint, rose, wintergreen, cellular complex blend, comforting blend, detoxification blend, digestion blend
Vomiting - basil, black pepper, cardamom, cassia, clove, dill, fennel, geranium, ginger, melaleuca, melissa, patchouli, peppermint, sandalwood, cellular complex blend, cleansing blend, comforting blend, detoxification blend, digestion blend
Yeast - See *Candida*

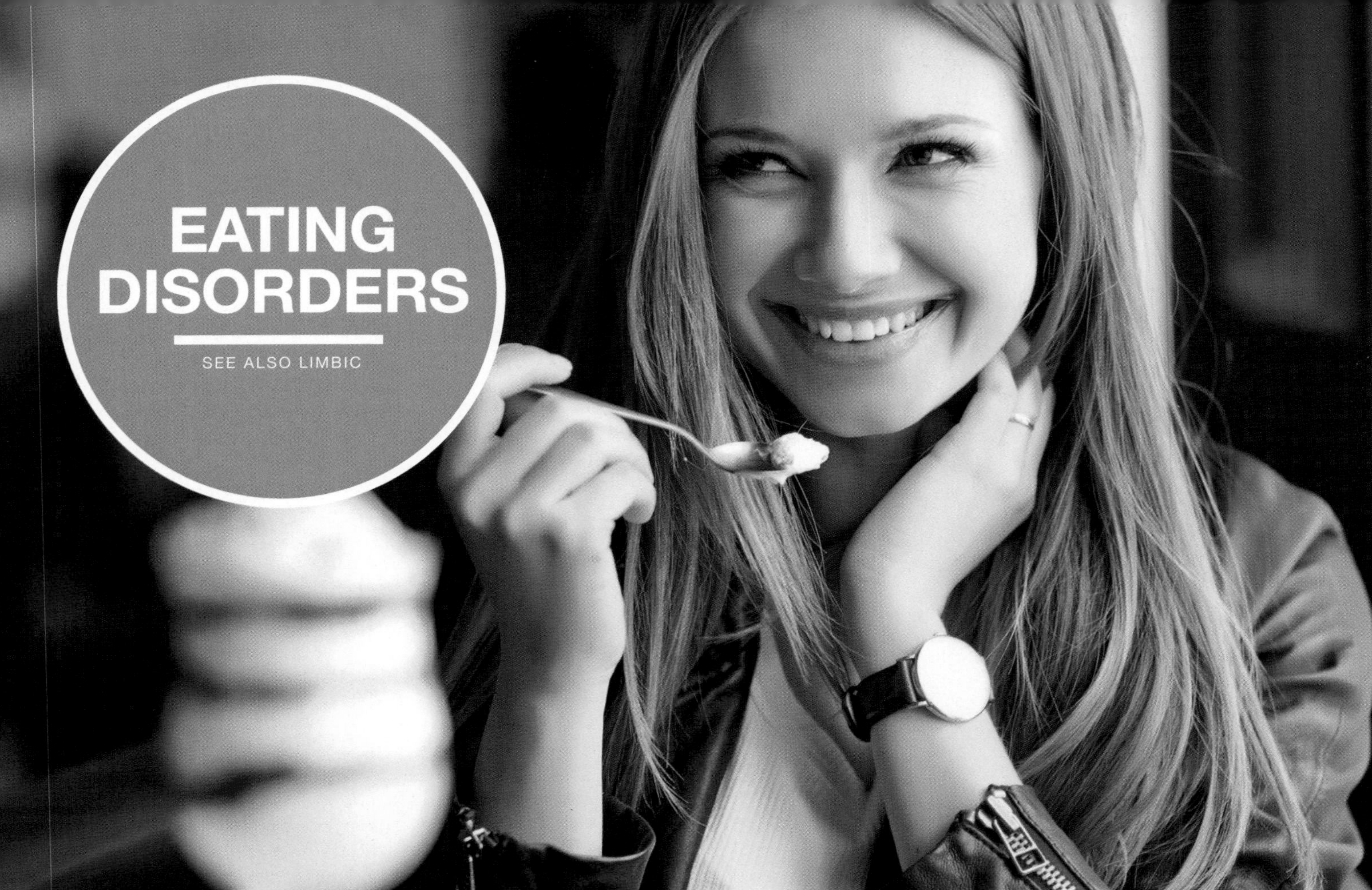

EATING DISORDERS comprise a group of serious disruptions in eating behavior and weight regulation that adversely impact physical, psychological, and social well being. The most common are anorexia nervosa, bulimia nervosa, and binge-eating disorder. While an individual may start by simply eating more or less food than normal, the tendency increases until he or she is eating portions outside of a healthy range and the urge to manage weight or food intake spirals out of control. While the majority of those with eating disorders are women, men have them also. An exception is binge-eating disorder, which appears to affect almost as many men as women.

Eating disorders are often accompanied by depression, substance abuse, or anxiety disorders. While they can become life-threatening if proper care is not received, it is important to remember that they are treatable medical illnesses. Such treatments usually involve psychotherapy, nutrition education, family counseling, medications, and may include hospitalization.

Anorexia nervosa is characterized by an obsession with food and being thin, even to the point of near starvation. Symptoms of this disorder may include refusal to eat and denial of hunger, intense fear of weight gain, excessive exercising, flat mood or lack of emotion, irritability, fear of eating in public, social withdrawal, trouble sleeping, menstrual irregularities or loss of menstruation (amenorrhea), constipation, abdominal pain, dry skin, irregular heart rhythms.

Alternating episodes of binging and purging are the primary symptoms of bulimia nervosa. During these episodes, an individual typically eats a large amount of food in a short duration and then tries to expel the extra calories through vomiting or excessive exercise. Additional symptoms may include eating to the point of discomfort or pain, laxative use, an unhealthy focus on body shape and weight, going to the bathroom after eating or during meals, abnormal bowel function, damaged teeth and gums, and swollen salivary glands in the cheeks.

Even though eating disorders manifest as a physical condition with physical consequences, many experts in the field believe that they actually originate from an individual's mental or emotional state. Many individuals with eating disorders may suffer from low self-esteem or self-worth or even feel helpless and thus choose to control something that is in their immediate control (the food that does or does not go into their body). Due to the unique direct relationship between emotional and physical well being with eating disorders, natural remedies can be a very effective part of treatment, since they can support individuals emotionally as they work with professionals to learn new habits and ways of coping.

Essential oils have a powerful effect in the brain. Aromas have direct access through the olfactory senses which connect directly to glands and areas such as the hypothalamus and amygdala, allowing oils to initiate rapid responses both physically and emotionally in the brain and the rest of the body. Inhalation and aromatic exposure are powerful methods of impacting the brain with essential oils. Oils offer an extremely effective way of supporting the body with eating disorders.

TOP SOLUTIONS

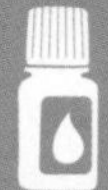

SINGLE OILS

Grapefruit - helps heal relationship with body and curb emotional eating (pg. 104)

Patchouli - supports restoring connection to and acceptance of body (pg. 121)

Bergamot - balances hormones and promotes sense of self-worth (pg. 79)

Cinnamon - balances glucose levels and metabolism; promotes sense of safety (pg. 86)

By Related Properties

For definitions of the properties listed below and more oil options, see Oil Properties Glossary (pg. 435) and Oil Properties (pg. 436).

Analgesic - basil, birch, cinnamon, clary sage, cypress, eucalyptus, frankincense, ginger, helichrysum, jasmine, lavender, lemongrass, melaleuca, oregano, ravensara, white fir, wintergreen

Antidepressant - bergamot, cinnamon, clary sage, frankincense, geranium, lavender, lemon, lemongrass, patchouli, rose, sandalwood, wild orange, ylang ylang

Antispasmodic - black pepper, cardamom, cassia, clary sage, clove, cypress, fennel, ginger, helichrysum, jasmine, lavender, lemon, marjoram, melissa, peppermint, ravensara, rosemary, sandalwood, spearmint, vetiver, wintergreen

Calming - bergamot, black pepper, clary sage, coriander, geranium, juniper berry, lavender, oregano, roman chamomile, vetiver

Carminative - bergamot, cassia, clary sage, clove, dill, fennel, jasmine, juniper berry, lemongrass, patchouli, peppermint, sandalwood, spearmint, wintergreen

Energizing - basil, clove, grapefruit, lemongrass, peppermint, rosemary, wild orange

Grounding - clary sage, cypress, melaleuca, vetiver

Relaxing - cassia, cedarwood, clary sage, cypress, lavender, marjoram, ravensara, roman chamomile, ylang ylang

Stomachic - cardamom, cinnamon, clary sage, fennel, ginger, melissa, rosemary, wild orange, yarrow

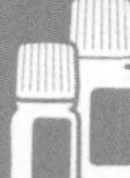

BLENDS

Metabolic blend - balances metabolism and insulin (pg. 157)

Grounding blend - balances emotions and promotes a feeling of tranquility (pg. 150)

Cleansing blend - encourages release of toxic emotions (pg. 144)

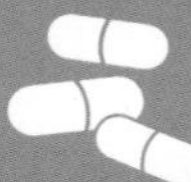

SUPPLEMENTS

Cellular vitality complex, defensive probiotic, **digestive blend softgels (pg. 173)**, essential oil omega complex, **food enzymes (pg. 177)**, fruit & vegetable supplement powder, phytoestrogen multiplex, **whole food nutrient supplement (pg. 183)**

Related Ailments: Anorexia Nervosa (AN) [Weight], Avoidant/restrictive Food Intake Disorder (ARFID), Binge Eating Disorder (BED), Bulimia Nervosa (BN) [Weight], Night Eating Syndrome (NES) [Sleep, Weight], Pica, Purging Disorder, Rumination Disorder

USAGE TIPS: Best methods of use for eating disorders

- **Aromatic:** Smell oils of choice, whether diffused, inhaled directly from bottle, swiped under nose, worn as a perfume/cologne, or placed on clothing, bedding, jewelry. Place oils in hands, rub together, cup over nose, inhale. Have on hand for immediate use.
- **Internal:**
  - › Drink oils to satisfy cravings or compulsions by placing a few drops in water.
  - › Plan ahead for typical cravings by taking supportive oils in a capsule prior to when urges hit.
  - › For more instant effects, licking a drop off back of hand to help pacify craving.
  - › Apply oils to roof of mouth (place oil on pad of thumb and then place pad on roof of mouth).
- **Topical:** Apply under nose, behind ears, to base of skull (especially in suboccipital triangles) and forehead, on roof of mouth (closest location to the amygdala; place on pad of thumb, then suck on thumb); for daily grounding, apply to bottoms of feet.

Conditions

Abdominal pain - cardamom, ginger, lavender, digestion blend; see *Digestive & Intestinal*

Abuse, history of, healing from - frankincense, melissa, roman chamomile; see *Mood & Behavior*

Anger - basil, bergamot, cedarwood, frankincense, helichrysum, roman chamomile, rose, calming blend, focus blend, grounding blend; see *Mood & Behavior*

Anorexia - bergamot, black pepper, cardamom, cinnamon, coriander, frankincense, ginger, grapefruit, melissa, patchouli, roman chamomile, rose, vetiver, calming blend, comforting blend, invigorating blend, joyful blend, reassuring blend

Anxiety - bergamot, clary sage, frankincense, tangerine, vetiver, wild orange, calming blend, focus blend, grounding blend; see *Mood & Behavior*

Appetite, lack of/refusal to eat - fennel, cardamom, metabolic blend; see *Digestive & Intestinal*

Apathetic/emotionally flat/lack of emotion - lime, ylang ylang; see *Mood & Behavior*

Appetite, loss of control - ginger, metabolic blend; see *Digestive & Intestinal*

Binging/overeating until "stuffed" - basil, cedarwood, cinnamon, ginger, grapefruit, peppermint, thyme, joyful blend, metabolic blend

Bulimia - arborvitae, bergamot, cinnamon, grapefruit, melissa, patchouli, digestion blend, metabolic blend

Cold, frequently being - cassia, cinnamon, ginger, oregano, patchouli; see *Cardiovascular*

Constipation - cardamom, cilantro, fennel, ginger, lavender, lemongrass, detoxification blend, digestion blend; see *Digestive & Intestinal*

Control, feeling out of, of behavior - See *Mood & Behavior*

Dehydration - cypress, juniper berry; see *Urinary*

Denial of hunger - cardamom, fennel, metabolic blend

Depression - bergamot, cinnamon, grapefruit, wild orange, ylang ylang, joyful blend, women's blend; see *Mood & Behavior*

Digestive issues - cardamom, fennel, ginger, peppermint, lavender, digestion blend; see *Digestive & Intestinal*

Dry skin - arborvitae, cedarwood, frankincense, geranium, lavender, melaleuca, sandalwood, anti-aging blend; see *Integumentary*

Emotionality/overly emotional - cypress, geranium

Excessive exercising - cypress, patchouli, vetiver, cleansing blend, grounding blend

Expressing/managing emotions/feelings, difficulty - focus blend, grounding blend, see *Mood & Behavior*

Family patterns/runs in family - lemon, white fir

Fear of eating in public - cardamom, wild orange, calming blend, metabolic blend

Guilt - bergamot, coriander, geranium, lemon, white fir, cleansing blend, repellent blend, respiration blend, skin clearing blend

Gum damage - clove, myrrh, anti-aging blend; see *Oral Health*

Helpless - cedarwood, clove, ginger, tangerine, white fir, digestion blend, invigorating blend, protective blend, tension blend

Hormone imbalance - See *Men's* or *Women's Health*

Impatient - basil, joyful blend, women's monthly blend, respiration blend, tension blend

Intense fear of gaining weight - cypress, melissa, juniper berry

Irregular heartbeat (arrhythmia) - basil, lavender, ylang ylang; see *Cardiovascular*

Irritability - coriander, jasmine, roman chamomile, rose, tangerine; see *Mood & Behavior*

Loneliness - marjoram, cedarwood, frankincense, myrrh, roman chamomile, anti-aging blend, cleansing blend, invigorating blend

Low blood pressure - basil, cardamom, helichrysum, lavender, lime, rosemary, cellular complex blend, cleansing blend; see *Cardiovascular*

Low self-esteem/self-worth - bergamot, cassia, grapefruit, jasmine, lemon, patchouli, rose, spearmint, tangerine, metabolic blend; see *Mood & Behavior*

Menstrual irregularities or loss of menstruation (amenorrhea) - clary sage, geranium, fennel, juniper berry, rosemary, ylang ylang, monthly blend for women; see *Women's Health*

Obsessive/compulsive - oregano, calming blend, grounding blend; see *Mood & Behavior*

Out of sync with natural urges of body - thyme

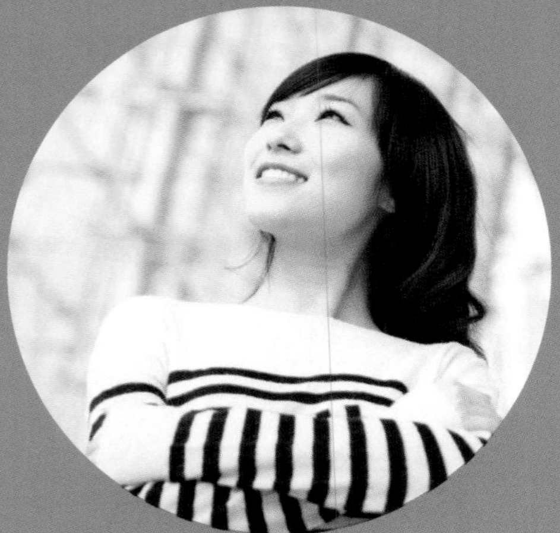

People-pleasing - black pepper, cinnamon, lavender, lime, peppermint, cleansing blend

Perfectionistic - cypress, melissa, tangerine, grounding blend, repellent blend

Preoccupation with food - cypress, grapefruit, lavender, vetiver, joyful blend

Purging urge - douglas fir, lime, patchouli, rose, tangerine, wintergreen, detoxification blend, metabolic blend

Self image, distorted/negative - bergamot, grapefruit, spearmint, metabolic blend

Shame/uncomfortable in own "skin" or body - grapefruit, patchouli, metabolic blend

Shame - bergamot, cypress, **douglas fir,** frankincense, thyme, protective blend

Shame, body - grapefruit, patchouli, metabolic blend

Social withdrawal - cassia, cinnamon, cedarwood, frankincense, ginger, myrrh, spearmint

Sores, throat and mouth - frankincense, lemon, melaleuca, melissa, myrrh, thyme, cellular complex blend, respiration blend; see *Oral Health*

Sores, scars, calluses on knuckles or hands - frankincense, geranium; see *Integumentary*

Stress - frankincense, jasmine, lavender, lime, ylang ylang, wild orange, calming blend, invigorating blend, joyful blend; see *Stress*

Swollen salivary glands in cheeks - marjoram, vetiver, cleansing blend, invigorating blend, joyful blend, tension blend

Teeth damage - birch, clove, helichrysum, wintergreen, protective blend; see *Oral Health*

Trouble sleeping - lavender, vetiver, calming blend, cellular complex blend; see Sleep

Vomiting, addiction to forcing - douglas fir, fennel, ginger, grapefruit, lavender, digestion blend, metabolic blend

Remedies

ANOREXIC ASSIST
2 drops vetiver
4 drops bergamot
Combine and diffuse around meal times or during emotional vulnerability.

BULIMIA OR ANOREXIA: Place one drop of bergamot, grapefruit oils and digestion blend under tongue each morning. Inhale oils of choice (choose what aroma is most impacting) throughout day. Can be inhaled from bottle, diffused or worn. Additionally, take a few drops during day internally in water or in a capsule. Choose from bergamot, cinnamon, grapefruit, melissa, patchouli, thyme, digestion blend, and metabolic blend. Combine or use individually.
Suggestions:
- Drink 2 drops cinnamon + 3 drops grapefruit in glass of water
- Wear 3 drops patchouli + 2 drops bergamot as a perfume on wrists, neck, etc.
- Combine 2 drops cinnamon, 3 drops melissa, 2 drops thyme, 3 metabolic blend in a capsule and consume.

OVEREATING CONTROL
2 drops black pepper
2 drops ginger
2 drops grapefruit
2 drops lemon
2 drops peppermint
Apply to bottoms of feet or take in a capsule before eating. Additionally, diffuse any of the oils.

KILL SUGAR CRAVINGS
Choose one or more as needed:
- Use 1-3 drops of basil (smell)
- Cinnamon (lick, drink)
- Grapefruit (drink, smell)
- Thyme (capsule) and/or
- Metabolic blend (drink, capsule)

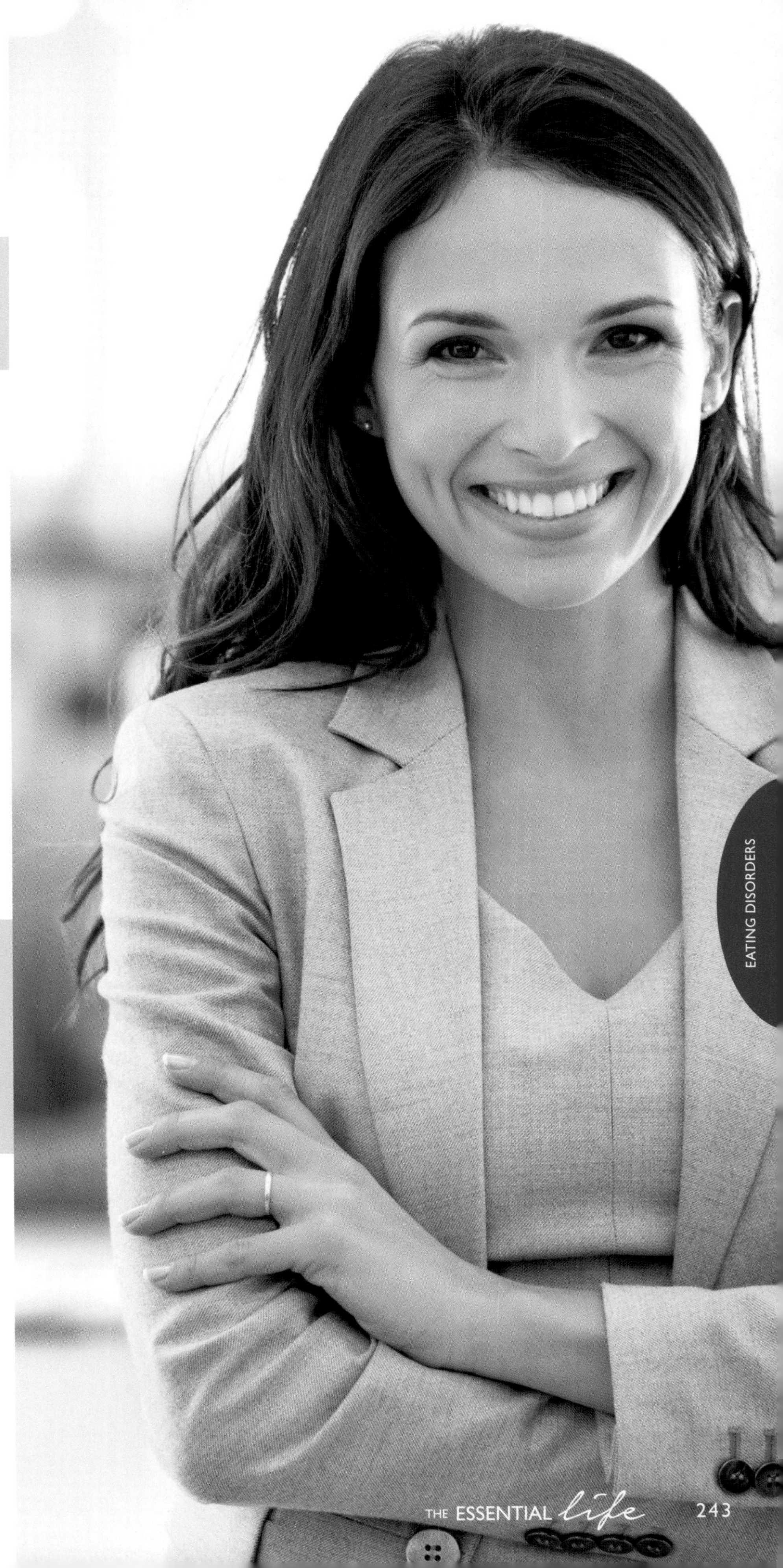

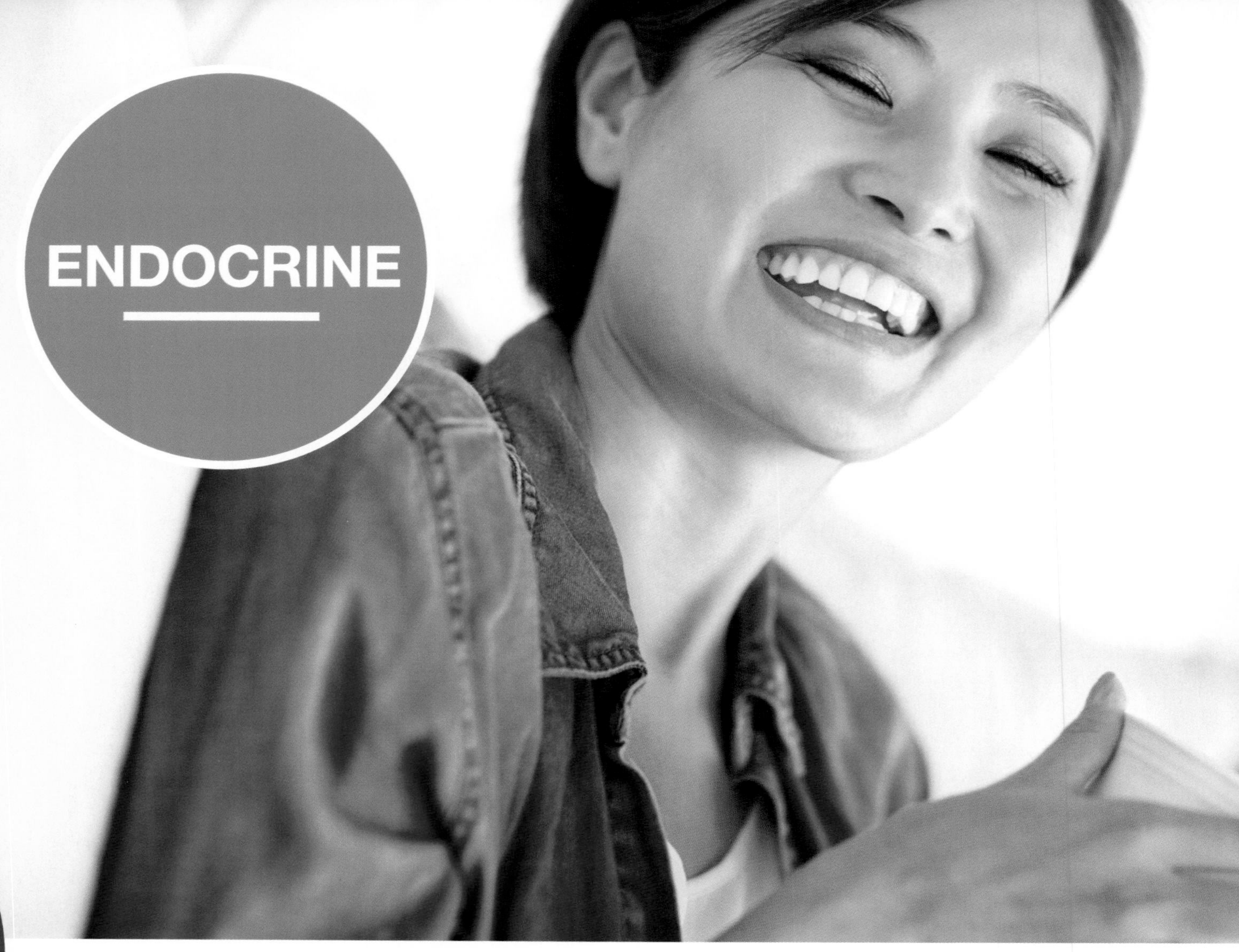

THE ENDOCRINE SYSTEM consists of glands in the body that produce and secrete hormones directly into the circulatory system. The hormones are carried to targeted organs and tissues where they bind only to cells with necessary specific receptor sites. The endocrine system is responsible for bodily functions and processes such as cell growth, tissue function, sleep, sexual and reproductive functions, metabolism, blood sugar management, how the body responds to injuries and stress, energy, water and electrolyte balance, and more. It basically tells the cells in the body exactly what to do.

The glands of the endocrine system include the pituitary gland (the master gland which helps regulate the other glands within the endocrine system), pineal gland, thyroid and parathyroid glands, adrenal glands, hypothalamus, thalamus, pancreas, gastrointestinal tract and reproductive glands (ovaries/testicles). Many organs that are part of other body systems (such as the liver, kidneys and heart) also secrete hormones, and this is recognized as a secondary endocrine function. The exocrine system also secretes hormones, but uses glands with ducts – such as sweat glands or salivary glands – to deliver these secretions.

Endocrine disorders are common, and include such conditions as obesity, thyroid malfunction, and diabetes. Endocrine disorders typically occur when hormone levels are too high or too low, a condition that can be caused by unregulated hormone release, cellular messaging problems (lack of response to signaling), when endocrine glands are not operating at full capacity, or when important organs/tissues become enlarged or malfunctioned. Stress, electrolyte or fluid imbalances in the blood, infection, tumors, and medication can also affect endocrine function. Hypofunction of endocrine glands means there isn't enough endocrine activity, whereas hyperfunction refers to too much activity; both types of imbalance can cause serious problems.

Because of the unique delivery system of the endocrine system (sending hormones to targeted organs & tissues via the circulatory system), essential oils can be especially beneficial since they use the same delivery system! Essential oils are able to profoundly benefit cells they encounter throughout the body as they circulate. There are also specific oils that have been shown to be incredibly supportive with certain gland/organ functions. Individuals can work together with their medical providers, when necessary, to consider the benefits of natural solutions as well as modern medical treatment options.

TOP SOLUTIONS

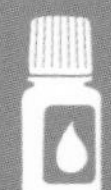

SINGLE OILS

Frankincense and sandalwood - for pineal, pituitary, and hypothalamus support (pg. 100)

Geranium and ylang ylang - hormone/glandular and adrenal support (pgs. 102 & 139)

Clove and lemongrass - for thyroid support (pgs. 90 & 112)

Rosemary - stimulates glands and brain function; adrenal support (pg. 127)

By Related Properties

For definitions of the properties listed below and more oil options, see Oil Properties Glossary (pg. 435) and Oil Properties (pg. 436).

Anti-inflammatory - arborvitae, basil, cassia, cinnamon, clary sage, clove, eucalyptus, fennel, helichrysum, jasmine, lemongrass, myrrh, patchouli, peppermint, rosemary, spikenard
Calming - basil, black pepper, cassia, frankincense, juniper berry, melissa, oregano, roman chamomile, tangerine
Detoxifier - arborvitae, cilantro, geranium, lime
Regenerative - clove, coriander, helichrysum, sandalwood, wild orange
Relaxing - cedarwood, clary sage, geranium, marjoram, myrrh, white fir
Sedative - basil, bergamot, coriander, geranium, lavender, melissa, patchouli, rose, spikenard, ylang ylang
Stimulant - basil, cardamom, cinnamon, coriander, dill, ginger, grapefruit, myrrh, spearmint, white fir
Uplifting - bergamot, clary sage, grapefruit, lemon, tangerine
Vasodilator - lemongrass, marjoram, rosemary, thyme

Related Ailments:

- **Adrenal:**
  Addison's Disease [located in Autoimmune], Adrenal Fatigue/Exhaustion, Cortisol Imbalance, Cushing's Syndrome
- **Pancreas:**
  Pancreas, Pancreatitis; for all other pancreas ailments related to blood sugar management, see the following section, Blood Sugar
- **Thyroid:**
  Goiter, Night sweats [Immune & Lymphatic, Women's Health], Grave's Disease [located in Autoimmune], Hashimoto's Disease [located in Autoimmune], Hyperthyroidism, Hypothyroidism, Silent Thyroiditis, Thyroid
- **Additional Endocrine Ailments:**
  Acromegaly, Endocrine System, Glands, Growth Problems, Melatonin Imbalances/Insufficiencies, Parathyroid, Pineal, Pituitary, Precocious Puberty, Schmidt's Syndrome (adrenals, thyroid) [located in Autoimmune], Thymus, Turner Syndrome

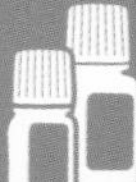

BLENDS

Cellular complex blend - nerve repair; glandular support (pg. 143)

Detoxification blend - adrenal and glandular support (pg. 146)

Women's blend - glandular support and mood stabilizer (pg. 168)

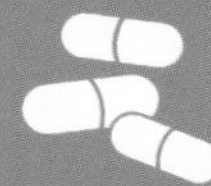

SUPPLEMENTS

Cellular vitality complex, children's chewable, **energy & stamina complex (pg. 174)**, essential oil cellular complex, **essential oil omega complex (pg. 175)**, liquid omega-3 supplement, whole food nutrient supplement

General Gland Support

Adrenal: basil, geranium, rosemary, ylang ylang, detoxification blend, invigorating blend
Glandular sluggishness - clove, cellular complex blend
Hypothalamus - cardamom, cedarwood, clove, frankincense, sandalwood, focus blend, grounding blend
Pancreas - basil, cassia, cinnamon, coriander, dill, eucalyptus, fennel, geranium, ginger, grapefruit, helichrysum, jasmine, lavender, lemon, lemongrass, oregano, rosemary, wild orange, ylang ylang, calming blend, metabolic blend, protective blend, uplifting blend
Parathyroid - basil, clary sage, clove, geranium, ginger, melissa, roman chamomile, grounding blend, women's monthly blend
Pineal - arborvitae, basil, cedarwood, frankincense, helichrysum, lavender, sandalwood, anti-aging blend, grounding blend
Pituitary - basil, cedarwood, frankincense, geranium, sandalwood, ylang ylang, cleansing blend, invigorating blend, protective blend
Thalamus - clary sage, frankincense, jasmine, melissa, vetiver, cleansing blend
Thymus - clary sage, lemongrass, protective blend, respiration blend; see *Immune & Lymphatic*
Thyroid - clove, lemongrass, geranium, myrrh, cellular complex blend, cleansing blend, protective blend

USAGE TIPS: For endocrine support, a variety of methods can be successful. Suggestions:

- **Internal:** Consume selected oils in capsule, under tongue, or place in water to drink.
- **Topical:** Apply selected oils directly over location of gland or the bottoms of feet on reflex points (see *Reflexology*) twice daily. Use a carrier oil to prevent sensitivity.
- **Aromatic:** Diffuse 5-10 drops of oils of choice, or inhale from product bottle or self-made blend, apply a few drops to clothing, or other inhalation methods.

ENDOCRINE

Conditions

ADRENAL:

Adrenal cortex, sluggish - basil, cinnamon, frankincense, geranium, rosemary, cellular complex blend, protective blend
Adrenal fatigue/exhaustion - basil, black pepper, geranium, ginger, rosemary, wild orange, ylang ylang, comforting blend, detoxification blend, invigorating blend, reassuring blend; see *Energy & Vitality*
Constantly feeling sick - bergamot, lemon, cellular complex, detoxification blend, protective blend; see *Immune & Lymphatic*
DHEA levels - clary sage, frankincense, geranium, lavender, roman chamomile, ylang ylang, women's blend
Difficulty concentrating - cedarwood, vetiver, focus blend; see *Focus & Concentration*
Mild depression - basil, bergamot, geranium, jasmine, lavender, joyful blend; see *Mood & Behavior*
Trouble sleeping - lavender, marjoram, vetiver; see *Sleep*
Weight gain - ginger, grapefruit, lemon, metabolic blend; see "Thyroid" below, *Weight*

PANCREAS:

Blood sugar issues (too high/too low) - See *Blood Sugar*
Balance cortisol levels - basil, clove, lavender, rosemary, wild orange, ylang ylang
Eyesight, poor/vision - coriander, frankincense, geranium, helichrysum, lemongrass, sandalwood, anti aging blend, cellular complex blend
Hunger pains - fennel, peppermint; see *Digestive & Intestinal*
Low sex drive - basil, clary sage, wild orange, ylang ylang, women's blend; see *Intimacy*
Obesity - cinnamon, fennel, ginger, grapefruit, peppermint, metabolic blend; see *Weight*
Pancreatic duct, congestion/blocked - cardamom, clary sage, helichrysum, rosemary
Pancreas, congested - grapefruit, detoxification blend, inspiring blend; see *Detoxification*
Pancreas sluggish/under-active - black pepper, helichrysum, lime, inspiring blend
Pancreas support - cinnamon, dill, fennel, frankincense, geranium, ginger, inspiring blend, uplifting blend
Pancreatitis - basil, cinnamon, coriander, lemon, marjoram, rosemary, thyme, cellular complex blend, detoxification blend, metabolic blend, protective blend; see *Immune & Lymphatic*
Urinary issues associated with pancreatic/blood sugar imbalances - See *Blood Sugar, Urinary*

THYROID:

Body temp, cold - black pepper, cinnamon, clove, eucalyptus, ginger, rosemary, metabolic blend, protective blend; see *Cardiovascular* "Warming" property
Cold intolerance - black pepper, cinnamon, eucalyptus; see *Cardiovascular* "Warming" property
Compromise - basil
Constipation - cardamom, ginger, peppermint, digestion blend; see *Digestive & Intestinal*
Grave's disease - frankincense, ginger, lemongrass, rosemary, metabolic blend; see *Autoimmune*
Hashimoto's - ginger, frankincense, lemongrass, myrrh, rosemary, cellular complex blend, protective blend; see *Autoimmune*
Hair falling out - arborvitae, cedarwood, clary sage, douglas fir, eucalyptus, geranium, frankincense, juniper berry, roman chamomile, rosemary, sandalwood, wintergreen, ylang ylang, cellular complex blend, women's blend; see *Integumentary*
Heat intolerance - eucalyptus, peppermint, tension blend
Hyperthyroid - cedarwood, clary sage, clove, frankincense, geranium, ginger, jasmine, juniper berry, lavender, lemon, lemongrass, myrrh, peppermint, rosemary, sandalwood, ylang ylang, cellular complex blend
Hypothyroid - bergamot, black pepper, cedarwood, clove, frankincense, geranium, ginger, lemongrass, myrrh, peppermint, spearmint, cellular complex blend, detoxification blend
Overheated/night sweats/hot flashes - cedarwood, clary sage, eucalyptus, ginger, lemon, lime, peppermint, massage blend, tension blend, women's blend, women's monthly blend; see "Hypothyroid" above, *Blood Sugar, Women's Health*
Thyroid hormones, false - lemongrass, myrrh; see *Candida*

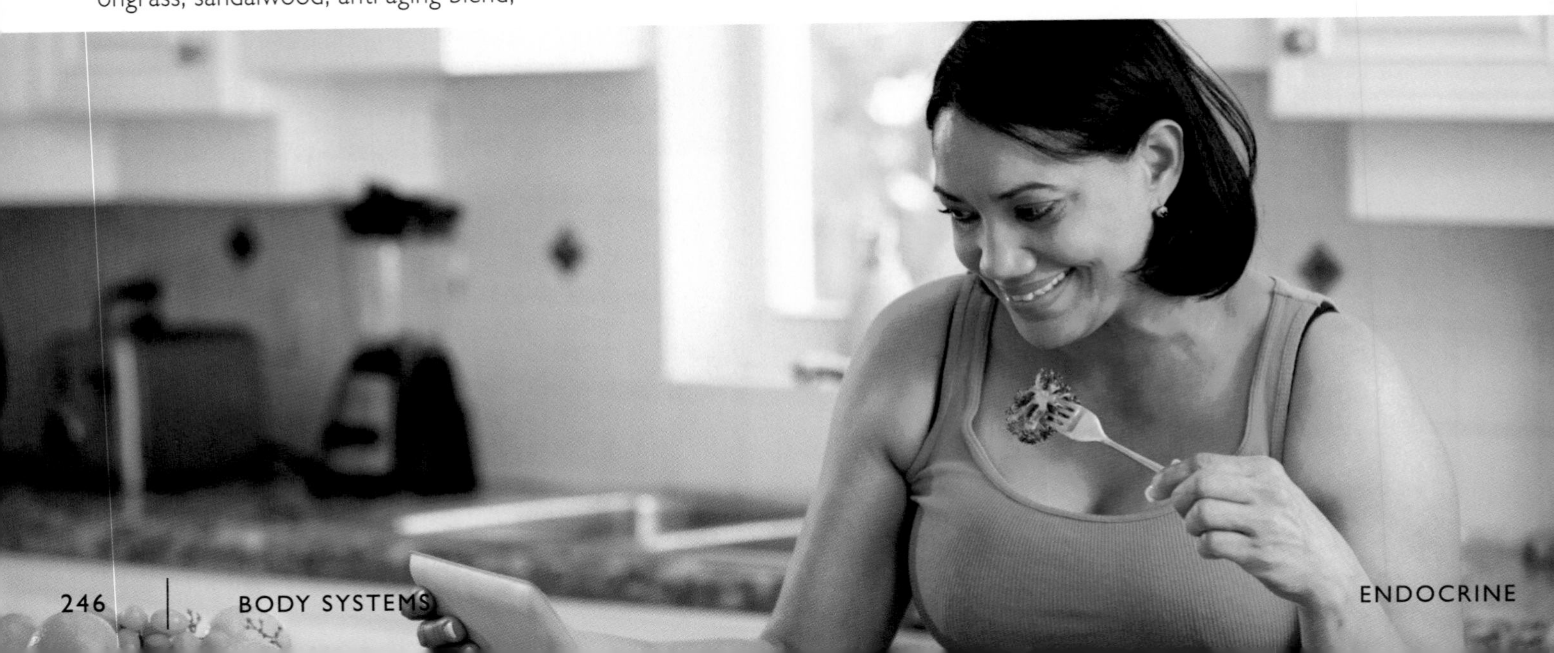

Remedies

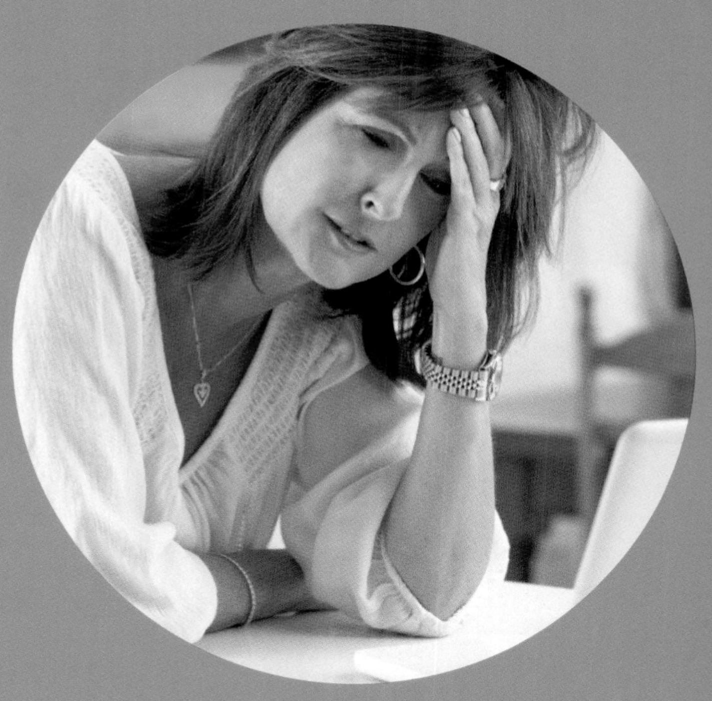

GLANDULAR HEALTH BASIC PROGRAM

- Supplement daily with:
  whole food nutrient complex
  essential oil omega complex
  energy & stamina complex
- Choose from the following for additional support:
  essential oil cellular complex and/or cellular complex blend
  metabolic blend
- Consider candida program - see *Candida*

ADRENAL ENERGY PUMP UP - use energy & stamina complex 2 capsules twice per day.

ADRENAL AID
3 drops clove
4 drops lemon
3 drops frankincense
7 drops rosemary
Combine in a 5ml bottle/roller bottle, fill remainder with carrier oil. Apply over kidneys (on both sides of back just below rib cage), follow with a warm, damp washcloth as a compress.

SIMPLE ADRENAL SUPPORT
2 drops basil internally in water one to two times per day or massage in 1 drop on back of neck.

PANCREATIC PROMOTER
30 drops basil
25 drops vetiver
25 drops cypress
Combine in 10ml roller bottle, fill remainder with carrier oil. Apply over pancreas (on abdomen just below sternum) morning and evening for pancreatic support.

THYROID BOOST
20 drops clove
20 drops myrrh
25 drops frankincense
15 drops lemongrass
Combine in a 10ml roller bottle, fill remainder with carrier oil. Apply at least once daily over thyroid (on both sides of neck just below Adam's apple).

INTERNAL THYROID ASSIST

- Take essential oil cellular complex morning and evening (may be combined with the thyroid boost treatment).
- Take 2 drops each frankincense, clove, peppermint, 1 drop each myrrh, lemongrass oils in a capsule three times per day.

THYROID CALMER
1 drop myrrh
1 drop lemongrass
Layer a base of carrier oil on thyroid area (on both sides of neck just below Adam's apple) and then massage oils on top. Apply to bottoms of feet focusing on base of big toe.

THYROID REMEDIES

- Use one of following recipes in 10ml roller bottle. Initially, apply directly to thyroid area and/or bottoms of feet two to four times per day to boost activity. As progress is made, apply once or twice per day.
  - Recipe #1: 10 drops myrrh, 10 drops lemongrass, 2-3 drops clove, 2-3 drops peppermint; add carrier oil to fill.
  - Recipe #2: 25 drops each lemongrass, clove, peppermint; fill remainder with carrier oil.
- Other variations:
  - Apply 1 drop of any single oil alone or combine with one or two others to thyroid area twice per day. Use with carrier oil.
    Choose from:
    - Clove, frankincense, lemongrass, myrrh, anti-aging blend
    - OR trade off weekly - first week lemongrass and myrrh; second week geranium and grounding blend; repeat.

ENERGY & VITALITY

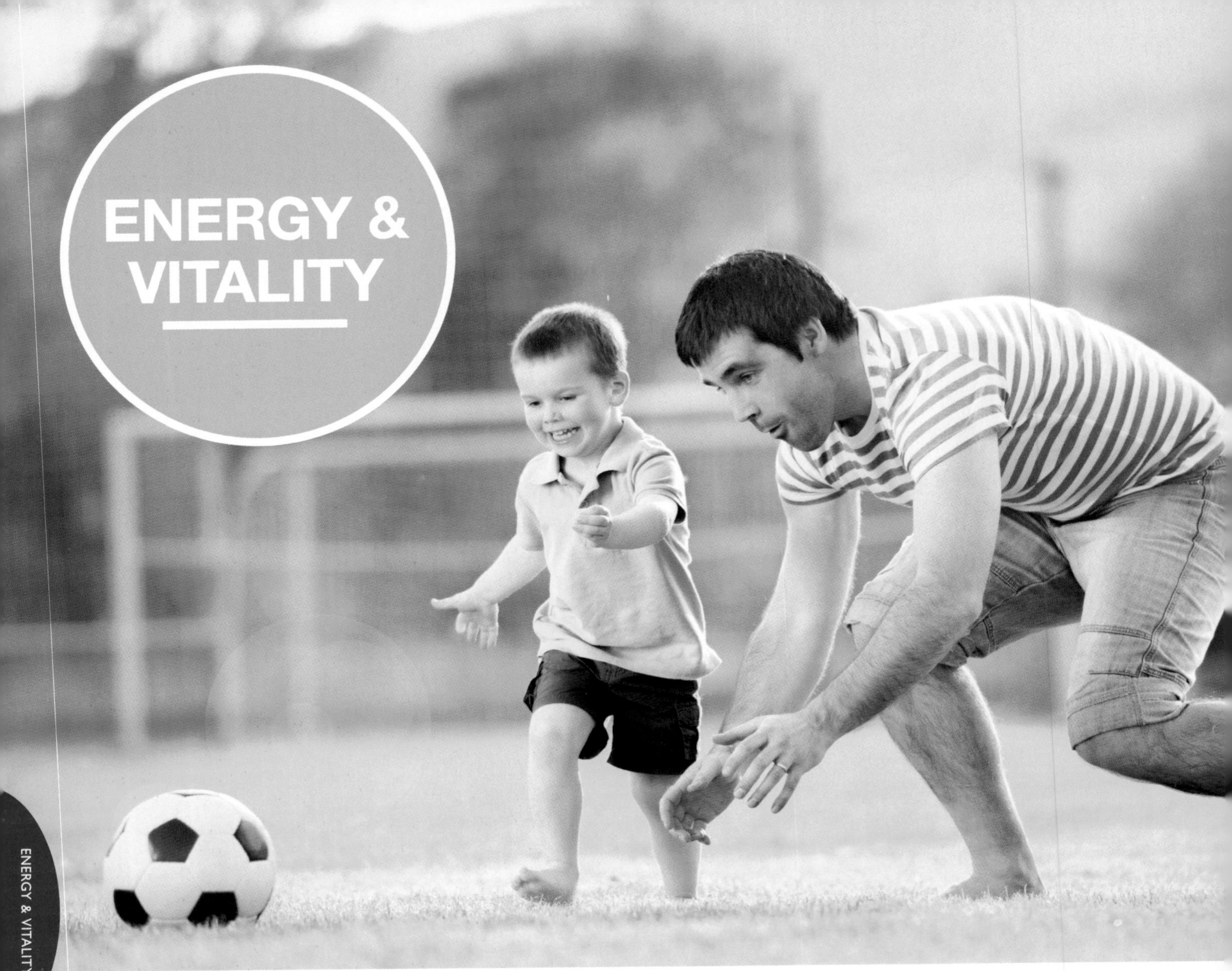

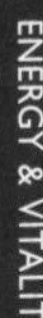

LACK OF ENERGY or diminished vitality can be described as tiredness, weariness, lethargy or fatigue and can contribute to symptoms like depression, decreased motivation, or apathy. Lack of energy can be a normal response to inadequate sleep, overexertion, overworking, stress, lack of exercise, or even boredom. When lack of energy is part of a normal response, it's often resolved with adequate rest and sleep, stress management, and good nutrition.

Persistent lack of energy that does not resolve with routine self-care may be an indication of an underlying physical or psychological disorder. Common causes may include allergies and asthma, anemia, cancer and its treatments, chronic pain, heart disease, infection, depression, eating disorders, grief, sleeping disorders, thyroid problems, medication side effects, alcohol use, or drug use.

Observing patterns and symptoms of lack of energy may be helpful in discovering its cause. Persistent fatigue with no clear diagnosis may result from chronic fatigue syndrome, which can start with a flu-like illness and may not be relieved with rest. Other symptoms, such as cognitive difficulties, long-term exhaustion and illness after activity, muscle or joint pain, sore throat, headache, and tender lymph nodes, are common. Lack of energy by itself is rarely an emergency and can be addressed successfully with effective supplementation and natural solutions. However, if it develops suddenly or is accompanied by other serious symptoms, it may require immediate evaluation to avoid serious complications.

Resolving issues of lack of energy and fatigue can be simple. First considerations include a focus on rest, proper diet, nutrition and supplementation, and balanced blood sugar. Certain essential oils are very effective partners to creating and supporting energy. Basil oil, for example, is superb for overall energy and vitality (if used in higher amounts has the opposite effect - calming). Lemongrass has an overall whole-body stimulating effect. Lavender helps balance body systems where energy might be squandered unnecessarily in one area. Any citrus oil and blend is considered refreshing, uplifting, and rejuvenating. And one of the most popular choices for an immediate, invigorating effect is peppermint oil.

TOP SOLUTIONS

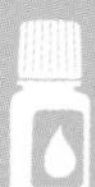

SINGLE OILS

Basil - stimulating and reviving (pg. 76)
Peppermint - invigorating and energizing (pg. 122)
Wild orange - uplifting and rejuvenating (pg. 136)
Lemon - cleansing and refreshing (pg. 110)
Lime - energizing and enlivening (pg. 113)

By Related Properties

For definitions of the properties listed below and more oil options, see Oil Properties Glossary (pg. 435) and Oil Properties (pg. 436).

Antidepressant - basil, bergamot, clary sage, coriander, dill, frankincense, geranium, jasmine, lemongrass, oregano, sandalwood, wild orange, ylang ylang
Energizing - basil, clove, cypress, grapefruit, lemongrass, rosemary, white fir, wild orange
Immunostimulant - cassia, cinnamon, clove, eucalyptus, frankincense, ginger, lemon, lime, melaleuca, melissa, rosemary, spearmint, vetiver, white fir, wild orange
Invigorating - grapefruit, lemon, peppermint, spearmint, wild orange, wintergreen
Refreshing - cypress, geranium, grapefruit, lemon, lime, melaleuca, peppermint, wild orange, wintergreen
Restorative - basil, frankincense, lime, patchouli, rosemary, sandalwood, spearmint
Stimulant - arborvitae, basil, bergamot, birch, black pepper, cardamom, cedarwood, cinnamon, clove, coriander, cypress, dill, eucalyptus, fennel, ginger, grapefruit, juniper berry, lime, melaleuca, myrrh, patchouli, rosemary, spearmint, thyme, vetiver, white fir, wintergreen, ylang ylang

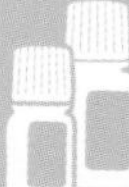

BLENDS

Invigorating blend - rejuvenating and energizing (pg. 153)
Respiration blend - invigorating and reviving (pg. 162)
Encouraging blend - stimulating, renewing, and strenghtening (pg. 148)
Inspiring blend - promotes excitement, passion and joy (pg. 152)
Joyful blend - uplifting and energizing (pg. 154)
Cleansing blend - refreshing and cleansing (pg. 144)

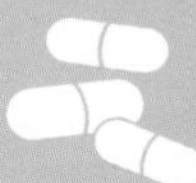

SUPPLEMENTS

Cellular vitality complex (pg. 171), children's chewable, essential oil cellular complex, essential oil omega complex, **energy & stamina complex (pg. 174)**, **whole food nutrient supplement (pg. 183)**

Related Ailments: Chronic Fatigue, Exhaustion, Fatigue, Poor Endurance, Scurvy

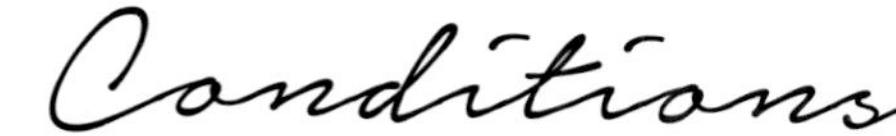

Conditions

Adrenal exhaustion/fatigue - basil, rosemary, invigorating blend; see *Endocrine (Adrenals)*
Alertness, decreased/drowsiness – frankincense, ginger, lemon, lemongrass, lime, peppermint, rosemary, basil, ylang ylang, white fir, focus blend, grounding blend; see *Focus & Concentration*
Debility - cinnamon, douglas fir, ginger, helichrysum, lavender, lemon, lime, cleansing blend, detoxification blend, protective blend
Energy, lack of - basil, black pepper, cardamom, cinnamon, coriander, cypress, eucalyptus, ginger, grapefruit, jasmine, juniper berry, lemon, lime, melissa, patchouli, peppermint, rosemary, thyme, sandalwood, white fir, wild orange, cleansing blend, encouraging blend, invigorating blend, protective blend, renewing blend, respiration blend
Exhaustion/fatigue - arborvitae, basil, cinnamon, douglas fir, eucalyptus, jasmine, lemon, lime, peppermint, rosemary, sandalwood, wild orange, wintergreen, ylang ylang, cellular complex blend, cleansing blend, detoxification blend, encouraging blend, invigorating blend, metabolic blend, respiration blend
Hyperactivity/restlessness/wound up - cedarwood, coriander, frankincense, lavender, patchouli, roman chamomile, vetiver, calming blend, grounding blend, focus blend; see *Focus & Concentration*
Jet lag - geranium, grapefruit, patchouli, peppermint, cellular complex blend, encouraging blend; see *Sleep*
Lethargy/lack of motivation - douglas fir, grapefruit, helichrysum, jasmine, lemon, lime, lemongrass, spearmint, cleansing blend, encouraging blend, invigorating blend, respiration blend
Nervous exhaustion - arborvitae, basil, cedarwood, cinnamon, coriander, ginger, grapefruit, helichrysum, lemongrass, patchouli, rosemary, encouraging blend, respiration blend, tension blend
Oxygen, lack of - frankincense, peppermint, respiration blend; see *Respiratory*
Weakness, physical after illness - basil, douglas fir, frankincense, thyme, cleansing blend, detoxification blend, protective blend

USAGE TIPS: For best success in support optimal energy and vitality
- **Internal:** Consume energy-producing oils, products (e.g. energy & vitality complex); for oils, place a few drops of selected oils (e.g. citrus oils) in a capsule for systemic or on-going support. Also, drinking oils in water or dropping under the tongue is effective.
- **Topical** & **Aromatic:** Rubbing selected and energy-producing oils on tired/sore shoulders, neck, back, legs and feet is invigorating, improves circulation, blood flow and oxygen levels in the body both by aroma and topical sensation.

Remedies

BRING THE ZING
Use grapefruit oil alone or in combination with frankincense oil, geranium oil, and/or bergamot oil. Diffuse, inhale, apply to bottoms of feet, back of neck. Dilute as desired.

DAILY ROUTINE FOR SUPPORTING HEALTHY ENERGY LEVELS

- Rub 1-2 drops of grounding blend on bottoms of feet morning and night.
- Consume 3-5 drops of frankincense under tongue morning and night.
- Use a daily supplement routine to create long-term results with the following: cellular vitality complex, essential oil omega complex, energy & stamina complex, whole food nutrient supplement, defensive probiotic, essential oil cellular complex.
- Add a favorite citrus oil to drinking water; consume throughout day.
- Use any of the blends below to create and support increase in energy and vitality.
- Rub 2-3 drops of essential oil cellular complex blend, followed by lavender oil, on bottoms of feet at night prior to sleep.

ENERGY BOOST
6 drops metabolic blend
3 drops peppermint
3 drops wild orange
Take oils in capsule as needed or desired.

INVIGORATING BLAST
1 drops frankincense
1 drops peppermint
2 drops wild orange
Inhale from cupped hands, massage on the back of neck.

MID AFTERNOON SLUMP BUSTER
15 drops peppermint
20 drops wild orange oil
Combine in 15ml roller bottle; fill remainder with carrier oil; apply to the back of neck, rub up into base of the skull, swipe across forehead near hairline, inhale.

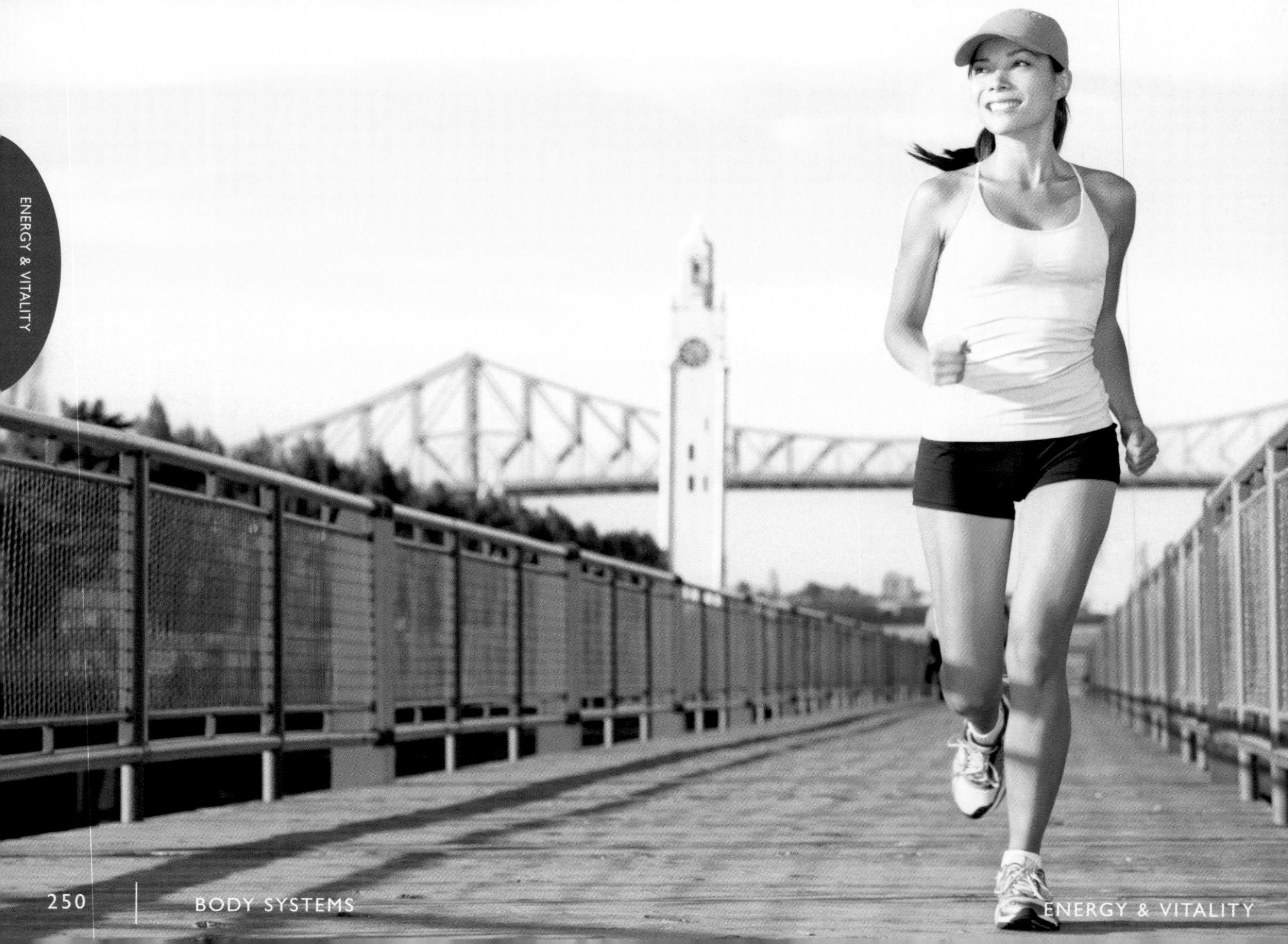

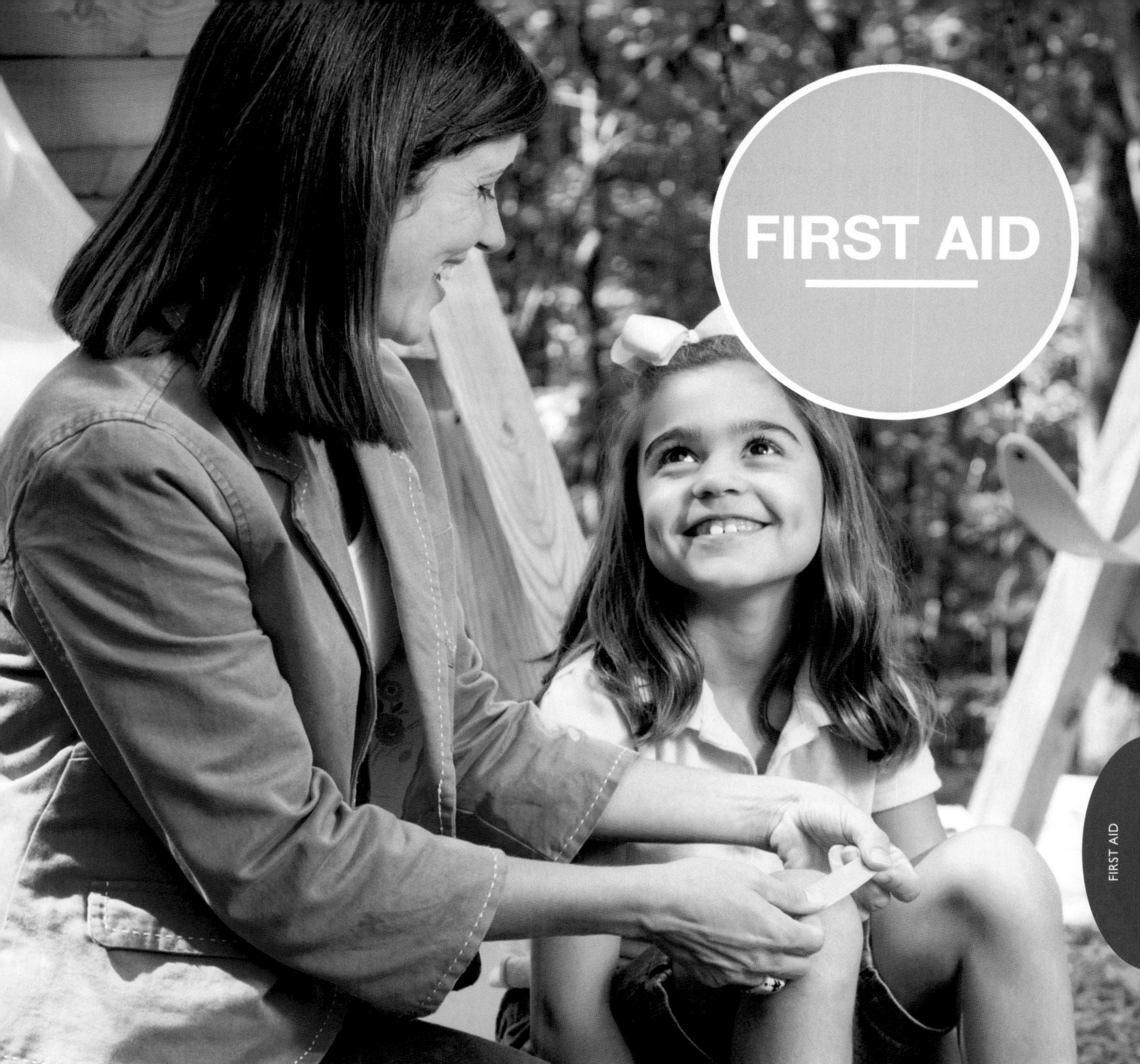

FIRST AID RESPONSE is required whenever there is an injury, illness, or an emergency situation that must be immediately addressed. Situations requiring first aid can include insect bites and stings, snake bites, scratches and cuts, bleeding and hemorrhaging, burns, bruises, shock, sudden vertigo, heart issues, breathing issues, fever, food poisoning, sprained muscles, broken and dislocated bones, heat exhaustion and sunstroke, hypothermia, and more.

In these situations it is important to have basic equipment readily available, such as antibiotic ointments, adhesive bandages, splints, etc., and to know how to respond in the event emergency personnel are required.

Essential oils and natural remedies make a great addition to complete any first aid kit. Particular oils have powerful antibiotic properties, help lower or raise body temperature, assist the respiratory system, help to settle nausea and other digestive problems, address burns, help to slow or stop bleeding, and more. Best of all, if the lids are secure and the first aid kit is kept in temperatures under 120 degrees F, the oils typically last much longer than over-the-counter medications.

When assembling a first aid kit, it is important to consider lifestyle and risk factors for specific activities (ie hiking, camping, boating, traveling, etc.), and to use common sense to anticipate future needs. See below for lists of ideas for both single and blend essential oil and supplemental suggestions.

TOP SOLUTIONS

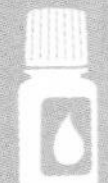

SINGLE OILS

Clove - powerful analgesic for numbing wounds (pg. 90)
Frankincense - universal healing properties, wound antiseptic/analgesic/healing, anti-scarring (pg. 100)
Helichrysum - stop bleeding; wound repair/healing, powerful pain reliever (pg. 105)
Lavender - antihistamine activity; wound, burn care, shock treatment; bite/sting recovery (pg. 108)
Lemon - sanitize, neutralize acid; universal for immune, skin, respiratory needs (pg. 110)
Lemongrass - connective tissue repair, sore muscle/cramp relief (pg. 112)
Marjoram - muscle repair, digestive/eliminative support, sore muscle/cramp relief (pg. 114)
Melaleuca - gentle/powerful wound antiseptic, antimicrobial activity (pg. 116)
Oregano - anti-inflammatory, powerful antibacterial/antiviral (pg. 120)
Peppermint - cooling, burn care, pain reliever; relieve nausea, vomiting (pg. 122)

By Related Properties

For definitions of the properties listed below and more oil options, see Oil Properties Glossary (pg. 435) and Oil Properties (pg. 436).

Analgesic - arborvitae, basil, bergamot, birch, black pepper, cassia, cinnamon, clary sage, clove, cypress, eucalyptus, fennel, frankincense, ginger, helichrysum, juniper berry, lavender, lemongrass, marjoram melaleuca, oregano, peppermint, ravensara, rosemary, white fir, wild orange, wintergreen
Anti-allergenic - geranium, helichrysum
Anticonvulsant - clary sage, fennel, geranium, lavender, tangerine
Antihemorrhagic - geranium, helichrysum, myrrh
Anti-infectious - arborvitae, basil, cardamom, cedarwood, cinnamon, clove, cypress, eucalyptus, frankincense, geranium, lavender, marjoram, melaleuca, myrrh, patchouli, roman chamomile, rosemary
Anti-inflammatory - bergamot, black pepper, cassia, cinnamon, clove, cypress, eucalyptus, fennel, frankincense, ginger, jasmine, lemongrass, melaleuca, myrrh, patchouli, peppermint, rosemary, sandalwood, spikenard, wintergreen
Antiseptic - arborvitae, bergamot, black pepper, cedarwood, cinnamon, clove, frankincense, ginger, grapefruit, helichrysum, juniper berry, lemon, marjoram, melaleuca, myrrh, oregano, rosemary, tangerine, thyme, vetiver, wild orange, ylang ylang
Antispasmodic - basil, cardamom, cassia, cinnamon, clove, eucalyptus, fennel, helichrysum, lavender, lemon, marjoram, peppermint, rosemary, sandalwood, spearmint, thyme, vetiver, wintergreen, yarrow, ylang ylang
Calming - bergamot, black pepper, clary sage, coriander, frankincense, geranium, juniper berry, lavender, patchouli, roman chamomile, tangerine, vetiver
Hypotensive - clary sage, dill, lavender, lemon, yarrow, ylang ylang
Insect repellent - arborvitae, birch, cedarwood, cinnamon, eucalyptus, geranium, lemongrass, patchouli, thyme, vetiver, ylang ylang
Vasoconstrictor - helichrysum, peppermint,
Warming - birch, black pepper, cassia, cinnamon, clary sage, clove, eucalyptus, ginger, lemongrass, marjoram, oregano, peppermint, thyme, wintergreen

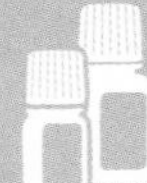

BLENDS

Calming blend - for shock, trauma recovery (pg. 142)
Cellular complex blend - antitrauma, cellular, cognitive support (pg. 143)
Cleansing blend - antiseptic properties; sanitize, bug bite/sting recovery (pg. 144)
Detoxification blend - anti-allergenic, blood, cleansing, anti-infectious support (pg. 146)
Digestion blend - excellent to resolve nausea, vomiting (pg. 147)
Massage blend - for injured tissue recovery; sore muscle/cramp relief (pg. 155)
Protective blend - immune protection, analgesic (pg. 158)
Repellent blend - bug repellent (pg. 161)
Skin clearing blend - antiseptic, wound care (pg. 163)
Soothing blend - bone/pain relief support; sore muscle/cramp relief (pg. 164)

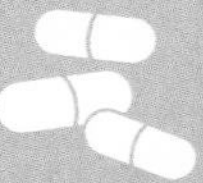

SUPPLEMENTS

Bone support complex, **energy & stamina (pg. 174), polyphenol complex (pg. 181)**

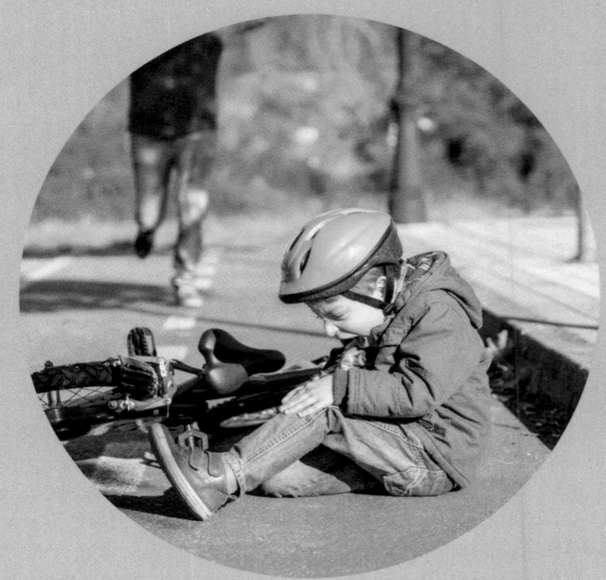

Related Ailments: Bee Sting, Chiggers, Fainting, Heat Exhaustion, Heat Illness/Dehydration, Heat Stroke, Hypothermia, Injury, Insect Bite, Insect Repellent, Mosquito Bites, Shock, Snake Bites, Tick Bites, Wasp Sting

FIRST AID

Conditions

Allergies to insect bite or sting - basil, cilantro, cinnamon, lavender, lemon, melaleuca, melissa, peppermint, thyme, cleansing blend, detoxification blend, protective blend, repellent blend, respiration blend; see *Allergies*

Bites, insect - arborvitae, basil, cinnamon, coriander, eucalyptus, frankincense, lavender, lemon, lemongrass, melaleuca, patchouli, roman chamomile, thyme, ylang ylang, cleansing blend, inspiring blend, reassuring blend

Bleeding/hemorrhaging - cypress, frankincense, geranium, helichrysum, lavender, lime, myrrh, rose, wild orange, comforting blend; see *Cardiovascular*

Blood vessels, broken - cypress, frankincense, geranium, helichrysum, lemon, lime, cleansing blend, detoxification blend; see *Cardiovascular*

Breathing, shortness of breath - eucalyptus, frankincense, peppermint, encouraging blend, respiration blend; see *Allergies*, "Allergies to insect bite or sting" above, *Respiratory*

Bruising - arborvitae, cypress, clove, fennel, geranium, grapefruit, helichrysum, lavender, oregano, roman chamomile, white fir, ylang ylang, cellular complex blend, cleansing blend, detoxification blend, inspiring blend, invigorating blend, reassuring blend, soothing blend or rub

Burns - clove, eucalyptus, frankincense, geranium, helichrysum, lavender, myrrh, peppermint, anti-aging blend, inspiring blend

Cellulitis - lime, oregano (internally), protective blend; see *Immune & Lymphatic, Integumentary*

Chills (shock) - basil, ginger, grapefruit, lemon, melaleuca, melissa, myrrh, peppermint, roman chamomile, rosemary, wild orange, wild orange, ylang ylang, grounding blend, encouraging blend, invigorating blend, metabolic blend, protective blend

Cuts/wounds, cleaning - cassia, cedarwood, cypress, frankincense, juniper berry, lavender, lemon, lemongrass, melaleuca (superb disinfectant), myrrh, skin clearing blend, protective blend, reassuring blend

Cuts/wounds, healing - basil, black pepper, cypress, douglas fir, eucalyptus, frankincense, geranium, helichrysum (clean wound before applying, as it seals up the wound rapidly), lavender, lime, melaleuca (superb disinfectant), peppermint, sandalwood, vetiver, anti-aging blend, invigorating blend, reassuring blend, skin clearing blend

Cuts/wounds, pain (numbing) - black pepper, cassia, clove, eucalyptus, frankincense, helichrysum, melaleuca, protective blend

Dizziness/lightheaded - geranium, ginger, peppermint, cellular complex blend, detoxification blend, grounding blend, tension blend, soothing blend, women's blend

Drop in blood pressure (allergic reaction) - cypress, helichrysum, lavender, peppermint, rosemary, thyme, white fir, ylang ylang; see *Allergies*, "Allergies to insect bite or sting" above

Fainting - basil, peppermint, rosemary, encouraging blend, grounding blend, invigorating blend

Food poisoning - black pepper, cinnamon, clove, ginger, juniper berry, lemon, melaleuca, oregano, thyme, cleansing blend, detoxification blend, digestion blend, protective blend

Heat exhaustion - basil, bergamot, black pepper, eucalyptus, lemon, lime, peppermint, soothing blend, tension blend

Hypothermia - birch, cassia, cinnamon, clove, cypress, eucalyptus, ginger, lemongrass, marjoram, oregano, patchouli, peppermint, thyme, wild orange, wintergreen, cellular complex blend, massage blend, protective blend

Insect repellent - arborvitae, basil, bergamot, cedarwood, cypress, douglas fir, eucalyptus, geranium (mosquito), lavender (flies, gnat, midge, mosquito), lemongrass, lime, patchouli, rosemary, cleansing blend, inspiring blend, renewing blend, repellent blend

Infections - juniper berry, melaleuca, oregano, cleansing blend, protective blend; see *Immune & Lymphatic*

Itching, excessive - cilantro, lavender, lemon, melaleuca, melissa, patchouli, vetiver, wild orange, anti-aging blend, detoxification blend, metabolic blend; see *Integumentary*

Lice - geranium, melaleuca, rosemary, thyme, repellent blend; see *Parasites*

Mites (i.e. chiggers, scabies) - See *Parasites*

Mosquito bites - arborvitae, juniper berry, lavender, melaleuca, roman chamomile, cleansing blend; see "Bites, insect" above

Motion sickness - bergamot, ginger, peppermint, digestion blend, uplifting blend; see *Digestive & Intestinal*

Nausea/vomiting - basil, bergamot, cardamom, cassia, clove, coriander, fennel, ginger, lavender, melissa, digestion blend; see *Digestive & Intestinal*

Nosebleeds - cypress, helichrysum, geranium, lavender, lemon, lime; see *Cardiovascular*

Poison - black pepper, juniper berry, lemongrass, inspiring blend

Poison ivy - lavender, lemon, melaleuca, anti-aging blend

Poison oak - clove, lavender, rose, vetiver, anti-aging blend, inspiring blend

Shivering/low body temp - see "Hypothermia" above

Shock - bergamot, coriander, douglas fir, frankincense, geranium, helichrysum, lavender, marjoram, melaleuca, melissa, peppermint, roman chamomile, melissa, tangerine, vetiver, wild orange, ylang ylang, calming blend, cellular complex blend, comforting blend, encouraging blend, focus blend, reassuring blend, tension blend

Snake bite - basil, clove, coriander, helichrysum, frankincense, geranium, melaleuca, patchouli, sandalwood, cleansing blend

Spider bite - basil, juniper berry, lavender, melaleuca, roman chamomile, thyme, cleansing blend, protection blend

Stinging nettle - clove, lemon (neutralizes acid), cleansing blend, invigorating blend

Stings - basil, cinnamon, clove, lavender, lemon, lime, melaleuca, roman chamomile, thyme, cleansing blend

Sunburn - eucalyptus, frankincense, helichrysum, lavender, peppermint, sandalwood, anti-aging blend

Sunstroke/heatstroke - dill, douglas fir, eucalyptus, lavender, lemon, peppermint, rosemary, detoxification blend, tension blend

Tick bites - lavender, melaleuca (addresses concern of tick regurgitating harmful bacteria into bite site before removing insect); see *Parasites*

Trauma - cypress, frankincense, geranium, juniper berry, myrrh, anti-aging blend, calming blend, cellular complex blend, cleansing blend, encouraging blend, grounding blend, repellent blend; see "Shock" above

Remedies

SPIDER BITE RECOVERY: Combine basil, cleansing blend, rosemary, and lemon to take "sting" away and reduce inflammation. When helichrysum is added at end of treatment, the bite location is encouraged to heal faster and leave little to no scar.

OWIE SPRAY
5 drops lemon
10 drops melaleuca
10 drops lavender
5 drops helichrysum
Add to 4-ounce glass spray bottle and fill with purified water.

NATURAL FIRST AID SPRAY
5 drops lavender
3 drops melaleuca
2 drops cypress
Place oils in a spray bottle with 1/ 2 teaspoon salt and 8 ounces of distilled water. Spray on before applying bandages. Repeat several times a day for three days.

HEAT EXHAUSTION RECOVERY:
Place 2-4 drops of lemon oil in drinking water and sip to rehydrate.
Place 1 drop of peppermint oil in drinking water and sip to cool down.
Combine the two as desired.

USAGE TIPS: For first aid success

- **Topical:**
  - Apply oils directly to area(s) of concern such as on cuts, bruises, bites, stings, injury sites and burns whenever possible. Otherwise, get as close as possible to site or use bottoms of feet as alternative location.
  - For acute situations, apply frequently, even every couple minutes as needed for pain relief, to stop bleeding, etc. Clean site (e.g. with melaleuca) prior to stopping bleeding and sealing up a cut site with helichrysum.
  - To cool or raise body temperature, place cooling or warming oils on back of neck, down spine, bottoms of feet, or spray on an oil/water (cooling only) mixture (shake first). For sunburn, apply to site.
- **Aromatic:** Use for emotional support for times like shock or trauma by offering immediate inhalation from a bottle or drops placed on hands. Create continue inhalation with a diffuser or by topical application that allows for ongoing exposure.
- **Internal:** for any allergic response, place a drop of anti-histamine oil (e.g. lavender) under tongue for older children/adults or bottoms of feet for any age (dilute for infants/toddlers); inhale as well. For nausea/vomiting place oil(s) on abdomen, lick off back of hand, drop in mouth, and/or bottoms of feet.

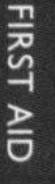

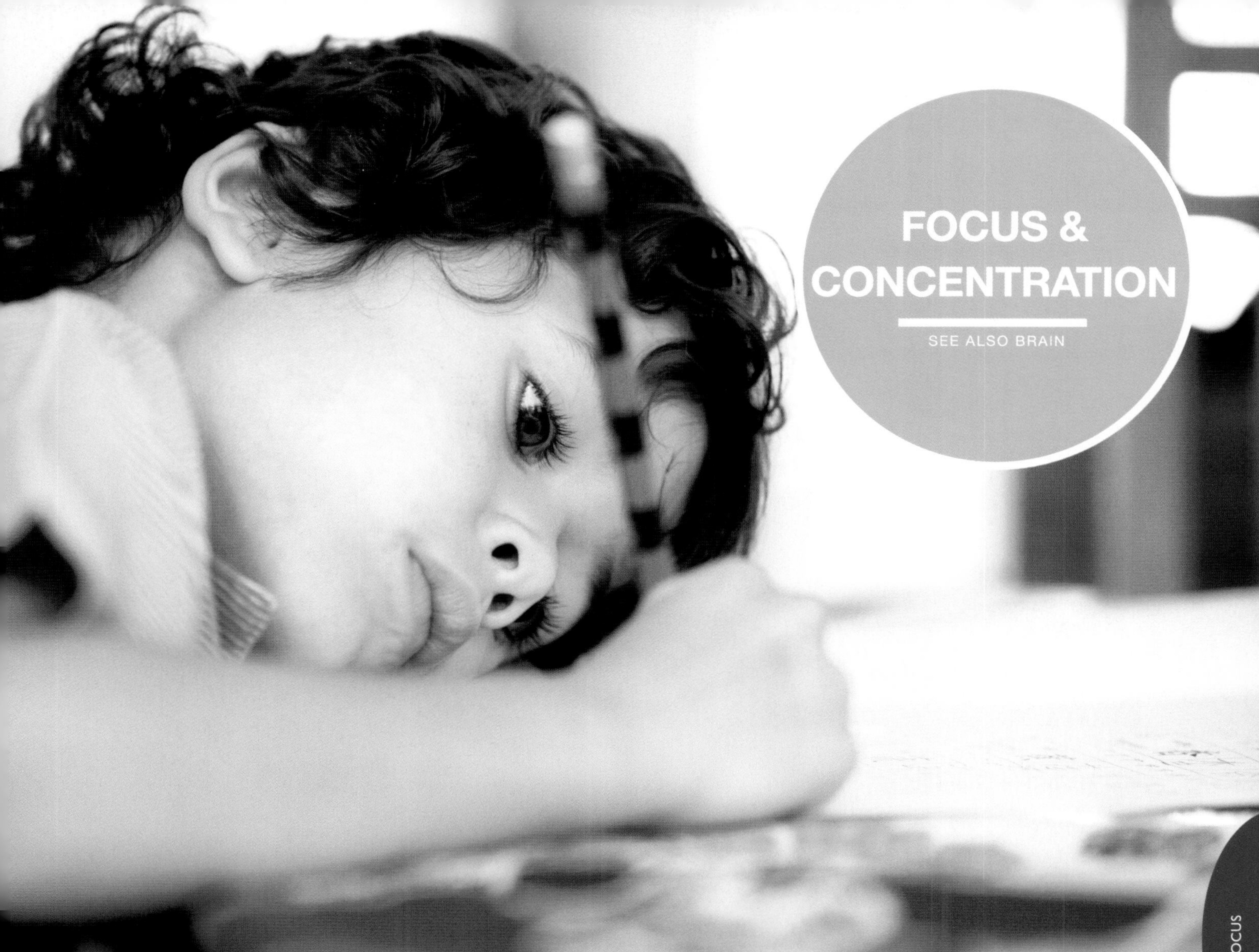

FOCUS & CONCENTRATION

SEE ALSO BRAIN

THE ABILITY TO FOCUS requires adequate neural connections in the brain to process incoming sensory data (sights, sounds, smells, etc.). When the brain is unable to assimilate this data, the stimuli becomes overwhelming or "noisy," and symptoms such as frustration, irritation, and even fatigue can occur. An increasing number of Individuals of any age are experiencing a decreasing ability to focus and concentrate. It is important to consider factors that contribute to the decline of optimal focus and concentration in order to reverse or prevent this trend.

Given the innate complexity of the human brain, it is not surprising that issues of focus and concentration and contributing factors are vast. Tiredness or lack of sleep, stress, hormonal changes (such as during pregnancy or puberty), medication side effects, alcohol, drugs, chronic illness, infection, brain injury, anxiety, depression, bipolar disorder, and emotional trauma are just a few that impact neural connections necessary to make sense of the vast sensory stimuli the brain receives moment to moment. For example, individuals with ADHD consistently struggle to "think over the noise" in their brains as stimuli come in without the necessary processing ability to make sense of it all.

The very nature of the brain's structure allows for improvements in function and ability. To summarize this complex process in a simple way, the more neurons available to make connections with other neurons, the easier and more efficient focus and learning will be. While traditional medicine and neurological specialists contribute great expertise to the science of improving brain activity, there are a myriad of natural remedies that can greatly impact and benefit brain activity, specifically in the area of focus and concentration.

When an individual inhales an essential oil (or other aroma) the olfactory bulb is activated and directly links to brain processes that stimulate and encourage neural connections. The simple act of diffusing an essential oil like lavender in the classroom, or inhaling peppermint from a bottle, can have immediate and effective impact on the learner. Simple yet powerful suggestions through both single oils or blends and remedies have demonstrated that essential oils and nutritional support are powerful tools for improving focus, concentration, and much more!

TOP SOLUTIONS

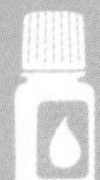

SINGLE OILS

Roman chamomile - reduces anxiety, promotes confidence (pg. 125)
Vetiver - promotes focus, concentration, mental performance (pg. 134)
Lavender - supports mental adaptability, performance (pg. 108)
Clary sage - supports a calm, clear, focused mind (pg. 88)
Cedarwood - calms mind, supports improved mental performance (pg. 84)

By Related Properties

For definitions of the properties listed below and more oil options, see Oil Properties Glossary (pg. 435) and Oil Properties (pg. 436).

Antidepressant - bergamot, frankincense, lemon, melissa, ravensara, roman chamomile, tangerine, wild orange
Antifungal - arborvitae, bergamot, cedarwood, cinnamon, clary sage, coriander, melaleuca, myrrh, oregano, sandalwood, tangerine, thyme; see *Immune & Lymphatic*, see *Candida*
Antioxidant - bergamot, clove, helichrysum, grapefruit, juniper berry, lemon, lemongrass, melaleuca, rosemary, patchouli, tangerine, thyme
Calming - cedarwood, clary sage, coriander, fennel, jasmine, lavender, patchouli, roman chamomile, sandalwood, vetiver
Energizing - basil, bergamot, cinnamon, cypress, ginger, rosemary, wild orange
Grounding - cedarwood, frankincense, vetiver, ylang ylang
Invigorating - lemon, lime, lemongrass, peppermint, wild orange
Neuroprotective - frankincense, myrrh, roman chamomile, sandalwood
Refreshing - any citrus oil, melaleuca,
Relaxing - cypress, geranium, roman chamomile
Sedative - bergamot, cedarwood, clary sage, frankincense, lavender, melissa, patchouli, roman chamomile, vetiver
Stimulant - arborvitae, basil, bergamot, black pepper, cardamom, cedarwood, cinnamon, coriander, cypress, dill, eucalyptus, ginger, grapefruit, juniper berry, lime, melaleuca, rosemary, spearmint, vetiver, wintergreen
Uplifting - bergamot, grapefruit, lime, melissa, wild orange

Related Ailments: ADD or ADHD [Brain], Concentration, Confusion, Focus, Hyperactivity [Mood & Behavior], Mental strength/clarity, Poor Concentration

BLENDS

Calming blend - relaxes the mind (pg. 142)
Focus blend - calms and stimulates the mind (pg. 149)
Encouraging blend - promotes motivation, mental stimulation and movement (pg. 148)
Grounding blend - promotes a grounded state of mind (pg. 150)

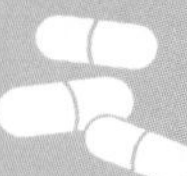

SUPPLEMENTS

Bone nutrient complex, cellular vitality complex, defensive probiotic, detoxification blend softgels, detoxification complex capsules, energy & stamina complex, essential oil cellular complex, **essential oil omega complex (pg. 175)**, food enzymes, whole food nutrient supplement, **liquid omega-3 supplement (pg. 178)**

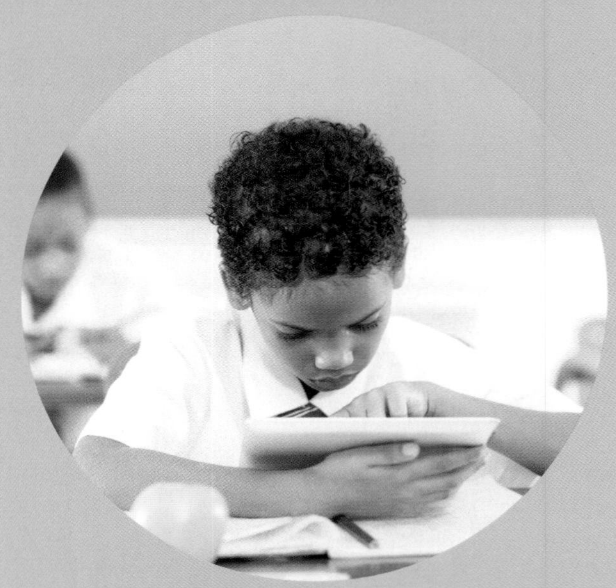

USAGE TIPS: For best methods of use for focus and concentration consider:

- **Aromatic:** Choose to diffuse 5-10 drops of oils of choice, inhale from product bottle or self-made blend, apply a few drops to clothing, bedding, or any other method that supports inhalation for oils to enter brain via nose and olfactory system.
- **Topical:** Apply on forehead, under nose, back of neck (especially in suboccipital triangles), roof of mouth (place oil on pad of thumb, place on roof, "suck").

Conditions

EMOTIONAL STATES:

(See *Mood & Behavior* for additional emotional support)

Afraid/unadventurous - black pepper, patchouli, ravensara

Agitated - arborvitae, bergamot, patchouli, calming blend, focus blend, grounding blend, soothing blend

Angry - bergamot, cardamom, cedarwood, frankincense, geranium, helichrysum, roman chamomile, calming blend, grounding blend, focus blend

Antisocial - bergamot, black pepper, cedarwood, oregano, patchouli

Anxious - basil, cedarwood, frankincense, juniper berry, patchouli, vetiver, calming blend, focus blend, grounding blend

Apathetic/lacking of motivation - birch, black pepper, cardamom, frankincense, jasmine, juniper berry, melissa, patchouli, rose, vetiver, wild orange, ylang ylang, encouraging blend, focus blend, grounding blend, joyful blend, respiration blend

Defensive - ginger, lemon, melaleuca, patchouli, wintergreen, protective blend, repellent blend, soothing blend, tension blend, women's monthly blend

Depressed - bergamot, jasmine, patchouli, roman chamomile, vetiver, wild orange, ylang ylang, inspiring blend, invigorating blend, joyful blend

Easily bugged/bothered - lemongrass, rose, white fir, ylang ylang, repellent blend

Fearful - frankincense, juniper berry, ravensara, wild orange, ylang ylang, calming blend, detoxification blend, grounding blend, protective blend, respiration blend

Frustrated - cardamom, ylang ylang, calming blend, focus blend

Hypersensitive - lavender, melissa, roman chamomile, rosemary, vetiver

Obsessed/preoccupied - cedarwood, frankincense, jasmine, oregano, sandalwood, vetiver, calming blend, focus blend

Performance stress/stage fright - bergamot, patchouli, ravensara, rose, wild orange, ylang ylang, respiration blend

Shy/timid/unsure - bergamot, cassia, clove, ginger, jasmine, juniper berry, melissa, patchouli, ravensara, spearmint, yarrow, ylang ylang, encouraging blend, focus blend, inspiring blend, respiration blend

Stubborn/willful - birch, ginger, lemongrass, melaleuca, oregano, wintergreen

Unsafe/vulnerable, feeling - bergamot, cardamom, cilantro, cinnamon, ginger, jasmine, oregano, ravensara, roman chamomile, ylang ylang, calming blend, massage blend, protective blend, repellent blend, respiration blend, women's blend

MENTAL STATES:

Attention deficit - lavender, vetiver, focus blend

Autistic - basil, bergamot, clary sage, frankincense, geranium, lemon, peppermint, rosemary, vetiver, anti-aging blend, calming blend, cellular complex, focus blend, grounding blend, soothing blend

Brain fogged - arborvitae, bergamot, douglas fir, eucalyptus, frankincense, juniper berry, lavender, lemon, lime, peppermint, roman chamomile, encouraging blend, focus blend

Brain oxygen, lack of - cedarwood, cypress, eucalyptus, frankincense, ginger, lemon, melaleuca, patchouli, peppermint, sandalwood, vetiver, inspiring blend, protective blend; see "Antioxidant" property

Chemicaly stressed/imbalanced - See *Brain*

Concentration/focus, lack of - cedarwood, douglas fir, eucalyptus, frankincense, lavender, lemon, lime, marjoram, patchouli, peppermint, sandalwood, vetiver, encouraging blend, focus blend

Confusion/disorganized - frankincense, sandalwood, vetiver, white fir, wintergreen, encouraging blend, grounding blend, joyful blend

Coping skills, lack of - bergamot, clove, eucalyptus, ginger, juniper berry, lavender, oregano, rosemary, wintergreen, calming blend, focus blend, grounding blend, invigorating blend, joyful blend, soothing blend, tension blend

Daydreamer - cedarwood, frankincense, peppermint, ravensara, rosemary, vetiver, ylang ylang, encouraging blend, massage blend, respiration blend

Dendrite and neuron support - vetiver

Distracted/bored easily - frankincense, peppermint, roman chamomile, vetiver, wild orange, encouraging blend

Environmental tension - lemon, wintergreen, yarrow

Equilibrium/balance, lack of - arborvitae, frankincense, lavender, spearmint, rosemary, ylang ylang, detoxification blend, focus blend, grounding blend, invigorating blend

Fatigued - basil, cassia, cinnamon, coriander, ginger, lemon, thyme, cellular complex blend, detoxification blend, encouraging blend, metabolic blend; see *Energy & Vitality*

Fixated - black pepper, lemongrass, tangerine, ylang ylang

Hyperactive/restlessness/wound up - coriander, frankincense, lavender, lemon, ravensara, roman chamomile, vetiver, calming blend, grounding blend, respiration blend

Impulsive/acting without thinking - white fir, grounding blend

Learning difficulties - cedarwood, patchouli, peppermint, vetiver, ylang ylang, focus blend, grounding blend

Left brain, lack of activity - lemon

Mentally fatigued - basil, bergamot, cardamom, douglas fir, frankincense, lavender, lemon, lemongrass, peppermint, ravensara, rose, rosemary, sandalwood, spearmint, white fir, ylang ylang, comforting blend, encouraging blend, inspiring blend, invigorating blend, respiration blend, reassuring blend

Mentally sluggishness - basil, eucalyptus, peppermint, rosemary, white fir, encouraging blend

Mentally strained/stressed - bergamot, cedarwood, grapefruit, lavender, roman chamomile, spearmint, white fir, anti-aging blend

Memory, lack of/unreliable/poor sense of time - bergamot, douglas fir, lemon, lemongrass, lime, juniper berry, melissa, peppermint, focus blend, inspiring blend, joyful blend

Memory, poor - frankincense, ginger, peppermint, rosemary, sandalwood, inspiring blend, focus blend

Memory, loss of short term - basil, cedarwood, peppermint, rosemary, ylang ylang, calming, grounding blend

Neurotransmitter production capacity, compromised - fennel, ginger

Oxygen deprived (brain) - cedarwood, cypress, eucalyptus, frankincense, ginger, lemon, melaleuca, patchouli, peppermint, sandalwood, vetiver, protective blend; see "Antioxidant" above

Restless/figidity/squirming - lavender and vetiver, ravensara, calming blend, grounding blend, invigorating blend, respiration blend

Right brain, lack of activity - douglas fir, roman chamomile, wild orange

Sensory systems, closed/blocked - birch, wintergreen, encouraging blend

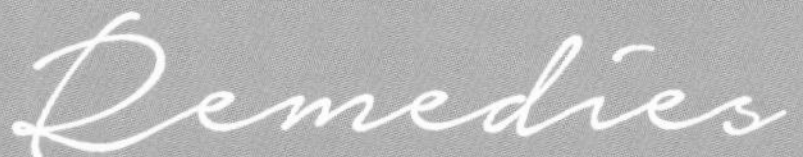

CONCENTRATION: Apply vetiver on feet or base of neck; for school children that need help during the school day, place a drop of oil on collarbone area so body heat will "diffuse" during day; apply oil to top of hand or on a necklace with a pendant made to diffuse oils for easy access to smell all day. If aroma is offensive, add an oil such as wild orange over top of vetiver to "deodorize" as desired.

FOCUS SUPPORT: Blend 2-4 drops frankincense or grapefruit with a few drops of carrier oil and massage temples.

FOCUS, MEMORY, RECALL
- Option #1: Combine frankincense with wild orange or peppermint; inhale or sniff.
- Options #2: In a 1/3 ounce roller bottle combine 20 drops each of wild orange, peppermint; fill the rest of the bottle with fractionated coconut oil and apply
- Option #3: Combine 1-2 drops each cedarwood, lavender, and vetiver and apply. Recipe can also be used in a 10ml roller bottle with a carrier oil. Place 7-13 drops of each oil depending on user's preference of aromas.

FRUSTRATION/ANGER: Use oils and blends that calm - helichrysum, lavender, ylang ylang, grounding blend, calming blend; apply to feet, back of neck, behind ears, behind knees; diffuse.

HEALTHY TOUCH: Allow individual to choose their favorite oils (up to three) by smelling for preference or make a personal blend; massage feet prior to bedtime then cover them with warm, weighted blankets.

HYPERACTIVITY: Apply grounding blend to the feet and calming blend and/or lavender to the base of the neck, or on and behind the ears; healthy touch can be a welcomed calming support for an individual, and the action of applying oils can create a calming effect.

PEACE AND CALM: Combine 10 drops of lavender, 20 drops of vetiver, and 10 drops of calming blend in a 10 ml roller bottle; top off with fractionated coconut oil; apply to feet, back of neck or head; diffuse or inhale; use at least two times per day.

"CHILL PILL"
10 drops clary sage
15 drops bergamot
20 drops grapefruit
25 drops wild orange
15 drops frankincense
10 drops lemon
Diffuse or apply topically at the base of the skull, back of the neck, along the spine, behind the ears, over the heart, and on the wrist.

MOTIVATION POWER
3 drops basil
3 drops grapefruit
2 drops bergamot
2 drops sandalwood
1 drop rosemary
1 drop ylang ylang
Combine oils and diffuse.

CALM AND CONFIDENT
8 drops vetiver
4 drops ylang ylang
2 drops frankincense
2 drops roman chamomile
2 drops clary sage
2 drop marjoram
1 drop ginger
Combine oils in a 10 ml roller bottle. Fill remainder of bottle with fractionated coconut oil. Rub behind ears, on occipital triangle area, bottoms of feet, and/or down the spine before bedtime and as needed.

MELLOW OUT
10 drops roman chamomile
10 drops lavender
10 drops wild orange
2 drops marjoram
2 drops frankincense
Combine oils in a 10 ml roller bottle. Fill remainder of bottle with fractionated coconut oil. Rub behind ears, on suboccipital triangle area, bottoms of feet, and/or down the spine before bedtime and as needed.

FIDGET FIXER
3 drops cedarwood
6 drops grounding blend
2 drops frankincense
2 drops lavender
Combine oils in a 10 ml roller bottle. Fill remainder of bottle with fractionated coconut oil. Apply to ears, forehead, back of neck, down spine, bottoms of feet; massage into tissue to enhance absorption. If desired, drops can be multiplied by two or three to increase intensity of blend. Consider age, size, need, and tolerance of the intended user to determine strength desired.

IMPROVED CONCENTRATION
2 drops cedarwood
2 drops lavender
1 drop roman chamomile
1 drop sandalwood
1 drop vetiver
Combine and apply to feet.

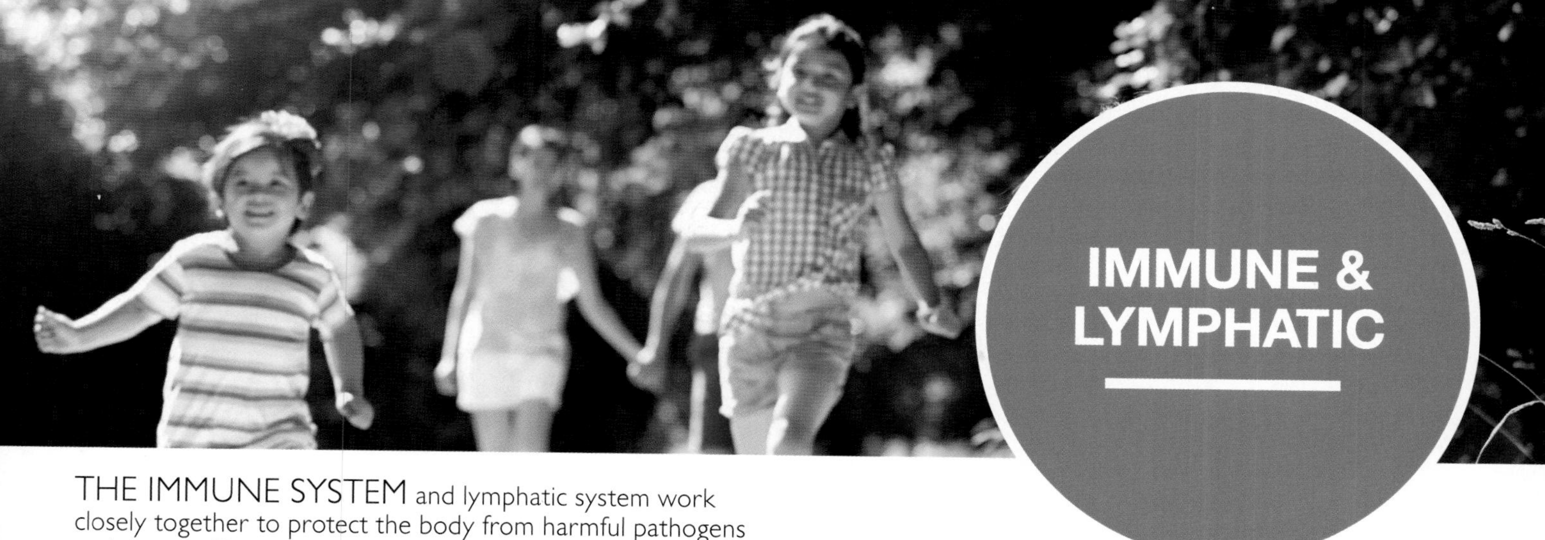

THE IMMUNE SYSTEM and lymphatic system work closely together to protect the body from harmful pathogens and disease. These systems include white blood cells, bone marrow, the spleen, tonsils, adenoids, appendix, thymus, lymph, and lymph nodes. A healthy immune response consists of the body's ability to properly identify a pathogen and engage in a series of responses designed to prevent pathogens from entering targeted cells/tissues.

The immune system consists of:

- The innate immune system–prevents pathogens from entering the body; it also provides a generalized response that destroys any pathogens that bypass the barriers.
- The adaptive immune system–analyzes the pathogen so the body can respond with an army of protective cells created specifically to destroy that particular pathogen. This system also supports the immune system by delivering nutrients to the cells and removing toxins and waste products.

The lymphatic system includes:

- Bone marrow–creates T-cells and creates and grows B-cells to maturation. B-cells travel via the blood system to destroy any lurking pathogens. T-cells, which attack pathogens and any toxic molecules, travel to the thymus, where they mature and later join the B-cells. These T-cells and B-cells are lymphocytes that travel in lymph.
- Lymph–a watery fluid, yellowish in color, that carries white blood cells. It circulates through tissues and picks up unwanted fats, bacteria, and other substances and filters it through the lymphatic system.

The first line of defense is the innate immune system, which includes physical barriers, such as skin, fingernails, mucous membranes, tears, and earwax that help prevent invaders from entering the body, and chemical barriers, such as fatty acids, stomach acid, proteins, and secretions that naturally help destroy pathogens.

When pathogens are undeterred by the innate immune response, the adaptive immune system, which is more complex than the innate, processes the pathogen in a way that allows it to design specific immune cells to combat it effectively. Then it produces huge numbers of those cells to attack the pathogen and any toxic molecules it creates. The cells that carry out this specific immune response are called lymphocytes and are created and delivered by the lymph system.

As part of the adaptive immune system response, humans have sophisticated defense mechanisms that include the ability to adapt over time to recognize specific pathogens more efficiently. This is accomplished by creating immunological memory after the initial response is rendered, leading to an enhanced response to subsequent encounters with that same pathogen.

Certain lifestyle choices can either provide great strength or can seriously weaken immune response. Nutrition is a key factor in a healthy immune system; if cells don't have the energy they need to provide critical safeguards for the body, pathogens can more easily penetrate and multiply. Detoxification is another critical activity that helps promote the body's natural defenses; many times when an individual gets sick it is simply the body's way to naturally eliminate toxins.

Natural essential oils, which have a chemical footprint compatible with the human body, have the unique ability to help the immune system bring itself to balance because they are lipophilic (soluble in fat) and thus are able to penetrate the cell membrane. Viruses are also lipophilic. Most pure essential oils are naturally drawn to the inside of the cell to help the body eradicate threats within the cell.

Interestingly, when essential oils are adulterated because the oil is synthetic (created in a laboratory), the signal molecule approaching the cell is the mirror-image of what it should be and thus is limited in the support it can give the body.

Note that for threats that exist outside the cell, namely, bacterial infections, essential oils can assist in warding off such risks. Oregano essential oil, for example, also has hydrophilic properties that allow it to effectively target threats that exist in the extracellular fluid (outside the cell). Knowledge of these powerful properties can help individuals provide effective reinforcements for the immune system.

Additional consideration for immune support:
When threats to the body from various pathogens are combined with a weakened immune system, illness can occur. Ideally, one would target pathogens within the body while simultaneously strengthening the immune system. The Oil Touch technique discussed in the introduction to this book accomplishes both objectives. The Oil Touch technique is a systematic application of eight different essential oils that serves to strengthen the immune system, eliminate pathogens, reduce stress, and bring the body into homeostasis, enabling the body to function more optimally. See Oil Touch technique, page 14.

TOP SOLUTIONS

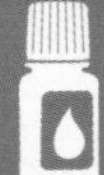

SINGLE OILS

Melaleuca - fights bacteria and viruses (pg. 116)
Cinnamon - fights bacteria and viruses (pg. 86)
Black pepper - supports digestion and boosts immunity (pg. 81)
Thyme - fights bacteria and viruses (pg. 133)

By Related Properties

For definitions of the properties listed below and more oil options, see Oil Properties Glossary (pg. 435) and Oil Properties (pg. 436).

Antibacterial - arborvitae, basil, black pepper, cassia, cedarwood, cilantro, cinnamon, clove, coriander, dill, eucalyptus, frankincense, geranium, ginger, lemongrass, lime, marjoram, melaleuca, melissa, myrrh, oregano, peppermint, ravensara, rosemary, tangerine, thyme, ylang ylang
Antifungal - arborvitae, cassia, cedarwood, cinnamon, coriander, cypress, eucalyptus, fennel, ginger, lemon, lemongrass, melaleuca, myrrh, oregano, rosemary, tangerine, wild orange
Anti-infectious - bergamot, cardamom, cinnamon, cypress, eucalyptus, frankincense, geranium, melaleuca, myrrh, roman chamomile, rose, rosemary
Anti-inflammatory - arborvitae, bergamot, black pepper, cardamom, cinnamon, clary sage, clove, coriander, fennel, frankincense, helichrysum, lavender, melissa, oregano, peppermint, roman chamomile, spikenard, wintergreen
Antimicrobial - arborvitae, basil, cassia, cilantro, cypress, fennel, frankincense, helichrysum, lavender, lemongrass, melissa, patchouli, ravensara, thyme
Antioxidant - black pepper, cassia, cinnamon, clove, frankincense, grapefruit, helichrysum, lemon, lime, melaleuca, oregano, vetiver, wild orange
Antiseptic - basil, bergamot, cardamom, cedarwood, clary sage, cypress, geranium, ginger, helichrysum, jasmine, lavender, lemon, lime, marjoram, melissa, myrrh, peppermint, ravensara, rosemary, spearmint, thyme, vetiver, wild orange, wintergreen
Antiviral - basil, cassia, clove, eucalyptus, ginger, helichrysum, melaleuca, melissa, myrrh, peppermint, rose, thyme, white fir
Immunostimulant - arborvitae, cassia, cinnamon, clove, eucalyptus, fennel, frankincense, ginger, lemon, lime, melaleuca, melissa, oregano, ravensara, rosemary spearmint, thyme, vetiver, white fir, wild orange
Stimulant - arborvitae, basil, cardamom, cedarwood, clove, cypress, dill, eucalyptus, fennel, grapefruit, melaleuca, myrrh, spearmint, vetiver, wintergreen, ylang ylang
Warming - birch, black pepper, cassia, cinnamon, clary sage, clove, eucalyptus, ginger, lemongrass, marjoram, oregano, peppermint, thyme, wintergreen

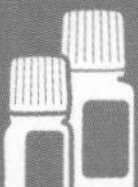

BLENDS

Protective blend - stimulates immune system and fights bacteria/viruses (pg. 158)
Detoxification blend - supports proper detoxification (pg. 146)
Cellular complex blend - manages abnormal cell activity and stimulates immune system (pg. 143)
Cleansing blend - disinfects and sanitizes (pg. 144)

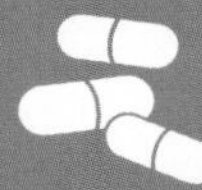

SUPPLEMENTS

Bone support complex, cellular vitality complex, children's chewable, **defensive probiotic (pg. 172)**, detoxification complex, essential oil cellular complex, essential oil omega complex, food enzymes, **GI cleansing softgels (pg. 178), protective blend softgels (pg. 181)**, protective blend lozenges, seasonal blend softgels, whole food nutrient supplement

Related Ailments: Adenitis, AIDS or HIV, Anthrax, Antiseptic, Bacteria, Body Temperature Issues, Chemical Sensitivity Reaction [Allergies], Chest Infections, Chicken Pox, Cholera, Common Cold, Conjunctivitis (Pink Eye), Cystitis, Cytomegalovirus Infection, Dengue Fever, E. Coli, Ebola, Epstein-Barr, Ehrlichiosis, Fever, Flu, H.Pylori, Hand Foot & Mouth Disease, Hepatitis, Herpes Simplex, Infection, Legionnaires' Disease, Listeria Infection, Lockjaw (Tetanus), Lyme Disease, Measles, Meningitis, Mesenteric Lymphadenitis, Mold, Mononucleosis, MRSA, Mumps, Plague, Polio [Nervous], Q Fever, Radiation Damage [Cellular Health], Rubella [Integumentary], Sepsis, Shigella Infection, Shingles, Staph Infection, Strep Throat [Oral Health], Tularemia, Typhoid, Virus

USAGE TIPS: For most effective use of essential oils for immune and lymphatic benefits:

- **Topical:** Apply oils topically on bottoms of feet, especially on back side of toes, rub oils down the spine and/or on any specific area of concern. Use Oil Touch technique.
- **Internal:** Take oils in capsule, place a drop(s) under or on tongue near back of throat or sip from a glass of water.
- **Aromatic:** Diffuse for associated respiratory symptoms and to clear pathogens from air.
- **Surfaces:** Sanitize surfaces with essential oil(s) mixed with water and emulsifier.

Remedies

LYME DISEASE

LYME DISEASE SUPPORT

Important facts regarding chemistry of essential oils for – Lyme protocol:

- Oregano - 60-90% carvacrol, kills bacteria, interrupts communication stream (quorum sensing) between harmful bacteria
- Thyme - 55% thymol, 10% carvacrol; protective agent for neurological tissue in brain
- Clove - 85% eugenol, controls symptoms, kills bacteria
  Carvacrol, eugenol, thymol are the most effective compounds for destroying pathogens; more powerful when used together
- Cassia - 80-90% cinnamaldehyde; Co2 inhibitor, antibacterial
- Cinnamon - 50% cinnamaldehyde; Co2 inhibitor, antibacterial
- Melissa - 65% aldehydes, 35% sesquiterpenes; antiviral, antibacterial; disrupts microorganism communication, immunostimulant, anti-inflammatory; antidepressant
  Protective blend contains cinnamon, clove, wild orange, eucalyptus, rosemary
- Frankincense - analgesic, anti-inflammatory, effective for pain management
- Patchouli - 63% sesquiterpenes; antioxidant, relief from secondary neurological effects in chronic Lyme

LYME DISEASE BOMB RECIPE

2 drops cinnamon or clove
2 drops cassia
2 drops oregano or thyme (alternate; use oregano in ten-day cycles; take break for twenty days)
2 drops frankincense
Place in a capsule; consume two times per day. Dilute with carrier oil if necessary or desired. Add melissa, protective blend, and/or GI cleansing softgels as needed.

LYME DISEASE INTENSE RESOLVE BLEND

3 drops oregano
3 drops thyme
3 drops clove
3 drops cassia or cinnamon
2 drops protective blend
2 drops melissa
2 drops frankincense
Place oils in capsule and take once or twice daily for two weeks depending upon intensity of symptoms. Rest from the blend for one week. Repeat this pattern until symptoms are gone for at least two months.

For greater intensity or for more chronic situations, use:

Topical application option (can do while taking a break from internal use or instead of): Apply 2 drops lemongrass + 1 drop oregano to the bottom of each foot before bed. Add melissa and/or protective blend, and/or other above suggested oils as needed.

NOTE: If rash or other discomfort occurs, reduce amount of oils being used or take a break until resolved. Consider improving intestinal elimination, removing certain foods from diet (foods that encourage microorganism growth), drink more water.

ADDITIONAL LYME SUPPORT

- Get an Oil Touch technique weekly. See page 14 in this book.
- Apply patchouli to bottoms of feet twice per day to support nervous system. Can add other oils as desired. Consider frankincense and wild orange.
- Supplementation program - consider the following - do a minimum of a four-month program :
- Basic: whole food nutrient supplement, essential oil omega complex
- Digestive/intestinal support: food enzymes, detoxification complex (mild detox support as well), GI cleansing softgels, defensive probiotic
- Anti-inflammatory/pain relief: cellular vitality complex or polyphenol complex
- Cell vitality: essential oil cellular complex
- Immune support: protective blend softgels AM and PM
- GI cleanse: Consider a focused cleanse followed by probiotic support: GI cleansing softgels and defensive probiotic.

See *Candida* for a superb detox program that is beneficial for Lyme Disease.

PAIN REMEDY

10 drops lavender
8 drops grounding blend
8 drops soothing blend
8 drops rosemary
6 drops lemongrass

- Combine above oils in 10ml roller bottle; fill remainder with carrier oil. Apply topically directly to painful joints and bottoms of feet several times each day as needed.
- Apply 1-3 drops each protective blend, melissa, frankincense, and patchouli to bottoms of feet.

- **Sleep support ideas** (see *Sleep*):
  Apply 3 drops vetiver, 3 drops juniper berry, and 3 drops lavender to the bottoms of feet.

- **Better by morning:**
  Rub one drop each basil and lemon at night behind ears to clear symptoms of physical illness by morning.

- **Muscle range of motion support** (see *Muscular, Skeletal*):
  Apply a few drops of bergamot and cypress topically.

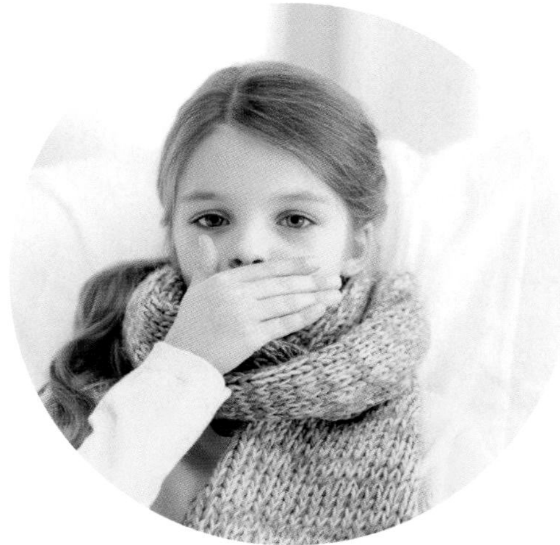

SKIN WOUND ANTISEPTIC

6 drops lavender
5 drops melaleuca
2 drops roman chamomile
1 ounce aloe vera gel
Blend in a glass bottle or bowl. Apply using cotton swab to affected areas of skin.

COLD & FLU DRINK

2 drops lavender
2 drops lemon
2 drops peppermint
2 drops melaleuca
Mix oils in ½ cup water. Add another ½ cup water, stir, and drink.

COLD & FLU BOMB

5 drops protective blend
5 drops melaleuca
3 drops oregano
Place in an empty capsule and swallow. Repeat every three to four hours while symptoms last.

SEASONAL WINTER-TO-SPRING BLEND

2 drops oregano
2 drops black pepper
4 drops grapefruit
Rub on the bottoms of feet five consecutive nights. Helps protect against seasonal and environmental elements.

SEASONAL SUMMER-TO-FALL BLEND

3 drops clove
2 drops white fir
4 drops lemon
Rub on the bottoms of feet five consecutive nights. Helps protect against seasonal and environmental elements.

HIV/AIDS SUPPORT

INITIAL CLEANSE:

- Add 2-4 drops of lemon in water daily (in glass container only).
- Take 3-4 drops each of protective blend, oregano or melissa, and peppermint in a capsule daily for ten days followed by five days of defensive probiotic. This process can be repeated monthly as needed.
- Dietary restrictions are important. Avoid processed foods, refined sugars; increase fresh fruits and vegetables.

ONGOING SUPPORT:

- Consume 2-4 drops of lemon in water daily (in glass container only).
- Take 3-4 drops each of frankincense, protective blend, melaleuca, rosemary in capsule daily
- Take whole food nutrient supplement, cellular vitality complex, essential oil omega complex daily
- Rub 2-3 drops each of grounding blend and protective blend on bottoms of feet twice a day (morning & night). Can also apply 2-4 drops of lavender for stress relief or sleep aid at night.
- Rub 1-2 drops frankincense on base of neck daily.
- Diffuse joyful blend during day for energy and calming blend at night for relaxation.
- Apply a hot compress for fifteen minutes after lightly massaging oils into back along the spine area for desired comfort and relief.
- For any other specific issue, refer to the respective Body System or Focus Area sections.

Perform the Oil Touch technique once a week. See *Oil Touch technique*. Benefits include:

- Strengthening the immune system
- Relieving stress and depression

Conditions

Abnormal cellular activity - frankincense, cellular complex blend; see *Cellular Health*
AIDS/HIV - arborvitae, cinnamon, clove, helichrysum, melissa, myrrh, rosemary, thyme, cellular complex, protective blend
Airborne germs and bacteria - arborvitae, cedarwood, eucalyptus, white fir, cleansing blend, protection blend, respiration blend; see "Antimicrobial" property
Allergies - See *Allergies*
Bacteria - arborvitae, basil, black pepper, cassia, cedarwood, cilantro, cinnamon, clove, coriander, dill, eucalyptus, frankincense, geranium, ginger, lemongrass, lime, marjoram, melaleuca, melissa, myrrh, oregano, peppermint, ravensara, rosemary, tangerine, thyme, ylang ylang, cellular complex blend, cleansing blend, detoxification blend, protective blend, renewing blend
Bacteria, staph - arborvitae, cinnamon, helichrysum, melissa, rosemary, uplifting blend; see "Antibacterial" property
Boils/carbuncles - eucalyptus, frankincense, lavender, marjoram, myrrh, sandalwood, anti-aging blend
Body temperature issues, too cold - See "Warming" property
Body temperature issues, too hot - bergamot, black pepper, eucalyptus, lemon, peppermint
Catch colds/get sick easily - see "Weakened/suppressed immune system" above
Cellulitis - cardamom, juniper berry, melaleuca, oregano, sandalwood, see "Antibacterial" property
Chills - basil, black pepper, cinnamon, ginger, protective blend; see "Warming" property
Cholera - cinnamon, eucalyptus, rosemary, detoxing blend, protective blend, respiration blend; see "Antibacterial" property
Cold, chronic - basil, cardamom, cypress, detoxification blend, protective blend
Cold/flu - cedarwood, cinnamon, clove, eucalyptus, frankincense, ginger, juniper berry, lavender, lemon, lime, melaleuca, peppermint, rose, rosemary, sandalwood, thyme, wild orange, protective blend, respiration blend; see "Antiviral" property
Cold/flu, reduce aches/pains from - black pepper, cypress, cedarwood, coriander, oregano, peppermint, thyme, white fir, wild orange, massage blend, protective blend, respiration blend, soothing blend, tension blend
Cold sores - arborvitae, basil, bergamot,

IMMUNE & LYMPHATIC

clove, fennel, geranium, helichrysum, lavender, lemon, melaleuca, melissa, myrrh, oregano, wild orange, detoxification blend, protective blend; see "Antiviral" property, *Oral Health*

Common Cold - see "Cold/flu" above

Conjunctivitis/pinkeye - clary sage, douglas fir, frankincense, melaleuca, jasmine, melissa, rosemary, corrective ointment; see "Antibacterial" property

Contagious diseases - clove, cinnamon, ginger, juniper berry, cellular blend, protective blend; see "Antibacterial, Anti-infectious, Antimicrobial, Antiviral" properties

Earache - basil, cypress, ginger, helichrysum, lavender, inspiring blend, invigorating blend, respiration blend, soothing blend; see *Respiratory*

Epidemics - basil, douglas fir, ginger, juniper berry, lemon, cellular complex, protective blend

Fever - arborvitae, basil, birch, black pepper, cardamom, cypress, eucalyptus, ginger, helichrysum, juniper berry, lavender, lemon, lemongrass, lime, patchouli, roman chamomile, rose, spearmint, wild orange, wintergreen, inspiring blend, renewing blend, tension blend

Fever blisters - see "Cold sores" above

Flu - see "Cold/flu" above

Fungus/candida - arborvitae, basil, cassia, cedarwood, cilantro, cinnamon, clove, coriander, lemongrass, marjoram, melaleuca, myrrh, oregano, patchouli, rosemary, spearmint, thyme; see *Candida*

Germs - grapefruit, lemon, lime, wild orange, cleansing blend, invigorating blend, protective blend; see "Antimicrobial, Antiseptic" properties

Glands, swollen - cardamom, cypress, douglas fir, frankincense, ginger, lemon, melaleuca, rosemary, sandalwood, cleansing blend, grounding blend, protective blend, respiration blend

Herpes simplex - basil, bergamot, clove, eucalyptus, frankincense, helichrysum, lavender, lemon, melaleuca, melissa, myrrh, oregano, peppermint, rose, sandalwood, comforting blend, protective blend; see "Antiviral" property

Illness prevention - clove, cinnamon, oregano, thyme, protective blend

Illness recovery - cinnamon, douglas fir, juniper berry, lemon, lemongrass, wild orange, metabolic blend

Immune, weakness - cinnamon, clove, douglas fir, frankincense, melaleuca, sandalwood, ylang ylang, cellular complex blend, detoxification blend, invigorating blend, protective blend, repellent blend

Infection - black pepper, cardamom, cassia, cinnamon, clove, lavender, melaleuca, melissa, oregano, thyme, wintergreen, protective blend; see "Antibacterial, Anti-infectious, Antimicrobial, Antiviral" properties

Infectious diseases - bergamot, cassia, lemongrass, rosemary, melissa, oregano, thyme, renewing blend; see "Antibacterial, Anti-infectious, Antimicrobial, Antiviral" properties

Leprosy - arborvitae, cedarwood, frankincense, melissa, myrrh, peppermint, sandalwood, thyme, cellular complex blend

Lymph, congestion/stagnation - birch, cassia, cypress, douglas fir, frankincense, geranium, grapefruit, lavender, lemon, lemongrass, lime, sandalwood, tangerine, wintergreen, cleansing blend, encouraging blend, inspiring blend, invigorating blend, respiration blend; see *Respiratory*

Malaria - bergamot, cardamom, cinnamon, douglas fir, eucalyptus, lemon, lemongrass, melaleuca, thyme, detoxification blend, respiration blend; see *Parasites*

Measles - clove, coriander, thyme, wild orange, thyme, cellular complex blend, protective blend; see "Antiviral" properties

Microorganisms (bacterial/viral) - black pepper, cinnamon, clove, lemongrass, melaleuca, thyme, oregano, protective blend

MRSA - cinnamon, clove, frankincense, geranium, lemon, melaleuca, melissa, oregano, peppermint, thyme, cellular complex blend, protective blend; see "Antibacterial" property

Mumps - basil, cinnamon, lemon, melaleuca, rosemary, cellular complex blend, detoxification blend, protective blend

Night sweats - ginger, lime, peppermint, cellular complex blend, detoxification blend, digestion blend; see *Women's Health, Endocrine (Thyroid)*

Parasites - See *Parasites*

Paralysis, facial - frankincense, ginger, helichrysum, juniper berry, marjoram, myrrh, cellular complex blend

Rheumatic fever - arborvitae, basil, coriander, eucalyptus, ginger, melissa, wintergreen

Rubella - basil, clove, coriander, lemon, melaleuca, oregano, thyme, metabolic blend

Ringworm - geranium, melaleuca, oregano, roman chamomile, thyme, skin clearing blend; see *Integumentary*

Scurvy - cypress, geranium, ginger, helichrysum, lemon, lemongrass, detoxification blend

Sore throat - cinnamon, lemon, melaleuca, melissa, myrrh, oregano, thyme, protective blend, respiration blend

Spleen - bergamot, cardamom, clary sage, lemon, rose

Spleen, congestion - cinnamon, fennel, helichrysum, lemon, sandalwood, focus blend

Spleen obstruction - basil, ginger, frankincense, marjoram, melissa

Staph - cinnamon, frankincense, geranium, lemon, melaleuca, melissa, oregano, peppermint, thyme, cleansing blend, protective blend, skin clearing blend

Strep - cinnamon, frankincense, lemon, oregano, protective blend, respiration blend

Sexually transmitted disease

- **Chlamydia** - arborvitae, basil, clove, melaleuca, thyme, protective blend
- **Gonorrhea** - basil, frankincense, melaleuca, rosemary, sandalwood
- **Syphilis** - black pepper, frankincense, melaleuca, melissa, myrrh, rosemary

Stomach flu (viral gastroenteritis) - arborvitae, thyme, oregano, cellular complex blend, detoxification blend, protective blend; see "Antiviral" property

Strep throat - cardamom, cinnamon, eucalyptus, lemon, melaleuca, oregano, thyme, protective blend, respiration blend; see "Antibacterial" property

Throat, sore - cinnamon, geranium, lavender, lemon, lime, oregano, thyme, inspiring blend, protective blend, respiration blend; see *Respiratory*

Tonsillitis - cinnamon, eucalyptus, frankincense, ginger, lavender, lemon, melaleuca, myrrh, roman chamomile, protective blend, respiration blend; see *Oral Health*

Typhoid fever - basil, cinnamon, clove, eucalyptus, lemon, melaleuca, oregano, peppermint, detoxification blend, protective blend

Virus - arborvitae, bergamot, black pepper, cassia, cinnamon, clove, eucalyptus, frankincense, helichrysum, marjoram, melaleuca, melissa, myrrh, oregano, patchouli, peppermint, rosemary, thyme, comforting blend, encouraging blend, protective blend; see "Antiviral" property

Viral, hepatitis - basil, cedarwood, clove, geranium, myrrh, rosemary, detoxification blend, encouraging blend

Virus, spinal - melaleuca, melissa, thyme, wintergreen; see "Antiviral" property

Weakened/suppressed immune system - frankincense, melaleuca, myrrh, thyme, protective blend, renewing blend

White blood cells (leukocytes), low count/lack of formation - frankincense, lavender, lemon, lime, myrrh

Zoonosis - cedarwood, eucalyptus, frankincense, melaleuca, myrrh, thyme, protective blend

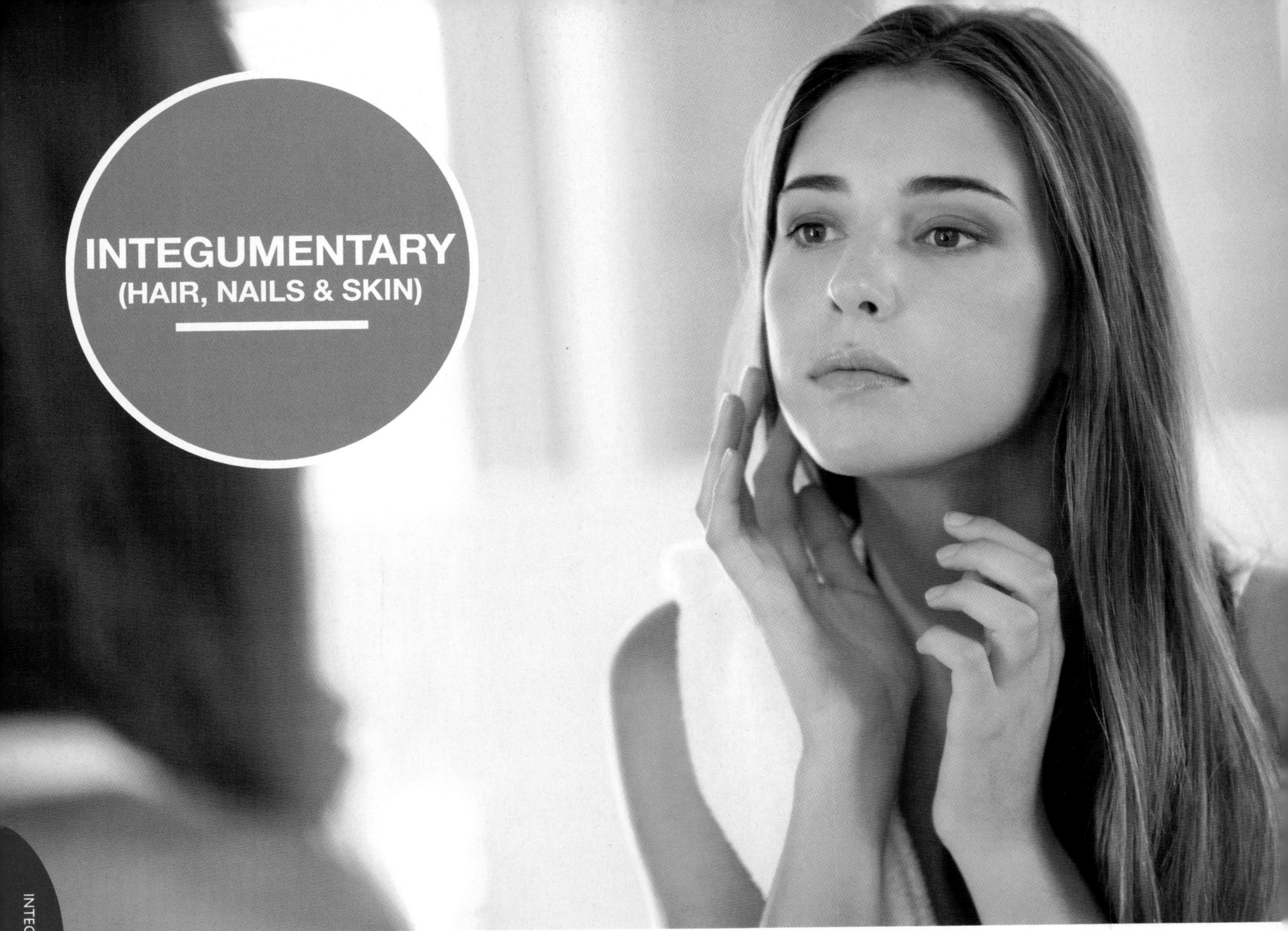

INTEGUMENTARY
(HAIR, NAILS & SKIN)

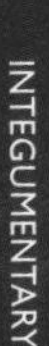

THE INTEGUMENTARY SYSTEM consists of the skin, hair, and nails. On the broadest scale, this system supports immune function and regulates homeostasis, as it constitutes the body's first line of defense against things that would disrupt its delicate balance and registers external stimuli through sensory receptors that communicate touch, pain, and pressure.

With a surface area averaging eighteen square feet, the skin is the largest organ of the body. It has two layers: the inner layer is called the dermis. The epidermis, or outer layer, consists of several strata that produce keratin, which gives strength and elasticity to the skin; melanin, which gives it its color; Merkel's cells, which facilitate touch reception; and Langerhans' cells, which produce antigens to support the immune system. And as a living organ, deep-level cells continually divide and push older cells to the surface to be worn off—millions every day—leaving behind a new epidermis every five to seven weeks.

The skin protects the internal organs, guards against infection, regulates temperature change and hydration levels through perspiration, and stores water, fat, and glucose. It excretes waste, generates vitamin D when exposed to ultraviolet light, and secretes melanin to protect against sunburn. It also has the capacity to form new cells to repair minor cuts and abrasions.

The array of dermatological conditions that may afflict people ranges from warts, eczema, acne, and moles to psoriasis, vitiligo, and a variety of skin cancers. Hair and nail conditions can be unsightly, uncomfortable, or even painful. Since many skin, hair, and nail conditions are an outward reflection of other imbalances going on inside the body, it is important to focus on detoxing, cleansing, and supplementing vital nutrition to the cells and internal organs in addition to essential oil applications that can easily target the area of concern.

Natural solutions are very effective and can be used as a first line of defense toward various integumentary conditions. If problems or conditions persist or cause concern, proper medical attention should be sought. Keep in mind that natural solutions can be used safely together with medical treatments if the latter become necessary. Many essential oils that are beneficial for integumentary support are diverse in the number of conditions they can impact. Some oils are more obvious choices, such as lavender and geranium with their marvelous healing properties. Other oils target more of the underlying factors. For example, birch oil is great used in ointments, creams, and compresses, especially for inflamed skin (eczema, boils, dermatitis, psoriasis, ulcers, etc.). There are a diverse number of oils and solutions that can be realized.

TOP SOLUTIONS

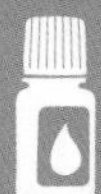

SINGLE OILS

Lavender - supports healing and maintaining healthy tissue (pg. 108)
Sandalwood - promotes regeneration and toning (pg. 128)
Geranium - regenerates tissue and tones skin (pg. 102)
Frankincense - invigorates skin, reduces inflammation (pg. 100)
Helichrysum - regenerates tissue and reduces scarring (pg. 105)

By Related Properties

For definitions of the properties listed below and more oil options, see Oil Properties Glossary (pg. 435) and Oil Properties (pg. 436).

Analgesic - arborvitae, basil, black pepper, cassia, cinnamon, coriander, cypress, eucalyptus, fennel, frankincense, ginger, juniper berry, lavender, melaleuca, peppermint, rosemary, white fir
Antifungal - arborvitae, cassia, cinnamon, clary sage, coriander, dill, ginger, helichrysum, lemongrass, melaleuca, patchouli, ravensara, spearmint, thyme
Anti-infectious - cedarwood, cinnamon, clove, cypress, frankincense, geranium, lavender, marjoram, melaleuca, roman chamomile, rosemary
Anti-inflammatory - arborvitae, basil, birch, black pepper, cedarwood, cinnamon, clove, coriander, fennel, frankincense, ginger, lavender, lime, myrrh, patchouli, spearmint, spikenard, wintergreen, yarrow
Antimicrobial - basil, cardamom, cinnamon, clary sage, cypress, dill, frankincense, helichrysum, lemon, lemongrass, myrrh, oregano, rosemary, thyme
Antimutagenic - cinnamon, ginger, lavender, lemongrass
Antiseptic - bergamot, birch, clary sage, clove, fennel, frankincense, ginger, grapefruit, juniper berry, lavender, marjoram, melaleuca, myrrh, oregano, ravensara, sandalwood, spearmint, vetiver, white fir, wintergreen, yarrow, ylang ylang
Antiviral - arborvitae, basil, cassia, clove, dill, eucalyptus, ginger, helichrysum, lime, melissa, myrrh, ravensara, rose, white fir
Astringent - cassia, cedarwood, clary sage, cypress, geranium, grapefruit, helichrysum, lemon, myrrh, sandalwood, wintergreen, yarrow
Cytophylactic - arborvitae, frankincense, geranium, lavender, rosemary, tangerine
Deodorant - bergamot, clary sage, cypress, eucalyptus, geranium, lavender, lemongrass, patchouli, spikenard, white fir
Insect repellent - arborvitae, birch, cedarwood, cinnamon, eucalyptus, geranium, lemongrass, patchouli, thyme, vetiver, ylang ylang
Regenerative - basil, cedarwood, clove, coriander, geranium, jasmine, lavender, lemongrass, melaleuca, myrrh, patchouli, sandalwood, wild orange
Revitalizer - coriander, juniper berry, lemon, lemongrass, lime
Tonic - arborvitae, basil, basil, birch, cardamom, clary sage, coriander, cypress, fennel, frankincense, geranium, ginger, grapefruit, lavender, lemon, lime, marjoram, myrrh, patchouli, roman chamomile, rose, rosemary, sandalwood, tangerine, thyme, wild orange, ylang ylang

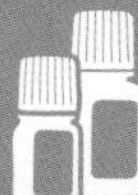

BLENDS

Anti-aging blend - restores and tones skin (pg. 141)
Skin clearing blend - cleanses skin and reduces inflammation (pg. 163)

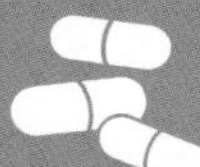

SUPPLEMENTS

Bone support complex, cellular vitality complex, defensive probiotic, **essential oil omega complex (pg. 175)**, detoxification complex, food enzymes, GI cleansing softgels, **liquid omega-3 supplement (pg. 178)**, whole food nutrient supplement

Related Ailments: Acne, Actinic Keratosis, Age Spots, Bags Under Eyes, Baldness, Bed Sores, Blisters, Blisters from Sun, Boils, Brittle Nails, Burns, Calluses, Chapped Skin, Clogged Pores, Cold Sores, Corns, Cuts, Cyst [Cellular Health], Dandruff, Dehydrated Skin, Dry Hair, Dry Hands, Dry Lips, Dry Skin, Eczema, Excessive Perspiration, Fragile Hair, Genital Warts, Hair Loss, Head Lice, Hernia (incisional), Ichthyosis Vulgaris, Impetigo [Immune], Infected Wounds, Ingrown Toenail, Itching [Allergies], Lichen Nitidus, Moles [Cellular Health], Oily Hair, Oily Skin, Plantar Warts, Poison Ivy [Allergies], Psoriasis, Rashes [Allergies], Ringworm, Rosacea, Scabies, Scarring, Sebaceous Cyst, Skin Ulcers, Stevens-Johnson Syndrome, Stretch Marks [Pregnancy], Sunburn, Swimmer's Itch [Candida], Tissue Regeneration [Cellular Health, Muscular], Ulcers – Leg and Varicose [Cardiovascular], Vitiligo, Warts, Wounds, Wrinkles

USAGE TIPS: For best support of hair, skin and nails:

- **Topical:** Apply oils directly to hair, scalp, nails, and skin. Use a carrier oil to dilute and reduce sensitivity to skin when necessary, especially with infants, elderly, and compromised skin.
- **Internal:** Consume specified oils by either capsule or under tongue. Gut health is a major component of integumentary health. See *Digestive & Intestinal, Candida*.

Conditions

HAIR:

Dandruff - cedarwood, cypress, lavender, patchouli, rosemary, thyme, wintergreen, cleansing blend, detoxification blend, joyful blend, uplifting blend

Dirty - lemon, lime, cleansing blend, invigorating blend

Dry - geranium, lavender, rosemary, sandalwood, spikenard, wintergreen, joyful blend, respiration blend

Dull - lemongrass, lime (has mild bleaching action), melaleuca, rosemary, repellent blend, respiration blend

Fragile - clary sage, geranium, lavender, lime, roman chamomile, sandalwood, thyme, wintergreen, respiration blend

Greasy/oily/brittle - basil, cedarwood, cypress, juniper berry (scalp), lavender, lemon, melaleuca, peppermint, rosemary, thyme, joyful blend, renewing blend, respiration blend

Growth, poor - cedarwood, clary sage, geranium, ginger, grapefruit, lavender, lemon, rosemary, thyme, ylang ylang, encouraging blend, joyful blend, invigorating blend

Lice - clove, melaleuca, rosemary, detoxification blend, invigorating blend, repellent blend; see *Parasites*

Loss - arborvitae, cedarwood, clary sage, cypress, eucalyptus, grapefruit, juniper berry, lavender, roman chamomile, rosemary, thyme, wintergreen, ylang ylang, invigorating blend, respiration blend

Scalp, itchy/flaky - cedarwood, lavender, rosemary, wintergreen, detoxification blend, renewing blend

Split ends - cedarwood, clary sage, lavender, rosemary, ylang ylang, detoxification blend

NAILS:

Brittle Nails - cypress, eucalyptus, grapefruit, lemon, lavender, marjoram, oregano, roman chamomile, rosemary, anti-aging blend, detoxification blend; see Cardiovascular

Fungus - arborvitae, basil, clove, eucalyptus, geranium, oregano, lemongrass, melaleuca, detoxification blend, invigorating blend, skin clearing blend; see Candida

Hangnail - basil, black pepper, cilantro, coriander, lavender, rosemary, sandalwood, ylang ylang, respiration blend

Missing (injury) - eucalyptus, frankincense, myrrh, joyful blend, protective blend, repellent blend

Ridges - eucalyptus, melaleuca, thyme, detoxification blend, joyful blend

Ripped/split - eucalyptus, geranium, lemon, melaleuca, skin clearing blend, joyful blend, invigorating blend

Soft/weak - eucalyptus, grapefruit, lemon, lime, white fir, cleansing blend, invigorating blend

Swelling/red/tender - lemongrass, melaleuca, myrrh, thyme, detoxification blend, protective blend

Yellowed/infected - eucalyptus, frankincense, lemon, melaleuca, myrrh, thyme, detoxification blend, joyful blend, massage blend, protective blend

INTEGUMENTARY

SKIN:

NOTE: See *First Aid* for Bites & Stings; *Allergies* for Hives, Rashes, etc. for additional suggestions.

Acne - arborvitae, bergamot, birch, cardamom, cedarwood (astringent), clary sage, clove, coriander, cypress, frankincense, geranium, grapefruit, helichrysum, juniper berry, lavender, lemon, lemongrass, melaleuca, myrrh, patchouli, rosemary, sandalwood, spearmint, vetiver, white fir, wintergreen, yarrow, ylang ylang, anti-aging blend, cellular complex blend, cleansing blend, renewing blend, skin clearing blend

Aging/age spots - basil, coriander, fennel, frankincense, geranium, helichrysum, lavender, lemon, lime, myrrh, roman chamomile, rose, sandalwood, vetiver, anti-aging blend, cellular complex blend, women's blend

Athlete's foot - arborvitae, cardamom, clove, lavender, lemongrass, melaleuca, myrrh, oregano, massage blend, metabolic blend; see *Candida*

Appearance, poor/dull - basil, cedarwood, douglas fir, fennel, frankincense, geranium, lemon, lemongrass, lime, myrrh, sandalwood, wild orange, anti-aging blend, skin clearing blend

Bags under eyes - arborvitae, cedarwood, dill, frankincense, geranium, helichrysum, juniper berry, lavender, melaleuca, myrrh, roman chamomile, sandalwood, wild orange, anti-aging blend, detoxification blend

Blister, friction/heat/liquid-filled - eucalyptus, lavender, myrrh, massage blend

Body odor - arborvitae, cilantro, coriander, douglas fir, eucalyptus, lemongrass, patchouli, tangerine, detoxification blend, joyful blend, repellent blend, women's blend

Boils/carbuncles - bergamot, frankincense, helichrysum, lavender, marjoram, myrrh, roman chamomile, sandalwood, anti-aging blend, repellent blend

Bruises - arborvitae, cypress, clove, fennel, geranium, helichrysum, lavender, oregano, roman chamomile, white fir, ylang ylang, cellular complex blend, cleansing blend, detoxification blend, invigorating blend, massage blend, soothing blend or rub

Bumps - clary sage, frankincense, patchouli, wild orange, detoxification blend, metabolic blend

Burn - eucalyptus, frankincense, geranium, helichrysum, lavender, marjoram, myrrh, roman chamomile, anti-aging blend; see *First Aid*

Callus - cypress, douglas fir, lavender, oregano, roman chamomile, white fir, skin clearing blend

Capillaries, broken - geranium, lemon; see *Cardiovascular*

Cell renewal - arborvitae, basil, cedarwood, lavender, frankincense, helichrysum, jasmine, lemongrass, lime, melaleuca, myrrh, patchouli, rosemary, sandalwood, spearmint, thyme, wild orange, anti-aging blend, cellular complex blend

Cellulitis - geranium, juniper berry, cellular complex blend, digestion blend

Chapped/cracked/dry/peeling - jasmine, lavender, myrrh, patchouli, sandalwood, spearmint, cleansing blend, corrective ointment, renewing blend

Circulation, poor - geranium, lemongrass, marjoram, rose

Collagen, lack of - helichrysum, lemongrass, sandalwood

Corns - arborvitae, clove, grapefruit, lemon, peppermint, ylang ylang, cellular complex blend, invigorating blend, repellent blend

Cuts/wounds - basil, bergamot, cardamom, cinnamon, dill, eucalyptus, frankincense, geranium, grapefruit, helichrysum, juniper berry, lavender, lemongrass, marjoram, melaleuca, myrrh, rose, sandalwood, thyme, vetiver, protective blend

Damaged - arborvitae, basil, cedarwood, cilantro, cypress, frankincense, geranium, helichrysum, lemongrass, lime, sandalwood, wild orange, anti-aging blend, cellular complex blend

Dermatitis - geranium, helichrysum, patchouli, thyme, joyful blend, skin clearing blend

Diseased - birch, cedarwood, geranium, lavender, oregano, thyme, wintergreen, detoxification blend

Eczema/psoriasis - arborvitae, birch, bergamot, cedarwood, douglas fir, geranium, helichrysum, juniper berry, lavender, melissa, myrrh, oregano, patchouli, peppermint, roman chamomile, rosemary, spearmint, thyme, wintergreen, ylang ylang, renewing blend, skin clearing blend

Facial, thread veins - rose, anti-aging blend

Fine lines or cracks - lavender, sandalwood, vetiver, anti-aging blend, cellular complex blend

Flushed - wild orange, cleansing blend, respiration blend

Fungus - arborvitae, cedarwood, clove, frankincense, lavender, melaleuca, myrrh, patchouli, roman chamomile, thyme, detoxification blend, skin clearing blend; see *Candida*

Growth, small/fleshy/rough/grainy - fennel, grapefruit, thyme, detoxification blend, joyful blend, metabolic blend, skin clearing blend

Heels, cracked - myrrh, vetiver, renewing blend, women's blend, corrective ointment

Hemorrhoids - cypress, geranium, helichrysum, myrrh, patchouli, roman chamomile, sandalwood, detoxification blend, digestion blend, massage blend

Hernia, incision - basil, geranium, helichrysum, lemongrass, protective blend

Impetigo - vetiver, geranium, lavender, oregano, detoxification blend, women's blend

Infection - arborvitae, cassia, cinnamon, clove, eucalyptus, frankincense, juniper berry, melissa, oregano, patchouli, peppermint, rose, sandalwood, thyme, protective blend

Inflammation/redness - cedarwood, geranium, jasmine, juniper berry, lavender, helichrysum, peppermint, roman chamomile, rose, sandalwood, wild orange, ylang ylang, anti-aging blend, calming blend, cellular complex blend, protective blend

Itching - cilantro, lavender, melaleuca, patchouli, peppermint, roman chamomile, sandalwood, vetiver, detoxification blend, metabolic blend

Lips, chapped/cracked/dry/peeling - cedarwood, jasmine, lavender, myrrh, sandalwood, women's blend, corrective ointment

Moles - frankincense, geranium, juniper berry, lavender, oregano, sandalwood, wild orange, cellular complex blend, detoxification blend, joyful blend, repellent blend, skin clearing blend

Oily - bergamot, cedarwood, coriander, frankincense, geranium, grapefruit, jasmine, sandalwood, vetiver, wild orange, ylang ylang, renewing blend, respiration blend, skin clearing blend, uplifting blend

Pores, blocked - cedarwood, sandalwood, anti-aging blend, cellular complex blend, skin clearing blend

Pores, enlarged - lemongrass, sandalwood, anti-aging blend, cellular complex blend, skin clearing blend

Perspiration, excessive - cypress, douglas fir, lemongrass, peppermint, detoxification blend

Perspiration, lack of - arborvitae, basil, black pepper, cypress, ginger, melaleuca, wild orange, detoxification blend

Pigmentation, excess - basil, cedarwood, lavender, lemon, sandalwood, spearmint, ylang ylang, anti-aging blend, invigorating blend, women's blend

Pigmentation, lack of - bergamot, cedarwood, douglas fir, sandalwood, vetiver, anti-aging blend, cellular complex blend

Radiation wounds - arborvitae, basil, cedarwood, clove, frankincense, geranium, helichrysum, jasmine, lavender, melaleuca, myrrh, patchouli, rosemary, sandalwood, thyme, wild orange, anti-aging blend, cellular complex blend

Rashes - frankincense, lavender, melaleuca, roman chamomile, sandalwood, vetiver, anti-aging blend, calming blend, cleansing blend, detoxification blend, metabolic blend, women's monthly blend; see *Candida*

Ringworm - cardamom, clove, geranium, lemongrass, melaleuca, oregano, roman chamomile, thyme, invigorating blend, skin clearing blend

Rough, dry, scaly cracked - cedarwood, jasmine, lavender, myrrh, roman chamomile, women's blend, corrective ointment

Sagging - basil, coriander, frankincense, geranium, grapefruit, helichrysum, jasmine, juniper berry, lime, melaleuca, myrrh, sandalwood, anti-aging blend, cellular complex blend, invigorating blend

Scabs - arborvitae, basil, birch, coriander, eucalyptus, frankincense, geranium, helichrysum, juniper berry, lavender, lemon, lemongrass, lime, spearmint, anti-aging blend, joyful blend, invigorating blend

Scarring - cypress, geranium, frankincense, helichrysum, lavender, rose, sandalwood, vetiver, anti-aging blend

Sensitive/tender - arborvitae, frankincense, ginger, helichrysum, jasmine, lavender, marjoram, melaleuca, rosemary, wild orange, cellular complex blend, joyful blend, repellent blend, women's blend

Skin disorders - arborvitae, black pepper, cilantro, coriander, frankincense, geranium, helichrysum, oregano, rosemary, tangerine, wild orange, anti-aging blend

Skin tags - cedarwood, coriander, geranium, lavender, oregano, sandalwood

Sores - lavender, myrrh, patchouli, sandalwood, spearmint, cleansing blend, protective blend

Stretch marks - arborvitae, douglas fir, frankincense, geranium, lavender, myrrh, sandalwood, anti-aging blend, massage blend, women's monthly blend

Sunburns - arborvitae, helichrysum, lavender, marjoram, myrrh, peppermint, cellular complex blend, massage blend

Sunburns, prevent (sunscreen) - arborvitae, helichrysum

Tightened/hardened - frankincense, patchouli, cellular complex blend, cleansing blend, detoxification blend

Tone, lack of/imbalanced - basil, cypress, frankincense, lemon, lemongrass, rose, sandalwood, ylang ylang, anti-aging blend, invigorating blend

Ulcers (open crater, red, tender edges) - cedarwood, coriander, frankincense, geranium, helichrysum, lavender, lemongrass, melaleuca, myrrh, wild orange, anti-aging blend

UV radiation - clove, coriander, myrrh, sandalwood, cellular complex blend

Varicose ulcer - cedarwood, coriander, frankincense, geranium, cellular complex blend, massage blend

Varicose veins - bergamot, cardamom, cypress, geranium, helichrysum, lemon, lemongrass, rosemary, cellular complex blend, digestion blend, massage blend

Vitiligo - bergamot, sandalwood, vetiver, anti-aging blend, cellular complex blend, detoxification blend, women's blend

Warts - arborvitae, cedarwood, cinnamon, clove, frankincense, lemon, lemongrass, lime, melissa, oregano, thyme, cellular complex blend, massage blend, renewing blend

White patches on skin, inside mouth - bergamot, black pepper, frankincense, melaleuca, myrrh, sandalwood

Wounds, weeping (yellow/green pus) - bergamot, clary sage, frankincense, helichrysum, melaleuca, wild orange

Wrinkles - arborvitae, douglas fir, fennel, geranium, grapefruit, frankincense, helichrysum, jasmine, lavender, myrrh, roman chamomile, rose, sandalwood, white fir, wild orange, anti-aging blend, renewing blend

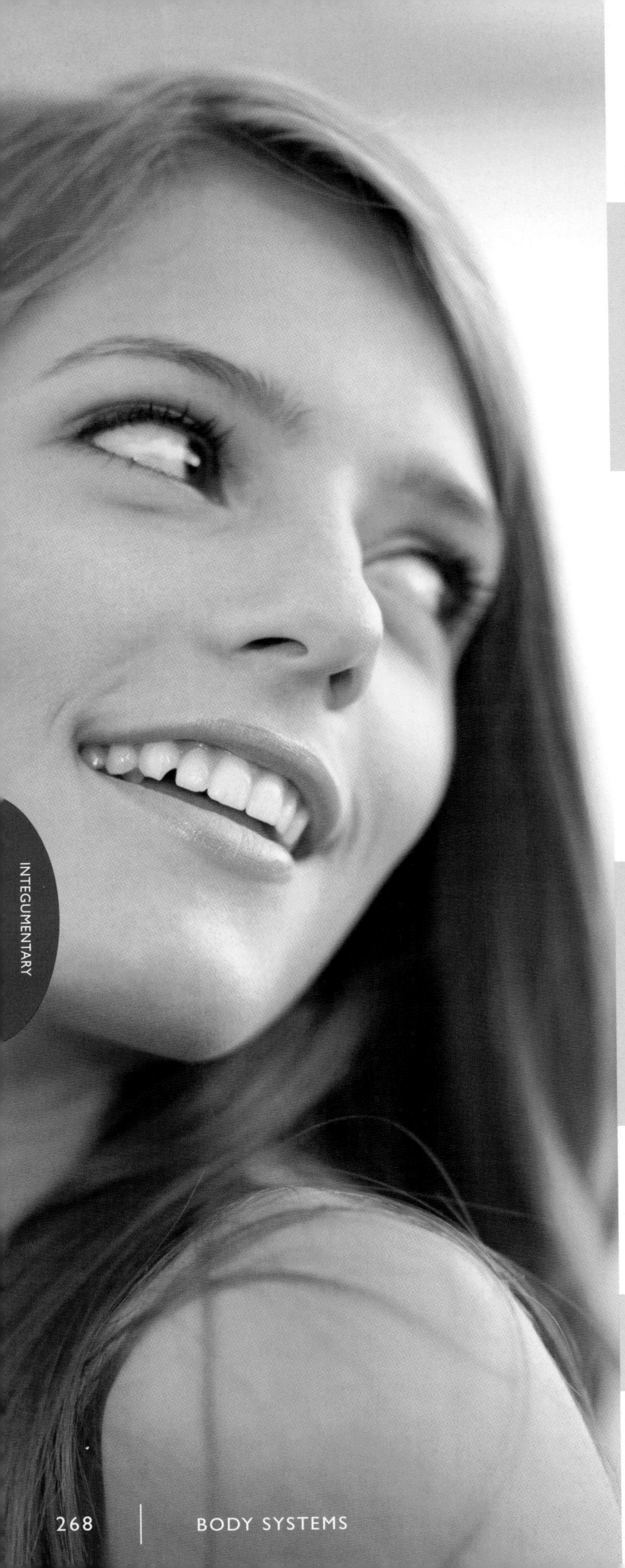

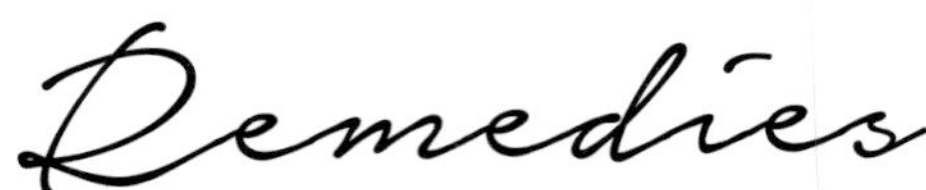

Remedies

SKIN:

DERMATITIS/ECZEMA BLEND
10 drops frankincense
10 drops lavender
10 drops melaleuca
10 drops helichrysum
3 drops lemongrass
4 drops juniper berry
5 drops geranium
45 drops fractionated coconut oil
Add ingredients to spray bottle and apply as needed.

GRAPEFRUIT EXFOLIATING SCRUB - to boost circulation and tone skin (Do not use this scrub on sensitive or inflamed skin)
30ml fractionated coconut oil
3 ounces fine sea salt
10 drops of grapefruit essential oil

- Pour carrier oil into a glass bowl for blending, add grapefruit oil, mix slightly; then add sea salt in stages, stirring until a thick paste is formed. Add more carrier oil if a looser consistency is desired.
- Once prepared, mixture keeps for six months; place contents in dark jar to preserve qualities of grapefruit oil. Make note of date it was made.
- Application: massage scrub in circular motion directly onto skin. Rinse with warm water.

SKIN TONE AND TEXTURE HEALTH
Add in the following order:
10 drops helichrysum
6 drops lavender
8 drops lemongrass
4 drops patchouli
5 drops myrrh
Add to roller bottle, top with 1 ounce carrier oil; gently shake to mix before each use. Apply to desired areas of skin three to four times daily.

SUNBURN REMEDY
25 drops lavender
25 drops helichrysum
25 drops peppermint
Add to 10ml roller or spray bottle; fill with carrier oil and apply gently to sunburn.

WART
Use 1 drop or less oregano oil (depending on size of area) twice daily for two weeks.

WOUND CARE - heal and prevent infection
Apply 1 drop melaleuca to affected area to clean wound; apply corrective ointment.

NAILS:

ANTIFUNGAL NAIL BLEND

5 drops melaleuca
1 drop cinnamon
2 drops lavender
½ ounce carrier oil
Mix and apply around and under affected nails two to three times per day until gone. Avoid contact with eyes.

HANGNAIL: Apply 1 drop arborvitae to area of concern, massage.

NAIL GROWTH: combine 1 drop of grapefruit essential oil with 10ml of carrier oil. Massage blend into nail bed, then with upward strokes towards nail tip

NAIL SOAK AND CUTICLE CURE - to stimulate circulation and promote healthy shine
4 drops lavender
2 drops bay leaf
3 drops sandalwood
½ ounce carrier
Soak in formula for ten minutes, buff, moisturize.

NAIL STRENGTHENER TREATMENT

2 drops lemon
2 drops frankincense
2 drops myrrh
2 drops fractionated carrier
Combine in glass bowl. Dip fingernails in blend; massage. Use twice per week.

NOURISH YOUR NAILS

15 drops lavender
10 drops lemon
4 drops myrrh
2 tablespoons fractionated coconut oil or choice of carrier oil
Mix in 2-ounce glass bottle with a dropper lid; fill remainder of bottle with carrier oil. Shake vigorously for two minutes. Warm to body temp. Let sit 24 hours. Apply 1 drop of mixture per nail; massage in each nail for one minute. Follow with a moisturizer.

SPLIT OR DAMAGED NAIL REPAIR

4 drops sandalwood
2 drops women's monthly blend
1 drops wild orange
1 tablespoon carrier oil
Soak nail in formula each night; massage in thoroughly to promote absorption; wipe off excess with tissue; follow with moisturizer. Add 1 drop myrrh oil to formula three times per week.

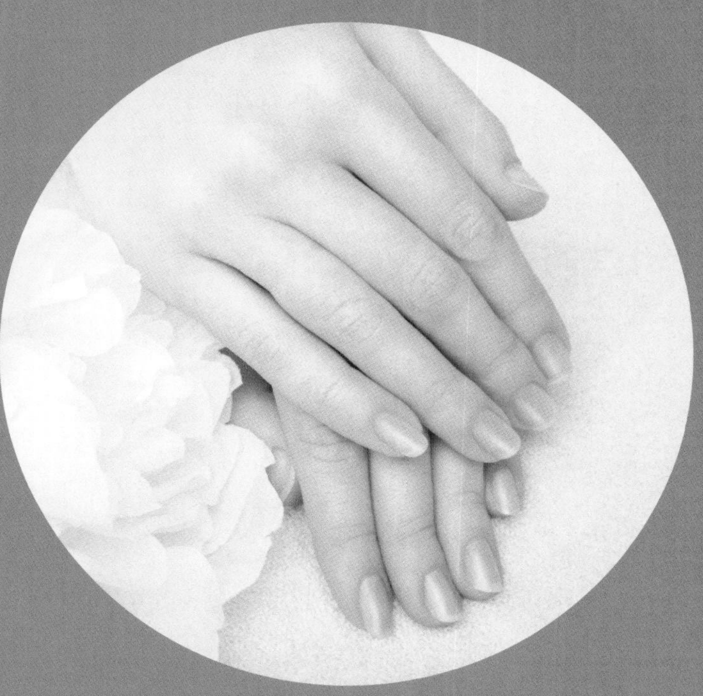

HAIR:

GREASY HAIR RESOLVE: Grapefruit oil rids scalp of impurities and residual styling products without drying out hair. It also promotes hair growth and helps rejuvenate hair.
1 teaspoon natural shampoo
1 drop of grapefruit essential oil
Combine shampoo and grapefruit oil; massage gently into scalp with fingertips. Rinse.

HAIR GROWTH: Add 2 drops of grapefruit essential oil to 8ml (just under one tablespoon) of jojoba and stir the blend. Massage the liquid into your scalp, using a circular motion with your fingertips. Leave on for thirty minutes and then wash your hair with a gentle shampoo.

HAIR LOSS REMEDY OPTIONS: Use 5 drops each of cedarwood, cypress, lavender, rosemary oils; add to 2 ounces of a natural shampoo and use when shampooing.
Blend with 2 drops of each oil listed above with 2 tablespoons of fractionated coconut oil. Massage into scalp, cover with a shower cap, and let sit for a few hours or overnight; shampoo and condition.

More intense blend: Combine 8 drops rosemary + 10 drops lavender + 10 drops sandalwood + 10 drops cedarwood + 10 drops melaleuca oils with 3 ounces of natural shampoo; work oils into scalp several times a week and let sit for twenty minutes prior to shampooing.

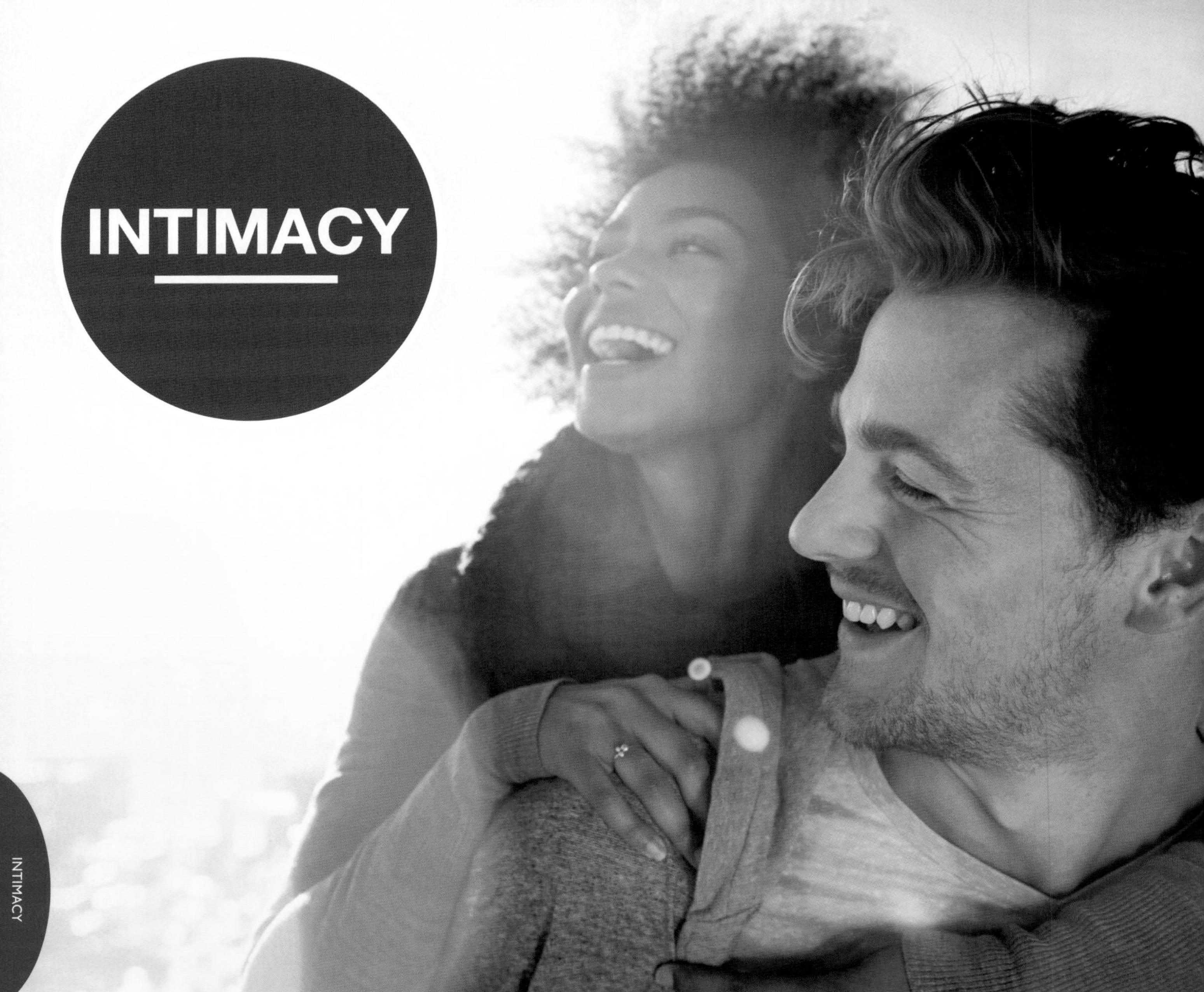

ALL HUMANS have a basic need to love and feel loved; intimate relationships that include a sexual component help to fulfill this need.If a couple desires to improve their emotional intimacy, they can attend seminars, read books, or go to marriage counseling to get some ideas. Because of past experiences and current health concerns, physical intimacy can have inherent challenges including low sex drive, exhaustion/fatigue, aches and pains, chronic illness, hemorrhoids, yeast infections, endometriosis, vaginal dryness, impotence, lack of nitric oxide, oxytocin production, and more.

At times, individuals may be interested in an aphrodisiac, which is a substance that enhances or stimulates passion and sexual arousal. An aphrodisiac can also help reduce physical, psychological, or emotional conditions that interfere with passion and sexual arousal. Certain essential oils have long been praised for their aphrodisiac qualities. One of the reasons why they are so effective is that their natural chemical composition works quickly on the circulatory, endocrine, and reproductive systems when applied to the skin (usually diluted).

Additionally, essential oils are an effective aphrodisiac because their aromatic qualities affect mood, thought, and feelings via olfaction; once inhaled, the odor molecules register a response in the limbic portion of the brain, which is also responsible for sexual behavior and memory and can influence the body's sexual response.

Essential oils can produce desired effects for oneself and/or one's partner. Most aphrodisiac essential oils work by raising the body temperature through their warm and rich aromas. Once the body has reached an ideal temperature, the sensual and euphoric properties of essential oils are most effective.

Essential oils can also help balance hormones, reduce fatigue and exhaustion, help support the body's physical health, and promote emotional wellness, which in turn promotes emotional and physical intimacy. Additionally, certain essential oil applications can help individuals relax and "get in the mood."

TOP SOLUTIONS

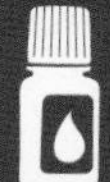

SINGLE OILS

Jasmine - enhances mood and libido, euphoric (pg. 106)

Ylang ylang - supports a healthy libido and endocrine function (pg. 139)

Patchouli - improves circulation, raises body temperature, enhances mood (pg. 121)

Clary sage - supports the endocrine system, enhances libido (pg. 88)

Bergamot - balances hormones, enhances libido (pg. 79)

By Related Properties

For definitions of the properties listed below and more oil options, see Oil Properties Glossary (pg. 435) and Oil Properties (pg. 436).

Anaphrodisiac - arborvitae, marjoram (avoid if interested in libido enhancement)
Antidepressant - bergamot, cinnamon, coriander, dill, frankincense, geranium, grapefruit, jasmine, lavender, lemon, lemongrass, patchouli, ravensara, sandalwood, wild orange, ylang ylang
Aphrodisiac - black pepper, cardamom, cinnamon, clary sage, clove, coriander, jasmine, juniper berry, patchouli, peppermint, ravensara, rose, rosemary, sandalwood, spearmint, thyme, vetiver, wild orange, ylang ylang
Calming - basil, bergamot, black pepper, cassia, clary sage, coriander, frankincense, geranium, jasmine, juniper berry, lavender, oregano, patchouli, sandalwood, tangerine, vetiver, yarrow
Energizing - basil, clove cypress, grapefruit, lemongrass, rosemary, white fir, wild orange
Grounding - basil, cedarwood, clary sage, cypress, melaleuca, vetiver, ylang ylang
Invigorating - grapefruit, lemon, peppermint, spearmint, wild orange, wintergreen
Relaxing - basil, cassia, cedarwood, clary sage, cypress, fennel, geranium, lavender, marjoram, myrrh, ravensara, roman chamomile, white fir, ylang ylang
Rubefacient - bergamot, birch, juniper berry, lavender, lemon, rosemary, vetiver, white fir
Sedative - bergamot, cedarwood, coriander, frankincense, geranium, juniper berry, lavender, marjoram, melissa, roman chamomile, rose, sandalwood, spikenard, vetiver, ylang ylang
Stimulant - basil, bergamot, birch, black pepper, cinnamon, clove, cypress, dill, eucalyptus, fennel, ginger, grapefruit, juniper berry, lime, myrrh, patchouli, rosemary, spearmint, vetiver, white fir, ylang ylang
Uplifting - bergamot, cedarwood, clary sage, cypress, lemon, lime, melissa, sandalwood, wild orange
Vasodilator - lemongrass, marjoram, rosemary, thyme
Warming - birch, cassia, cinnamon, clary sage, ginger, wintergreen

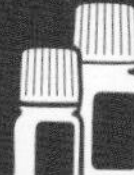

BLENDS

Women's blend - support healthy libido (pg. 168)

Inspiring blend - promotes passion, excitement and joy (pg. 152)

Joyful blend - uplifts mood, energizes (pg. 154)

Massage blend - supports circulation, relieves tension (pg. 155)

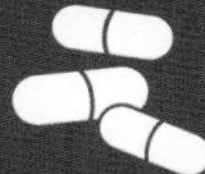

SUPPLEMENTS

Cellular vitality complex, detoxification blend softgels, detoxification complex, **energy & stamina complex (pg. 174)**, essential oil cellular complex, essential oil omega complex, GI cleansing softgels, **polyphenol complex (pg. 181)**, whole food nutrient supplement

USAGE TIPS: For best results to support optimal intimacy

- **Aromatic:** Set the mood by diffusing oils of choice that are calming, warming and arousing to both parties.
- **Topical:** Enjoy using specified oils to obtain desired results. When in sensitive areas be sure to use a carrier oil.

Remedies

ACTIVATE HER APHRODITE
4 drops ylang ylang
2 drops clary sage
2 drops geranium
2 drops patchouli
2 drops sandalwood
1 drop bergamot
Combine and store in a glass bottle. Apply to pressure points, or diffuse.

APHRODISIAC AROMA AROUSER: Combine 12 drops sandalwood oil, 5 drops ylang ylang, 1 drop cinnamon, 1 drop jasmine oil. Apply on back of neck and behind ears. Dilute with a carrier oil if desired or necessary for sensitive skin.

BODY WARMER
2 drops rose or geranium
3 drops sandalwood
2 drops ylang ylang
3 drops clary sage
In a 2-ounce glass bottle, combine oils, swirl, fill with carrier oil. Use as a massage oil to warm the body temperature and create arousal.

DREAMMAKER BLEND: Combine 25 drops frankincense, 20 drops bergamot, and 15 drops roman chamomile oil in a 10ml roller bottle; fill remainder with carrier oil. Apply topically.

ECSTASY EXTENDER MASSAGE BLEND
Combine 2 drops geranium oil with 1 drop each cinnamon, ginger, lemongrass, and peppermint oil in a 2-ounce glass bottle with a orifice reducer; fill remainder with fractionated coconut oil. Blend supports reaching and prolonging climax. Use 10-15 drops at a time and massage lightly on genitals.

KISS AND MAKE UP: Combine 6 drops clove, 2 drops lemon oil, and 2 drops frankincense. Use blend to "diffuse" an argument or calm a partner. Diffuse or apply topically with a carrier oil.

LET'S GET IT ON - a men's formula
6 drops sandalwood
4 drops ylang ylang
2 drops clary sage
2 drops wild orange
Combine and apply to pressure points, or diffuse.

MOOD MAKER: Combine 1 drop each cinnamon, patchouli, rosemary, sandalwood, white fir, and ylang ylang oil. Diffuse to set the mood.

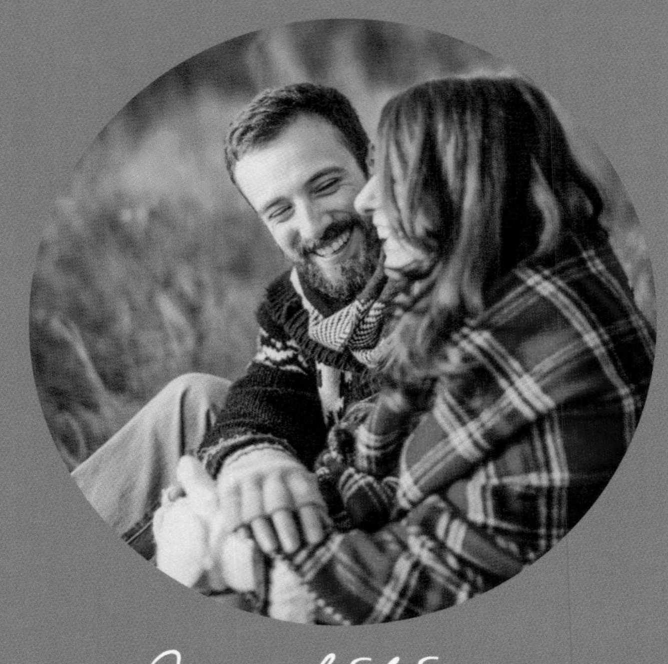

Conditions

Depressed - bergamot, rose, wild orange, ylang ylang, encouraging blend, joyful blend, women's monthly blend; see *Mood & Behavior*
Emotional issues, female sexuality - clary sage, jasmine, roman chamomile, rose, ylang ylang, encouraging blend, women's blend; see *Mood & Behavior*
Endometriosis - basil, clary sage, frankincense, ginger, lemon, rosemary,, sandalwood, thyme, ylang ylang, metabolic blend; see *Women's Health*
Exhaustion/fatigue - arborvitae, bergamot, cinnamon, cypress, grapefruit, peppermint, wild orange, cellular complex blend, detoxification blend, encouraging blend, inspiring blend; see *Energy & Vitality*
Frigidity - cinnamon, rose, ylang ylang, inspiring blend, reassuring blend; see *Mood & Behavior*
Headache - cinnamon, frankincense, geranium, lavender, peppermint, rose, wintergreen, tension blend; see *Pain & Inflammation*
Hemorrhoids - cypress, helichrysum, myrrh, roman chamomile, sandalwood, detoxification blend, digestion blend; see *Cardiovascular*
Impotence - cinnamon, clary sage, cypress, geranium, ginger, rose, sandalwood, ylang ylang, cleansing blend, comforting blend, inspiring blend, massage blend, women's blend; see *Men's Health*
Lack of confidence - bergamot, cedarwood, jasmine, lime, melissa, rose, focus blend, invigorating blend; see *Mood & Behavior*
Lack of nitric oxide - cinnamon, Oil Touch technique
Oxytocin production - clary sage, fennel, geranium, myrrh, ylang ylang
Sex drive, excessive - arborvitae, marjoram
Sex drive, low (low libido) - black pepper, cardamom, cassia, cinnamon, clary sage, clove, coriander, geranium, ginger, jasmine, juniper berry, patchouli, peppermint, ravensara, roman chamomile, rose, rosemary, sandalwood, spearmint, thyme, vetiver, wild orange, ylang ylang, comforting blend, inspiring blend, reassuring blend, renewing blend, uplifting blend, women's blend; see *Men's Health* and *Women's Health*
Tension - geranium, ginger, jasmine, lavender, lemongrass, peppermint, rose, wild orange, wintergreen, ylang ylang, calming blend, tension blend; see *Muscular*
Vaginal dryness - clary sage, grounding blend
Warming, localized - bergamot, birch, cassia, cinnamon, clary sage, juniper berry, lavender, lemon, rosemary, vetiver, white fir, wintergreen; see *Cardiovascular*
Yeast infection - basil, clary sage, coriander, frankincense, lemon, melaleuca; see *Candida*

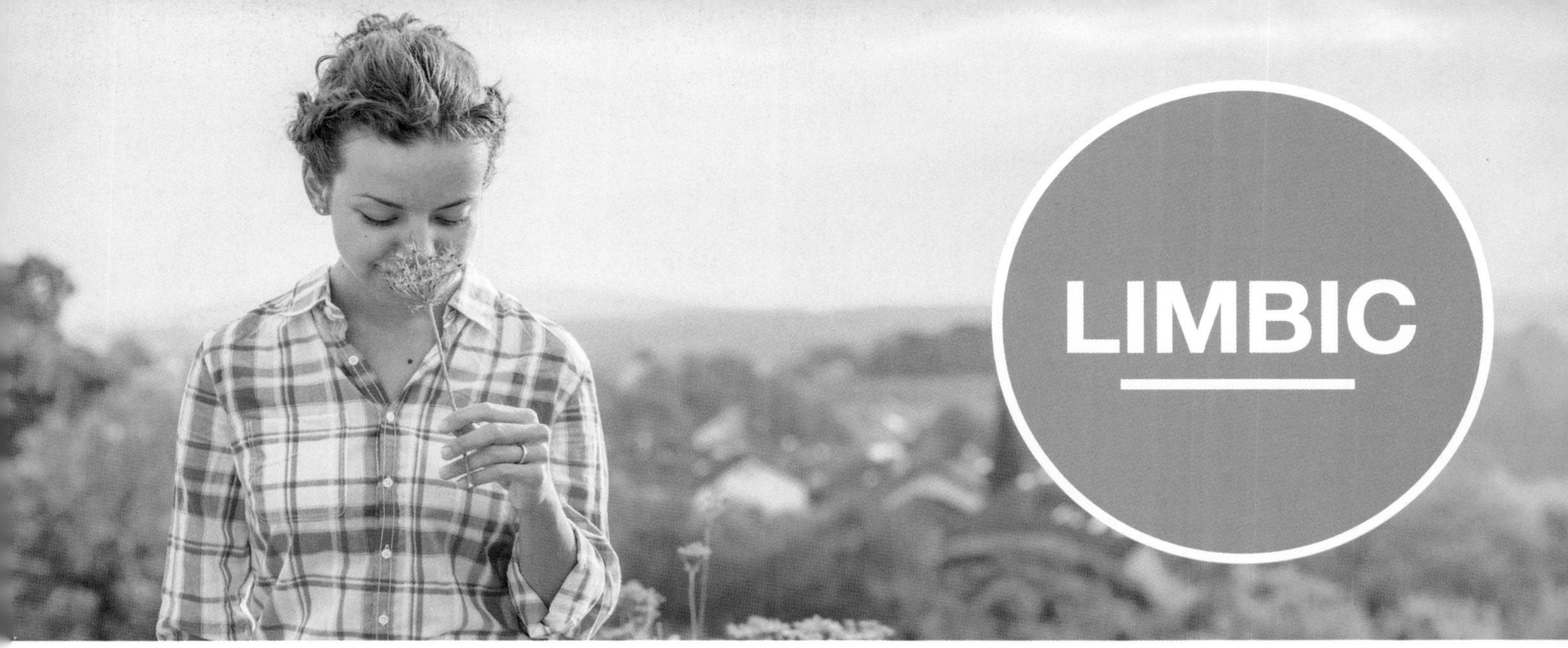

LOCATED IN THE CENTER of both hemispheres of the brain just under the cerebrum, the limbic system includes the amygdala, hippocampus, hypothalamus, olfactory cortex, and thalamus. The limbic system is a busy part of the brain, responsible for regulating both our emotional lives and higher mental functions such as learning, motivation, formulating and storing memories, controlling adrenaline and autonomic response, and regulating hormones and sexual response, sensory perception (optical and olfactory), and motor function.

Since the limbic system is involved in so many of the body's activities, and because it works so closely with several other systems, the actual anatomical parts of the limbic system are somewhat controversial. It is the reason there is pleasure in activities such as eating and sexual intimacy, and why stress manifests in the physical body and directly impacts health.

The limbic system is directly responsible for the processes of intercellular communication that affect how an individual responds to situations and all sensory stimuli and forms and stores memories about those situations and the resulting emotions. The limbic system works closely with the endocrine system to help with hormone regulation. It partners with the autonomic nervous system, the part of the body responsible for the "fight-or-flight" response, that helps the body recuperate during periods of rest, that regulates heart rate and body temperature, and that controls gastrointestinal functions. It also works with the nucleus accumbens, the pleasure center of the brain which is involved with sexual arousal and euphoric response to recreational drugs.

Deep in the core of the limbic system lies the amygdala, which is involved in many of the limbic activities listed above. It serves as the "watchtower," evaluating situations to help the brain recognize potential threats and prepare for fight-or-flight reactions. One of the ways it performs its duties is through the sense of smell. Aromas, via the olfactory system, have a quick, unfiltered route to the amygdala where emotions and memories are stored. Why? Because the sense of smell is necessary for survival.

The sense of smell is one of the more complex and discerning senses and is ten thousand times more powerful than our sense of taste. Aromas have a direct and profound effect on the deepest levels of the body systems, emotions, and psyche. Interestingly, we have only three types of receptors for sight, but an amazing one hundred distinct classes of smell receptors. We can distinguish an infinite number of smells even at very low concentrations. It is the ONLY sense linked directly to the limbic brain. The response is instant and so are the effects on the brain's mental and emotional responses and our body chemistry.

Herein lies the power and beauty of using essential oils for limbic health. Their aromas are one hundred to ten thousand times more concentrated and more potent than the solid form of a plant. Due to their unique ability to bypass the blood-brain barrier and their concentrated aromatic compounds, pure essential oils can provide significant benefits to individuals who desire to improve limbic system function.

When inhaled, essential oils enter the olfactory system and directly affect the amygdala and therefore impact mood and emotional response; thus they can be beneficial in reprogramming the significance that individuals have attached to past experiences and can initiate rapid responses both physically and emotionally in the brain and the rest of the body. Inhalation of essential oils with the resulting aromatic exposure is the most effective method of impacting the brain.

It is important to know that many apparently physical and seemingly unrelated symptoms are associated with limbic system imbalance because activities of the limbic system are so deeply integrated with other body systems. For any other related condition not listed in this section, see the corresponding body system in which the symptom tends to occur. For example, chronic fatigue - see *Energy & Vitality*; anxiety, depression, or irritability - see *Mood & Behavior*.

Specific sections in this book are complementary to the topic of limbic health. See *Addictions, Eating Disorders*, and *Mood & Behavior* following this section and *Emotional Usage* later in the book.

TOP SOLUTIONS

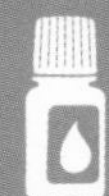

SINGLE OILS

Melissa - reduces depression and supports trauma recovery (pg. 118)

Juniper berry - helps release fears, trauma, and nightmares (pg. 107)

Frankincense - balances brain activity; supports a sense of protection, safety and releases traumatic memories (pg. 100)

Patchouli - sedates, grounds, stabilizes; supports central nervous system (pg. 121)

By Related Properties

For definitions of the properties listed below and more oil options, see Oil Properties Glossary (pg. 435) and Oil Properties (pg. 436).

Antidepressant - frankincense, lavender, melissa, vetiver
Calming - frankincense, melissa, patchouli, sandalwood, vetiver
Grounding - cedarwood, clary sage, cypress, vetiver, ylang ylang
Relaxing - cedarwood, clary sage, cypress, lavender, myrrh, ravensara, roman chamomile, white fir, ylang ylang
Sedative - bergamot, cedarwood, clary sage, frankincense, lavender, melissa, patchouli, rose, sandalwood, vetiver, ylang ylang

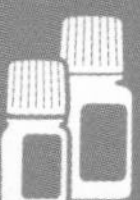

BLENDS

Calming blend - calms feelings of fear, anger, jealousy, and rage (pg. 142)

Uplifting blend - brings feelings of cheerfulness, optimism and positivity (pg. 166)

Encouraging blend - stimulates self-belief, courage and confidence (pg. 148)

Joyful blend - stabilizes mood and promotes courage and cheerfulness (pg. 154)

Grounding blend - calms an overactive mind; promotes sense of connectivity (pg. 150)

Related Ailments: Electrical Hypersensitivity Syndrome, Focal Brain Dysfunction (brain injury), Gulf War Syndrome, Hallucinations, Hypersexuality (excessive sex drive), Obsessive Compulsive Disorder, Post Traumatic Stress Disorder (PTSD)

Examples of other ailments that are associated with limbic imbalance:
Chronic Fatigue Syndrome - see *Energy & Vitality*
Fibromyalgia - see *Muscular*
Food Sensitivity - see *Allergies*
Chronic Pain - see *Pain & Inflammation*

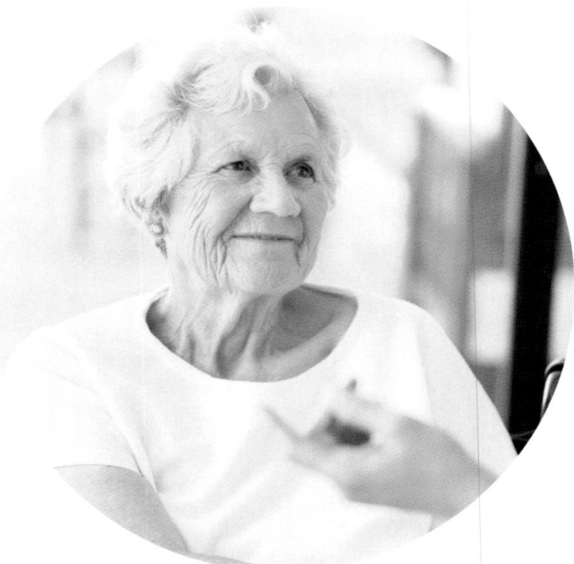

Conditions

Bipolar disorder - bergamot, cedarwood, frankincense, lavender, melissa, vetiver, calming blend, grounding blend, invigorating blend, joyful blend; see *Mood & Behavior*

Delusions (false belief) - clary sage, frankincense, juniper berry, helichrysum, patchouli, vetiver, encouraging blend, grounding blend, inspiring blend, joyful blend, soothing blend

Environmental sensitivity (in addition to removing the stressors) - lemongrass, ylang ylang, calming blend, cellular complex blend, grounding blend

Excessive sex drive - arborvitae, marjoram

Hallucinations - cedarwood, cilantro (small amounts), clove, coriander (small amounts), frankincense, juniper berry, melissa, myrrh, sandalwood, thyme, vetiver, cellular complex blend, focus blend, grounding blend

Nightmares - cinnamon, clary sage, cypress, dill, eucalyptus, geranium, grapefruit, juniper berry, lavender, melissa, roman chamomile, white fir, wild orange, vetiver, ylang ylang, calming blend, grounding blend, joyful blend; see *Sleep*

Obsessive/compulsive thoughts/behaviors - bergamot, black pepper, cypress, frankincense, geranium, lavender, patchouli, sandalwood, vetiver, ylang ylang, calming blend, focus blend, grounding blend, joyful blend, renewing blend

Overreacting - cedarwood, clary sage, melissa, roman chamomile, sandalwood, vetiver, wintergreen, grounding blend, protective blend, repellent blend

Psychiatric conditions (not a substitute for medical care) - jasmine, melissa, patchouli, sandalwood, calming blend, focus blend, grounding blend, joyful blend

PTSD/Stress, traumatic (past, present) - cedarwood, frankincense, helichrysum, jasmine, lavender, melissa, patchouli, roman chamomile, sandalwood, vetiver, wild orange, ylang ylang, calming blend, encouraging blend, grounding blend, invigorating blend, joyful blend, renewing blend, soothing blend; see *Stress*

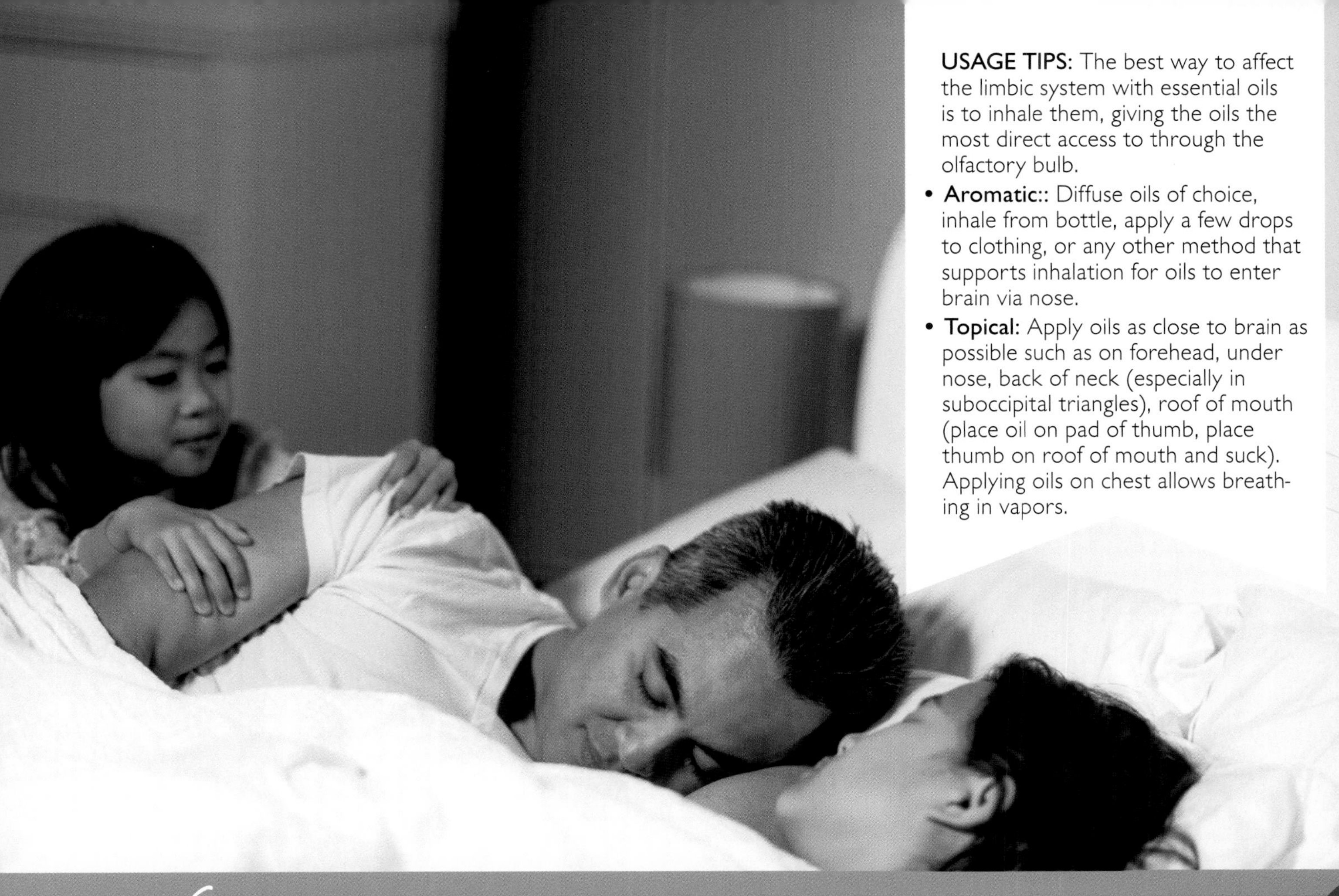

USAGE TIPS: The best way to affect the limbic system with essential oils is to inhale them, giving the oils the most direct access to through the olfactory bulb.

- **Aromatic::** Diffuse oils of choice, inhale from bottle, apply a few drops to clothing, or any other method that supports inhalation for oils to enter brain via nose.
- **Topical:** Apply oils as close to brain as possible such as on forehead, under nose, back of neck (especially in suboccipital triangles), roof of mouth (place oil on pad of thumb, place thumb on roof of mouth and suck). Applying oils on chest allows breathing in vapors.

Remedies

BIPOLAR BLENDS: Best used aromatically (inhale, diffuse); topically on back of neck, on wrists.

- Recipe #1: 3 drops bergamot and 2 drops clary sage
- Recipe #2: 1 drop lavender oil, 1 drop ylang ylang oil and 3 drops grapefruit
- Recipe #3: 2 drops frankincense, 1 drop lemon and 2 drops jasmine

POST TRAUMATIC STRESS BLEND: Combine 2 drops each cedarwood, frankincense, sandalwood, lavender, vetiver oils with a small amount of carrier oil and apply to back of neck, forehead, and bottoms of feet.

RELEASING OBSESSIONS & COMPULSIONS: In a 5 ml roller bottle, place 20 patchouli + 30 grounding blend (or other oils as desired) and apply behind ears, on wrists, bottoms of feet two or three times daily. If aroma is inviting, drop 2-3 drops of each individual oil on palms of hands, cup over nose, and inhale deeply.

NIGHTMARES BE GONE

- Dilute 1 drop juniper berry with 1 teaspoon fractionated coconut oil for children. Apply to back of neck, forehead, behind ears, bottoms of feet
- Diffuse juniper berry in bedroom at bedtime.

CLEAR MINDED
3 drops frankincense
3 drops ylang ylang
2 drops cedarwood
2 drops melissa
5 drops wild orange
Combine oils in a 10ml roller bottle and fill remainder of bottle with fractionated coconut oil. Roll onto forehead, back of neck, and inside of wrists.

RESET ENTHUSIASM : Combine 1 drop ylang ylang and 3 drops wild orange.

OH HAPPY DAY! Diffuse joyful blend throughout the day to promote a sense of joy and well-being.

OBSESS NO MORE: Apply focus blend to back of neck and forehead to support mind in letting go of obsessive thoughts and focusing instead on what really matters.

PEACEFUL PERFUME
3 drops ylang ylang
2 drops geranium
1 drop patchouli
1 drop juniper berry
Combine oils in a 10ml roller bottle; fill remainder with fractionated coconut oil. Roll onto forehead, back of neck, and inside of wrists.

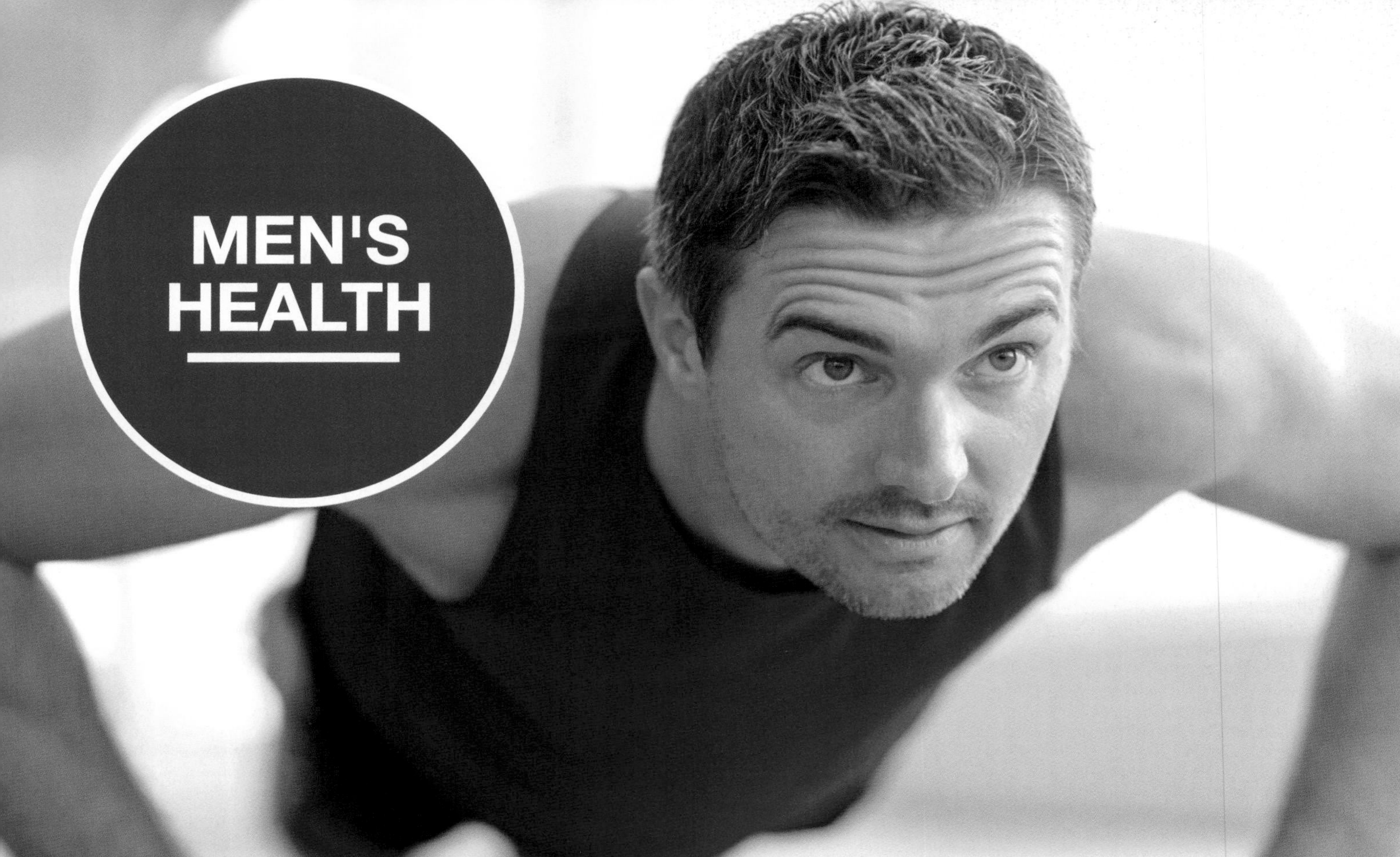

MEN'S HEALTH encompasses issues that are unique to men as well as those that are particularly common and challenging for the male gender.

The primary sex organs in the male reproductive system have dual functions. The testes produce sperm and the hormone testosterone. The penis allows sperm access to the female reproductive system during intercourse and also serves an excretory function for urine. Testosterone is primarily secreted by the testicles in men, and small amounts are also secreted by the adrenal glands. It is the principal male sex hormone and an anabolic steroid. It is responsible for the development of the testes and prostate as well as secondary sex characteristics, including increased muscle and bone mass, body hair, and a deeper voice. Testerone levels gradually decrease over a man's lifetime.

The prostate located beneath the bladder and connects the bladder and seminal vesicles to the penis. It produces part of the seminal fluid that is alkaline, which helps lengthen the life of sperm as they enter the vagina. It also has involuntary muscles that contract to expel the sperm during ejaculation. Normally it is a little larger than a walnut in size, but the cells that make up the prostate continue to multiply throughout a man's life. The enlarged organ can become a problem (benign prostatic hyperplasia) if it pinches off the urethra that runs through it, causing difficulty in emptying the bladder. Symptoms include urgency to urinate, hesitancy, frequency, incontinence, and an inability to completely empty the bladder. This can also lead to infection, stones, damaged bladder and kidneys, and erectile dysfunction. As men age they are at greater risk for prostate cancer as well. Next to skin cancer, prostate cancer is the most common cancer in men.

Sexual health is important for a healthy lifestyle. The ability for a man to participate in intercourse depends on hormones, the brain, nerves, and blood vessels that supply the penis. For an erection to occur all these mechanisms need to be in place. Erectile dysfunction or impotence can be caused by a complication in any of these areas and may be attributed to diabetes, peripheral vascular disease, smoking, medications, prostate cancer, and more.

As far as general health goes, compared to women, men make more risky or unhealthy choices, smoke and drink more, and put off making health decisions. Some of the most common health issues men deal with are heart disease, high blood pressure, liver disease, influenza and pneumococcal infection, skin cancer, and diabetes (which can contribute to impotence and low testosterone levels, which can in turn contribute to depression and anxiety). Regardless of the cause, many men suffer from depression that goes untreated. This can be a byproduct of a decline in physical health. Self confidence is often at stake when a man does not feel healthy. It is common for men to hide negative emotions as they continue to function on a daily basis.

Since men are independent by nature, empowering themselves with knowledge and practical application of natural remedies can help them reduce health risks while managing mood and helping the body maintain better overall health.

TOP SOLUTIONS

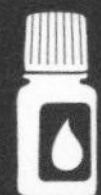

SINGLE OILS

Frankincense - promotes longevity, supports brain and prostate health (pg. 100)
Melaleuca - fights bacteria and fungus with antiseptic action (pg. 116)
Juniper berry - supports urinary and prostate health, wound healing (pg. 107)
Cardamom - supports digestive, muscular, and respiratory health (pg. 82)
Lemon - detoxifies and has an alkalizing effect (pg. 110)

By Related Properties

For definitions of the properties listed below and more oil options, see Oil Properties Glossary (pg. 435) and Oil Properties (pg. 436).

Anti-inflammatory - arborvitae, basil, bergamot, birch, black pepper, cardamom, cassia, cedarwood, cinnamon, coriander, cypress, dill, eucalyptus, frankincense, geranium, ginger, helichrysum, jasmine, lavender, lemongrass, lime, melaleuca, melissa, myrrh, oregano, patchouli, peppermint, roman chamomile, sandalwood, spearmint, spikenard, wild orange, wintergreen
Cardiotonic - cassia, cypress, ginger, lavender, marjoram
Restorative - basil, frankincense, lime, patchouli, rosemary, sandalwood, spearmint
Steroidal - basil, bergamot, birch, cedarwood, clove, fennel, patchouli, rosemary, thyme

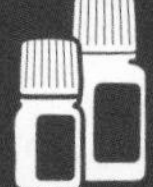

BLENDS

Grounding blend - makes great cologne, aftershave; brain support (pg. 150)
Protective blend - supports cardiovascular and immune health (pg. 158)
Detoxification blend - supports urinary, prostate; prevents hair loss (pg. 146)
Cellular complex blend - assists with cellular repair and longevity (pg. 143)

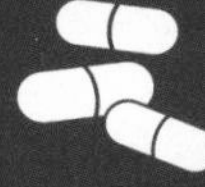

SUPPLEMENTS

Cellular vitality complex (pg. 171), energy & stamina complex (pg. 174), essential oil cellular complex (pg. 174), essential oil omega complex (pg. 175), polyphenol complex (pg. 181), whole food nutrient supplement (pg. 183)

Related Ailments: Abnormal Sperm Morphology, Erectile Dysfunction, Impotence, Infertility, Libido (low) for Men, Prostate, Prostate Problems, Prostatitis, Testes, Testosterone (low)

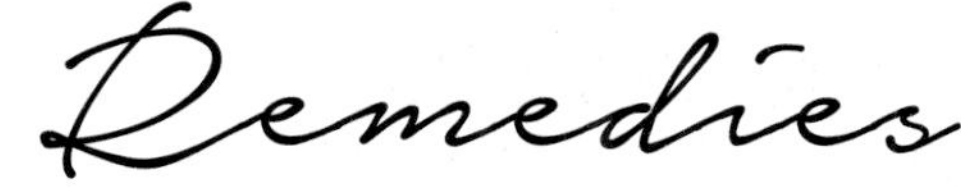

Remedies

GIDDY UP (**for erectile dysfunction**): Restore: Apply anti-aging blend to genital area two to three times daily.
- Encourage and stimulate hormonal balance: 1 drop sandalwood, 2 drops clary sage, and 1 drop ylang ylang. Apply topically on lower abdomen; diffuse; take internally in a gel capsule.
- Circulation support: Apply 1-2 drops cypress or massage blend to inner thighs and lower abdomen.
- Anxiety and stress relief: Diffuse 1-2 drops of basil, lavender, or ylang ylang. Inhale in cupped hand, put a few drops on pillow.
- Support healthy nutrition: Take essential oil omega complex, whole food nutrient supplement.

PROSTATE RELIEF
- Apply 2-3 drops of grounding blend to bottoms of feet morning and evening before sleep.
- Consume 1-2 essential oil cellular complex blend softgels two to three times daily at mealtimes.
- Apply 2-3 drops cellular complex blend topically on feet (focusing on heel area), lower abdomen, and inner thigh. Add 2-3 drops of juniper berry on abdomen area. Dilute with carrier oil for sensitive skin. Apply morning and night.
- Consume 3-5 drops of frankincense under tongue morning and evening.

HAIR STAY THERE
24 drops rosemary
18 drops cedarwood
14 drops geranium
12 drops peppermint
8 drops lavender
40 drops carrier oil
Combine in 5ml bottle. Apply daily before bed or just after shower. Put 4-7 drops in palm of hand, dip fingertips, gently massage throughout scalp, paying special attention to thinning or balding spots.

EARTHY SPICE COLOGNE
18 drops bergamot
13 drops white fir
10 drops clove
8 drops lemon
Combine into 10ml roller bottle, top off with carrier oil, apply to pulse points.

LIME DELIGHT COLOGNE
2 drops lime
1 drop vetiver
Rub vetiver over heart, layer lime over top, dilute with carrier oil for sensitive skin.

AFTERSHAVE: Use anti-aging blend in a roller bottle and add 1-2 drops frankincense and lavender for sensitive skin relief. Rub together in palm, then apply gently to the neck and face in an upward motion.

Conditions

Baldness - cedarwood, cypress, geranium, lavender, rosemary, thyme, ylang ylang, comforting blend, detoxification blend, women's blend

Dihydrotestosterone, levels too high (male pattern baldness, enlarged prostate) - see "Testosterone (DHT), high" below

Estrogen dominance - basil, clove, lemongrass, thyme, cleansing blend

Genital warts - arborvitae, frankincense, lemongrass, thyme, anti-aging blend, joyful blend

Hormones, imbalanced - frankincense, geranium, rosemary, ylang ylang, cellular complex blend, comforting blend, detoxification blend, uplifting blend, women's blend

Impotence - cassia, clary sage, clove, cypress, dill, douglas fir, ginger, jasmine, sandalwood, ylang ylang, cellular complex blend, detoxification blend, massage blend

Impatience - grounding blend; see *Mood & Behavior*

Infertility - basil, cinnamon, clary sage, geranium, jasmine, melissa, thyme, cellular complex blend, detoxification blend

Jock itch - cypress, lavender, melaleuca; see *Candida*

Prostate issues - basil, cinnamon, fennel, frankincense, helichrysum, jasmine, juniper berry, myrrh, rosemary, cellular complex blend, inspiring blend, uplifting blend

Prostate, congested - cinnamon, cypress, juniper berry, lemon, rosemary, cellular complex blend, detoxification blend, inspiring blend

Prostate, enlarged - fennel; see *Detoxification*

Prostate, inflamed - basil, cypress, douglas fir, eucalyptus, juniper berry, lavender, roman chamomile, rosemary, sandalwood, thyme, cellular complex blend, massage blend, protective blend

Prostate infection - oregano, thyme; see *Immune & Lymphatic*

Semen production, low - rose, cellular complex blend, cleansing blend, detoxification blend, women's blend

Sperm count, low - cedarwood, geranium, ginger, juniper berry

Testosterone, low - cassia, clary sage, ginger, myrrh, sandalwood, women's blend

Testosterone (DHT), high - juniper berry, rosemary, cellular complex blend

USAGE TIPS: Best results for men's health:

- **Get oils in, on and around you.** Start with a couple drops per day and go from there.
- **Use common sense.** Whether its taking oils in a capsule, glass of water, or under tongue for internal use; using as an aftershave, applying them to bottoms of feet or on an area of concern for topical use; smelling or diffusing them for aromatic purposes, enjoy the benefits to all aspect of men's health.

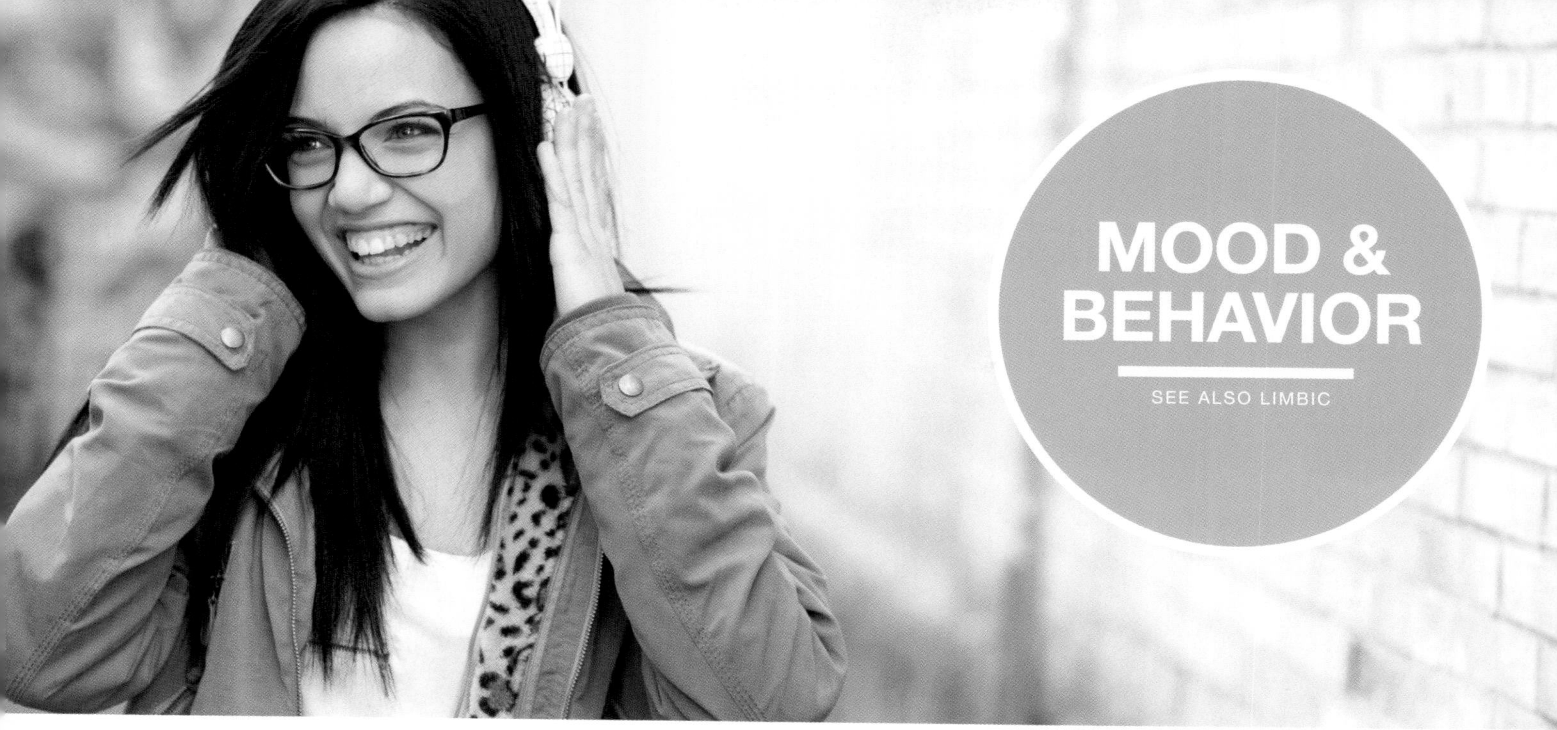

MOOD CHALLENGES and disorders are becoming more prevalent, especially in industrialized nations where computers, technology, and other conveniences have become a way of life. People are increasingly disconnected in their personal relationships, but they may have upward of half a million "friends" on social media sites, and it isn't uncommon to see teenagers texting each other, rather than conversing, while standing right next to each other!

Digestive issues and disorders are rampant, in part because of the refined and processed foods that many individuals eat. In recent years, scientists have discovered that there are more neurotransmitters in the gut than there are in the brain, and, among other things, healthy mood management depends on how well these neurotransmitters relay messages to each other. How can an individual hope to experience healthy moods if their cells are depleted of nutrition, their emotional needs for social connection are unmet, and if their neurotransmitters reside in an area with blockages and inflammation? The list of contributors to mood challenges is extensive.

The limbic system in the brain has glands that help relay and respond to emotions. It includes the amygdala, hippocampus, hypothalamus, and thalamus. The hippocampus, specifically, is involved in storing memories and producing emotions. It works effectively at full capacity when it is producing new neurons and solid nerve connections to assist with these key activities. When an individual experiences stress, the blood flow around the hippocampus changes – and individuals in their later years can often experience up to 20% loss in the nerve connections of the hippocampus, which can drastically affect mood and memory.

One of the challenges with balancing brain functions is that the brain is well-protected by a layer of high density cells called the blood-brain barrier that restricts passage of all but a small, select group of substances. This is actually a good thing; this layer of cells helps keep neurotoxins, viruses, and other invaders out of the control center of the body. Among the few substances that can bypass this barrier are natural fat-soluble substances such as sesquiterpenes, a compound found in many essential oils.

Since the brain is the origin and relayer of messages that produce emotions, and the brain functions on a chemical level, it stands to reason that natural remedies with strong chemical messages (signal or messenger molecules) can help balance and cleanse the very processes that need assistance. Essential oils can assist with cleansing and balancing the GI tract (see *Digestive & Intestinal*, *Detoxification* sections for further information), benefit brain functions, specifically those involving focus, concentration (see *Focus & Concentration*), mood, and memory with both aromatic and topical application.

When inhaled, natural aromatic compounds enter the olfactory system and pass the olfactory bulb, which leads directly to the limbic center of the brain. Oils can be inhaled by smelling directly from the bottle, rubbing a drop of essential oil in the palms of the hands and cupping over the nose, or by utilizing a diffuser (a device that disperses essential oils into the air.) Inhalation is the fastest way to get an essential oil into the body and has significant benefits on mood as it alters the chemical messages being relayed within the limbic system.

When applying essential oils topically to assist mood, it is important to get the oils as close to the limbic system as possible and apply them where they can best bypass the blood-brain barrier. Directly below the base of the skull, on both sides of the neck, there is an "indentation" that can be felt with the fingers. This area is called the suboccipital triangle, and when pure essential oils are applied here, they are able to enter the circulatory system of the brain prior to entering the circulatory system of the body. Oils may also be topically applied on the mastoid bones behind the ears, across the front of the forehead, directly under the nose, and may even be applied to the roof of the mouth (place oil on pad of thumb and then place on roof of mouth) for more direct access to the limbic system.

TOP SOLUTIONS

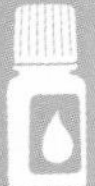

SINGLE OILS

Lavender - calms and relaxes, increases the ability to express feelings (pg. 108)

Wild orange - melts away anxiousness and energizes (pg. 136)

Cedarwood - grounds, promotes a sense of belonging and being connected socially (pg. 84)

Bergamot - helps increase self-confidence (pg. 79)

By Related Properties

For definitions of the properties listed below and more oil options, see Oil Properties Glossary (pg. 435) and Oil Properties (pg. 436).

Antidepressant - arborvitae, basil, bergamot, cinnamon, clary sage, coriander, dill, frankincense, geranium, grapefruit, jasmine, lavender, lemon, lemongrass, melissa, oregano, patchouli, ravensara, rose, sandalwood, wild orange, ylang ylang

Calming - bergamot, birch, black pepper, cassia, clary sage, coriander, fennel, frankincense, geranium, jasmine, juniper berry, lavender, melissa, oregano, patchouli, roman chamomile, sandalwood, tangerine, vetiver, yarrow

Energizing - basil, clove, cypress, grapefruit, lemongrass, rosemary, spearmint, white fir, wild orange

Grounding - arborvitae, basil, birch, cedarwood, clary sage, cypress, melaleuca, patchouli, vetiver, ylang ylang

Invigorating - grapefruit, lemon, peppermint, spearmint, wild orange, wintergreen

Relaxing - basil, cassia, cedarwood, clary sage, cypress, fennel, geranium, jasmine, lavender, marjoram, myrrh, ravensara, roman chamomile, white fir, ylang ylang

Sedative - basil, bergamot, cedarwood, clary sage, coriander, frankincense, geranium, jasmine, juniper berry, lavender, lemongrass, marjoram, melissa, patchouli, roman chamomile, rose, sandalwood, spikenard, vetiver, ylang ylang

Stimulant - arborvitae, basil, bergamot, birch, black pepper, cardamom, cedarwood, cinnamon, clove, coriander, cypress, dill, eucalyptus, fennel, ginger, grapefruit, juniper berry, lime, melaleuca, myrrh, patchouli, rosemary, spearmint, thyme, vetiver, white fir, wintergreen, ylang ylang

Uplifting - bergamot, cardamom, cedarwood, clary sage, cypress, grapefruit, lemon, lime, melissa, sandalwood, tangerine, wild orange, ylang ylang

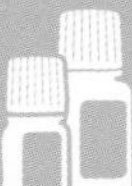

BLENDS

Invigorating blend - stimulates the mind and mood; encourages creativity (pg. 153)

Joyful blend - energizes, balances hormones; restores a sense of buoyancy (pg. 154)

Uplifting blend - promotes a cheerful, positive attitude (pg. 166)

Calming blend - encourages a restful state for mind and body (pg. 142)

Encouraging blend - stimulates belief, courage and confidence (pg. 148)

Grounding blend - promotes a state of balance and calm (pg. 150)

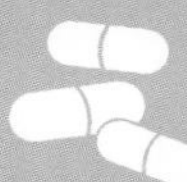

SUPPLEMENTS

Energy & stamina complex (pg. 174), essential oil cellular complex, **essential oil omega complex (pg. 175)**, food enzymes, **liquid omega-3 supplement (pg. 178)**, **phytoestrogen multiplex (pg. 180)**, whole food nutrient supplement

Related Ailments: Abuse trauma, Agitation, Agoraphobia, Anger, Anxiety, Apathy, Attachment Disorder (RAD), Depression, Emotional Trauma, Fear, Fear of Flying, Grief, Hysteria, Lack of Confidence, Mood Swings, Nervousness, Oppositional Defiant Disorder, Overwhelm, Panic Attacks, Seasonal Affective Disorder, Social Anxiety Disorder

USAGE TIPS: For best effect for mood and behavior

- **Aromatic:** Diffuse oils of choice, inhale from bottle, apply a few drops to clothing, or any other method that supports inhalation for oils to enter brain via nose.
- **Topical:** Apply oils as close to brain as possible such as on forehead, under nose, back of neck (especially in suboccipital triangles), roof of mouth (place oil on pad of thumb, place thumb on roof of mouth and suck). Applying oils on chest allows breathing in vapors.
- **Internal:** Place one to five drops of chosen oil in water to drink or take in a capsule, drop under tongue, lick a drop off back of hand, apply to roof of mouth (place oil on pad of thumb and then place pad on roof of mouth).

Conditions

Abandoned - birch, cilantro, clary sage, dill, frankincense, myrrh, focus blend, renewing blend
Abuse, healing from - frankincense, geranium, juniper berry, melissa, roman chamomile, ylang ylang, white fir, encouraging blend
Angry - bergamot, cardamom, cedarwood, frankincense, helichrysum, melissa, roman chamomile, rose, spearmint, thyme, wild orange, ylang ylang, calming blend, comforting blend, focus blend, grounding blend, protective blend, tension blend
Anxious - arborvitae, basil, bergamot, cedarwood, cilantro, clary sage, cypress, dill, douglas fir, frankincense, geranium, grapefruit, jasmine, juniper berry, lavender, lemon, lemongrass, lime, marjoram, melissa, patchouli, ravensara, roman chamomile, rose, sandalwood, tangerine, vetiver, wild orange, wintergreen, ylang ylang, calming blend, focus blend, grounding blend, tension blend, women's blend
Antisocial - black pepper, clove, oregano, lemongrass, patchouli, rosemary, spearmint, yarrow, cleansing blend
Apathetic/indifferent - basil, cardamom, eucalyptus, ginger, juniper berry, lemon, lime, melissa, patchouli, rosemary, vetiver, wild orange, ylang ylang, detoxification blend, encouraging blend, focus blend, joyful blend, respiration blend, uplifting blend
Betrayed/deceived - cardamom, cinnamon, lemon, juniper berry, marjoram, melissa, peppermint, rose, comforting blend, encouraging blend, women's blend
Blaming/bitter - arborvitae, cardamom, geranium, helichrysum, lemon, myrrh, ravensara, rosemary, oregano, thyme, wintergreen, cleansing blend, detoxification blend, skin clearing
Conflicted - clary sage, frankincense, geranium, juniper berry, patchouli, roman chamomile, rosemary, sandalwood, anti-aging blend, comforting blend, detoxification blend, women's blend
Confused - basil, cedarwood, cinnamon, clary sage, cypress, frankincense, ginger, jasmine, juniper berry, lemon, peppermint, patchouli, wild orange, encouraging blend, focus blend, invigorating blend, reassuring blend
Confidence, lack of/timid/self-rejection - bergamot, birch, coriander, dill, douglas fir, grapefruit, jasmine, juniper berry, melissa, patchouli, roman chamomile, rose, rosemary, spearmint, vetiver, yarrow, comforting blend, digestion blend, encouraging blend, focus blend, grounding blend, respiration blend, skin clearing blend, uplifting blend
Crying - cypress, frankincense, geranium, lavender, roman chamomile, rose, wild orange, white fir, ylang ylang, calming blend, comforting blend, grounding blend, joyful blend, uplifting blend
Denial/dishonest - birch, black pepper, cinnamon, coriander, grapefruit, juniper berry, lemongrass, marjoram, peppermint, thyme, cleansing blend, detoxification blend
Depressed/sad - basil, bergamot, cardamom, cinnamon, douglas fir, frankincense, geranium, grapefruit, helichrysum, jasmine, juniper berry, lavender, lemon, lemongrass, melissa, patchouli, peppermint, roman chamomile, rose, sandalwood, spearmint, rose, thyme, tangerine, vetiver, wild orange, ylang ylang, comforting blend, inspiring blend, invigorating blend, joyful blend, uplifting blend, women's monthly blend
Discernment, lack of/double-minded - arborvitae, basil, cinnamon, clary sage, frankincense, juniper berry, lavender, melissa, roman chamomile, rosemary, sandalwood, white fir
Disconnected - cedarwood, cinnamon, coriander, frankincense, marjoram, myrrh, rose, roman chamomile, white fir, wintergreen, vetiver, encouraging blend, grounding blend, joyful blend, women's blend
Distrusting/suspicious - black pepper, cedarwood, cilantro, eucalyptus, frankincense, lavender, marjoram, melaleuca, rose, spearmint, spikenard, white fir, encouraging blend, grounding blend, invigorating blend, respiration blend
Expression, lack of - birch, fennel, lavender, ravensara, roman chamomile, wild orange, inspiring blend, women's blend
Fearful/lack of courage - basil, bergamot, birch, black pepper, coriander, frankincense, jasmine, juniper berry, patchouli, ravensara, tangerine, wild orange, calming blend, comforting blend, detoxification blend, encouraging blend, grounding blend, protective blend, repellent blend
Frustrated - cardamom, lemongrass, rosemary, wintergreen, ylang ylang, calming blend, focus blend, women's blend
Grieving - bergamot, cedarwood, frankincense, geranium, helichrysum, marjoram, melissa, rose, sandalwood, tangerine, calming blend, grounding blend, joyful blend, soothing blend, respiration blend, women's blend
Heartbroken - clove, geranium, lime, spikenard, wild orange, ylang ylang, invigorating blend, joyful blend, women's blend
Hopeless - jasmine, lime, patchouli, rose, vetiver, wild orange, ylang ylang, joyful blend
Humiliated - bergamot, birch, cassia, fennel, grapefruit, myrrh, patchouli, ylang ylang, protective blend
Impatient - arborvitae, cardamom, cilantro, frankincense, grapefruit, lavender, lemongrass, marjoram, ravensara, roman chamomile, white fir, wintergreen, calming blend, tension blend
Indecisive - cassia, cinnamon, clove, marjoram, melaleuca, ravensara, rosemary, protective blend, detoxification blend, massage blend
Insecure/feeling unsafe or vulnerable - bergamot, clary sage, grapefruit, melaleuca, myrrh, ravensara, roman chamomile, yarrow, ylang ylang, massage blend, protective blend, respiration blend
Irritable/agitated - arborvitae, bergamot, coriander, geranium, lavender, lemon, roman chamomile, rose, wild orange, calming blend, comforting blend, renewing blend, repellent blend
Jealous - cinnamon, grapefruit, myrrh, patchouli, roman chamomile, rose, ylang ylang, white fir, calming blend
Melancholy - basil, bergamot, ginger, grapefruit, jasmine, lemon, lime, melissa, spearmint, tangerine, wild orange, invigorating blend, joyful blend
Night terrors/nightmares - juniper berry, melissa, roman chamomile, sandalwood, vetiver, joyful blend, protective blend, repellent blend
Obsessive/compulsive - arborvitae, clary sage, cedarwood, frankincense, grapefruit, jasmine, lavender, oregano, patchouli, roman chamomile, sandalwood, vetiver, ylang ylang, calming blend, focus blend, grounding blend, joyful blend
Overwhelmed/burdened - basil, clary sage, douglas fir, lemon, lemongrass, ravensara, rosemary, wild orange, ylang ylang, comforting blend, encouraging blend, focus blend, invigorating blend, joyful blend, tension blend
Over sensitive or reactive/defensive - clove, geranium, ginger, grapefruit, lavender, lemon, melaleuca, melissa, patchouli, roman chamomile, rosemary, vetiver, white fir, wintergreen, calming blend, protective blend, repellent blend, soothing blend, tension blend
Powerless, feeling - bergamot, cedarwood, cinnamon, coriander, dill, fennel, frankincense, ginger, grapefruit, jasmine, lime, melaleuca, rose, vetiver, white fir, wild orange, protective blend, women's blend
Rejected - bergamot, fennel, frankincense,

MOOD & BEHAVIOR

geranium, grapefruit, lime, myrrh, patchouli, invigorating blend, joyful blend, women's blend

Resentful - cardamom, frankincense, geranium, lemon, lemongrass, oregano, roman chamomile, thyme, cleansing blend

Restless - dill, lavender, lemon, patchouli, vetiver, white fir, calming blend, focus blend, grounding blend, reassuring blend, women's blend; see "Anxious" above

Selfish - arborvitae, cardamom, cedarwood, oregano, thyme, wild orange, wintergreen

Sexual Frustration - cinnamon, ylang ylang; see *Intimacy*

Shame, feel - bergamot, fennel, grapefruit, helichrysum, jasmine, lavender, oregano, vetiver, ylang ylang

Shocked - bergamot, frankincense, geranium, helichrysum, roman chamomile, focus blend; see *First Aid*

Sluggish/stuck - cypress, ginger, lemongrass, juniper berry, peppermint, rosemary, cellar complex blend, digestion blend, massage blend

Spiritual connection, lack of - cinnamon, frankincense, juniper berry, melissa, roman chamomile, sandalwood, spikenard, yarrow, joyful blend, renewing blend

Stiffnecked/arrogant - birch, cedarwood, cypress, lemongrass, oregano, thyme, wintergreen, massage blend, tension blend

Stubborn/willful/defiant/controlling - black pepper, cardamom, cedarwood, coriander, lemongrass, oregano, thyme, wintergreen, tension blend

Tense/uptight - basil, juniper berry, lavender, melissa, patchouli, vetiver, ylang ylang, calming blend, tension blend

Terror/panicked/hysterical - clary sage, jasmine, lavender, marjoram, melissa, patchouli, roman chamomile, spikenard, vetiver, wild orange, ylang ylang, calming blend, grounding blend, respiration blend

Traumatized - clove, frankincense, grapefruit, helichrysum, melissa, rose, spikenard, tangerine, vetiver, calming blend, grounding blend, reassuring blend, soothing blend

Weary/faint - cassia, cinnamon, lime, peppermint, rosemary, spearmint, wild orange, invigorating blend, joyful blend

Wounded, deep emotionally - birch, eucalyptus, frankincense, geranium, helichrysum, lime, myrrh, roman chamomile, rose, spikenard, white fir, anti-aging blend, cellular complex blend, encouraging blend, soothing blend, uplifting blend

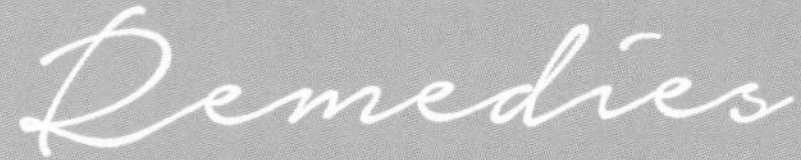

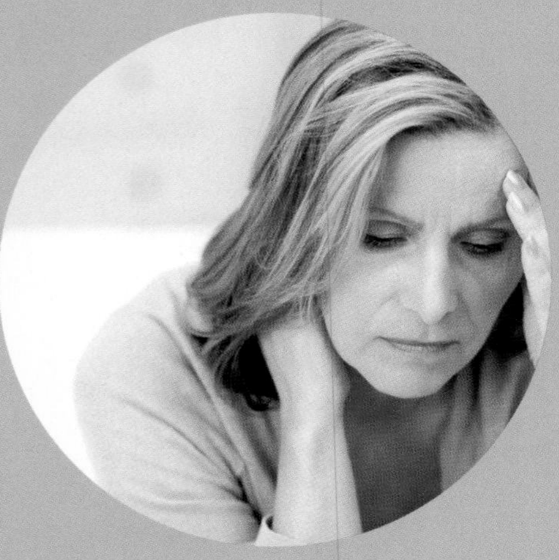

DIFFUSER BLENDS: Diffuse several times a day to manage issues and as needed for emotional support.

NOTE: Diffuser recipes can be made into topical blends. Place the oils for a particular blend into a roller bottle, multiplying the number of drops by approximately four; fill remainder with carrier oil and used on "perfume" points.

ORANGE YOU HAPPY
3 drops basil
3 drops wild orange

HEART'S DESIRES
3 drops jasmine
3 drops sandalwood
1 drop rose or geranium
1 drop sandalwood
1 drop wild orange or bergamot
1 drop ylang ylang

BRIGHTEN
3 drops bergamot
1 drop grapefruit
1 drop ylang ylang

REFRESH
2 drops bergamot
2 drops clary sage
1 drop frankincense

LIFT
3 drops bergamot or wild orange
2 drops clary sage
2 drops frankincense
1 drop jasmine or ylang ylang
1 drop lemon

UNCONDITIONAL LOVE
7 drop wild orange
4 drops frankincense
2 drops bergamot
1 drop ylang ylang
1 drop geranium
Combine in 10ml roller bottle; fill remainder with carrier oil; apply to pulse points, rub on neck, center of back, then cup hands together and inhale. For more potency, double the amount of oils in a 15ml bottle, fill remainder with carrier oil. Premix without carrier oil for use in a diffuser.

BETTER THAN BITTER AND BROODING
1 drop bergamot
1 drop helichrysum
1 drop roman chamomile
Put oil into palms, rub hands together vigorously, cup your hands together, and slowly inhale.

AGGRESSION-LESS (to reduce aggression)
4 drops bergamot
3 drops sandalwood
3 drops ylang ylang
2 drops lemon
2 drops white fir
Combine in 15ml bottle/roller bottle; fill with carrier oil. Put 4-5 drops in palms and rub on bottoms of feet and at base of rib cage over top of liver, cup hands together and slowly inhale.

NOT SO SAD: (reduce/eliminate effects of Seasonal Affective Disorder)
3 drops grapefruit
2 drops bergamot
Combine in hands, rub hands together and then rub on pulse points, back of neck into hairline and then slowly inhale. For a 5ml roller bottle blend and less intensity, follow same ratio, multiply by 4 for 12 and 8 drops respectively; fill with carrier oil; use throughout day.

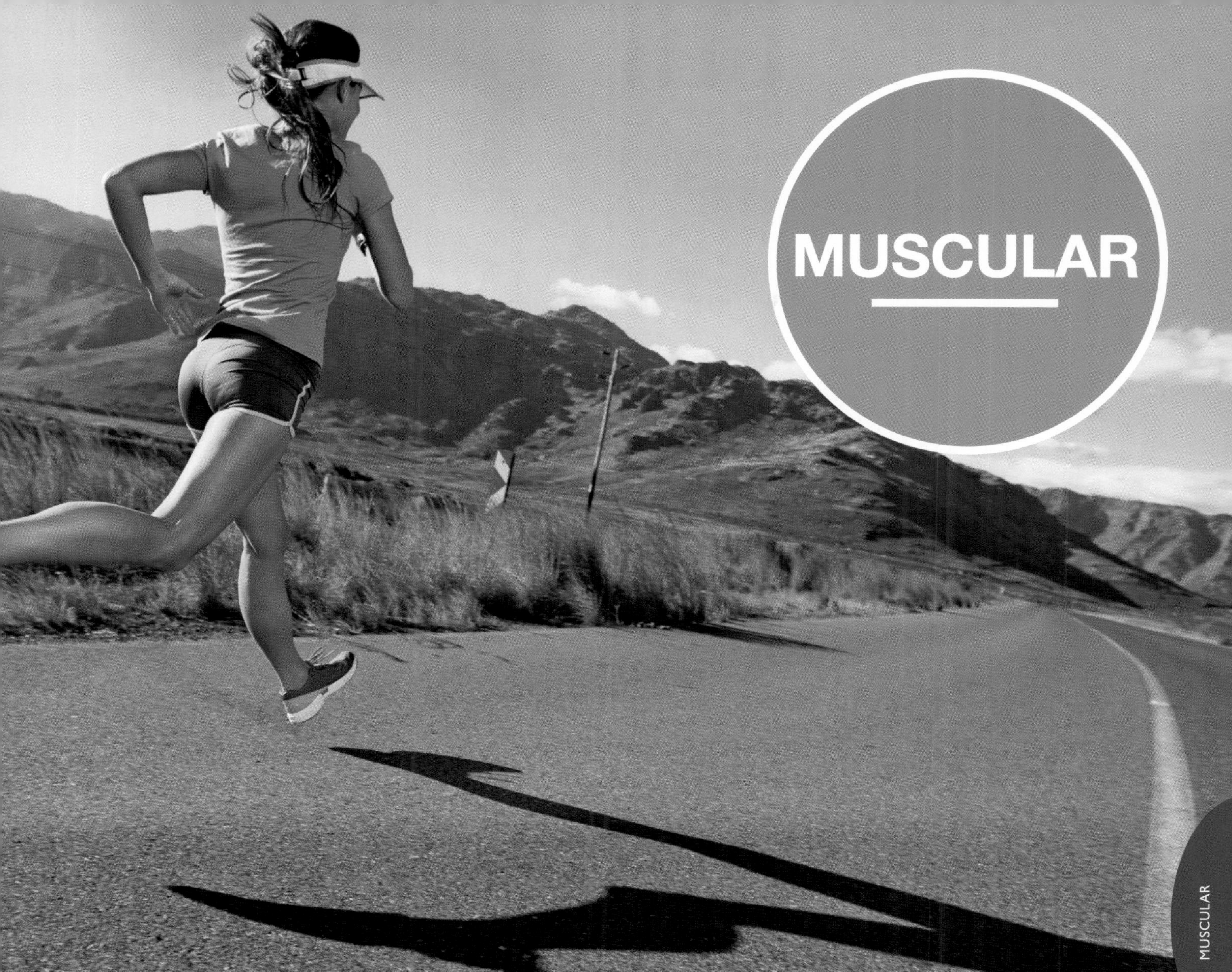

THE MUSCULAR SYSTEM consists of 650 muscles in three main categories: skeletal, smooth, and cardiac muscles. It is controlled by the nervous system via two pathways: somatic and autonomic. Only skeletal muscles fall into the somatic category, meaning that they are under voluntary control; these are the muscles attached to the skeleton. They are striated in appearance and provide strength, balance, posture, movement, and heat for the body.

Tendons are bands of fibrous tissue attached to the skeletal muscles that allow movement in the body. When a skeletal muscle contracts, it pulls on the tendon to which it is attached, causing the tendon to pull on the bone and resulting in movement. Ligaments, on the other hand, are the fibrous material that connects bone to bone and holds the skeletal structure together. Once injured, both require long healing times and are prone to weakness or re-injury. Rest is required, as scar tissue usually takes at least ninety days to form; once formed, the fibers can take up to another seven to nine months to reach maximum strength again.

Autonomic muscles contract and relax involuntarily and include both smooth and cardiac muscles. Smooth muscles are non-striated and are typically found in layers, one behind the other. They can be found in the walls of internal organs (excluding the heart), such as blood vessels, intestines, bladder, digestive system, and stomach. They are constantly at work, performing their functions throughout the body.

Cardiac muscles are specific to the heart and are also known as myocardium. These involuntary muscles contract to pump blood through the heart, then relax to allow blood to return after it has carried vital oxygen and nutrients to the body.

The muscular system is constantly in motion and supporting vital body functions. Essential oils have a unique ability to affect muscles and connective tissue and to support muscle function on a cellular level. Once oils are applied, users often experience near-instant relief. Minor issues and injuries are easily managed with either topical and internal application. For more serious muscle and tendon issues, professional medical care is appropriate. Traditional treatment methods can be enhanced and supported with essential oil and nutritional supplement solutions.

TOP SOLUTIONS

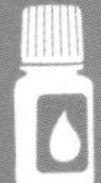

SINGLE OILS

Lemongrass - soothes muscle aches, supports connective tissue repair (pg. 112)
Cypress - promotes blood flow to muscle and connective tissue, reduces pain and spasms (pg. 93)
Marjoram - relaxes muscles and decreases spasms (pg. 114)
Ginger - reduces spasms and muscle aches and pain (pg. 103)

By Related Properties

For definitions of the properties listed below and more oil options, see Oil Properties Glossary (pg. 435) and Oil Properties (pg. 436).

Analgesic - basil, bergamot, birch, black pepper, cinnamon, clove, coriander, eucalyptus, fennel, frankincense, helichrysum, juniper berry, lavender, lemongrass, marjoram, melaleuca, oregano, peppermint, rosemary, white fir, wintergreen
Anticonvulsant - clary sage, fennel, geranium, lavender, tangerine
Anti-inflammatory - arborvitae, basil, birch, black pepper, cardamom, cassia, cedarwood, cinnamon, coriander, cypress, dill, eucalyptus, fennel, frankincense, geranium, ginger, helichrysum, jasmine, lavender, lemongrass, lime, melaleuca, melissa, myrrh, oregano, patchouli, peppermint, roman chamomile, rosemary, sandalwood, spearmint, spikenard, wild orange, wintergreen, yarrow
Antispasmodic - basil, bergamot, birch, black pepper, cardamom, cassia, cinnamon, clary sage, clove, coriander, cypress, dill, eucalyptus, fennel, ginger, helichrysum, jasmine, juniper berry, lavender, lemon, lime marjoram, melissa, patchouli, peppermint, ravensara, roman chamomile, rosemary, sandalwood, spearmint, tangerine, thyme, vetiver, wild orange, wintergreen, yarrow, ylang ylang
Energizing - clove, cypress, grapefruit, lemongrass, rosemary, white fir, wild orange
Relaxing - basil, cassia, cedarwood, clary sage, cypress, fennel, geranium, jasmine, lavender, marjoram, myrrh, ravensara, roman chamomile, white fir, ylang ylang
Regenerative - basil, cedarwood, clove, coriander, frankincense, geranium, helichrysum, jasmine, lavender, lemongrass, melaleuca, myrrh, patchouli, sandalwood, wild orange
Steroidal - basil, bergamot, birch, cedarwood, clove, fennel, patchouli, rosemary, thyme
Tonic - arborvitae, basil, bergamot, birch, cardamom, cedarwood, clary sage, coriander, cypress, eucalyptus, fennel, frankincense, geranium, ginger, grapefruit, juniper berry, lavender, lemon, lemongrass, lime, marjoram, melissa, myrrh, patchouli, roman chamomile, rose, rosemary, sandalwood, tangerine, thyme, vetiver, white fir, wild orange, yarrow, ylang ylang
Warming - birch, black pepper, cassia, cinnamon, clary sage, ginger, marjoram, peppermint, wintergreen

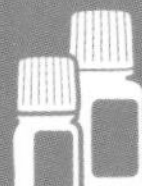

BLENDS

Massage blend - promotes circulation and relieves pain (pg. 155)
Soothing blend - soothes muscle and joint pain and inflammation (pg. 164)
Tension blend - soothes sore muscles and tissue; releases tension (pg. 165)
Cellular complex blend - helps with connective tissue repair and soothes pain (pg. 143)

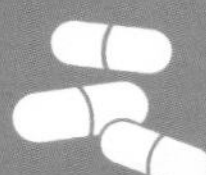

SUPPLEMENTS

Bone support complex (pg. 170), cellular vitality complex, detoxification complex, detoxification blend softgels, **energy & stamina complex (pg. 174)**, essential oil cellular complex, **essential oil omega complex (pg. 175)**, **polyphenol complex (pg. 181)**, whole food nutrient supplement

Related Ailments: Aches, Back Muscle Fatigue, Back Pain, Back Stiffness, Body Myositis, Bruised Muscles, Connective Tissue Trauma, Convulsions, Cramps/Charley Horse, Do Quervain's Tenosynovitis, Fibromyalgia, Frozen Shoulder, Growing Pains, Headache, Inflammatory Myopathies, Leg Cramps, Lumbago, Metabolic Muscle Disorders, Migraine, Muscle Pain, Muscle Spasms, Muscle Stiffness, Muscle Strains, Muscle Weakness, Muscular Dystrophy, Myasthenia Gravis, Myotonic Dystrophy, Neck Pain, Neuromuscular Disorders (drooping eyelids, double vision, slurred speech, difficulty swallowing, difficulty breathing), Over-exercised, Polymyositis, Rheumatism, Sore Feet, Sore Muscles, Sprains, Tendinitis, Tension, Tension Headache, Tissue Pain, Tissue Regeneration, Whiplash

Conditions

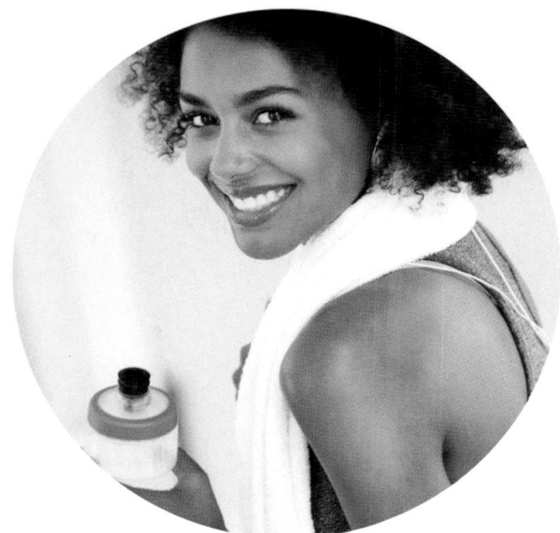

Bruising - birch, helichrysum, geranium, fennel, lavender, roman chamomile, white fir, massage blend

Circulation (increase) - basil, cypress, eucalyptus, lavender, marjoram, encouraging blend, massage blend, soothing blend, skin clearing blend; see *Cardiovascular*

Collagen, lack of - helichrysum, lemongrass, sandalwood

Connective tissue/fascia (tendons) - basil, birch, clary sage, clove, cypress, geranium, ginger, helichrysum, lavender, lemongrass, marjoram, oregano, peppermint, roman chamomile, rosemary, sandalwood, thyme, vetiver, white fir, wintergreen, massage blend, soothing blend, tension blend

Cramping/charley horse - arborvitae, basil, birch, black pepper, cardamom, cedarwood, cilantro, cinnamon, clary sage, clove, cypress, dill, grapefruit, jasmine, lavender, lemongrass, marjoram, peppermint, roman chamomile, rosemary, vetiver, white fir, wintergreen, detoxification blend, massage blend, reassuring blend, soothing blend, tension blend, uplifting blend

Fatigued/overused - basil, black pepper, cinnamon, cypress, douglas fir, eucalyptus, grapefruit, marjoram, peppermint, rosemary, thyme, white fir, cellular complex blend, detoxification blend, encouraging blend, massage blend

Fibromyalgia - basil, birch, clove, frankincense, marjoram, oregano, peppermint, ginger, helichrysum, lavender, roman chamomile, rosemary, thyme, white fir, wintergreen, cellular complex blend, detoxification blend, soothing blend

Headaches - frankincense, lavender, peppermint, wintergreen, soothing blend, tension blend, uplifting blend; see *Pain & Inflammation*

Headaches, migraine - basil, helichrysum, roman chamomile; see *Pain & Inflammation*

Heart - cassia, cinnamon, douglas fir, frankincense, geranium, marjoram, lavender, peppermint, rosemary, sandalwood, ylang ylang, massage blend

Hernia, inguinal - fennel, frankincense, ginger, helichrysum, lavender, vetiver

Inflammation, acute (with swelling, redness or pain) - basil, clary sage, clove, coriander, eucalyptus, frankincense, ginger, helichrysum, marjoram, peppermint, rosemary, sandalwood, white fir, wintergreen, massage blend, soothing blend, tension blend, uplifting blend; see *Pain & Inflammation*

Inflammation, chronic - basil, birch, cypress, eucalyptus, frankincense, marjoram, oregano, peppermint, patchouli, rosemary, sandalwood, vetiver, wintergreen, massage blend, soothing blend; see *Pain & Inflammation*

Injuries - birch, frankincense, helichrysum, lavender, lemongrass, myrrh, sandalwood, white fir, wintergreen, yarrow, massage blend, soothing blend

Muscle development - basil, birch, douglas fir, lemongrass, marjoram, rosemary, wintergreen, massage blend, soothing blend

Muscle, neuralgia - basil, douglas fir, eucalyptus, frankincense, lemongrass, marjoram, peppermint, rosemary, massage blend, soothing blend; see *Pain & Inflammation*

Neck pain - birch, cypress, eucalyptus, helichrysum, myrrh, peppermint, wintergreen, anti-aging blend, soothing blend, tension blend; see *Pain & Inflammation*

Numbness - arborvitae, basil, cypress, frankincense, ginger, lemongrass, patchouli, wintergreen, massage blend

Pain, burning/intense - cardamom, eucalyptus, frankincense, juniper berry, lime, oregano, cellular complex blend, detoxification blend, soothing blend, tension blend

Pain, dull/chronic - birch, helichrysum, lemongrass, marjoram, rosemary, wintergreen, anti-aging blend, massage blend, soothing blend; see *Pain & Inflammation*

Pain, sharp/acute - basil, birch, cypress, frankincense, ginger, lavender, lemongrass, marjoram, rosemary, vetiver, white fir, wintergreen, massage blend, soothing blend, tension blend; see *Pain & Inflammation*

Paralysis - basil, douglas fir, frankincense, ginger, lavender, lime, melissa, patchouli, peppermint, sandalwood, cellular complex blend, encouraging blend, massage blend, tension blend

Parkinson's disease - See *Brain, Addictions "Conditions Associated with Addictions"* - dopamine

Shoulder - basil, birch, cypress, helichrysum, marjoram, white fir, wintergreen, cellular complex blend, soothing blend

Spasms - basil, bergamot, black pepper, cypress, marjoram, melissa, peppermint, rosemary, thyme, encouraging blend, inspiring blend, massage blend, tension blend

Sprain/strain - birch, black pepper, clove, eucalyptus, frankincense, ginger, helichrysum, jasmine, lavender, lemongrass, marjoram, roman chamomile, rosemary, thyme, vetiver, white fir, wintergreen, massage blend, reassuring blend, soothing blend, tension blend

Tender tissues, swollen, red - frankincense, helichrysum, lemongrass, myrrh, wintergreen, detoxification blend, soothing blend, tension blend,

Tendons/tendonitis - lemongrass, white fir; see "Connective Tissue" above

Tension/stiffness, nervous - basil, bergamot, cedarwood, coriander, cypress, frankincense, ginger, grapefruit, helichrysum, lavender, lemongrass, marjoram, melissa, patchouli, peppermint, roman chamomile, rose, rosemary, sandalwood, vetiver, white fir, wild orange, wintergreen, ylang ylang, encouraging blend, inspiring blend, massage blend, reassuring blend, soothing blend, tension blend

Tingling - frankincense, ginger, white fir, cellular complex blend, soothing blend, tension blend

Trouble running and jumping - cellular complex blend, soothing blend

Walking on toes - white fir, cellular complex blend, detoxification blend, grounding blend

Weakness/loss of mass or tone/degeneration - basil, bergamot, birch, black pepper, clove, coriander, cypress, lavender, marjoram, melissa, rosemary, wintergreen, cellular complex blend, soothing blend, tension blend, women's blend

Whiplash - birch, coriander, frankincense, helichrysum, lemongrass, peppermint, white fir, soothing blend, tension blend

Remedies

FOOT LOVE
1 drop frankincense
2 drop of spearmint or peppermint
4 drop of rosemary
Stir oils into 1/4 cup Epsom salts; mix well, add to warm water in foot bath. Soak for 20 minutes.

ACHE-Y BRAKE-Y BATH (muscle relief)
4 drops white fir
4 drops frankincense
1 drop clove
Stir oils into ½ cup Epsom salts; mix well, add to hot bath water. Soak for 20 minutes.

MASSAGE IN A BOTTLE
Apply massage blend and/or soothing blend to any unhappy muscle. Reapply every thirty minutes for acute pain and twice per day for more chronic issues.

ANTI-SPAZ (for muscle spasms)
12 drops white fir
9 drops lemongrass
6 drops basil
Combine oils in 10ml roller bottle; fill remainder with carrier oil. Apply topically on or near affected area as needed.

COLD COMPRESS RELIEF RECIPES
Drop oils into small bowl of ¼ - ½ cup cold water. Dip wash-cloth onto to oils. Apply moistened directly to muscle.

- **Muscular Pain Relief:** 3 drops roman chamomile, 3 drops lavender
- **Muscle Inflammation Relief:** 3 drops peppermint, 3 drops yarrow
- **Pulled Muscle Relief:** 3 drops roman chamomile, 2 drops marjoram

READY ROLLERBALL RECIPES
Combine in a 5ml roller bottle; fill remainder with carrier oil. Apply to affected area as needed.

- **Leg Muscle Cramps**
  4 drops ginger
  8 drops black pepper
  8 drops cinnamon
- **Loosen Tight Muscles**
  4 drops ginger oil
  8 drops lavender
  8 drops rosemary
- **Muscle Spasm Relief**
  6 drops cypress
  3 drops lemongrass
  8 drops marjoram
  4 drops ginger
- **Soothe Aching Muscles**
  2 drops of cardamom
  4 drops lemongrass
  5 drops ginger
  6 drops lavender oil

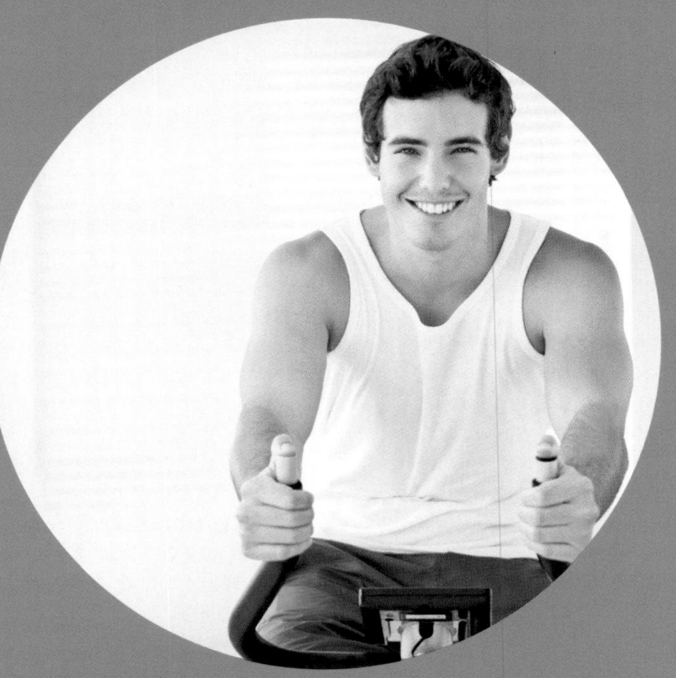

USAGE TIPS: For best results with muscles and connective tissue:

- **Topical:** Apply oils directly to area of concern, massage in thoroughly whenever possible. Drive oils in with heat, cold, or moisture. Use carrier oil as needed or desired. Layering multiple oils over affected area, placing them on tissue one at a time, is very effective. Any kind of cream or carrier barrier will slow absorption if placed on first and improve it if placed on last.
  - **Acute:** Apply often, every 20-30 minutes, until symptoms subside, then reduce to every two to six hours.
  - **Chronic:** Apply two to three times daily.
- **Internal:** Consume oils to support resolving inflammation in a capsule or under tongue.

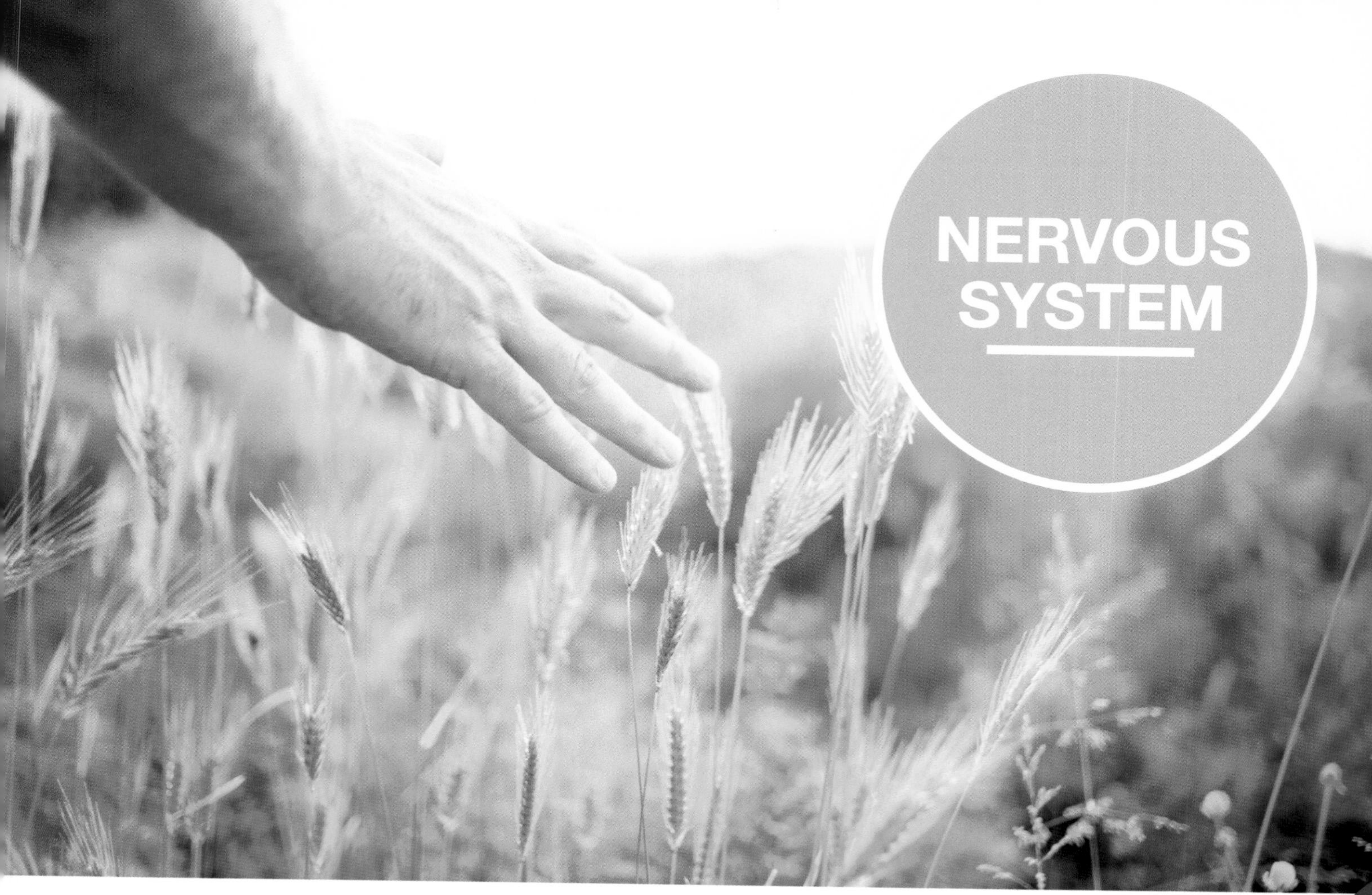

THE NERVOUS SYSTEM is a complex system of nerves and specialized cells that allows the body to transmit and receive messages. It serves as the body's primary control and communications center, responsible for transmitting and receiving messages between every other system in the body.

The sensory function involves transmitting data from sensory receptors, which register internal and external stimuli to the central nervous system (CNS), where it is processed by the brain. The CNS relies on the conscious and subconscious signals from the body's sensory receptors to make it aware of any threats. It is also charged with the higher functions of language, imagination, emotion, and personality.

When the CNS receives sensory input, a complex network of neurons in the brain and brain stem evaluates, categorizes, and files this information, making it available for decision-making and future retrieval. After the incoming sensory signals are evaluated, a signal is sent through the nerves of the peripheral nervous system (PNS) to effector cells, which release hormones or otherwise cause the body to respond to the stimulus.

The somatic nervous system (SNS), which is part of the PNS, directs the conscious, voluntary movements of the body. The autonomic nervous system (ANS), on the other hand, controls all the involuntary neurons, those that do not require conscious direction to function, such as cardiac, visceral, and glandular tissues.

The ANS is further divided into the sympathetic and parasympathetic systems. The sympathetic system is responsible for the body's fight or flight response which, when activated, increases respiration, heart rate, and adrenaline and stress hormone levels in the blood, while suppressing digestive functions. The parasympathetic system takes over when the body rests and digests. This system tries to undo what the sympathetic system does when it encounters a threat, e.g. decreasing respiration and heart rate, while increasing digestion and waste elimination.

The enteric nervous system (ENS) is yet another division of the autonomic nervous system and is in charge of regulating the digestive system. As mentioned above, it receives input from both the sympathetic and parasympathetic divisions of the ANS, instructing it what to do. The majority of the ENS's functions, however, are regulated independently, warranting the nickname "the second brain," and rightly so, for it alone boasts as many neurons as exist in the spinal cord.

Essential oils can facilitate the complex messaging that occurs throughout the nervous system. They help with homeostasis, circulation, and brain function (see Limbic System) as the brain interprets and sends out data.They even help the neurons transmitting and receiving messages to be more efficient due to their regenerative and soothing properties. They address root causes of ailments connected to the nervous system, helping improve symptoms because the body has support in helping itself.

TOP SOLUTIONS

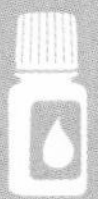

SINGLE OILS

Helichrysum - invigorates nerves and relieves pain (pg. 105)
Peppermint - stimulates nerves and supports repair (pg. 122)
Lemongrass - stimulates nerves and electrical system of body (pg. 112)
Patchouli - provides nerve protection and supports regeneration; removes toxins (pg. 121)
Basil - stimulates, energizes and restores nerves; relaxes tension (pg. 76)
Frankincense - provides nerve protection and supports regeneration (pg. 100)

By Related Properties

For definitions of the properties listed below and more oil options, see Oil Properties Glossary (pg. 435) and Oil Properties (pg. 436).

Analgesic - arborvitae, basil, bergamot, birch, cassia, cinnamon, clary sage, coriander, eucalyptus, fennel, frankincense, ginger, jasmine, juniper berry, lavender, lemongrass, marjoram, melaleuca, oregano, peppermint, ravensara, rosemary, white fir, wild orange, wintergreen
Anti-inflammatory - arborvitae, basil, bergamot, birch, black pepper, cardamom, cassia, cedarwood, cinnamon, coriander, cypress, dill, eucalyptus, fennel, frankincense, geranium, ginger, helichrysum, jasmine, lavender, lemongrass, lime, melaleuca, melissa, myrrh, oregano, patchouli, peppermint, roman chamomile, rosemary, sandalwood, spearmint, spikenard, wild orange, wintergreen, yarrow
Calming - bergamot, birch, black pepper, cassia, clary sage, coriander, fennel, frankincense, geranium, jasmine, juniper berry, lavender, melissa, oregano, patchouli, roman chamomile, sandalwood, tangerine, vetiver, yarrow
Grounding - basil, cedarwood, clary sage, cypress, melaleuca, vetiver, ylang ylang
Nervine - basil, clary sage, clove, helichrysum, juniper berry, lavender, lemongrass, melissa, patchouli, peppermint, rose, rosemary, thyme
Neuroprotective - frankincense, lavender roman chamomile, thyme, vetiver
Neurotonic - arborvitae, basil, bergamot, black pepper, clary sage, cypress, ginger, melaleuca
Regenerative - basil, cedarwood, clove, coriander, frankincense, geranium, helichrysum, lavender, lemongrass, melaleuca, myrrh, patchouli, sandalwood, wild orange
Relaxing - basil, cassia, cedarwood, cypress, fennel, geranium, jasmine, lavender, marjoram, myrrh, ravensara, roman chamomile, white fir, ylang ylang
Steroidal - basil, bergamot, birch, cedarwood, clove, fennel, patchouli, rosemary, thyme
Stimulant - arborvitae, basil, bergamot, birch, black pepper, cardamom, cedarwood, cinnamon, clove, coriander, cypress, dill, eucalyptus, fennel, ginger, grapefruit, juniper berry, lime, melaleuca, myrrh, patchouli, rosemary, spearmint, thyme, vetiver, white fir, wintergreen, ylang ylang

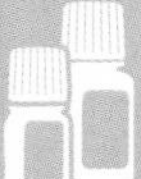

BLENDS

Focus blend - helps with mental focus and reduces inflammation (pg. 149)
Massage blend - increases circulation (pg. 155)
Soothing blend - invigorates and stimulates nerves (pg. 164)
Cellular complex blend - regenerates and protects nerves (pg. 143)
Anti-aging blend - regenerates nerves and increases clarity (pg. 141)

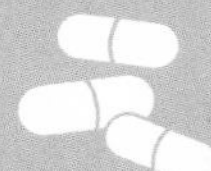

SUPPLEMENTS

Bone support complex, cellular vitality complex, energy & stamina complex, **essential oil cellular complex (pg. 174), essential oil omega complex (pg. 175)**, food enzymes, **liquid omega-3 supplement (pg. 178)**, polyphenol complex, whole food nutrient supplement

Targeted Nervous System Support

Autonomic nervous system - basil, bergamot, dill, fennel, lemon, calming blend, digestion blend, grounding blend
Central nervous system - basil, black pepper (circulation to nerves), frankincense, grapefruit, lavender, patchouli, peppermint, rosemary (stimulant), anti-aging blend, cellular complex blend
Parasympathetic nervous system - lavender, lemongrass (regulates), marjoram, patchouli, wild orange, calming blend, grounding blend, respiration blend, tension blend
Sympathetic nervous system - cedarwood, eucalyptus, fennel (stimulant), ginger, grapefruit (stimulant), peppermint, cellular complex blend

Related Ailments: Bell's Palsy, Blurred Vision, Carpal Tunnel Syndrome, Cataracts, Floaters, Glaucoma, Iris Inflammation, Macular Degeneration, Nervous Fatigue, Neuralgia, Neuritis, Neuropathy, Numbness, Multiple Sclerosis, Optic Neuritis, Ocular Rosacea, Phantom Pains, Poor Taste, Poor Vision, Porphyria, Retinitis Pigmentosa, Sciatica, Shock, Tourette Syndrome, Trigeminal Neuralgia, Uveitis, Xerophthalmia

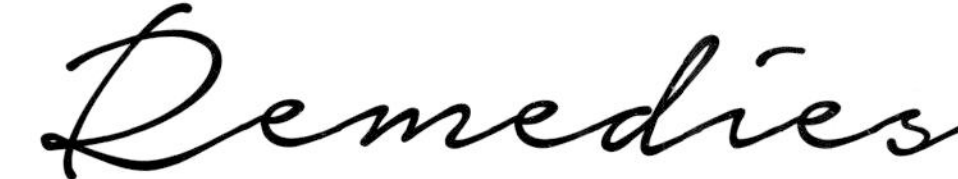

Remedies

INTERNAL NERVE BATH (nervous system cleanse: for brain and organ function):
4 drops frankincense
4 drops thyme
4 drops clove
Combine oils and take in a capsule daily.

BRAIN REVITALIZER
7 drops helichrysum
7 drops patchouli
6 drops sandalwood
5 drops roman chamomile
3 drops cypress
Combine in a 5ml roller bottle; fill remainder with carrier oil. Apply to mastoid bone behind ears, back of neck into hairline, and forehead, morning and night.

BRAIN DEFOGGER DAILY ROUTINE
- Use as directed cellular vitality complex, essential oil cellular complex, essential oil omega complex, energy & stamina complex, whole food nutrient supplement, defensive probiotic.
- Rub 1-2 drops of grounding blend on bottoms of feet morning and night.
- Place 4-5 drops of frankincense under tongue morning and night.
- Consume water with favorite citrus oil throughout day.
- Use "Mid-Afternoon Slump Buster" blend - see *Energy & Vitality*, use as needed for focus boost.
- Layer anti-aging blend and focus blend up back of neck into hairline morning and evening.

NERVE DAMAGE
14 drops frankincense
10 drops helichrysum
10 drops roman chamomile
8 drops vetiver
6 drops peppermint
Combine into 5mil roller bottle; fill remainder with carrier oil. Massage into spine or affected area daily.

SHINGLES SPRITZER
20 drops eucalyptus
20 drops marjoram
20 drops melaleuca
20 drops roman chamomile
20 drops protective blend
10 drops frankincense
Combine into 1-ounce spritzer bottle; fill remainder of bottle with half fractionated coconut oil and half distilled water. Spray affected area every twenty to thirty minutes. Shake bottle before each use.

SIMPLE SHINGLES REMEDY
Combine equal parts melaleuca and frankincense in 5-10ml roller bottle. Use NEAT (directly on skin without dilution).

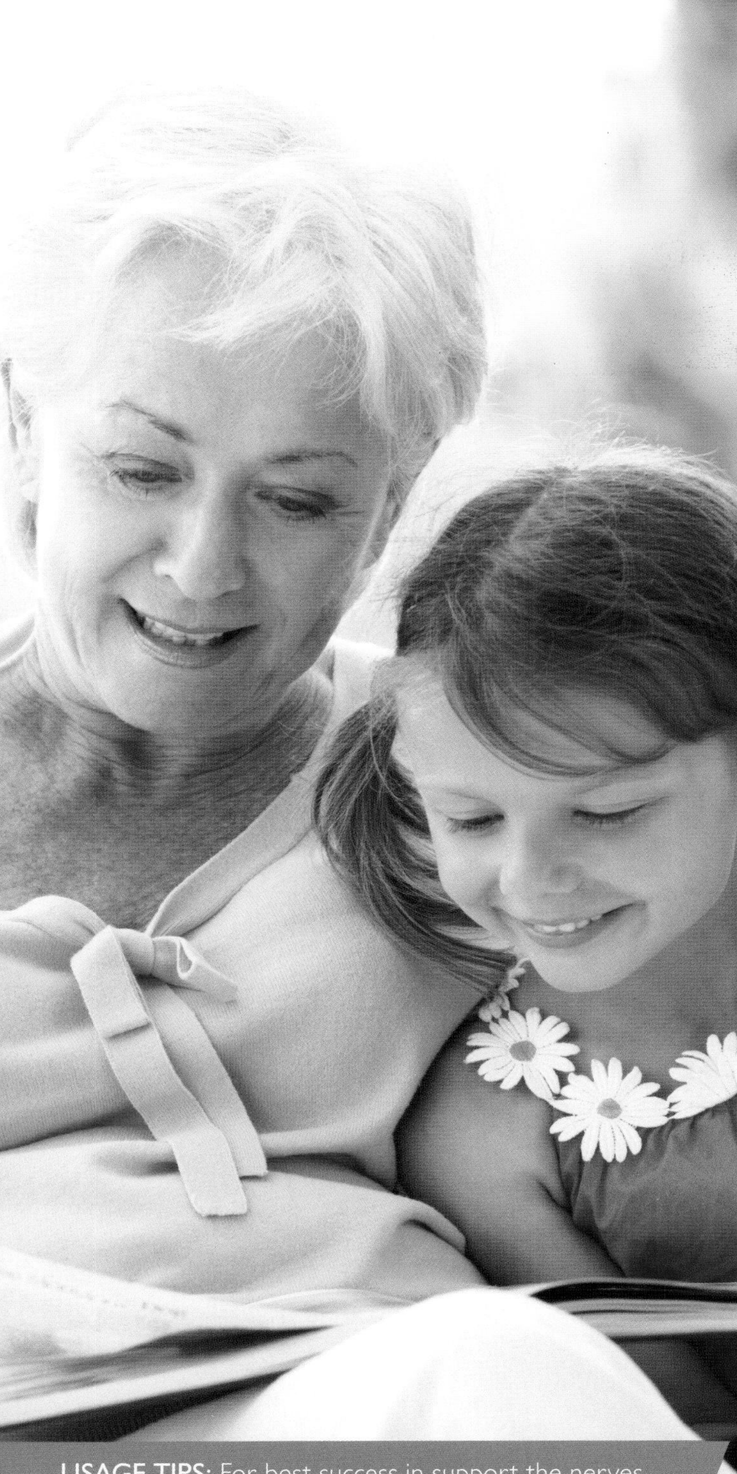

USAGE TIPS: For best success in support the nerves and nervous system
- **Topical:** Apply selected oil(s) directly to any area of concern remembering to use a carrier oil if necessary to prevent sensitivity.
- **Internal:** Consume oils in a capsule or under tongue to address nervous issues and bring a particular chemical message to affected areas.
- **Aromatic:** Inhaling from a preparation or diffusing selected oils can have direct impact on brain and nervous system via olfactory pathways.

Conditions

Carpal tunnel, pain/tingling - basil, cypress, ginger, lemongrass, marjoram, oregano, peppermint, cellular complex blend, massage blend, soothing blend; see *Skeletal*
Decreased ability to taste - black pepper, ginger, helichrysum, peppermint, soothing blend
Dendrites, lack of - vetiver
Dizziness - basil, black pepper, bergamot, clove, frankincense, ginger, juniper berry, peppermint, roman chamomile, tangerine, cellular complex blend, detoxification blend, invigorating blend, metabolic blend, women's blend
Dropsy - basil, black pepper, dill, frankincense, ginger, juniper berry, marjoram, myrrh, patchouli, peppermint, vetiver, wintergreen, calming blend, anti-aging blend, cellular complex blend, massage blend, protective blend, respiration blend
Eyes -
⚠ **CAUTION** - do not put oils in eyes; place oils on skin near eyes; use very small amounts, dilute with carrier oil; use reflex point on toes for eyes - consult Reflexology chapter in this book.
- **Dry, itchy, red/redness, tear duct (blocked), watery** - See *Respiratory*
- **Fatigue** - cypress, lavender
- **Optical nerve** - frankincense, juniper berry (regeneration), patchouli, anti-aging blend
- **Pain** - frankincense, lavender, melaleuca
- **Sensitivity to light/glare** - basil, frankincense, helichrysum, patchouli, roman chamomile, vetiver, anti-aging blend, cellular complex blend
- **Stinging/burning/scratching** - frankincense, helichrysum, lavender, patchouli, rosemary, cellular complex blend
- **Swollen** - cypress, frankincense
- **Vision, clouded/blurred/poor** - basil, bergamot, black pepper, clary sage, clove, cypress, frankincense, ginger, helichrysum, lemongrass, melaleuca, anti-aging blend, cellular complex blend
- **Vision, double in one eye** - clary sage, helichrysum, lavender, lemongrass
- **Vision, fading or yellowing of colors** - basil, black pepper, clary sage, cypress, frankincense, lavender, vetiver, cellular complex blend, massage blend
- **Vision, weak** - clove, frankincense, helichrysum, lemongrass, anti-aging blend

Headache - basil, frankincense, lavender, patchouli, peppermint, thyme, wintergreen, tension blend
Headache, migraine - frankincense, lavender, marjoram, melissa, peppermint, roman chamomile, spearmint, tension blend
Huntington's disease - See *Autoimmune*
Impaired gait, posture, and balance - frankincense, marjoram, patchouli, peppermint, thyme, anti-aging blend, grounding blend
Increased sensitivity to sound - helichrysum, anti-aging blend
Multiple sclerosis - bergamot, clove, cypress, frankincense, helichrysum, melissa, oregano, patchouli, peppermint, rosemary, anti-aging blend, cellular complex blend, comforting blend, focus blend; see *Autoimmune*
Myelin sheath, compromised - frankincense, patchouli, peppermint, rosemary, sandalwood, vetiver, anti-aging blend
Nausea - basil, bergamot, fennel, ginger, juniper berry, lavender, detoxification blend, digestion blend; see *Digestive & Intestinal*
Nerve, damaged - basil, ginger, helichrysum, lemongrass, patchouli, soothing blend
Nerve degeneration - basil, frankincense, geranium, helichrysum, juniper berry, patchouli, peppermint, anti-aging blend, detoxification blend, encouraging blend, focus blend, soothing blend
Nerve inflammation - cedarwood, clove, eucalyptus, frankincense, juniper berry, lavender, lemongrass, patchouli, peppermint, roman chamomile, vetiver, wintergreen, anti-aging blend, focus blend, soothing blend
Nerve, lack of tone - black pepper, cardamom, fennel, patchouli, peppermint, sandalwood, spearmint, renewing blend
Nerve pain (neuralgia) - basil, bergamot, birch, cedarwood, cinnamon, coriander, eucalyptus, frankincense, geranium, helichrysum, juniper berry, lavender, marjoram, patchouli, peppermint, roman chamomile, rosemary, wintergreen, anti-aging blend, soothing blend
Nerve problems - black pepper, cinnamon, grapefruit, lemon, lime, patchouli, peppermint, roman chamomile, rose , sandalwood, vetiver, invigorating blend, renewing blend, women's monthly blend
Nerve, virus - clove, frankincense, lemongrass, melissa, myrrh, cellular complex blend, encouraging blend
Nervous debility - coriander, ginger, grapefruit, helichrysum, patchouli, soothing blend

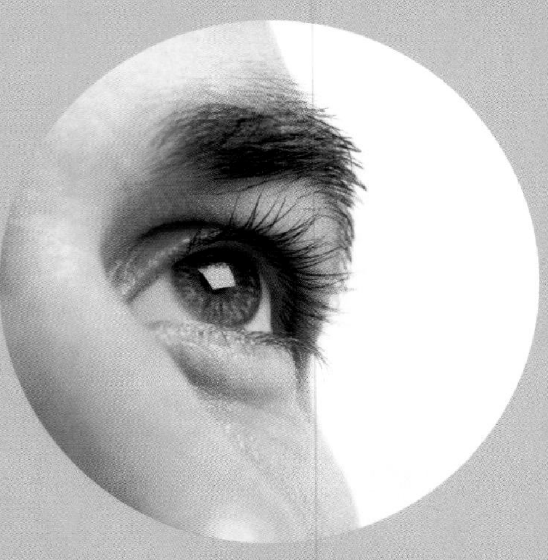

Nervous disorders - melissa, patchouli, roman chamomile, vetiver, soothing blend
Neurons, impaired activity - roman chamomile, vetiver, tension blend
Nervous tension - basil, bergamot, douglas fir, geranium, grapefruit, jasmine, lavender, melissa, roman chamomile, rose, sandalwood, vetiver, wild orange, ylang ylang, tension blend
Numbness/prickling/pain - basil, cypress, marjoram, peppermint, wintergreen, massage blend, tension blend, soothing blend
Paralysis - cardamom, cypress, douglas fir, frankincense, geranium, ginger, helichrysum, juniper berry, lemongrass, melissa, peppermint, sandalwood, cellular complex blend, cleansing blend, grounding blend, massage blend
Paralysis, side of face - helichrysum, marjoram, patchouli, peppermint, rose, rosemary, thyme, metabolic blend; see "Paralysis" above
Paralysis, temporary - frankincense, rosemary, massage blend
Sciatic, issues with - basil, birch, cardamom, cypress, frankincense, helichrysum, lavender, peppermint, sandalwood, thyme, wintergreen, comforting blend
Sedation, need - cedarwood, coriander, geranium, melissa, patchouli, wild orange, ylang ylang
Shock - bergamot, frankincense, geranium, helichrysum, peppermint, focus blend; see *First Aid*
Speech impediment - frankincense, rosemary, focus blend
Teeth grinding - frankincense, geranium, lavender, wild orange, calming blend, marjoram, roman chamomile; see *Parasites*

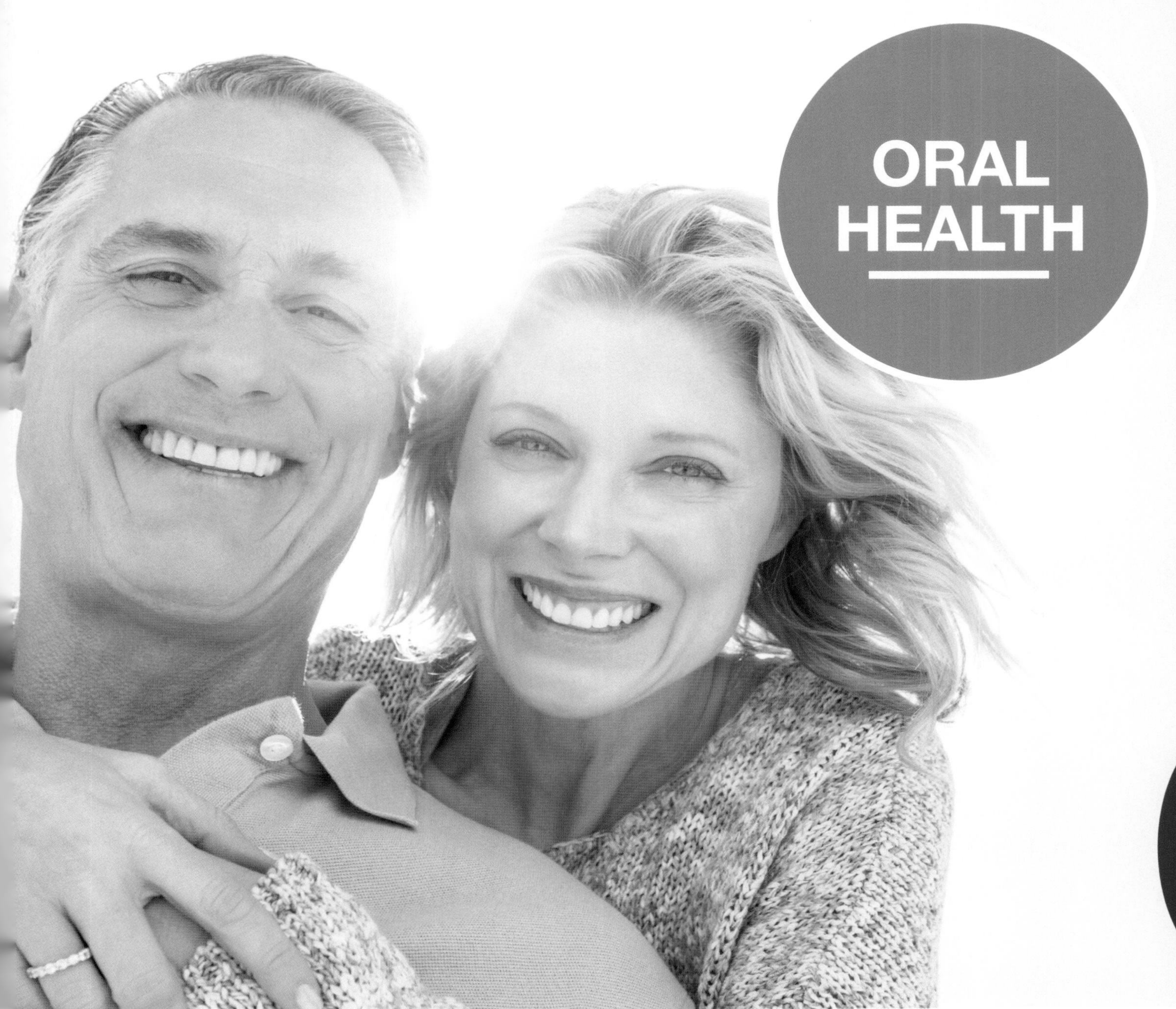

ORAL HEALTH

ALTHOUGH ORAL HEALTH is often treated separately from the body as a whole, the health of the oral cavity - the mouth and its tissues - impacts overall health. Poor oral health may be the cause of a more serious underlying disease process, or it may predispose an individual to other health conditions.

The mouth is colonized by hundreds of different bacterial species that inhabit dental plaque. These species adhere in layers to oral surfaces. They are not easily eliminated by the body's natural immune responses and must be mechanically removed. Bacteria increase tenfold when the mouth is not sufficiently cleaned.

A clean mouth contains several hundred billion bacteria, and this number increases when poor oral care exists. Using saliva and gingival fluid to supply their nutrients, bacteria inhabit all areas of the mouth, threatening oral and systemic health. Bacteria beneath the gums, or gingiva, have been reported to be involved in numerous systemic diseases. Oral health care, primarily proper cleaning and caution in the consumption of and ongoing exposure to intensely acidic and sugary foods (i.e. soda pop), contributes to a healthy lifestyle.

Essential oils are a particularly effective means of supporting oral health, partly because they are antibacterial and antifungal in nature. Clove oil helps to relieve oral pain, cinnamon and peppermint are effective against plaque and gum disease, melaleuca is soothing and helpful in eradicating canker sores, and lavender is soothing to sore muscles that result from teeth grinding. Oil pulling is also particularly beneficial to restoring and maintaining oral health. Specific essential oils can be chosen as part of that routine to target desired results. See *Detoxification* for further instruction.

TOP SOLUTIONS

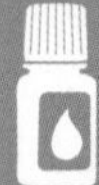

SINGLE OILS

Myrrh - fights gum disease, infections and sores; soothes gums (pg. 119)

Clove - protects nerves, soothes pain; prevents tooth decay (pg. 90)

Peppermint - freshens breath; reduces swelling, inflammation, and tenderness (pg. 122)

Wintergreen - protect nerves, soothes pain; prevents tooth decay (pg. 137)

By Related Properties

For definitions of the properties listed below and more oil options, see Oil Properties Glossary (pg. 435) and Oil Properties (pg. 436).

Analgesic - arborvitae, bergamot, black pepper, cassia, cinnamon, clove, coriander, cypress, eucalyptus, fennel, frankincense, ginger, jasmine, juniper berry, lavender, lemongrass, marjoram, melaleuca, oregano, ravensara, white fir, wild orange, wintergreen

Antibacterial - arborvitae, basil, bergamot, birch, black pepper, cardamom, cassia, cedarwood, cilantro, cinnamon, clary sage, clove, coriander, cypress, dill, eucalyptus, geranium, ginger, grapefruit, helichrysum, lemongrass, lime, marjoram, melaleuca, melissa, myrrh, oregano, patchouli, peppermint, ravensara, rosemary sandalwood, spearmint, spikenard, tangerine, thyme, wild orange, ylang ylang

Anti-infectious - arborvitae, bergamot, cardamom, cedarwood, cinnamon, clove, cypress, eucalyptus, frankincense, geranium, lavender, marjoram, melaleuca, myrrh, roman chamomile, rosemary

Anti-inflammatory - arborvitae, bergamot, birch, black pepper, cardamom, cassia, cedarwood, cinnamon, coriander, dill, eucalyptus, fennel, frankincense, geranium, ginger, helichrysum, jasmine, lavender, lemongrass, lime, melaleuca, myrrh, oregano, patchouli, peppermint, roman chamomile, rosemary, sandalwood, spearmint, spikenard, wild orange, wintergreen

Detoxifier - arborvitae, cassia, geranium, juniper berry, lemon, lime, rosemary

Immunostimulant - arborvitae, cassia, cinnamon, clove, eucalyptus, fennel, frankincense, ginger, lemon, lime, melaleuca, melissa, oregano, ravensara, rosemary spearmint, thyme, vetiver, wild orange

Related Ailments: Abscess [Integumentary], Bleeding Gums, Canker Sores, Cavities, Dental Infection, Dysphagia [Digestive & Intestinal], Gingivitis, Gum Disease, Hoarse Voice, Halitosis, Laryngitis, Mouth Ulcers, Plaque, Pyorrhea, Sore Throat [Respiratory], Teeth Grinding, Teething Pain, Tonsillitis, Toothache

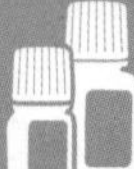

BLENDS

Protective blend - helps fight infection and bacteria; prevents tooth decay (pg. 158)

Cellular complex blend - protects nerves, soothes pain; prevents tooth decay (pg. 143)

Tension blend - reduces tension, inflammation, swelling, and pain in jaw (pg. 165)

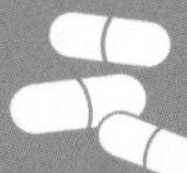

SUPPLEMENTS

Bone support complex (pg. 170), cellular vitality complex, detoxification softgels, essential oil omega complex, food enzymes, fruit & vegetable supplement powder, protective blend softgels, whole food nutrient supplement

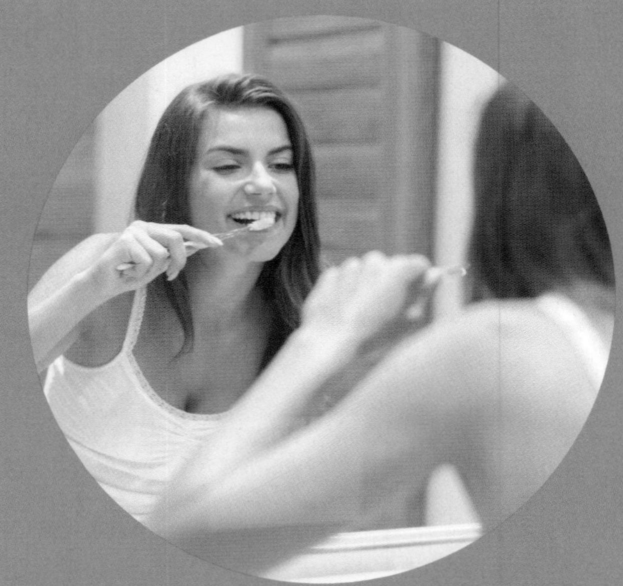

USAGE TIPS: For oral health support

- **Topical:** Apply oils directly to area of concern in mouth such as gums, teeth, tongue, sores, etc. To relieve pain, also apply pain-relieving oils to outside cheek/jaw area (can use a carrier oil as needed); apply frequently as needed for acute situations.
- **Internal:** Place oils on toothbrush and brush teeth with selected oils to affect surface of teeth. Ingest oils (e.g. lemon) to change pH (alkalize) in body/mouth which affects tooth and oral health.

Remedies

COLD SORE ROLLER BOTTLE
6 drops peppermint
6 drops melaleuca
1 drop helichrysum
2 drops clove
3 drops lavender
2 drops cinnamon
Add to a 5ml roller bottle Fill remainder of bottle with a carrier oil and apply to the area until healed and then one day more.

CANKER SORE REMEDY
1 drop melissa
2 drops geranium
2 drops helichrysum
2 drops black pepper
1 drop clove
Combine with 2 teaspoons fractionated coconut oil and apply as needed.

BRACES PAIN: Place helichrysum or tension blend on jaw; dilute with carrier oil if desired.

TMJ: Use calming blend or tension blend on neck and jaw.

MOUTHWASH
5 drops melaleuca
5 drops peppermint
3 drops clove
2 drops cinnamon
2 drops myrrh
Combine in a 4-ounce glass bottle. Fill remainder with purified water. Shake before use.

Conditions

Bleeding gums - cardamom, clove, dill, frankincense, helichrysum, lemon, lime, melaleuca, myrrh, oregano, patchouli, peppermint, rosemary, spearmint, thyme, wild orange, cellular complex blend, detoxification blend, protective blend
Bleeding, tooth extraction - cardamom, frankincense, helichrysum, lavender, lemon, lime, cellular complex blend, detoxification blend
Breath, bad (halitosis) - bergamot, cardamom, cilantro, juniper berry, lavender, patchouli, peppermint, spearmint, cellular complex blend, detoxification blend, digestion blend, metabolic blend, uplifting blend
Cankers - birch, black pepper, helichrysum, oregano, myrrh, wild orange, cellular complex blend, metabolic blend, protective blend
Cold sores - arborvitae, basil, bergamot, clove, fennel, geranium, lavender, lemon, marjoram, melaleuca, melissa, myrrh, oregano, wild orange, cellular complex blend, detoxification blend, protective blend
Fever blisters - see "Cold sores" above
Gum disease - cinnamon, clove, grapefruit, melaleuca, myrrh, protective blend
Gums, infection - basil, geranium, myrrh, rose, cellular complex blend, protective blend
Gums, inflammation - cinnamon, clove, melaleuca, myrrh, peppermint, comforting blend, protective blend
Gums, receding - clove, geranium, myrrh, cellular complex blend, protective blend
Gums, tender - cardamom, cinnamon, clove, frankincense, helichrysum, lavender, lemon, lime, melaleuca, myrrh, peppermint, rosemary, spearmint, thyme, wild orange, cellular complex blend, protective blend
Headache, jaw-related - basil, frankincense, lavender, marjoram, peppermint, wintergreen, calming blend, cellular complex blend, grounding blend, tension blend
Mouth, dry - frankincense, grapefruit, lemon, tangerine, wild orange
Mouth, infection - bergamot, cinnamon, clove, frankincense, helichrysum, lavender, lemon, lime, melaleuca, oregano, rosemary, thyme, cellular complex blend, protective blend
Mouth, injury/trauma - frankincense, helichrysum, myrrh, white fir, protective blend
Mouth ulcers and sores - basil, bergamot, cinnamon, clove, douglas fir, frankincense, geranium, helichrysum, lavender, lemon, marjoram, melaleuca, melissa, myrrh, oregano, wild orange, cellular complex blend, detoxification blend, protective blend
Pain with pressure of chewing/biting - helichrysum, myrrh, thyme, detoxification blend
Plaque - clove, grapefruit, lemon, lime, myrrh, tangerine, thyme, wild orange, detoxification blend, protective blend
Salivary glands, blocked/congested - cypress, grapefruit, lemon, lemongrass, cleansing blend, detoxification blend, invigorating blend, massage blend, protective blend
Swallowing, difficulty/inability/gagging - peppermint, rosemary
Swollen in face/cheek - basil, cypress, frankincense, lemon, peppermint, wintergreen, massage blend, soothing blend
Tartar - black pepper, coriander, lemon, lime, ravensara, tangerine, detoxification blend, metabolic blend, protective blend
Teeth grinding - frankincense, lavender, calming blend; see *Parasites*
Teeth, new spaces between - clary sage, frankincense, patchouli, cellular complex blend
Teeth, sensitivity to hot/cold - frankincense, helichrysum, lavender, myrrh, cellular complex blend, detoxification blend, protective blend
Tooth abscess - cinnamon, clove, frankincense, helichrysum, lavender, melaleuca, myrrh, rosemary, thyme, cellular complex blend, cleansing blend, protective blend
Throat, sore - cinnamon, helichrysum, lemon, melaleuca, myrrh, thyme, wild orange, cellular complex blend, protective blend, respiration blend; see *Respiratory*
Throat, tickling/raw - frankincense, helichrysum, rosemary, wild orange, protective blend
Tingling/burning sensation in mouth - grapefruit, lemon, detoxification blend
Tongue, indentations - protective blend
Tonsils, red/swollen/white patches - melaleuca, oregano
Toothache - bergamot, black pepper, clove, cinnamon, frankincense, grapefruit, helichrysum, lavender, myrrh, peppermint, roman chamomile, detoxification blend, protective blend
Tooth decay - birch, clove, melaleuca, wintergreen, protective blend
Tooth enamel, worn - white fir, wintergreen
Tooth, loose - bergamot, cinnamon, frankincense, lavender, myrrh, peppermint, rose, cellular complex blend
Tooth stains, black/brown/white - frankincense, lemon, lime, myrrh, wild orange, detoxification blend
Voice, weak, hoarse, or loss/laryngitis - basil, cardamom, cinnamon, eucalyptus, fennel, frankincense, ginger, jasmine, lavender, lemon, lemongrass, lime, myrrh, peppermint, rosemary, sandalwood, thyme, vetiver, ylang ylang, calming blend, cleansing blend, detoxification blend, invigorating blend, joyful blend, protective blend, respiration blend, tension blend

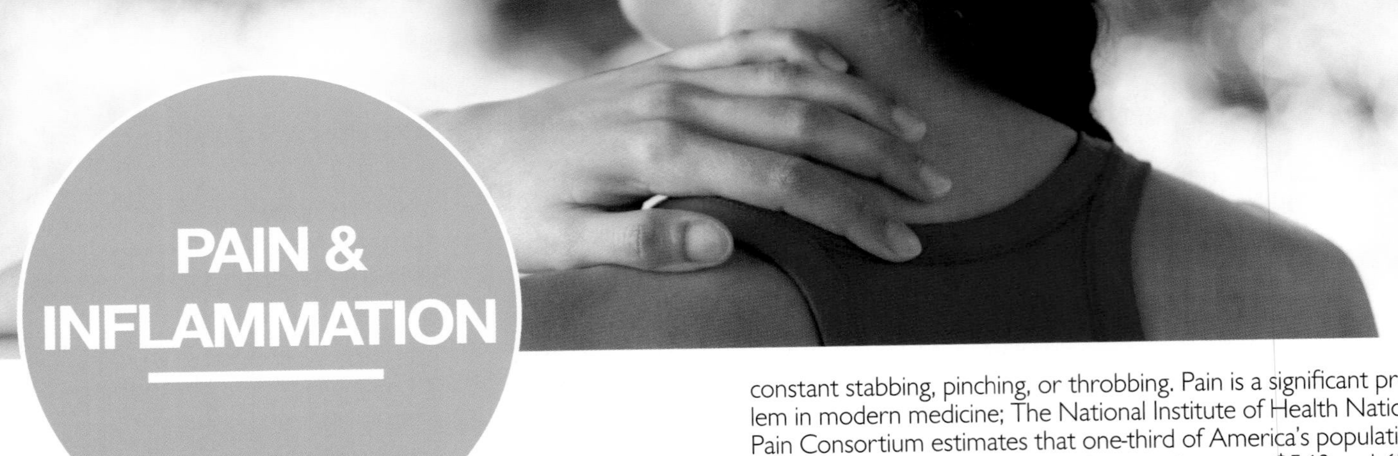

PAIN & INFLAMMATION

INFLAMMATION is the body's biological response to anything the body considers harmful, including pathogens, irritants, infection, allergens, injury, and pain. Healthy inflammation is part of the innate immune system (see Immune), which responds to pathogens with an "automatic" generalized response aiming to clear tissues and cells of harmful stimuli and initiate cellular repair. It works closely with the local vascular system to deliver the plasma and leukocytes that are the "first responders." Sometimes trying to reduce swelling too quickly can actually slow down the body's healing processes! Symptoms of inflammation can include swelling, redness, pain, heat, and at times, reduced function. Healthy inflammation is necessary for the body to prevent breakdown of body tissues due to pathogens or injury. Note that inflammation is not infection, but is part of the body's response to it.

There are two types of inflammation: acute and chronic. Acute inflammation occurs when there is a one-time trigger or event, and the body responds immediately to that trigger by moving plasma and leukocytes into the compromised tissues. Situations that can cause acute inflammation are intense physical training, cold or flu, an infected ingrown toenail, a scratch or cut, sore throat, appendicitis, etc.

Chronic inflammation is long-term inflammation and can occur because the body was unable to repair the initial cause of acute inflammation or because of an autoimmune response, in which the body mistakes healthy tissue as harmful and thus attacks healthy tissue on an ongoing basis. Conditions contributing to chronic inflammation include asthma, arthritis, any chronic condition, and any autoimmune condition.

While wounds, infections, and disease would not be able to heal without acute inflammation, chronic inflammation can cause a myriad of undesirable diseases or conditions that can include cancers, other chronic conditions, and hay fever. When chronic inflammation occurs, the type of cells at the site shift, and the result is the concurrent repair and destruction of the tissue. Inflammation must be regulated to serve as nature intended.

Cortisol, which is a hormone produced by the adrenal glands, is the most powerful anti-inflammatory substance in your body. When the adrenal glands become stressed or fatigued, insufficient amounts of cortisol are produced, resulting in increased inflammation. Therefore, proper care of the adrenal glands is a critical component to ensuring an appropriate inflammatory response.

Pain, which is very closely related to inflammation, can be slight, moderate or severe, and can manifest in a myriad of ways including constant stabbing, pinching, or throbbing. Pain is a significant problem in modern medicine; The National Institute of Health National Pain Consortium estimates that one-third of America's population deals with significant pain issues that cost between $560 and 635 billion dollars each year. Even worse than the monetary cost of pain is an assertion by England's chief medical officer who estimated that more than five million people in the UK develop chronic pain each year, but only two-thirds recover. Chronic pain, in addition to the extreme discomfort it causes, can lead to loss of ability to work or function in relationships, addiction to pain medications, and feelings of frustration and helplessness.

There are several ways to classify pain. These include:

- **Acute:** typically intense and short-lived, caused by an injury that heals in time and pain subsides
- **Chronic:** Ongoing, can be mild or intense
- Nociceptive: includes somatic and visceral pain
  - › Somatic: Includes all musculo-skeletal pain, includes sore/strained muscles, cuts on skin, etc.
  - › Visceral: Refers to internal organs and body cavities such as the thorax, abdomen and pelvis; includes cramping and aching sensations
- **Non-nociceptive:** Includes neuropathic and sympathetic
  - › Neuropathic: Refers to nerve pain that can be caused by nerves between tissues and the spinal cord, or between the spinal cord and the brain–sometimes referred to as pinched nerves; can also be caused by degenerative disease (i.e. stroke or loss of myelin sheath) or infection, as in the case of shingles
  - › Sympathetic: Refers to pain of the sympathetic nervous system (controls blood flow, etc.) which typically occurs after a fracture or soft-tissue injury. Though there are no specific pain receptors, the affected area can become extremely sensitive, causing the individual to forego use of the injured limb or area.
- **Referred pain:** When pain is felt in an area other than the original site of injury/infection, such as when the arm or back hurts in case of a heart attack

When considering how best to treat pain, medical professionals take into account the original site of pain, what other areas are affected, the type of pain, what activities lessen or worsen the pain, when pain is more aggravated, and the effect the pain has on an individual's mood and ability to function.

Responding to both inflammation and pain with natural remedies can be highly effective, since both these topics involve systematic bodily responses to injury or disease; natural remedies support the body in doing its job. When dealing with chronic injury and/or inflammation, it is important to participate in a wellness regimen that interrupts the continuation of chronic inflammation, so that the body can be liberated to properly address acute conditions that occur. Supplementation is critical so that cells and tissues have the nourishment they need to subdue more chronic conditions, and when the cells and tissues are well-nourished they respond readily to the powerful chemical influence of pure essential oils.

TOP SOLUTIONS

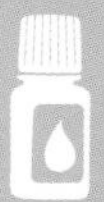

SINGLE OILS

Helichrysum - reduces pain; accelerates healing; chelates toxins (pg. 105)

Wintergreen - soothes aches and pain, warms; has a cortisone-like effect; supports bone healing (pg. 137)

Peppermint - reduces inflammation and pain, cools, invigorates, and stimulates (pg. 122)

Ginger - invigorates nerves, promotes circulation and healing to bones and muscles (pg. 103)

Black pepper - reduces inflammation, relieves pain, increases circulation (pg. 81)

Basil - calms nerves, improves circulation and healing; steroidal action (pg. 76)

By Related Properties

For definitions of the properties listed below and more oil options, see Oil Properties Glossary (pg. 435) and Oil Properties (pg. 436).

Analgesic - arborvitae, basil, bergamot, birch, black pepper, cassia, cinnamon, clary sage, clove, coriander, cypress, eucalyptus, frankincense, ginger, helichrysum, jasmine, juniper berry, lavender, lemongrass, marjoram, melaleuca, oregano, peppermint, rosemary, white fir, wild orange, wintergreen

Anti-inflammatory - arborvitae, basil, bergamot, birch, black pepper, cardamom, cassia, cedarwood, cinnamon, coriander, dill, eucalyptus, fennel, frankincense, geranium, ginger, helichrysum, jasmine, lavender, lemongrass, lime, melaleuca, melissa, myrrh, oregano, patchouli, peppermint, roman chamomile, sandalwood, spearmint, spikenard, wild orange, wintergreen, yarrow

Calming - bergamot, birch, black pepper, cassia, clary sage, coriander, fennel, frankincense, geranium, jasmine, juniper berry, lavender, melissa, oregano, patchouli, roman chamomile, sandalwood, tangerine, vetiver, yarrow

Neurotonic - arborvitae, basil, bergamot, black pepper, clary sage, cypress, ginger, melaleuca

Purifier - arborvitae, cinnamon, eucalyptus, grapefruit, lemongrass, lime, marjoram, melaleuca, oregano, wild orange

Relaxing - basil, cassia, cedarwood, clary sage, cypress, fennel, geranium, jasmine, lavender, marjoram, myrrh, ravensara, roman chamomile, white fir, ylang ylang

Sedative - basil, bergamot, cedarwood, clary sage, coriander, frankincense, geranium, jasmine, juniper berry, lavender, lemongrass, marjoram, melissa, patchouli, roman chamomile, rose, sandalwood, spikenard, vetiver, ylang ylang

Steroidal - basil, bergamot, birch, cedarwood, clove, fennel, patchouli, rosemary, thyme

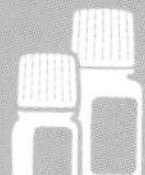

BLENDS

Soothing blend - invigorates nerves and reduces inflammation (pg. 164)

Cellular complex blend - protects cells against free-radical damage while supporting healthy cellular function and renewal (pg. 143)

Tension blend - soothes joints and tissues (pg. 165)

Massage blend - stimulates circulation and blood flow (pg. 155)

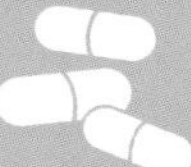

SUPPLEMENTS

Cellular vitality complex (pg. 171), defensive probiotic, **essential oil cellular complex (pg. 174)**, **essential oil omega complex (pg. 175)**, **polyphenol complex (pg. 181)**, whole food nutrient supplement

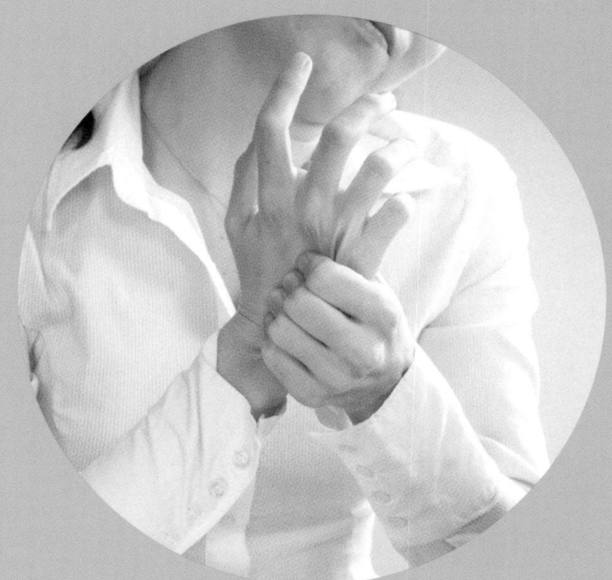

Related Ailments: Chronic pain, Inflammation, Pain, Rheumatic fever

For other ailments of Pain & Inflammation, see the appropriate section. For example *Autoimmune, Brain, Cellular Health, Digestive & Intestinal, Endocrine, Immune & Lymphatic, Muscular, Nervous, Skeletal, Urinary*. Pain and inflammation can occur in any region or part of the body.

Conditions

GENERAL:

Emotional cause - basil, bergamot, cardamom, frankincense, geranium, patchouli, calming blend, women's blend; see *Mood & Behavior*

Inflammation - birch, bergamot, cardamom, cassia, cinnamon, clove, coriander, cypress, frankincense, geranium, jasmine, lavender, peppermint, roman chamomile, rosemary, wintergreen, cellular complex blend, joyful blend, massage blend, reassuring blend, renewing blend, soothing blend, tension blend, women's blend

Pain, acute/sharp - black pepper, clove, ginger, helichrysum, lavender, peppermint, rosemary, wintergreen, calming blend, cellular complex blend, massage blend, soothing blend, tension blend

Pain, chronic - birch, black pepper, cardamom, cilantro, cinnamon, clary sage, clove, coriander, cypress, eucalyptus, frankincense, ginger, helichrysum, juniper berry, lavender, lemon, lemongrass, marjoram, melaleuca, oregano, peppermint, roman chamomile, rosemary, sandalwood, vetiver, white fir, wintergreen, cellular complex blend, cleansing blend, comforting blend, detoxification blend, encouraging blend, massage blend, reassuring blend, soothing blend, tension blend, women's blend

Unexplained/undefined - arborvitae, frankincense, helichrysum, cellular complex blend, cleansing blend, detoxification blend, soothing blend, tension blend; see *Cellular Health*

VISCERA (organ pain):

Abdominal, lower or side/back - bergamot, black pepper, cardamom, clary sage, cypress, ginger, lemongrass, cleansing blend, detoxification blend; see *Urinary*

Abdominal, upper/mid - cardamom, cinnamon, fennel, frankincense, ginger, lavender, marjoram, peppermint, digestion blend; see *Digestive & Intestinal, Parasites*

Breathing issues - cardamom, cypress, douglas fir, eucalyptus, frankincense, peppermint, respiration blend, soothing blend; see *Respiratory, Skeletal*

Chest - marjoram, ylang ylang, anti-aging blend, massage blend; see *Cardiovascular*

Deep, glandular - basil, myrrh, anti-aging blend, cellular complex blend, detoxification blend, grounding blend; see *Endocrine* to address specific glandular issues

Illness/infection - cinnamon, helichrysum, melissa, peppermint, rosemary, protective blend; see *Immune & Lymphatic*

SOMATIC (skeletal muscular pain):

Backaches - basil, bergamot, birch, coriander, cypress, eucalyptus, frankincense, helichrysum, lavender, lemongrass, marjoram, peppermint, white fir, wintergreen, ylang ylang, cellular complex blend, massage blend, soothing blend; see *Skeletal*

Cramping/charley horse - arborvitae, basil, cypress, lemongrass, marjoram, peppermint, massage blend, soothing blend; see *Muscular*

Headache - basil, cardamom, cilantro, dill, frankincense, helichrysum, juniper berry, lavender, lemongrass, marjoram, peppermint, rose, rosemary, wintergreen, calming blend, cellular complex blend, grounding blend, inspiring blend, reassuring blend, renewing blend, soothing blend, tension blend, uplifting blend

Headache, migraine - basil, bergamot, clove, coriander, frankincense, helichrysum, lavender, melissa, patchouli, peppermint, marjoram, roman chamomile, rosemary, rose, spearmint, detoxification blend, inspiring blend, reassuring blend, tension blend, renewing blend, uplifting blend

Joints - birch, white fir, soothing blend; see *Skeletal*

Referred - frankincense, helichrysum, juniper berry, cellular complex blend, soothing blend, tension blend

Spinal conditions - birch, lemongrass, white fir, cellular complex blend, soothing blend; see *Skeletal*

Tissue damage/injury - birch, cedarwood, clary sage, frankincense, helichrysum, lemongrass, marjoram, myrrh, sandalwood, vetiver, soothing blend; see *First Aid* ·

NEUROPATHIC (damaged nerve fiber pain):

Facial nerve - arborvitae, basil, clary sage, clove, frankincense, patchouli, cellular complex blend, calming blend, soothing blend; see *Nervous*

Nerve damage - arborvitae, black pepper, clary sage, clove, frankincense, ginger, helichrysum, lavender, lemongrass, cellular complex blend, grounding blend, tension blend; see *Nervous*

Phantom pains - arborvitae, basil, cypress, frankincense, helichrysum, lavender, cellular complex blend, tension blend; see *Nervous*

Shooting/burning - arborvitae, basil, bergamot, black pepper, clary sage, clove, frankincense, helichrysum, juniper berry, lavender, patchouli, peppermint, roman chamomile, thyme, vetiver, cellular complex blend, inspiring blend, soothing blend

Spinal cord injury - arborvitae, basil, clary sage, frankincense, helichrysum, lemongrass, thyme, anti-aging blend, cellular complex blend, soothing blend, tension blend; see *Nervous*

Tingling/numbness - arborvitae, basil, black pepper, clary sage, clove, cypress, anti-aging blend, cellular complex blend, tension blend; see *Nervous*

USAGE TIPS: Best practices for essential oil use for relief from pain and inflammation

- **Topical:** Very effective for many situations especially when it is more structural; most importantly, apply oils directly to any area of concern remembering to use a carrier oil if necessary to prevent sensitivity. Apply often, every 20-30 minutes, until symptoms subside, then reduce to every two to six hours for acute pain. For chronic pain, apply two to three times daily. Layering is also very effective for using multiple oils at the same time; apply one at a time.
- **Internal:** Highly effective for more chronic or internal pain; place oils in a capsule or drop under tongue (hold for 30 seconds; swallow).

Remedies

ARTHRITIS RUB
Mix 2 drops each of wintergreen, lemongrass, frankincense, and eucalyptus oils with a small amount of fractionated coconut oil and massage into painful areas.

JOINT & ARTHRITIS PAIN RELIEF
4 drops juniper berry
3 drops marjoram
3 drops roman chamomile
3 drops ginger
3 drops helichrysum
Mix essential oils in roller bottle with 1 teaspoon carrier oil, shake, and use as needed. OR add essential oils to 1/2 cup Epsom salt, stir; use in hot bath.

MIGRAINE INTERRUPTER: Place 1-2 drops juniper berry oil and helichrysum oil on back of neck. Dilute if desired.

HEADACHE RESOLVE (also works to reduce swelling): Layer or mix prior to application 1-2 drops each cedarwood, peppermint, frankincense oils to areas of need. Reapply every thirty minutes until headache or swelling are gone. Dilute as desired.

HEADACHE BLEND
7 drops of peppermint
5 drops of lavender
5 drops of frankincense
Combine oils into a 5ml roller bottle. Fill bottle with fractionated coconut oil or other carrier oil. Apply as needed. Reapply every thirty minutes until relief is achieved.

PAIN AWAY (soothing blend for jaw, knee, foot pain): Immediately use helichrysum oil, soothing blend, and frankincense oil on site of pain. Reapply frequently (every twenty to sixty minutes) until relief is achieved. Continue to apply to support healing process.

SORE MUSCLE SALVE
1 tablespoon beeswax
4 tablespoons carrier oil
10-30 drops each of wintergreen, lemongrass, marjoram and/or lavender
Gently melt the beeswax with the carrier oil over very low heat, stirring frequently. Remove from heat, and allow to cool. While still soft, stir essential oils into mixture. Pour into small glass storage container. Cool completely before putting on lid. Apply to sore muscles or any aches or pains.

SORE MUSCLE SOAK
Mix 4 drops black pepper, 2 drops rosemary, 1 drop ginger into ½ cup Epsom salt. Add to a bathtub of hot water and soak for up to thirty minutes. Remember to drink lots of water while soaking and thereafter.

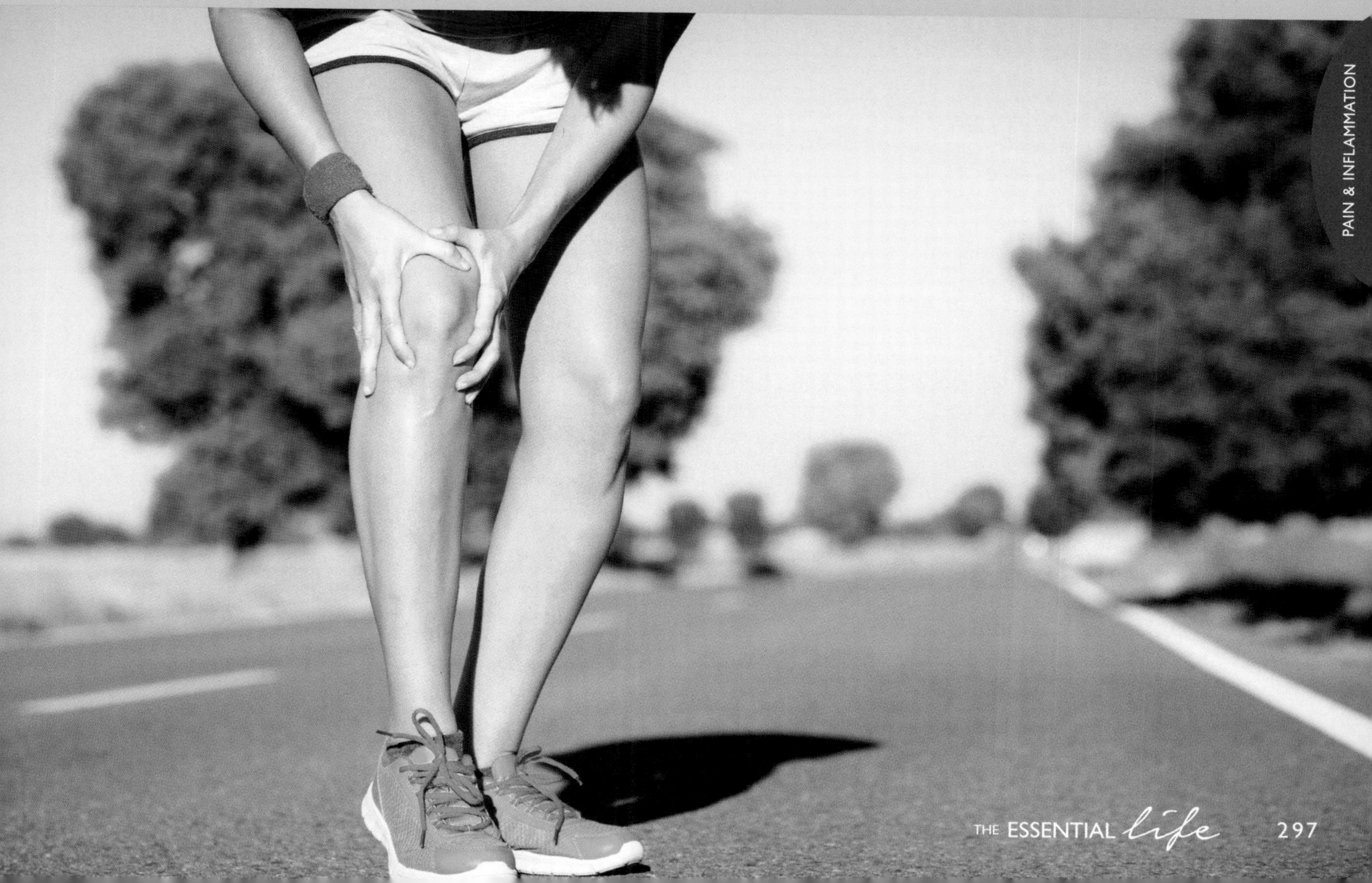

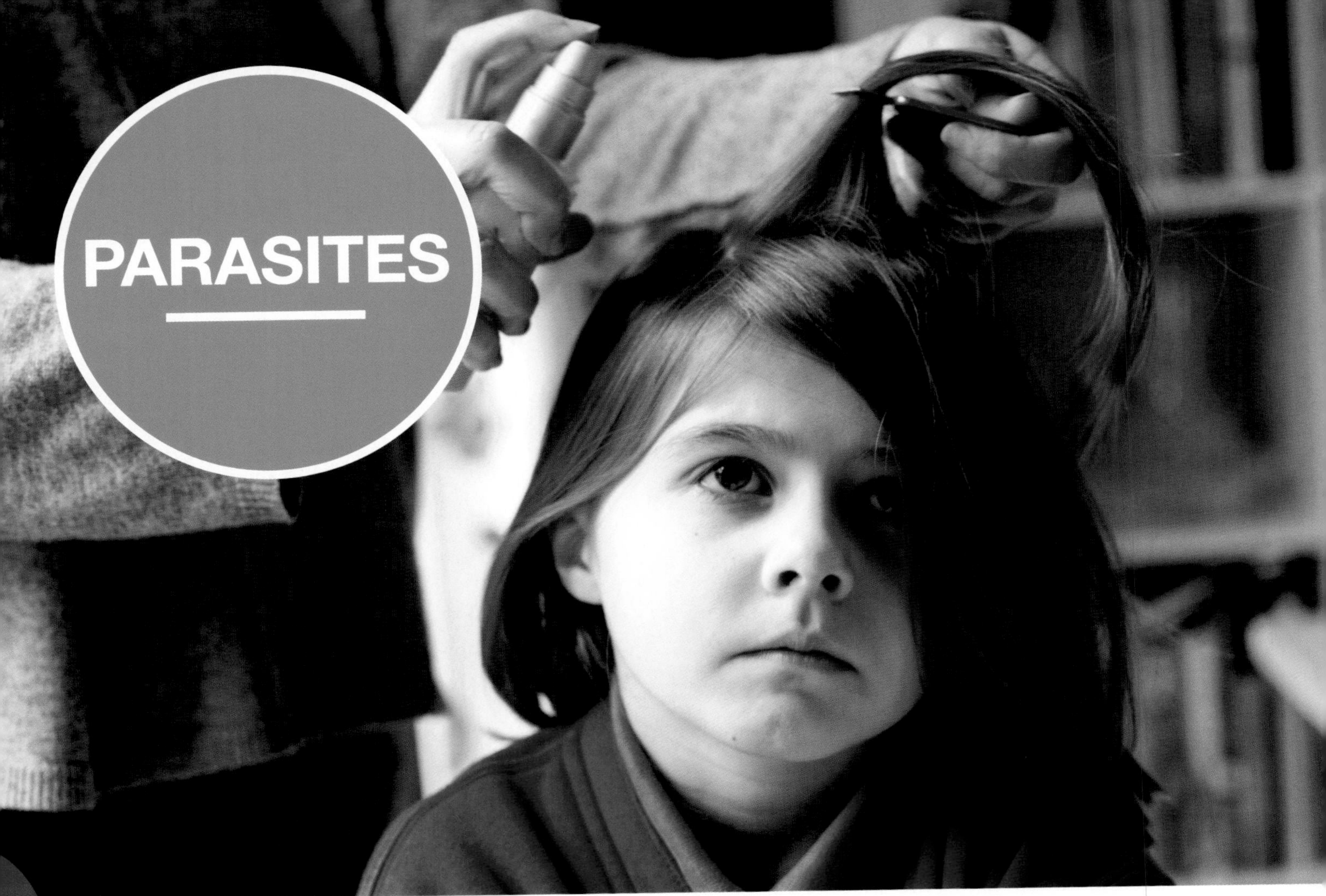

A PARASITE is an organism that lives on or in another organism, and gets food at the expense of its host. The majority of human parasites are microscopic (not visible to the naked eye), and contrary to common belief, can actually infest tissues all over the body – not just in the intestines. Not all parasites cause sickness, but those that do can cause incredible damage to the human body. Most parasites reproduce very quickly and infest human tissues and organs. There are over a thousand types of parasites, which can be broken down into six major categories:

1–Protozoa make up about 70 percent of parasites that invade humans. They are one-celled microscopic organisms that can quickly colonize the intestinal tract and from there move on to blood and other tissues and organs. A well-known protozoa parasite is Giardia lamblia.

2–Nematoda are worm-like, multicellular organisms that reproduce by laying eggs that typically grow in soil or within an intermediate host before infecting humans. Many people don't show signs of nematode infestation unless it is very heavy. Experts estimate that 75 percent of the world's population has some type of parasite infestation. Commonly known nematodes are roundworm, hookworm, and pinworm; nematodes typically infect the intestinal tract, blood, and tissues. Ascaris parasites are roundworms typically found in the intestines. Ascaris lumbricoides is probably the best known parasite in humans. Throughout their lifecycle, they infect various organs/tissues of the body that can include the intestines, the lungs, and the brain. When they infiltrate sensitive tissues, they can cause serious health problems.

3–Platyhelminthes. In this group, cestodes, or tapeworms, can be seen with the naked eye. The head attaches to the intestinal wall, and they feed on partially digested particles in the intestinal tract. As long as the head is intact, new tapeworms can grow. Beef, pork, fish, and dog tapeworms are well-recognized in the cestode category. Trematodes, also called flatworms or flukes, are leaf-shaped flatworm parasites that originate from infected snails. They can penetrate human skin or infiltrate a human host after the host has eaten an infected fish, plant, or crustacean. They can infect the intestines, blood, liver, and lungs. Common trematodes include Intestinal flukes, blood flukes, and liver flukes.

5–Acanthocephala, or thorny-headed worms, in their adult form, live in the intestines. They are considered by many to be the intermediary between nematodes and cestodes. They have elongated appendages with spines they use to pierce and attach to the organ walls of their hosts. Infections by acanthocephalans in humans are relatively rare.

6–Arthropoda are part of a classification called ectoparasites. This includes every kind of arthropod that receives its nourishment from other hosts (such as mosquitoes), but more specifically refers to the arthropods that burrow into and attach to the skin and remain for a time, such as chiggers, ticks, fleas, lice, scabies, and mites. Arthropods cause disease, and are common transmitters of pathogens that cause disease.

Certain dietary and lifestyle habits encourage parasitic invasion. Poorly and improperly digested food particles, mucus-forming foods, and sick/unhealthy tissue and organs encourage the proliferation of internal parasitic populations that rely on such substances or circumstances for their food. Unsanitary conditions, contact with infected individuals, certain outdoor activities such as walking barefoot in infested sand or soil, and even improper handwashing can bring exposure.

Symptoms of parasitic infestation are: diarrhea, constipation, gas, history of food poisoning, difficulty sleeping, difficulty staying asleep, skin irritations, unexplained skin rashes, hives, rosacea, eczema, teeth grinding (during sleep), pain or aching in muscles or joints, fatigue, exhaustion, depression, feelings of apathy, feeling satiated only after meals, iron-deficiency anemia. Since many of these symptoms are commonly associated with other conditions, it is important to work with a medical professional who can properly diagnose the presence of parasites.

The use of essential oils has at times been referred to as "intelligent medicine" because these oils have a unique ability to recognize what is supposed to be present in an organism and what should be eliminated. Parasites can be especially threatening due to their mobile nature (they move from tissue to tissue, wreaking havoc in their wake) and ability to reproduce so quickly. Essential oils should be considered as part of a well-planned approach to regain systemic balance after parasitic damage is discovered.

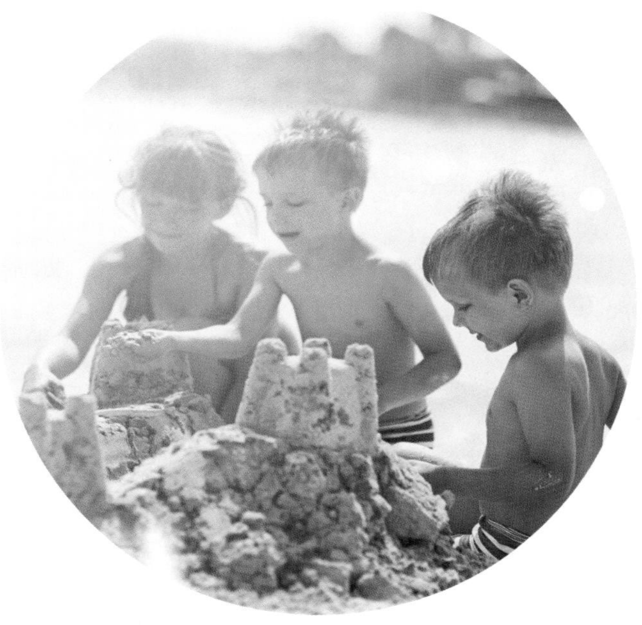

TOP SOLUTIONS

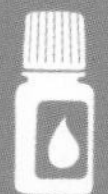

SINGLE OILS

Cinnamon (pg. 86), clove (pg. 90), lemongrass (pg. 112), oregano (pg. 120), roman chamomile (pg. 125), thyme (pg. 133) - to establish an unfriendly environment for parasites and encourage elimination

By Related Properties

For definitions of the properties listed below and more oil options, see Oil Properties Glossary (pg. 435) and Oil Properties (pg. 436).

Anti-parasitic (indicated for the treatment of parasitic diseases such as nematodes, cestodes, trematodes, and infectious protozoa) - bergamot, black pepper, cinnamon, clove, fennel, frankincense, juniper berry, lavender, melaleuca, oregano, roman chamomile, rosemary, thyme

Vermicide (a substance toxic to worms) - clove, lavender, oregano, wintergreen

Vermifuge (an agent that destroys or expels parasitic worms) - arborvitae, basil, bergamot, black cumin oil (skin clearing), cedarwood, cinnamon, clove, eucalyptus, fennel, geranium, lavender, lemon, melaleuca, peppermint, roman chamomile, rosemary, thyme, vetiver, wild orange, wintergreen

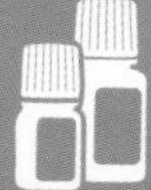

BLENDS

Cellular complex blend (pg. 143), cleansing blend (pg. 144) detoxification blend (pg. 146), digestion blend (pg. 147), protective blend (pg. 158), skin clearing blend (pg. 163) - to establish an unfriendly environment for parasites and encourage elimination

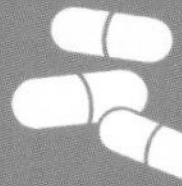

SUPPLEMENTS

Essential oil cellular complex, defensive probiotic, **detoxification complex (pg. 173)**, digestion blend softgels, food enzymes, **GI cleansing softgels** (pg. 178) (When conducting an intestinal parasite cleanse, it is essential to keep the intestinal tract moving so toxins do not remain in the body.)

Related Ailments: Ear Mites, Head Lice, Malaria [Immune & Lymphatic], Parasites, Pinworms, Worms

USAGE TIPS: For parasite elimination
The goal is to get oils to location(s) where parasite(s) lives (e.g. on skin or in gut). Consume or apply topically accordingly. Use a carrier oil to prevent sensitivity wherever needed.

Remedies

PARASITE INFECTION
2 drops cinnamon
4 drops clove
2 drops rosemary
3 drops oregano
3 drops lemon
3 drops melaleuca
Put into a capsule or dilute with water in a shot glass. Take twice a day for ten to fourteen days. If you suspect parasites or worms; drink lemon water several times a day for two weeks. Additional blend suggestions:
- Tapeworms - cinnamon + clove + cypress (combine); lemon + oregano + sandalwood; thyme
- Thorny-headed worms - combine: arborvitae, peppermint, thyme, wintergreen

MITES BE GONE: topical formula for humans (e.g. chiggers and scabies)
- Blend 4 drops of peppermint and 4 drops lavender with a teaspoon of carrier oil (recipe can be multiplied and stored in a small glass bottle for future use) and apply generously to all affected areas of skin at least twice per day, preferably after a bath. Do a patch test first to insure there is no skin reaction.
- To make the bath more effective, add 2 drops lavender and 2 drops rosemary mixed in a teaspoon of milk to encourage elimination of mites.
- To assist skin in recovery from dry, blotchy patches, apply lavender and myrrh, 2 drops of each per 1 teaspoon of carrier oil. Apply at least twice per day.

MITE CONTROL - for household invasion
Use eucalyptus, lemon, lavender, melaleuca, and peppermint oils. Eucalyptus and melaleuca are the most important oils in this blend, so be sure you use those even if you don't have the others. Blend 35 drops each of the above oils in 24 ounces of water in a spray bottle. Add 2 ounces witch hazel (optional). Generously spray carpets, beds, curtains, pillows, furniture, etc.

DUST MITES BEWARE!
- Clean mattress: put approximately 1 cup baking soda into a small mason jar with some kind of screen or multiple-hole-punctured lid (for sprinkling purposes) and add 4 to 5 drops of any of the following: eucalyptus, lemon, lavender, melaleuca, and/or peppermint (use your favorite scent) and give it a good shake! This is enough for a twin mattresses.
  - Sprinkle on mattress.
  - Leave for on for two hours.
  - Vacuum up residue.

  The baking soda not only draws out moisture and dirt, but it also deodorizes and leaves the mattress smelling fresh and clean. An oil like lavender promotes calm and peaceful sleep.
- While the baking soda works, it's a really great time to wash all the bed linens in HOT water. Add a few drops of any of the same oils. When drying pillows, add a tennis ball or two to help fluff them back up.

A study on the impact of essential oils on dust mites found that lemon oil immobilized 61 percent of dust mites after thirty minutes, and 80 percent were dead after two hours. Lavender oil immobilized 86 percent after thirty minutes and 87 percent were dead after two hours. Melaleuca oil immobilized 100 percent of the dust mites after thirty minutes, and were 100% dead after two hours.

Source: Williamson, E. M., Priestley, C. M., & Burgess, I. F. (2007). An investigation and comparison of the bioactivity of selected essential oils on human lice and house dust mites. Fitoterapia, 78(7-8), 521-525.

PARASITES

Conditions

Giardia - lavender, bergamot, cardamom, clove, frankincense, ginger, melaleuca, oregano, patchouli, rosemary, thyme, detoxification blend

Parasites, general - cinnamon, clove, lemongrass, oregano, protective blend

Parasites, intestinal worms - bergamot, clove, geranium, lemon, peppermint, roman, chamomile, thyme, detoxification blend, protective blend, skin clearing blend

Worms - basil, black pepper, cinnamon, clove, fennel, lavender, lemon, lemongrass, oregano, roman chamomile, thyme, renewing blend
- **Flukes** - clove, oregano, cleansing blend
- **Hookworms** - clove, thyme
- **Pinworms** - bergamot, clove, lemon, lemongrass, oregano, roman chamomile, thyme, protective blend
- **Roundworms** - cypress, geranium, oregano, sandalwood
- **Tapeworms** - cinnamon, clove, cypress, lemon, oregano, sandalwood, thyme
- **Thorny-headed worms** - arborvitae, peppermint, thyme, wintergreen

Fleas - cedarwood, eucalyptus, lavender, lemon, lemongrass, peppermint, cleansing blend

Lice, head - arborvitae, cedarwood, cinnamon, clove, eucalyptus, geranium, lavender, melaleuca, oregano, rosemary, thyme, detoxification blend, invigorating blend, repellent blend

Lice, pubic or crab - melaleuca, rosemary

Mites, ear - basil, cedarwood, lavender, melaleuca, oregano, rosemary, clove, cleansing blend, focus blend

Scabies (caused by Sarcoptes scabiei mite) - bergamot, cinnamon, clove, frankincense, lavender, melaleuca, oregano, peppermint, roman chamomile, rosemary, thyme, cellular blend, cleansing blend, soothing blend, protective blend, skin clearing blend, uplifting blend

Trombiculosis (caused by chiggers mite) - clove, lavender, melaleuca, peppermint, thyme, vetiver, protection blend

Tick bites - eucalyptus, juniper berry, lavender, lemon, lemongrass, cleansing blend; see *First Aid*

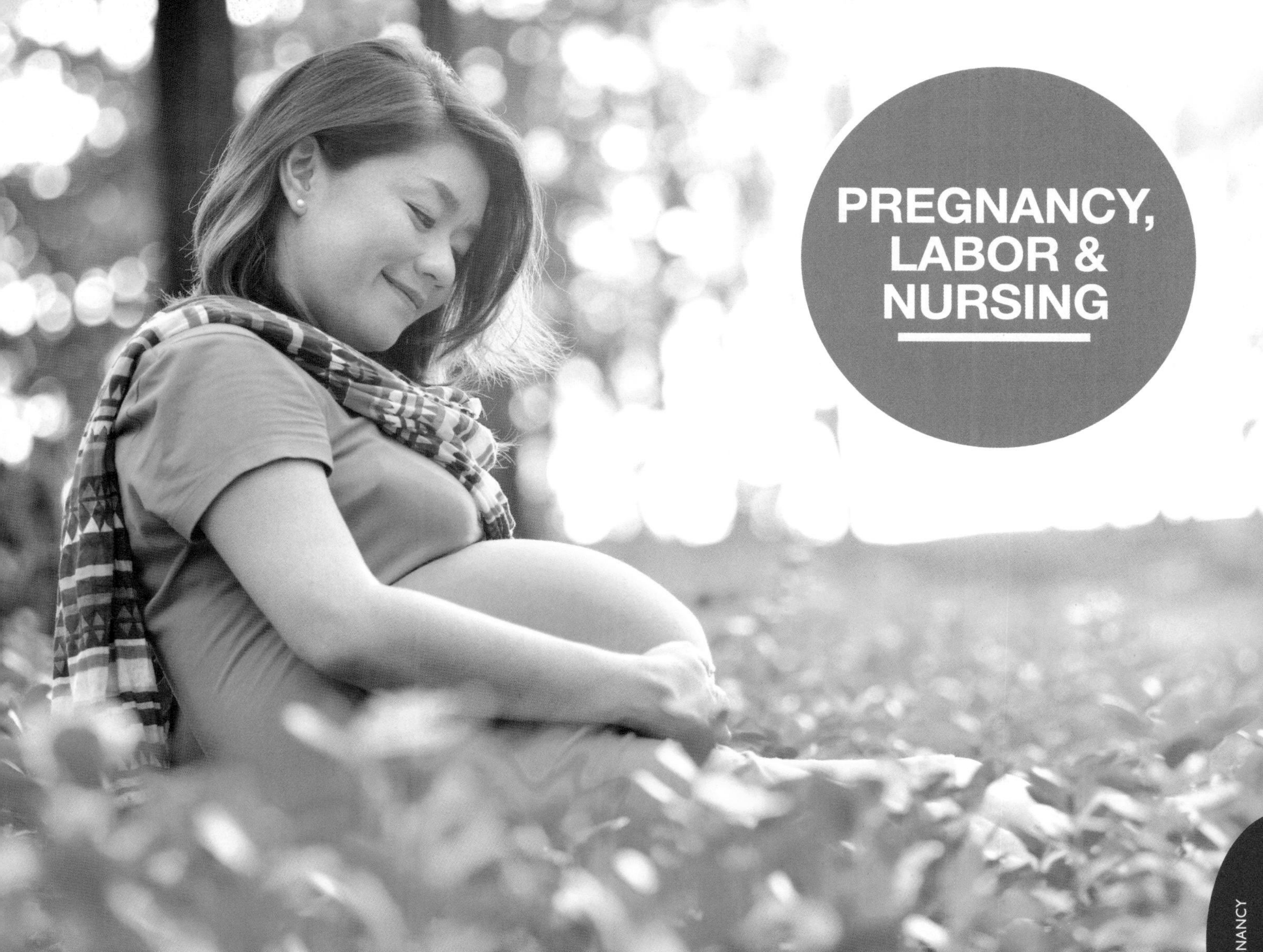

PREGNANCY, LABOR & NURSING

PREGNANCY can be a unique, exciting and joyous time in a woman's life. For a woman to become pregnant, she must release an egg from her ovary – ovulation. Next, the egg and sperm must meet and form a single cell – fertilization. Then pregnancy begins when and if the fertilized egg attaches to a woman's uterus and begins to grow – implantation.

The growing fetus depends entirely on its mother's healthy body for all needs. Pregnant women must take steps to remain as healthy and well nourished as they possibly can. After an approximate nine-month gestation period a woman's body begins the work of opening up and pushing the baby out into the world. This work is called labor.

Labor is a process by which the baby inside the womb adjusts itself to its surroundings and passes out of the uterus to be born as an infant into the world. Every labor is different. It can be long or short, very difficult or not. Each labor, however, follows a basic pattern:

- Contractions (labor pains) open the cervix
- The womb pushes the baby down through the vagina
- The baby is born, and then
- The placenta (afterbirth) is born

Once the baby is born it no longer receives nutrients from the umbilical cord. Breastfeeding is the normal way of providing young infants the nutrients they need for healthy growth and development. Typically most mothers can breastfeed, provided they have accurate information. Exclusive breastfeeding is recommended up to six months of age, with continued breastfeeding along with appropriate complementary foods as desired.

It is difficult to get all the proper vitamins and minerals needed in a normal diet, so supplementation is usually necessary both during pregnancy and while nursing. Taking whole food supplements is key. This makes the vitamins and minerals bioavailable to the body so it is better equipped to provide adequate nutrition for both mother and baby. Many synthetic or non-food based supplements are not able to be absorbed by the body and can sometimes cause more harm than good.

Essential oils can assist with some of the uncomfortable changes that take place in a woman's body during pregnancy, labor, and postpartum periods as well as during breastfeeding. The oils may be applied topically, diffused, or ingested for breast soreness, constipation, depression, fatigue, high blood pressure, nausea/ vomiting, sleep, stretch marks, swelling, and more.

TOP SOLUTIONS

pregnancy

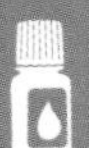

SINGLE OILS

Wild orange - energizes and lifts mood (pg. 136)
Ginger - relieves nausea and morning sickness (pg. 103)
Peppermint - relieves digestive upsets and supports memory (pg. 122)

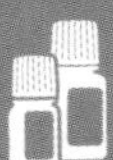

BLENDS

Soothing blend - soothes aches and pains (pg. 164)
Tension blend - relieves tension (pg. 165)
Metabolic blend - balances glucose levels and metabolism (pg. 157)
Digestion blend - supports digestion and relieves morning sickness (pg. 147)
Women's blend - balances hormones (pg. 168)

labor

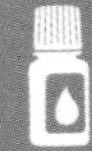

SINGLE OILS

Clary Sage - broad-spectrum support to labor process (pg. 88)
Jasmine - assists with labor and afterbirth (pg. 106)
Geranium - supports perineum, labor performance, mood and healing (pg. 102)
Lavender - calms and soothes mood and tissues (pg. 108)
Frankincense - lessens stress and trauma; promotes healing (pg. 100)
Basil - relieves pain; enhances labor performance (pg. 76)
Helichrysum - slows/stops bleeding and promotes healing (pg. 105)

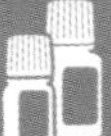

BLENDS

Grounding blend - improves coping capacity (pg. 150)
Tension blend - relieves tension (pg. 165)
Women's monthly blend - enhances labor performance (pg. 167)
Soothing blend - soothes aches and pains (pg. 164)

nursing

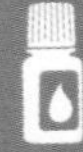

SINGLE OILS

Fennel - promotes milk production; prevents clogged ducts, infection, and thrush (pg. 98)
Ylang Ylang - alleviates tender breasts and depression (pg. 139)
Clary sage - promotes milk supply and hormone balancing; boosts mood (pg. 88)
Lavender - promotes milk production; prevents/heals tender sore breasts, nipples, and clogged milk ducts (pg. 108)

BLENDS

Women's blend - balances hormones and increases libido (pg. 168)
Joyful blend - supports mood and alleviates depression (pg. 154)

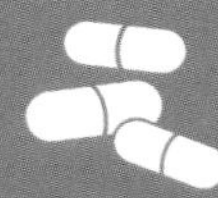

SUPPLEMENTS

Bone support complex (pg. 170), defensive probiotic (pg. 172), digestion blend softgels, essential oil cellular complex, **essential oil omega complex (pg. 175), food enzymes (pg. 177),** whole food nutrient supplement

By Related Properties

For definitions of the properties listed below and more oil options, see Oil Properties Glossary (pg. 435) and Oil Properties (pg. 436).

Analgesic - arborvitae, basil, bergamot, cassia, cinnamon, clary sage, fennel, frankincense, ginger, helichrysum, peppermint, rosemary, white fir, wintergreen
Antidepressant - bergamot, clary sage, frankincense, geranium, grapefruit, jasmine, lemon, melissa, patchouli, rose, sandalwood, wild orange, ylang ylang
Anticoagulant - clary sage, helichrysum, lavender
Antiemetic - basil, cardamom, cassia, clove, coriander, fennel, ginger, lavender, patchouli, peppermint
Antihemorrhagic - geranium, helichrysum, lavender, myrrh
Antispasmodic - basil, bergamot, black pepper, cardamom, cassia, cinnamon, clary sage, clove, cypress, eucalyptus, fennel, ginger, helichrysum, lavender, lemon, marjoram, patchouli, peppermint, roman chamomile, rose, rosemary, sandalwood, spearmint, tangerine, vetiver, wild orange, wintergreen, ylang ylang
Calming - bergamot, clary sage, fennel, frankincense, geranium, jasmine, lavender, patchouli, roman chamomile, sandalwood, tangerine, vetiver
Carminative - basil, bergamot, cardamom, cinnamon, clary sage, fennel, ginger, lavender, lemon, myrrh, patchouli, peppermint, roman chamomile, rosemary, sandalwood, spearmint, vetiver, wild orange, wintergreen
Digestive stimulant - basil, bergamot, black pepper, cardamom, cinnamon, coriander, fennel, frankincense, grapefruit, myrrh, patchouli, spearmint, wild orange
Energizing - basil, cypress, grapefruit, lemongrass, rosemary, white fir, wild orange
Galactagogue - basil, clary sage, dill, fennel, jasmine, lemongrass, wintergreen
Immunostimulant - arborvitae, cassia, cinnamon, clove, frankincense, ginger, lemon, lime, melaleuca, melissa, oregano, rosemary spearmint, thyme, vetiver, wild orange
Invigorating - grapefruit, lemon, peppermint, spearmint, wild orange, wintergreen
Regenerative - basil, cedarwood, clove, coriander, frankincense, geranium, helichrysum, jasmine, lavender, melaleuca, myrrh, patchouli, sandalwood, wild orange
Relaxing - basil, cassia, cedarwood, clary sage, cypress, fennel, geranium, jasmine, lavender, marjoram, myrrh, ravensara, roman chamomile, white fir, ylang ylang
Sedative - basil, bergamot, cedarwood, clary sage, frankincense, geranium, jasmine, lavender, marjoram, melissa, patchouli, roman chamomile, rose, sandalwood, tangerine, vetiver, ylang ylang
Stomachic - cardamom, cinnamon, clary sage, coriander, fennel, ginger, marjoram, peppermint, rosemary, tangerine, wild orange
Uplifting - bergamot, clary sage, grapefruit, lemon, lime, melissa, sandalwood, tangerine, wild orange, ylang ylang
Warming - birch, black pepper, cassia, cinnamon, clary sage, clove, eucalyptus, ginger, lemongrass, marjoram, oregano, peppermint, thyme, wintergreen

Remedies

Optimal Pregnancy and Post-pregnancy Success Suggestions

- **BASIC SUPPLEMENT PROGRAM**
  Benefits: basic nutrition, gut health, energy, stamina, emotional stability, regulate blood pressure, avoid postpartum depression, support proper digestion and absorption of nutrients, prepare for rich breast milk supply; prevent infection; ease leg/muscle/ligament cramps or spasms; support healthy connective tissue and skin, prepare cervix for birth
  - Whole food nutrient supplement - delivers multivitamins and minerals
  - Essential oil omega complex - supplies essential fatty acids
  - Food enzymes - provides digestive enzyme support
  - Defensive probiotic - provides and promotes prebiotics and probiotics
  - Bone support complex - supplies needed calcium, magnesium, and more

In addition to the above basic supplementation program, choose as needed:

- Prevent/overcome - use as often as needed; don't wait for upset, prevent if possible
  - Morning sickness - digestion blend, ginger, peppermint; support liver/gallbladder: apply topically - lemon, grapefruit, detoxification blend
  - Heartburn - digestion blend
- Stay calm, grounded - use one or more of following at least twice daily as needed:
  - Frankincense, wild orange, calming blend, grounding blend Balance metabolism, sugar cravings, appetite - choose one; use three times daily:
  - Grapefruit or metabolic blend
- Maintain optimal elimination and antioxidant support - use ? or more daily
  - Cellular complex blend, detoxification blend, lemon and/or other citrus oils
  - Gut cleanse - 2 drops each lemon, melaleuca, thyme at least two times a day for ten days, rest; take extra defensive probiotic
- Prevent/overcome leg/muscle/ligament cramps or spasms
  - Use as needed: cypress, lavender, marjoram, massage blend, soothing blend

PREGNANCY SWELLING RELIEF
3 drops ginger
2 drops cypress
2 drops lavender
Combine oils with 2 teaspoons carrier oil; massage into legs and feet.

NO MORE STRETCH MARKS BLEND
10 drops cypress
10 drops lavender
10 drops wild orange
10 drops invigorating blend
5 drops geranium
Place oils in a 10ml roller bottle; fill remainder with carrier oil. Use twice daily.

STRETCH MARK RELIEF
2 drops each of helichrysum, lavender, myrrh oil mixed with ½ - 1 teaspoon fractionated coconut oil (depending on surface area intended to cover) and apply to abdomen.

HEALING HEMORRHOIDS
20 drops helichrysum
20 drops geranium
20 drops arborvitae or cypress
10 drop peppermint
Make blend in 2-ounce glass bottle with an orifice-reduction seal; mix oils; fill remainder with carrier oil. Apply at least once or twice daily and/or after every bowel evacuation. For additional, more intense support if needed, 1 drop of each oil can be applied NEAT. Any burning sensation should subside within five to ten minutes, or apply carrier oil prior to oil application if desired.

THE FINAL COUNTDOWN ROLL-ON (reduces swelling and bleeding at labor)
10 drops clary sage
10 drops ginger
10 drops lavender
10 drops lemon
10 drops massage blend
Combine oils in 10ml roller bottle; fill remainder with carrier oil. Twice daily apply a thin layer of carrier oil to target areas to improve distribution of oils; then apply oils. Apply blend to low back and ankles every day during the last week of pregnancy. Massage into skin thoroughly.

JUMP START CONTRACTIONS
Apply 1-2 drops each of myrrh and clary sage oil to wrists and abdomen as well as on uterine and cervical reflex points under inside ankle bones once labor begins but has slowed/stalled.

INCREASE MILK SUPPLY SALVE
7 drops basil
6 drops clary sage
4 drops geranium
Combine 4 tsp fractionated coconut oil to 2 tsp beeswax (approx ⅛ stick).
Melt over low heat. Cool. While still soft, add oils to make a salve. Rub onto breasts throughout the day.

HELLO WORLD! - recovery for mom and baby; use as desired at least two times daily to support optimal recovery for mom and bonding with baby. Use any or all as desired, a drop or few at a time. Diffuse and/or use topically. A few drops of each:
- Fennel, frankincense, lavender, lemon, joyful blend

POSTPARTUM DEPRESSION BLENDS: Apply topically or diffuse. These are single-use quantities; multiply as desired.
- Recipe #1: 1 drop rose, 1 drop wild orange, and 3 drops sandalwood
- Recipe #2: 1 drop lavender, 3 drops grapefruit, and 1 drop ylang ylang
- Recipe #3: 1 drop bergamot, 1 drop grapefruit, 1 drop clary sage, 1 drop wild orange, and 3 drops frankincense

Conditions

PREGNANCY:

Appetite cravings/blood sugar imbalance - metabolic blend
Backache - peppermint, rosemary, massage blend, soothing blend
Bleeding - geranium, helichrysum, lavender, myrrh; see *Cardiovascular*
Blood pressure, high - eucalyptus, lavender, lemon, marjoram, ylang ylang
Breast tenderness - geranium, grapefruit, lavender, ylang ylang, women's monthly blend
Constipation - cilantro, fennel, ginger, lemon, lemongrass, marjoram, peppermint, detoxification blend, digestion blend; see *Digestive & Intestinal*
Cramps - arborvitae, basil, cypress, marjoram, massage blend, soothing blend
Depression - basil, bergamot, frankincense, geranium, lavender, lemon, melissa, patchouli, ravensara, rose, sandalwood, vetiver, wild orange, ylang ylang, grounding blend, invigorating blend, joyful blend, women's monthly blend; see *Mood & Behavior*
Energy, low/fatigue - cypress, grapefruit, lemon, peppermint, wild orange, invigorating blend, joyful blend; see *Energy & Vitality*
Headaches - frankincense, lavender, peppermint, wintergreen, soothing blend, tension blend
Heartburn/gas/bloating - peppermint, wild orange, digestion blend; see *Digestive & Intestinal*
Hemorrhoids - See "Varicose veins" below
Infection - lemon, melaleuca, oregano, protective blend
Labor, preterm/cramping - frankincense, lavender, marjoram, patchouli, roman chamomile, wild orange + ylang ylang, women's blend, women's monthly blend
Leg cramps - basil, cypress, lavender, lemongrass, marjoram, wintergreen, massage blend
Miscarriage, prevents - myrrh, patchouli, rose, anti-aging blend, joyful blend
Miscarriage, recovery - clary sage, frankincense, geranium, grapefruit, lavender, myrrh, patchouli, roman chamomile, rose, anti-aging blend, cellular complex blend, cleaning blend, detoxification blend, joyful blend, soothing blend, women's monthly blend
Miscarriage, process and recovery - clary sage, lavender, white fir, soothing blend, women's monthly blend
Morning sickness/nausea - arborvitae, bergamot, cardamom, coriander, fennel, geranium, ginger, lavender, lemon, peppermint, digestion blend, soothing blend
Muscles, sore - arborvitae, basil, birch, black pepper, clary sage, coriander, frankincense, geranium, helichrysum, juniper berry, marjoram, peppermint, white fir, wintergreen, massage blend, respiration blend, soothing blend
Preeclampsia - cinnamon, cypress, frankincense, ginger, lavender, marjoram, roman chamomile, calming blend, massage blend, metabolic blend
Postbirth healing - cypress, frankincense, helichrysum, geranium, lavender, myrrh, roman chamomile, protective blend
Progesterone, low - geranium, grapefruit, oregano, thyme
Skin, itching/pregnancy mask - geranium, lavender, roman chamomile, sandalwood, anti-aging blend
Sleep, restless/insomnia - frankincense, lavender, roman chamomile, wild orange, calming blend, grounding blend; see *Sleep*
Stretch marks - cypress, frankincense, geranium, lavender, myrrh, sandalwood, tangerine, wild orange, anti-aging blend, invigorating blend, renewing blend
Uterus, weak - clary sage, frankincense, ginger, jasmine, lemongrass, marjoram, cellular complex blend, renewing blend
Urinary tract infections - basil, cassia, cinnamon, cypress, lemon, lemongrass, melaleuca, oregano, thyme, protective blend
Varicose veins - bergamot, cardamom, cypress, geranium, helichrysum, lemon, lemongrass, melaleuca, patchouli, peppermint, rosemary, detoxification blend; see *Cardiovascular*
Water retention (edema)/blood pressure elevated - cypress, ginger, juniper berry, lavender, lemon, invigorating blend, massage blend; see *Cardiovascular, Urinary*

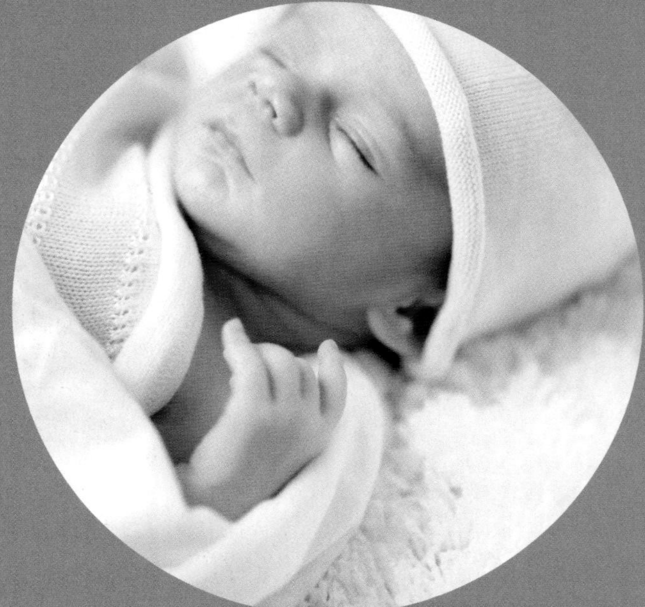

LABOR:

Afterbirth/placenta delivery - clary sage, geranium, jasmine, lavender
Bleeding - geranium, helichrysum, myrrh
Calm nerves, relax mind - basil, frankincense, lavender, calming blend, encouraging blend, grounding blend
Contractions, slow/weak/stalled labor - cinnamon, clary sage, fennel, jasmine, lavender, myrrh, detoxification blend, encouraging blend, grounding blend, joyful blend
Coping, poor/overwhelmed, low confidence/fearful mindset, mood issues - basil, clary sage, jasmine, geranium, lavender, peppermint, wild orange, calming blend, encouraging blend, grounding blend, invigorating blend, joyful blend, massage blend, soothing blend
Difficult - basil, cedarwood, clary sage, fennel, geranium, lavender, myrrh, rose, spearmint, calming blend, grounding blend, massage blend
Increase awareness, lift mood - basil, lavender, invigorating blend, joyful blend
Labor pains, management/lower back/support circulation - arborvitae, basil, birch, black pepper, clary sage, coriander, cypress, frankincense, geranium, helichrysum, juniper berry, lavender, marjoram, myrrh, white fir, wintergreen, calming blend, grounding blend, massage blend, reassuring blend, soothing blend
Overall support for optimal labor - basil, clary sage, geranium, reassuring blend, women's monthly blend

PREGNANCY

Overheated - birch, eucalyptus, peppermint, wintergreen
Pain - cypress, lavender, marjoram, soothing blend, tension blend
Perineum, prep/avoid episiotomy - frankincense, geranium, roman chamomile, sandalwood
Position of baby needs work - peppermint
Prep for labor - basil, clary sage, geranium, jasmine, women's monthly blend
Tension, excess - clary sage, geranium, lavender, massage blend, tension blend
Transition - basil, women's blend
Uterus, performance during labor - clary sage, frankincense, jasmine, myrrh, rose, joyful blend, women's monthly blend

POST-DELIVERY & NURSING:

After pains/uterine cramping that occurs while nursing - bergamot, birch, coriander, clary sage, frankincense, helichrysum, myrrh, women's blend
Breasts, tender - frankincense, geranium, grapefruit, lavender, ylang ylang; see *Women's Health*
Clogged milk ducts - fennel, lavender, patchouli, cleansing blend
Constipation - cilantro, douglas fir, fennel, ginger, lemon, lemongrass, marjoram, peppermint, detoxification blend, digestion blend; see *Digestive & Intestinal*
Depression, postpartum - bergamot, clary sage, frankincense, geranium, grapefruit, lavender, lemon, myrrh, roman chamomile, sandalwood, vetiver, wild orange, ylang ylang, calming blend, comforting blend, cellular complex blend, detoxification blend, grounding blend, invigorating blend, joyful blend, reassuring blend, women's blend; see *Mood & Behavior*
Engorgement - peppermint, massage blend, soothing blend
Episiotomy/healing from - black pepper, cypress, frankincense, helichrysum, myrrh, anti-aging blend
Infection (mastitis) - fennel, frankincense, lavender, melaleuca, patchouli, rosemary, wild orange, cleansing blend, invigorating blend; *for internal use to fight infection - cinnamon or clove, melaleuca, oregano, thyme
Milk production (lactation), lack of - basil, clary sage, dill, fennel, geranium, jasmine, lavender, lemongrass (avoid nipple area if applying topically); *avoid peppermint or blends with peppermint as it decreases milk supply
Milk production, to stop - peppermint
Nipple vasospasms (nipple compressed after nursing) - lime, women's blend
Nipples dry,cracked/sore (improper latch) - frankincense, geranium, lavender, myrrh, roman chamomile, sandalwood
Recovery from childbirth - clary sage, coriander, cypress, geranium, frankincense (soothe perineum or circumcision), helichrysum, jasmine (supports expulsion of placenta), lavender (supports expulsion of placenta; soothes perineum or circumcision), sandalwood, white fir, ylang ylang, calming blend (to overcome distress, deal with newness of breastfeeding), grounding blend (for emotional stability, recovery), anti-aging blend (cesarean-section recovery), women's blend
Sore nipples - frankincense, lavender, roman chamomile, detoxification blend
Thrush - clary sage, dill, fennel, frankincense, lemon, melaleuca, wild orange; see *Candida*

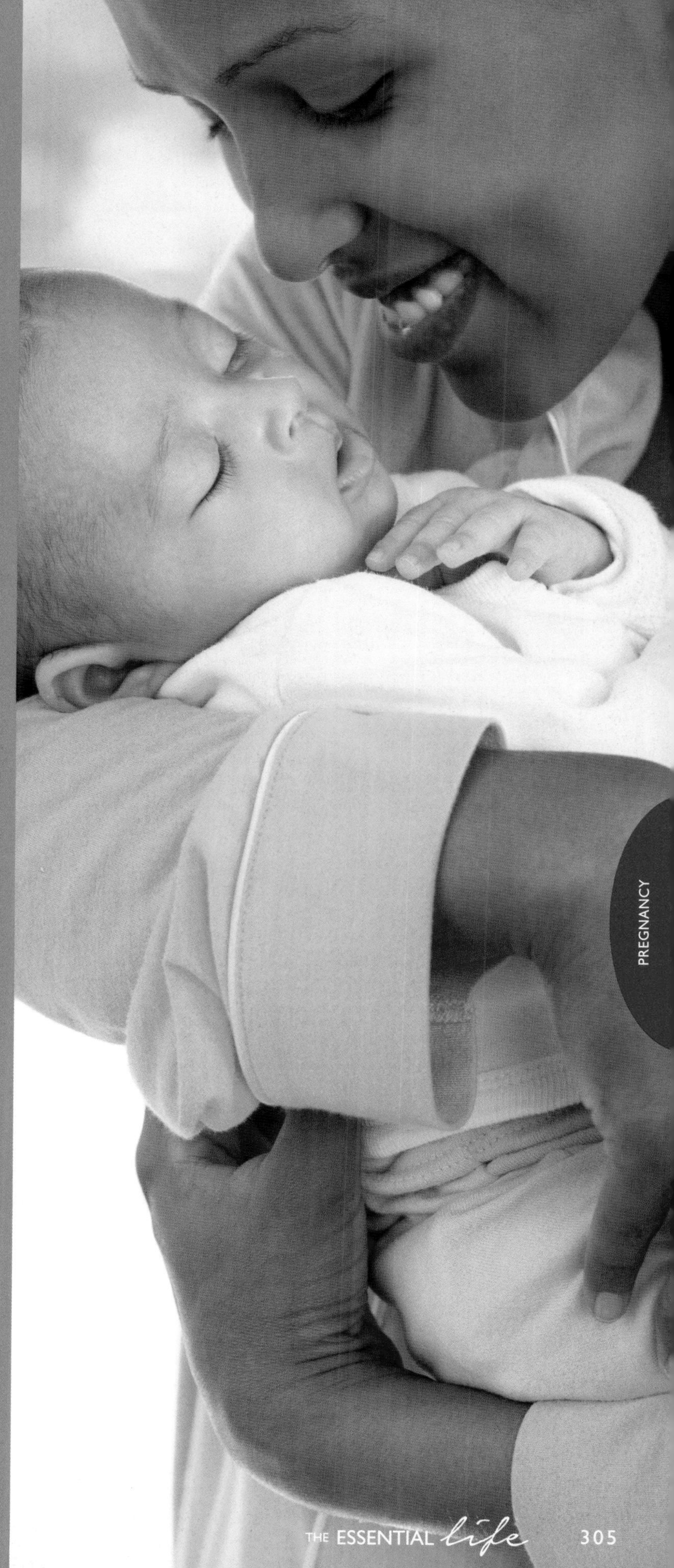

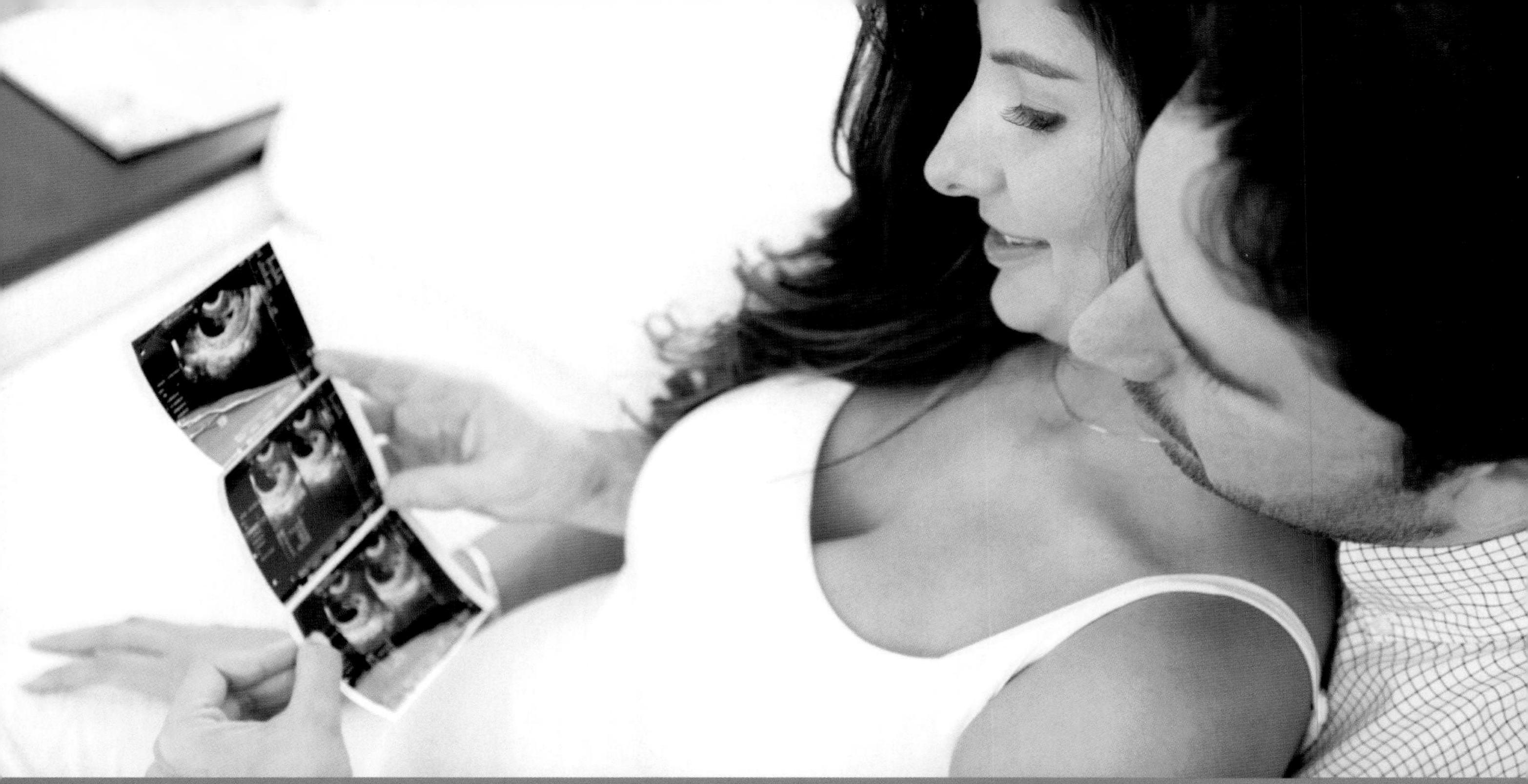

PREGNANCY

ESSENTIAL OIL USAGE FOR PREGNANT & NURSING WOMEN

There are differing opinions regarding essential use and safety during pregnancy as well as nursing. It is common to find warnings everywhere about which oils one should and should not use during pregnancy. The most commonly expressed concern is over the topical and internal use of essential oils.

When using essential oils that are laden with impurities there is a legitimate threat posed to a developing fetus. However, if the user has ensured they are using only pure, unadulterated essential oils, many of those concerns become unwarranted. It is recommended a pregnant women be under the care of a physician and/or midwife and consult with them prior to taking/using new products.

Here are a few safety guidelines to use when selecting oils for use during pregnancy:

1. **Use truly therapeutic, superior grade essential oils** that are certified as pure, potent, genuine and authentic and subjected to rigorous testing to ensure no harmful ingredients are present. Many products on the market contain synthetic components/ingredients and are to be avoided altogether.
2. **Be aware.** When using pure and potent oils, be aware of what they might do before using them. When using more powerful oils, use small amounts and dilute with a carrier oil.
3. **Be a wise steward.** The first three months are the time baby develops rapidly. Simply be more cautious during the first trimester.
4. **Pay attention to how the body responds** to dosages. As body weight increases, there may be a need to increase dosage accordingly. OR use less due to heightened sensitivity. Once again, pay attention to the body's responses. Consider using oils diluted (especially if particularly strong or "hot") as a habit during pregnancy versus using them NEAT (undiluted). The bottoms of the feet are an excellent conservative application location (commonly used with children). Another option is to do a patch test if concerned. Simply apply a single drop on skin and observe results prior to use.
5. **Use oils aromatically** as a safe method during pregnancy. They are excellent for boosting mood and energy and creating an uplifting environment. The also support stress and tension reduction and promote a good night's sleep.
6. **Consider the source.** When it comes to trying to decipher facts regarding essential oil use during pregnancy and nursing, human studies are not conducted. Rather animal studies, mainly on rats, are the source of the majority of information. During these studies inordinately high doses of essential oils are injected at levels that exceed human consumption and fail to duplicate the human experience. Frankly, no human would consume or use these quantities nor do they inject them as a form of use.
7. **Err on the side of safety.** In conclusion, use prudence, dilute, and avoid anything that simply doesn't feel right. Some oils will be better diluted such as the "hot" oils listed in the usage section located earlier in this book. Consult with healthcare practitioner about usage as desired or needed.

NOTE: The use of clary sage by women who have a history of preterm labor or miscarriage or are experiencing such should be avoided. The use of peppermint oil while nursing can limit milk production for some women and therefore it is recommended for them to reduce or stop usage while breastfeeding. Some women report that minor use is acceptable but advise avoiding regular use so as to avoid a significant decrease in milk production. Fennel, clary sage, or basil can counteract effects of peppermint on lactation as they increase milk supply.

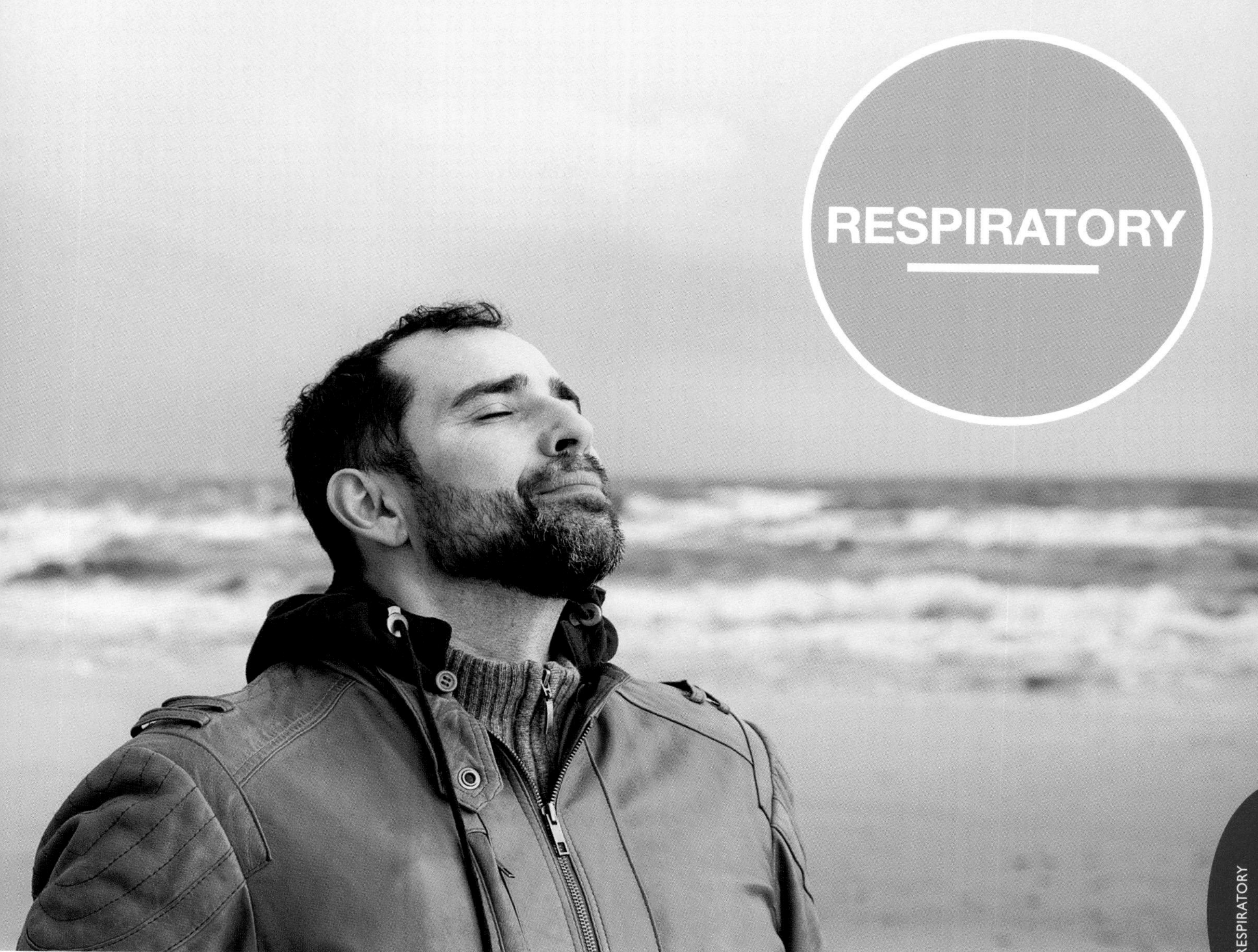

RESPIRATION is the process of inhaling, warming, filtering, controlling the humidity of, and exhaling air. Lungs exchange oxygen for carbon dioxide, and the heart pumps oxygenated blood to the rest of the body. Additionally, the cilia in the lungs secrete mucus as they move back and forth, carrying out of the lungs; dust, germs, and other matter, where it is expelled by sneezing, coughing, spitting, and swallowing.

Breathing is controlled by the diaphragm, located at the base of the ribcage. When the diaphragm contracts it pulls down on the thoracic cavity, causing the lungs to expand and air to be inhaled. When the diaphragm relaxes, the lungs retract and air is exhaled. The breathing process, one of the most basic and important functions performed by the body, often is taken for granted...until something goes wrong. For some individuals, breathing can be challenging, especially if they suffer from some type of respiratory condition or disease.

Respiratory disease is a broad term used to refer to a series of conditions that affect the respiratory system. Therefore, any condition that affects the lungs, bronchial tubes, upper respiratory tract, trachea, pleural cavity, or even nerves and muscles used for breathing can be termed as a respiratory disease.

Infection, histamine reaction, or prolonged irritation can negatively impact the respiratory system. A variety of ailments may result, ranging from mild allergies or stuffy nose to more severe asthma or diphtheria.

In general, a respiratory illness can have a debilitating effect on one's overall health. Many people mistake respiratory illnesses for other health problems, particularly when they experience an overall feeling of fatigue and malaise. Loss of appetite, indigestion, severe weight loss, and headaches are also quite common in respiratory diseases.

Medical attention and diagnosis is absolutely essential for any respiratory ailment that is severe or persistent. However, milder conditions can be easily resolved with the support of natural and simple home remedies. The scope of home remedies is vast. They can be used alone or in combination with conventional treatments.

TOP SOLUTIONS

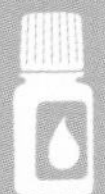

SINGLE OILS

Black pepper - reduces inflammation and mucus (pg. 81)
Eucalyptus - opens airways, supports proper respiratory function (pg. 98)
Peppermint - opens airways, expels mucus (pg. 122)
Rosemary - helps with many different respiratory issues (pg. 127)

By Related Properties

For definitions of the properties listed below and more oil options, see Oil Properties Glossary (pg. 435) and Oil Properties (pg. 436).

Anticatarrhal - basil, black pepper, clary sage, cardamom, eucalyptus, fennel, frankincense, helichrysum, oregano, rosemary, sandalwood, spearmint, white fir, wild orange
Anti-inflammatory - arborvitae, basil, bergamot, birch, black pepper, cardamom, cassia, cedarwood, cinnamon, coriander, cypress, dill, eucalyptus, fennel, frankincense, geranium, ginger, helichrysum, jasmine, lavender, lemongrass, melaleuca, melissa, myrrh, oregano, patchouli, peppermint, roman chamomile, rosemary, sandalwood, spearmint, spikenard, wild orange, wintergreen
Antispasmodic - clary sage, roman chamomile
Decongestant - basil, cardamom, cassia, cypress, eucalyptus, ginger, grapefruit, lemon, lemongrass, melaleuca, patchouli, white fir
Expectorant - arborvitae, basil, black pepper, cardamom, cedarwood, clove, dill, eucalyptus, fennel, frankincense, ginger, helichrysum, jasmine, marjoram, melaleuca, myrrh, lemon, oregano, peppermint, ravensara, rosemary, sandalwood, thyme, white fir
Immunostimulant - arborvitae, basil, black pepper, cassia, cinnamon, clove, eucalyptus, fennel, frankincense, ginger, lemon, lime, melaleuca, melissa, oregano, ravensara, rosemary, sandalwood, spearmint, thyme, vetiver, white fir, wild orange
Mucolytic - basil, cardamom, cedarwood, clary sage, cinnamon, cypress, fennel, helichrysum, lemon, myrrh, sandalwood, wild orange
Steroidal - basil, birch, cedarwood, clove, fennel, patchouli, rosemary, thyme

Related Ailments: Acute Respiratory Distress Syndrome (ARDS), Anosmia, Asthma, Auditory Processing Disorder, Blocked Tear Duct, Breathing Problems, Bronchitis, Congestion, Cough, Croup, Cystic Fibrosis, Diphtheria, Dry Eyes, Dry Nose, Earache, Ear Infection (Otitis Media), Emphysema, Hearing in a Tunnel, Hearing Problems, Hiccups, Hyperpnea (increased deep and/or rapid breathing to meet demand following exercise, lack of oxygen, high altitude, as the result of anemia), Mucus, Nasal Polyp [Cellular Health], Nosebleed, Perforated Eardrum, Pleurisy, Pneumonia (viral, bacterial), Rhinitis [allergies], Sinus Congestion, Sinus Headache, Sinusitis (sinus infection), Sleep Apnea, Snoring, Stye (Eye), Swollen Eye, Tinnitus, Tuberculosis, Whooping Cough

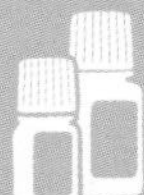

BLENDS

Cleansing blend - decongests (pg. 144)
Protective blend - fights respiratory infections, helps resolve respiratory issues (pg. 158)
Respiration blend - addresses a broad spectrum of respiratory issues (pg. 162)

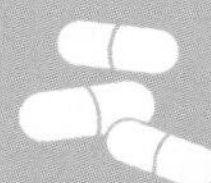

SUPPLEMENTS

Essential oil cellular complex, essential oil omega complex, food enzymes, **protective blend lozenges (pg. 181), defensive probiotic (pg. 172), respiration blend lozenges (pg. 182)**, whole food nutrient supplement

USAGE TIPS: Whether for preventative measures (to clear airborne pathogens and sterilize air) or to **resolve respiratory conditions**, essential oils are excellent for "clearing the air" in both the environment and the body's own respiratory system as well as addressing contributing factors such as poor digestion.

- **Aromatic:** Diffuse (using a diffuser) or inhale selected oils. For a quick treatment, drop oil(s) in hands, rub together, cup around nose and mouth area (can avoid touching face) and repeatedly, deeply inhale through mouth and nose. Additionally, use oils can be applied under the nose, on clothing or bedding, or on jewelry made for diffusing purposes or such to create long-lasting inhalation exposure.
- **Topical:** Rub oils on chest (for aromatic benefit as well), back, forehead (sinuses), and on back side of toes and ball of foot (reflex points for head and chest).
- **Internal:** Place drops of oils in a capsule or in water for systemic or chronic support.
- **Surfaces:** Make a spray mixing essential oils in water with witch hazel for surfaces such as countertops and door knobs for cleaning purposes will also support eradicating bacteria, viruses, fungi, or other harmful germs.

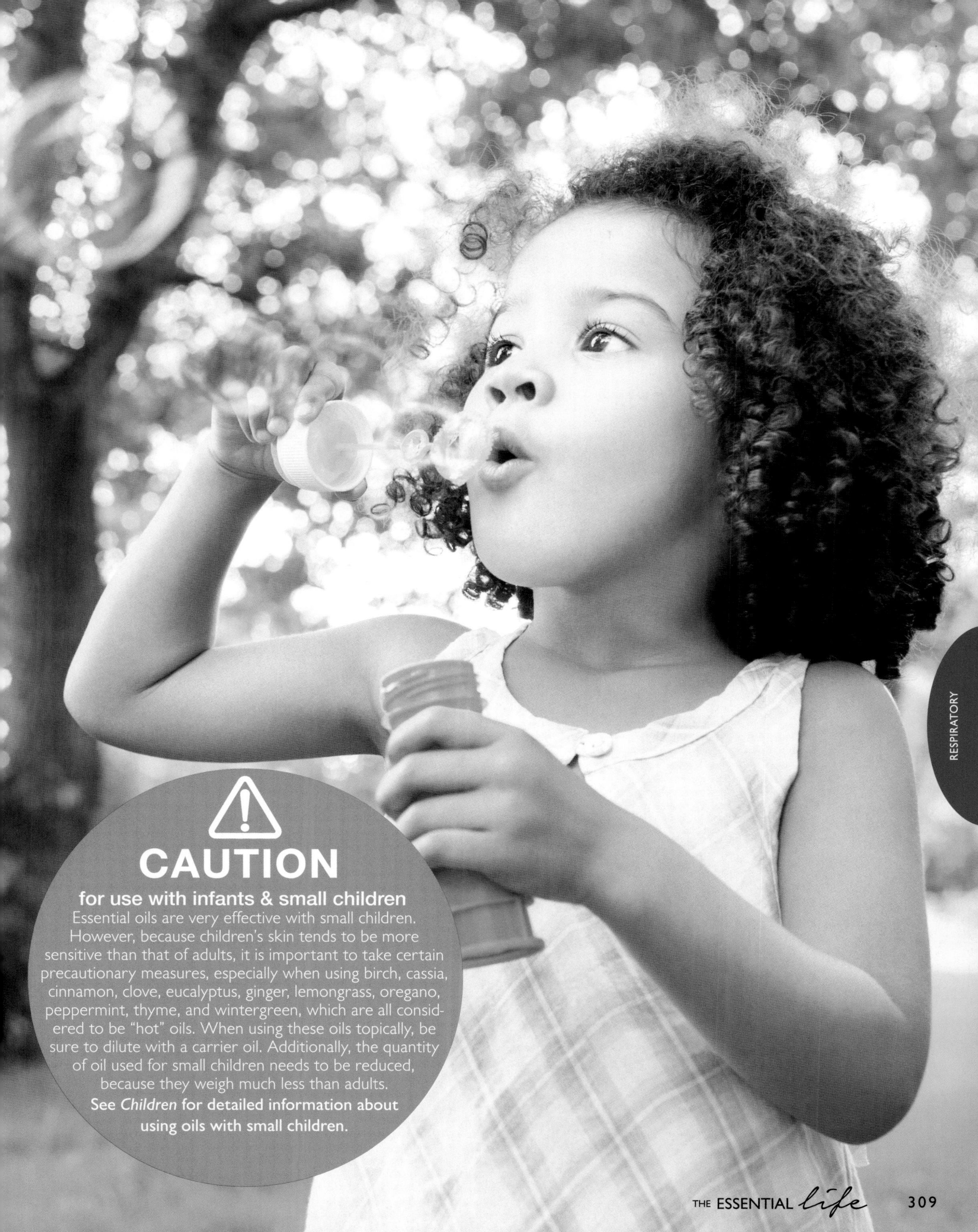

CAUTION

for use with infants & small children

Essential oils are very effective with small children. However, because children's skin tends to be more sensitive than that of adults, it is important to take certain precautionary measures, especially when using birch, cassia, cinnamon, clove, eucalyptus, ginger, lemongrass, oregano, peppermint, thyme, and wintergreen, which are all considered to be "hot" oils. When using these oils topically, be sure to dilute with a carrier oil. Additionally, the quantity of oil used for small children needs to be reduced, because they weigh much less than adults.

See *Children* for detailed information about using oils with small children.

Remedies

ALLERGY POWER TRIO
2 drops lavender
2 drops lemon
2 drops peppermint
Place drops of oil in 4-6 ounces of water. Drink. Repeat every thirty minutes as needed for relief.

GARGLE – salt, warm water, and 1-2 drops essential oil(s) of choice – at least twice per day

CLEAR THE AIR: (for any respiratory or lung specific issue) Add essential oils to diffuse into air to alleviate respiratory issues and snoring; use in a diffuser or cold-mist humidifier. Choose desired oils. Some suggested combinations:
Recipe #1: 3 drops frankincense and 3 drops respiration blend
Recipe #2: 5-10 drops respiration blend
Recipe #3: 5 drops protective blend
Recipe #4: 1 drop white fir, 2 drops wild orange and 2 drops cinnamon
Recipe #5: 2 drops cardamom, 2 drops rosemary and 2 drops lime

ALL STEAMED UP: (using moist air to support respiratory resolve): Using a humidifier, steam from a pan or sauna, or steam from a shower, add a few drops of desired essential oils such as respiration blend or eucalyptus to hot water and inhale. If possible, drape a towel over head and source of steam, breathe for fifteen minutes three times a day.

HOT TEA: Drop a few drops of an essential oil in warm water, slowly inhale steam, then sip water when cool to relieve throat and breathing issues. Here are some options: cinnamon, clove, eucalyptus, lemon, oregano, rosemary, thyme.

SORE THROAT/LARYNGITIS REMEDY: Add 1 drop ginger and 3 drops lemon to a teaspoon of honey. Can be added to warm water to drink or placed in a spoon and licked.

CLEAR RESPIRATORY INFECTION: Diffuse oregano, breathe in at close range for 15-20 minutes with eyes closed.

FLU-BUSTING, LUNG-STIMULATING SMOOTHIE
1 cup orange juice
½ cup lemon juice
½ cup chopped pineapple
1 tablespoon raw honey
1 tablespoon coconut oil
1 piece of ginger (2" long up to 1" thick) or 1-2 drops of ginger
¼ tsp cayenne pepper
1-2 drops peppermint
Blend and enjoy.

PINK EYE: Mix 1 drop each lavender and melaleuca with a few drops of carrier oil. Apply small amount of mixture around eye area. Avoid the eye itself. Additionally, apply oil mixture to crooks of toes.

COUGH BUSTER RUB
¾ cup virgin coconut oil
¾ cup fractionated coconut oil
4 tablespoons beeswax
Melt in glass container (double boiler or glass jar in a pot of water)
Remove from heat and add:
2 tablespoon Vitamin E
80 drops basil
80 drops frankincense
80 drops lime
80 drops marjoram
30 drops peppermint
10 drops eucalyptus
10 drops rosemary
10 drops lemon
5 drops cardamom
Mix and let cool. Rub on chest as needed.

HOMEMADE COUGH SYRUP
1/ 2 cup honey
8 drops peppermint
8 drops lemon
8 drops lavender
8 drops frankincense
3 drops clove
3 drops wild orange
1 drop cinnamon
Mix and take 1 teaspoon every three hours as needed.

SINGER'S OR SPEAKER'S VOICE RECOVERY SPRAY
8 drops lemon
8 drops protective blend
4 drops peppermint
2 drops myrrh
1 drop oregano
1 drop clove
1 drop sandalwood
Add all oils to 15ml glass spray bottle. Add distilled water, shake. Spray on back of throat frequently (every 20-60 minutes) to obtain desired results.

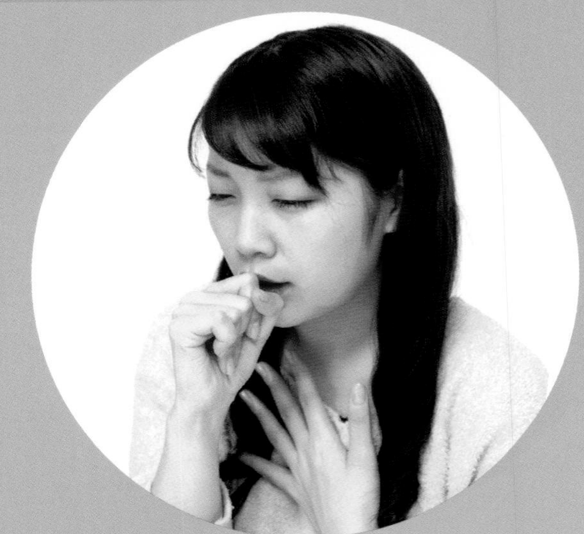

Conditions

BRONCHIAL

Infection (i.e. bronchitis) - cardamom, cedarwood, clary sage, clove, eucalyptus, frankincense, lavender, lime, marjoram, oregano, peppermint, rosemary, spearmint, thyme, comforting blend, protective blend, reassuring blend, renewing blend, respiration blend, respiration blend lozenges

Inflammation - basil, cardamom, cedarwood, clove, cypress, rosemary, spearmint, white fir, wild orange, respiration blend, respiration blend lozenges

BREATHING, GENERAL NEED TO IMPROVE - cinnamon, eucalyptus, patchouli, peppermint, thyme, cleansing blend, encouraging blend, respiration blend, uplifting blend, respiration blend lozenges

Closed off - arborvitae, cardamom, eucalyptus, lemongrass, ravensara, rosemary, white fir, calming blend, respiration blend

Constricted/tight airways - birch, cinnamon, clove, douglas fir, eucalyptus, frankincense, helichrysum, lavender, lemon, marjoram, myrrh, peppermint, rosemary, thyme, white fir, wild orange, wintergreen, calming blend, cellular complex blend, comforting blend, encouraging blend, inspiring blend, respiration blend, respiration blend lozenges

Difficulty (hyperpnea) - cardamom, clary sage, patchouli, peppermint, cleansing blend, respiration blend

Labored - cinnamon, ylang ylang, calming blend, cleansing blend

Rapid - melissa, calming blend, cellular complex blend

Shortness of breath/breathlessness/difficulty breathing (dyspnea) - cinnamon, eucalyptus, frankincense, patchouli, peppermint, cellular complex blend, cleansing blend, reassuring blend, respiration blend

Shortness of breath/breathlessness/discomfort while lying down (orthopnea) - melaleuca, roman chamomile, ylang ylang, cleansing blend

Shortness of breath/breathlessness with exertion or during exercise or activity - myrrh, oregano, wintergreen, ylang ylang, cleansing blend, detoxification blend, reassuring blend, respiration blend, women's blend

Sleep apnea - eucalyptus, lemongrass, peppermint, rosemary, thyme, wintergreen, cleansing blend, grounding blend, protective blend, respiration blend, women's blend

Wheezing - birch, cinnamon, clary sage, clove, eucalyptus, fennel, frankincense, helichrysum, lavender, lemon, marjoram, myrrh, peppermint, rosemary, thyme, white fir, wintergreen, cleansing blend, calming blend, protective blend, respiration blend, women's blend

CONGESTION (respiratory), mucus/sputum/phlegm, catarrh (nose, throat) - frankincense, comforting blend, encouraging blend, renewing blend

Thick mucus - bergamot, birch, cardamom, cassia, cypress, eucalyptus, lemon, myrrh, thyme, wild orange, cellular complex blend, cleansing blend, inspiring blend, invigorating, metabolic blend, protective blend, reassuring blend, renewing blend

Yellow, green mucus - basil, cilantro, eucalyptus, ginger, lemongrass, protective blend, women's blend

Clear mucus - black pepper, cardamom, clove, eucalyptus, ginger, lavender, lemon, melissa, sandalwood, cleansing blend

Chronic discharge of mucus - basil, eucalyptus, wintergreen

General - cardamom, cassia, clary sage, cypress, dill, douglas fir, eucalyptus, fennel, frankincense, ginger, helichrysum, jasmine, lemon, lime, marjoram, myrrh, patchouli, peppermint, rosemary, white fir, detoxification blend, digestion blend, inspiring blend, protective blend, respiration blend

COUGH, GENERAL - arborvitae, cardamom, cedarwood, douglas fir, eucalyptus, frankincense, ginger, helichrysum, jasmine, juniper berry, melaleuca, oregano, thyme, white fir, wild orange, comforting blend, detoxification blend, protective blend, respiration blend, respiration blend lozenges

Barking (i.e. croup) - basil, bergamot, cinnamon, grapefruit, lemon, lemongrass, marjoram, oregano, patchouli, sandalwood, thyme, wild orange, cellular complex blend, digestion blend, protective blend, respiration blend

Chronic - cardamom, cassia, cinnamon, eucalyptus, helichrysum, lemon, melissa, oregano, rosemary, thyme, protective blend

Dry - eucalyptus, frankincense, lavender, white fir, ylang ylang, respiration blend, women's blend

Heavy mucus - arborvitae, cinnamon, clary sage, eucalyptus, fennel, frankincense, ginger, lemon, melaleuca, myrrh, oregano, wintergreen, comforting blend, digestion blend, encouraging blend, inspiring blend, invigorating blend

Moist (sputum-producing) - eucalyptus, ginger, lemon, oregano, cleansing blend, metabolic blend, protective blend

Persistent/spastic (i.e. whooping cough) - basil, cardamom, cassia, clary sage, cypress, frankincense, helichrysum, lavender, melissa, oregano, roman chamomile, rosemary, sandalwood, thyme, calming blend, cleansing blend, reassuring blend, renewing blend

Coughing up blood - cardamom, eucalyptus, geranium, helichrysum, lavender, myrrh, oregano, rose, wild orange, wintergreen, cleansing blend, protective blend, women's blend; see "Lung - infections" below (consider radon poisoning)

GERD - See *Digestive & Intestinal*

Worsens with activity/from exposure to irritant - ginger, ylang ylang, cleansing blend, protective blend

EARS

Auditory processing challenges - helichrysum, cleansing blend, women's blend; see *Brain*

Earache/pain - basil, clary sage, cypress, fennel, ginger, helichrysum, lavender, melaleuca, peppermint, roman chamomile, wild orange, detoxification blend, inspiring blend, invigorating blend, metabolic blend, protective blend, soothing blend

Eardrum, perforated - patchouli, cleansing blend, protective blend

Ear, infection - basil, helichrysum, lavender, lemon, melaleuca, rosemary

Ear mites - basil, cedarwood, myrrh, wild orange, digestion blend, focus blend; see *Parasites*

Hearing problems - basil, clary sage, frankincense, helichrysum, lemon, melaleuca, patchouli, metabolic blend, soothing blend, tension blend

Ringing/noise in the ear (tinnitus) - arborvitae, helichrysum, juniper berry, cleansing blend, detoxification blend, repellent blend

EYES

⚠ CAUTION: do not put oils in eyes; place oils on skin in areas around eyes, using very small quantities; use high dilution with carrier oil; additionally or alternatively use reflex point on toes for eyes - see *Reflexology.*

Dry - lavender, sandalwood

Itchy - oregano, patchouli, wild orange, cellular complex blend, detoxification blend, invigorating blend

Stringy mucus in or around eyes - clary sage, fennel, melaleuca, cellular complex blend

Tear duct, blocked - eucalyptus, frankincense, lemongrass, melaleuca, cleansing blend

Watery/teary - arborvitae, basil, black pepper, frankincense, lime, patchouli, wild orange, anti-aging blend, cellular complex blend, cleansing blend, detoxification blend, massage blend, protective blend

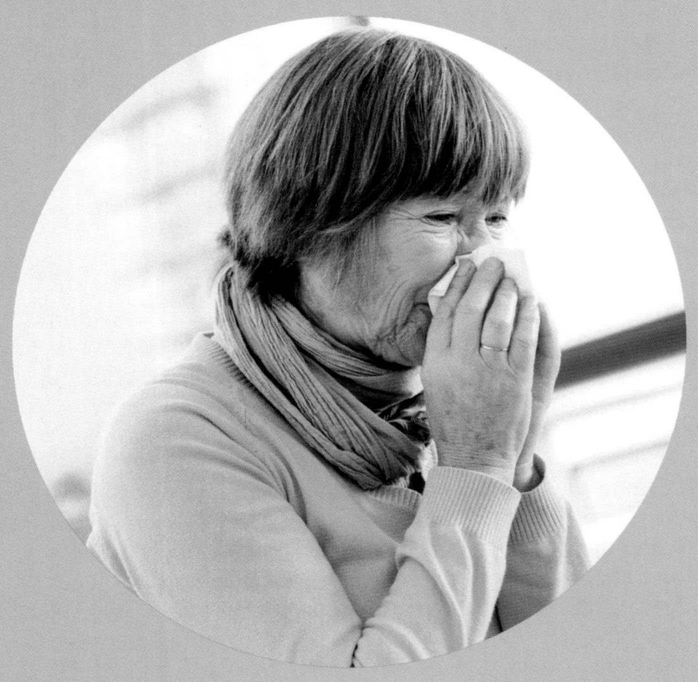

GENERAL RESPIRATORY

Infection, general respiratory - black pepper, cardamom, cinnamon, eucalyptus, frankincense, lemon, melissa, oregano, ravensara, rose, encouraging blend, protective blend, renewing blend

Inflammation - birch, black pepper, coriander, cypress, eucalyptus, ginger, marjoram, melaleuca, melissa, myrrh, rose, peppermint, spearmint, metabolic blend, respiration blend, protective blend

Virus - cassia, cinnamon, clove, eucalyptus, melissa, oregano, ravensara, rosemary, thyme, protective blend, respiration blend

LUNG

Infection (i.e. pneumonia) - black pepper, cedarwood, cinnamon, eucalyptus, frankincense, juniper berry, lavender, oregano, ravensara, rose, sandalwood, thyme, vetiver, comforting blend, protective blend

Problems/conditions - basil, bergamot, birch, cardamom, cinnamon, douglas fir, eucalyptus, fennel, frankincense, ginger, lemon, lemongrass, melaleuca, melissa, oregano, peppermint, rosemary, sandalwood, thyme, white fir, wild orange, wintergreen, cleansing blend, encouraging blend, respiration blend, uplifting blend

NOSE

Bleeding - cypress, geranium, helichrysum, lavender, calming blend, cellular complex blend, cleansing blend, massage blend, protective blend, soothing blend

Inflammation - basil

Itchy - lavender, lemon, lemongrass, cleansing blend, protective blend

Nasal polyps - cinnamon, frankincense, lemongrass, oregano, sandalwood, invigorating blend, protective blend, repellent blend, soothing blend

Postnasal drip - cinnamon, lavender, lemon, cleansing blend, protective blend

Runny - lavender, lemon, peppermint, cleansing blend, detoxification blend, women's blend

Smell, decreased/loss of - arborvitae, basil, peppermint, detoxification blend, protective blend, tension blend

Sneezing - coriander, cilantro, lavender, lemon, peppermint, cleansing blend, detoxification blend, women's blend

Stuffy - cardamom, cassia, dill, eucalyptus, fennel, frankincense, ginger, jasmine, lemon, lime, marjoram, myrrh, patchouli, peppermint, rosemary, white fir, detoxification blend, digestion blend, protective blend, respiration blend

SINUS - bergamot, douglas fir, eucalyptus, helichrysum, lemon, melissa, peppermint, rosemary, sandalwood, white fir, digestion blend, renewing blend, respiration blend

Facial, forehead pain/pressure tenderness, swelling and pressure around eyes, cheeks, nose, or forehead - cinnamon, lemongrass, peppermint, thyme, cleansing blend, protective blend

Infection/inflammation - basil, cedarwood, clove, eucalyptus, helichrysum, melissa, peppermint, rosemary, white fir

Pain in teeth - arborvitae, lavender, lemon, myrrh, calming blend, cellular complex blend, cleansing blend, protective blend

THROAT

Dry - cypress, grapefruit, lemon, lime, peppermint, wild orange, cleansing blend, detoxification blend, respiration blend, respiration blend lozenges

Sore, infection - basil, cardamom, cinnamon, eucalyptus, lemon, lemongrass, lime, myrrh, myrrh + lemon, oregano, patchouli, rosemary, sandalwood, thyme, cleansing blend, detoxification blend, protective blend, protective blend lozenges

Swollen, glands - lavender, lemon, peppermint, metabolic blend

VOICE

Hoarse - cinnamon, eucalyptus, fennel, ginger, jasmine, lemon, lemongrass, peppermint, ylang ylang, cleansing blend, protective blend

Loss of (laryngitis) - cinnamon, frankincense, ginger, jasmine, lavender, lemon, lime, sandalwood, thyme, cleansing blend, detoxification blend, tension blend

OTHER RESPIRATORY ISSUES

Airborne germs/bacteria, fights - arborvitae, cassia, cedarwood, cinnamon, clove, eucalyptus, grapefruit, lavender, lemon, melaleuca, thyme, white fir, cleansing blend, protective blend, respiration blend

Chest pain - douglas fir, consider cardiac association - see *Cardiovascular*

Smoking, quit - See *Addictions*

Hiccups - basil, peppermint, sandalwood

Mouth, dry - lemon, lemongrass, tangerine, vetiver, wild orange, invigorating blend, metabolic blend, protective blend, women's blend

Pleura, inflammation of - birch, cypress, lemon, melissa, rosemary, thyme

Snoring - eucalyptus, geranium, patchouli, peppermint, cleansing blend, detoxification blend, respiration blend, protective blend

Taste, loss of - cinnamon, helichrysum, lemongrass, lime, tangerine, cleansing blend

Breath, bad - patchouli, peppermint, ylang ylang, cellular complex blend, digestion blend, digestion blend softgels

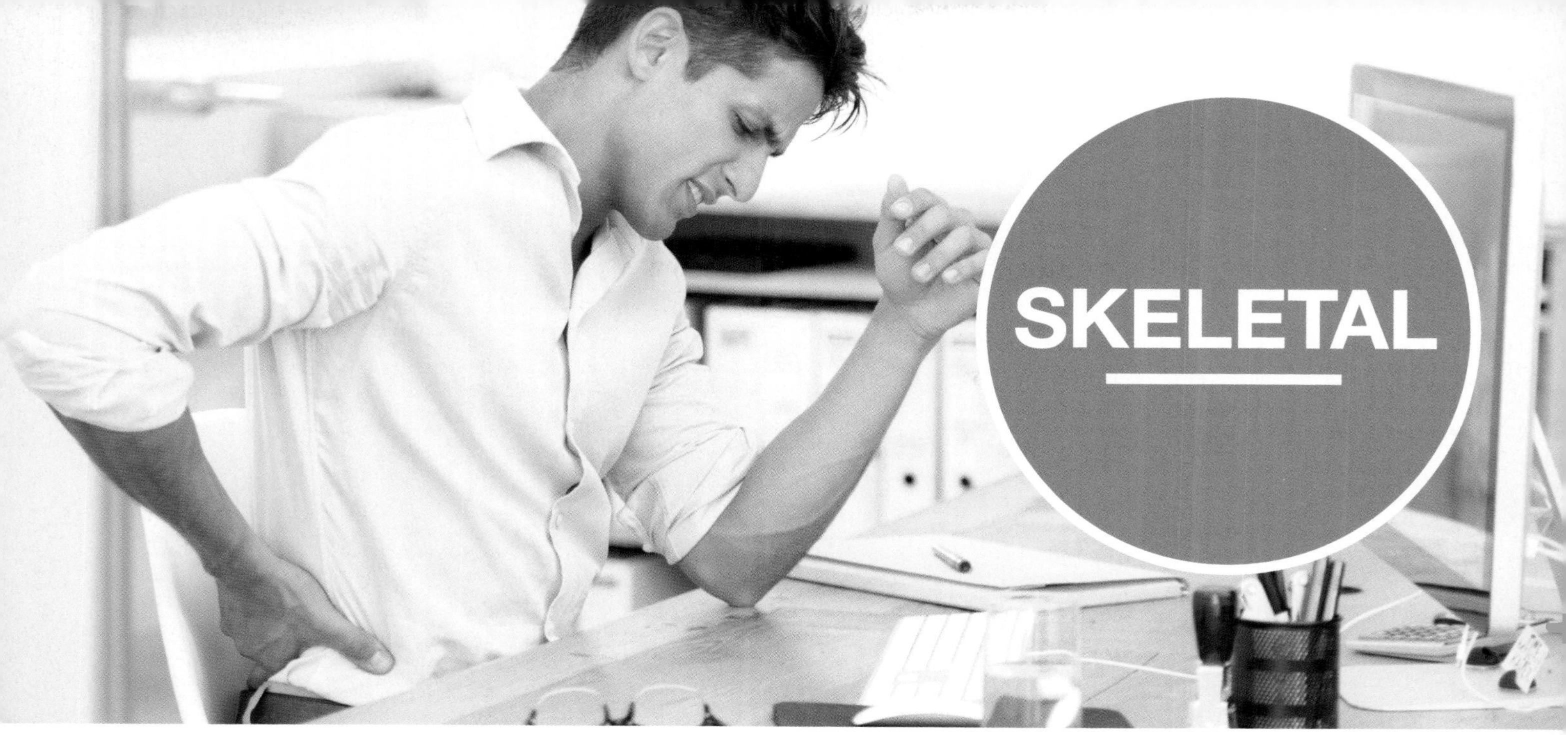

THE BODY'S SKELETAL STRUCTURE comprises the framework upon which all other organs and tissues depend for proper placement and coordination. But bones are not inert material; they are alive, and they need blood and oxygen to metabolize nutrients and produce waste. They respond to external stresses by changing shape to accommodate new mechanical demands. The skeleton is often referred to in terms analogous to a tree: the trunk, or torso, supports the limbs, and so on. This system accounts for about 20 percent of the body's overall weight.

The backbone, also called the spine or vertebral column, is made up of twenty-four moveable bone segments called vertebrae and is divided into three sections. The top seven are cervical vertebrae, which support the cranium, or skull. The thoracic vertebrae, twelve in all, comprise the mid-back area and support the ribs. The lower back, or lumbar spine, consists of five vertebrae that connect to the pelvis at the sacrum. Each vertebra is stacked upon another and is separated and cushioned by intervertebral discs held in place by tendons and cartilage. Through a channel formed by a hole in each of the stacked vertebrae runs the spinal cord, off of which branch root nerves. This nerve network enables the communication between the brain, the muscles,and the organs of the body system.

In addition to providing a structure to keep other body systems from lying in a heap on the floor, the skeleton protects the softer body parts. The cranium fuses around the brain, forming helmet-like protection. The vertebrae protect the spinal cord from injury. And the rib cage creates a barrier around the heart and lungs. Similarly, the majority of hematopoiesis, or the formation of blood cells, occurs in the soft, red marrow inside bones themselves.

Ligaments connect bones to each other and help to stabilize and move joints. They are composed essentially of long, elastic collagen fibers, which can be torn or injured if overworked. Gentle stretching before any strenuous activity protects the ligaments and prevents injury to joints and muscles. If ligaments are injured, healing can take ninety days and up to nine months for the fibers to regain their maximum strength.
The skeleton's dynamic functions are facilitated by a simple yet sophisticated network of levers, cables, pulleys, and winches actuated by muscles and tendons. When muscles contract, they shorten their length, thus drawing in an adjacent bone that pivots around a connecting joint, much like the boom, stick, and hydraulic lever system of a backhoe.

Since the skeletal system is in a constant state of use, it also undergoes perpetual repair and rejuvenation. It is therefore vulnerable, as is any body system, to imbalance and disease. The joints, in particular, are susceptible to damage due to constant friction, impact, and leverage. As we grow older, we may also experience challenges stemming from calcium or other mineral deficiencies—calcium being the primary material of which bones are made.

Proper pH balance in the body supports a strong skeletal structure. When pH balance is off and the body is too acidic, the blood is compelled to take minerals from the bones and organs, which can cause disease and depletion in the skeletal system. Sugar, refined and processed foods, and overconsumption of meat and dairy make the body more acidic throwing off the pH balance. Certain essential oils like dill, lemon, fennel, or lemongrass can help reduce acidity by creating a more alkaline environment. Maintaining an alkaline environment helps promote healing. Similarly, adequate nourishment with bioavailable vitamins, minerals, and trace minerals helps to maintain a proper pH balance in the blood. Adequate, high-quality supplementation will manage any chronic inflammation, and a topical use of anti-inflammatory essential oils will support joint health.

When there is a skeletal injury, the use of essential oils can accelerate the healing process and recovery time. For example, in the case of a broken bone, oils such as wintergreen and birch have been demonstrated to be useful in relieving and resolving inflammatory conditions and supporting injury recovery. Additionally, lemongrass essential oil supports the healing of any connective tissue damage.

TOP SOLUTIONS

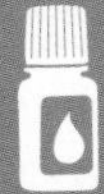

SINGLE OILS

Lemongrass - enhances connective tissue repair (pg. 112)

Wintergreen - reduces aches, pains, and inflammation; stimulates bone repair (pg. 137)

Birch - reduces inflammation and stimulates bone repair (pg. 80)

Helichrysum - relieves pain and inflammation; accelerates bone repair (pg. 105)

White fir - eases bone and joint pain; reduces inflammation (pg. 135)

By Related Properties

For definitions of the properties listed below and more oil options, see Oil Properties Glossary (pg. 435) and Oil Properties (pg. 436).

Analgesic - arborvitae, basil, bergamot, birch, black pepper, cassia, cinnamon, clary sage, clove, coriander, cypress, eucalyptus, fennel, frankincense, ginger, helichrysum, juniper berry, lavender, lemongrass, marjoram, melaleuca, oregano, peppermint, ravensara, rosemary, white fir, wild orange, wintergreen
Antiarthritic - arborvitae, cassia, ginger, white fir
Anti-inflammatory - arborvitae, basil, bergamot, birch, black pepper, cardamom, cassia, cedarwood, cinnamon, coriander, cypress, dill, eucalyptus, fennel, frankincense, geranium, ginger, helichrysum, jasmine, lavender, lemongrass, lime, melaleuca, melissa, myrrh, oregano, patchouli, peppermint, roman chamomile, rosemary, sandalwood, spearmint, spikenard, wild orange, wintergreen, yarrow
Anti-rheumatic - birch, cassia, clove, coriander, cypress, eucalyptus, ginger, juniper berry, lavender, lemon, lemongrass, lime, oregano rosemary, thyme, white fir, wintergreen, yarrow
Regenerative - basil, cedarwood, clove, coriander, frankincense, geranium, helichrysum, jasmine, lavender, lemongrass, melaleuca, myrrh, patchouli, sandalwood, wild orange
Steroidal - basil, bergamot, birch, cedarwood, clove,

Related Ailments: Amyotrophic lateral sclerosis, Ankylosing Spondylitis, Arthritis Pain [Pain & Inflammation], Bone Pain, Bone Spurs, Broken Bone, Bunions, Bursitis, Calcified Spine, Cartilage Injury, Chondromalacia Patella, Club foot, Deteriorating Spine, Ganglion Cyst, Gout, Herniated Disc, Joint Pain, Knee Cartilage Injury, Myelofibrosis, Osgood-Schlatter Disease, Osteoarthritis [Pain & Inflammation], Osteomyelitis [Immune], Osteoporosis, Paget's Disease, Plantar Fasciitis [Muscular], Rheumatism, Scoliosis, Shin Splints, Spina Bifida [Nervous], Tennis Elbow [Muscular], TMJ

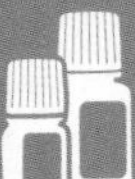

BLENDS

Soothing blend - soothes, relaxes, and relieves aches and pains; helps with after injuries/surgery healing (pg. 164)

Tension blend - helps relieve and resolve tension, soreness, and stiffness (pg. 165)

Cellular complex blend - reduces/resolves inflammation and regenerates tissue (pg. 143)

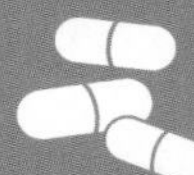

SUPPLEMENTS

Bone support complex (pg. 170), cellular vitality complex, defensive probiotic, digestion blend softgels, essential oil cellular complex, **essential oil omega complex (pg. 175)**, food enzymes, **polyphenol complex (pg. 181)**, whole food nutrient supplement

USAGE TIPS: For best results with skeletal and connective tissue issues:

- **Topical:** Apply oils directly to area of concern for structural issues and in the case of injury, massage in thoroughly whenever possible. Drive oils in with heat, cold, or moisture. Use carrier oil as needed or desired. Layering multiple oils over affected area, placing them on tissue one at a time, is very effective. Any kind of cream or carrier oil will slow absorption if placed on first and improve it if placed on last.
  - **Acute:** Apply often, every 20-30 minutes, until symptoms subside, then reduce to every two to six hours.
  - **Chronic:** Apply two to three times daily.
- **Internal:** Consume oils (to support resolving inflammation and bone repair) in a capsule or under tongue. place oils in a capsule or drop under tongue (hold for 30 seconds; swallow).

Remedies

BROKEN BONE FIX MIX
7 drops frankincense
6 drops white fir
2 drops wintergreen
11 drops helichrysum
4 drops lemongrass
Combine oils in 10ml roller bottle; fill remainder with carrier oil. Apply topically on or near affected area every two hours for two days and every four hours for the next three days. If it isn't possible to apply to area of concern, utilize sympathetic response and rub opposite arm, leg, etc.

BONE SPUR RESOLVE
5 drops frankincense
6 drops cypress
7 drops wintergreen
5 drops marjoram
4 drops helichrysum
Combine in a 10ml roller bottle, fill remainder with carrier oil. Apply topically on or near affected area morning and evening. Continue for an additional two weeks after spur is gone.

EASE-E-FLEX (for joint pain & inflammation)
15 drops frankincense
20 drops soothing blend
4 drops lavender
Combine in a 10ml roller bottle; fill remainder with carrier oil. Apply topically on or near affected area as needed

CONNECT REPAIR (for carpal tunnel, tendon, ligaments)
15 drops lemongrass
15 drops helichrysum
10 drops basil
10 drops ginger
10 drops lavender
10 drops marjoram
Combine in 10ml roller bottle; fill remainder with carrier oil. Apply topically to affected area.

OH MY ACHING BACK
10 drops frankincense
10 drops helichrysum
4 drops cypress
4 drops white fir
2 drops peppermint
2 drops wintergreen
Add to 10ml roller bottle and fill remainder with carrier oil. Use along back/spine area as needed for pain. For chronic issues, apply at least morning and night.

RHEUMATIC PAIN
2 drops spikenard
2 drops lavender
4 drops ginger
4 drops white fir
Combine in a 5ml roller bottle; fill remainder with carrier oil. Apply to affected area(s) as needed.

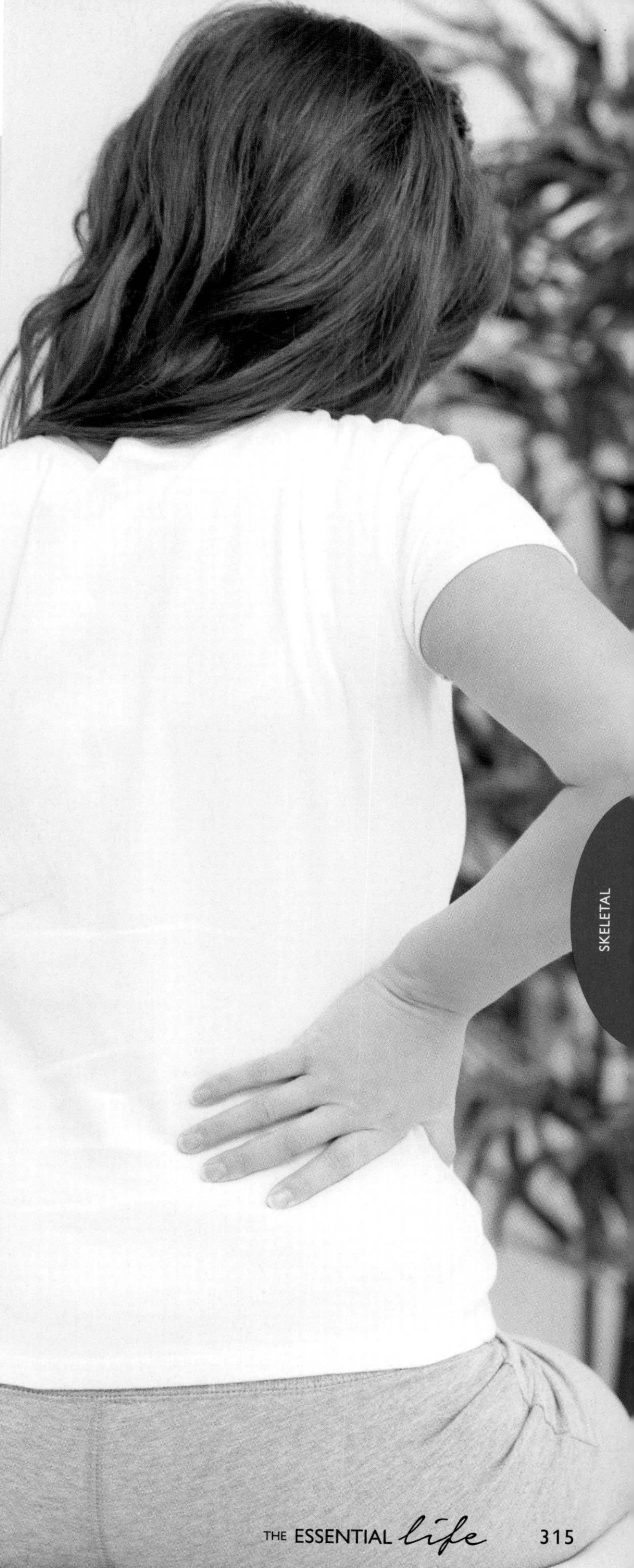

Conditions

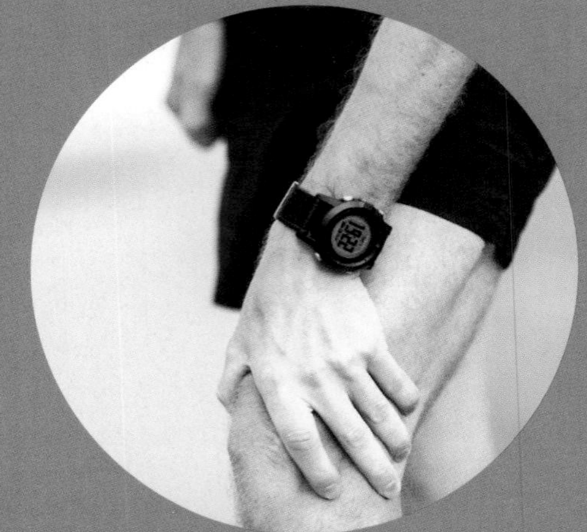

Aching pain in/around ear - arborvitae, basil, bergamot, black pepper, cedarwood, cilantro, cinnamon, clary sage, clove, cypress, eucalyptus, ginger, helichrysum, myrrh, oregano, white fir, wintergreen, cellular complex blend, massage blend, soothing blend, women's blend

Arthritis - basil, black pepper, cypress, eucalyptus, frankincense, ginger, lavender, lemongrass, marjoram, wintergreen, comforting blend, massage blend, reassuring blend, renewing blend, soothing blend, uplifting blend; see *Pain & Inflammation*

Back/lower back, pain - birch, eucalyptus, frankincense, lavender, lemongrass, peppermint, sandalwood, wintergreen, comforting blend, massage blend, soothing blend; see *Pain & Inflammation*

Bones, tender - birch, geranium, helichrysum, juniper berry, myrrh, roman chamomile, wintergreen, cellular complex blend, cleansing blend, protective blend, soothing blend

Bones, bruised - basil, birch, clary sage, frankincense, helichrysum, wintergreen, cellular complex blend, protective blend, soothing blend

Bones, breaking easily - basil, birch, clove, helichrysum, myrrh, oregano, white fir, wild orange, wintergreen, cellular complex blend, soothing blend

Bones, broken - birch, cypress, ginger, helichrysum, white fir, wintergreen, soothing blend

Bones, bumps under skin on - birch, cypress, marjoram, myrrh, oregano, rosemary, white fir, wintergreen, cellular complex blend, massage blend, soothing blend

Bones, porous - birch, clove, peppermint, white fir, wintergreen

Bones, spurs - basil, cypress, eucalyptus, frankincense, helichrysum, ginger, peppermint, wintergreen, massage blend

Bunions - basil, cypress, eucalyptus, ginger, lemongrass, thyme, wintergreen, massage blend

Breathing difficulty - cardamom, cypress, douglas fir, eucalyptus, marjoram, myrrh, oregano, peppermint, white fir, wintergreen, massage blend, respiration blend, soothing blend, tension blend; see *Respiratory*

Cartilage, inflamed/injured - basil, birch, coriander, eucalyptus, helichrysum, lemongrass, marjoram, peppermint, sandalwood, white fir, wintergreen, soothing blend; see *Pain & Inflammation*

Cartilage, generate - helichrysum, sandalwood, white fir

Chewing difficulty - basil, clary sage, frankincense, oregano, white fir, wintergreen, cellular complex blend, massage blend, soothing blend, tension blend

Club foot - arborvitae, basil, ginger, helichrysum, lavender, peppermint, roman chamomile, rosemary

Connective tissue/fascia (ligaments) - basil, birch, clary sage, helichrysum, ginger, lemongrass, sandalwood, white fir, soothing blend, skin clearing blend

Connective tissue (ligaments), injured/weak/damaged/aches and pains - birch, clove, cypress, geranium, ginger, helichrysum, lavender, lemongrass, marjoram, oregano, peppermint, roman chamomile, rosemary, thyme, white fir, wintergreen, soothing blend, tension blend

Frozen shoulder - basil, birch, lemongrass, oregano, peppermint, white fir, wintergreen, soothing blend

Headaches - basil, clary sage, clove, eucalyptus, frankincense, geranium, helichrysum, lavender, myrrh, oregano, peppermint, roman chamomile, spearmint, thyme, white fir, wintergreen, cellular complex blend, protective blend, soothing blend, tension blend

Hearing loss - basil, birch, clary sage, helichrysum, oregano, white fir, tension blend

Inflamed/deteriorating/disc - birch, clary sage, eucalyptus, peppermint, thyme, white fir, wintergreen, cellular complex blend, massage blend, protective blend, soothing blend

Inflammation - basil, birch, clove, eucalyptus, frankincense, ginger, peppermint, roman chamomile, sandalwood, vetiver, wintergreen, white fir, renewing blend, soothing blend, tension blend, uplifting blend

Joint, clicking - birch, marjoram, myrrh, wintergreen, cellular complex blend, protective blend, soothing blend

Joint, grinding sensation - bergamot, birch, rosemary, white fir, wintergreen, cellular complex blend, cleansing blend

Joint, inflammation - arborvitae, basil, bergamot, cardamom, cedarwood, cinnamon, clove, coriander, cypress, douglas fir, eucalyptus, frankincense, ginger, helichrysum, lavender, lemon, marjoram, peppermint, roman chamomile, rosemary, thyme, vetiver, white fir, wild orange, wintergreen, cellular complex blend, detoxification blend, soothing blend

Joint, locking - basil, birch, clary sage, helichrysum, marjoram, white fir, wintergreen, cellular complex blend, massage blend, protective blend, soothing blend

Joint, pain/stiffness - arborvitae, basil, birch, black pepper, cardamom, cinnamon, coriander, douglas fir, eucalyptus, geranium, lemongrass, thyme, white fir, wintergreen, massage blend, soothing blend

Joint, swollen/warm/red/tender - eucalyptus, frankincense, lavender, roman chamomile, massage blend, soothing blend

Ligament strain - frankincense, lemongrass, marjoram, white fir, soothing blend

Rheumatism - basil, birch, douglas fir, eucalyptus, ginger, lavender, lemongrass, spikenard, thyme, white fir, cellular complex blend, massage blend, renewing blend, soothing blend, uplifting blend; see *Pain & Inflammation*

Rheumatoid arthritis - basil, bergamot, birch, cardamom, cypress, douglas fir, frankincense, ginger, lavender, lemon, marjoram, wintergreen, massage blend, soothing blend, tension blend

Sciatic issues - See *Nervous*

Shoulder, frozen - basil, birch, lemongrass, oregano, peppermint, cellular complex blend, white fir, wintergreen, soothing blend

Shoulder, rotator cuff - birch, white fir, wintergreen, soothing blend, tension blend

Shin splints - basil, frankincense, helichrysum, lavender, lemongrass, marjoram, myrrh, patchouli, wintergreen, massage blend, soothing blend

Stiff/limited range of motion - birch, frankincense, marjoram, white fir, wintergreen, soothing blend or rub, tension blend

Vertebral misalignment - helichrysum, marjoram, rose, white fir, massage blend, soothing blend

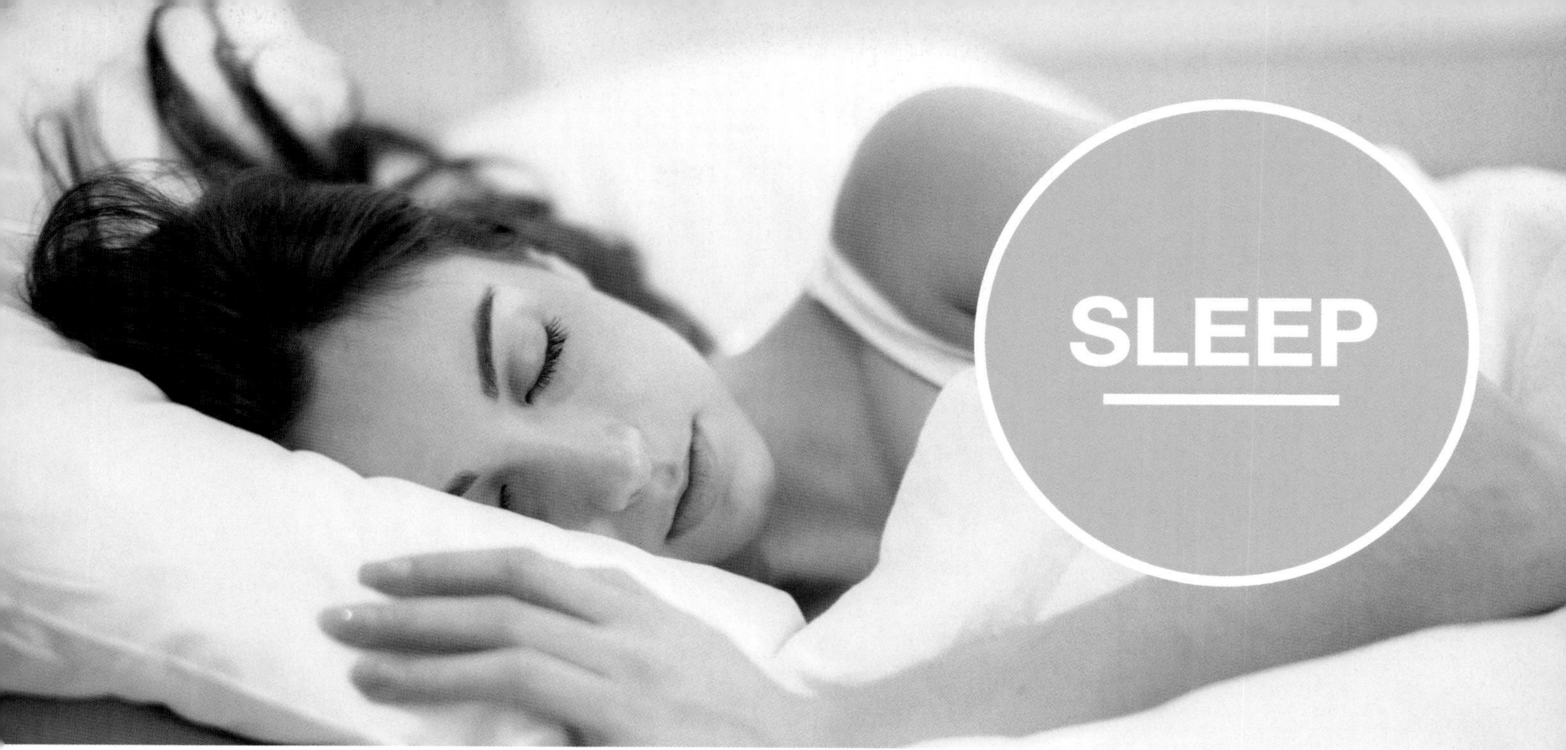

SLEEP DESCRIBES the period when the body ceases to engage in most voluntary bodily functions, thus providing an opportunity for the body to focus on restoration and repair. During this time, conscious brain activity is fully or partially suspended, a state that contributes to restoring and maintaining emotional, mental, and physical health. In recent years, doctors and organizations such as the National Sleep Foundation have encouraged the wide acceptance of sleep as one of the three pillars of health, together with nutrition and exercise.

All sleep can be divided into two states: REM and Non-REM. REM is an acronym for Rapid Eye Movement sleep, and represents a period when brain waves have fast frequency and low voltage, similar to brain activity during waking hours. However, during REM sleep all voluntary muscles cease activity except those that control eye movements. Dreams take place during REM sleep. It is the period of sleep where the body is in a deeply subconscious state, and much healing, repair, and restoration occurs.

Non-REM sleep can be further subdivided into three stages: Stage N1 sleep is the state between wakefulness and sleep; it is very light, and some people don't even recognize they are asleep during this stage. Stage N2 is a true deep sleep. Stage N3 is deep sleep or delta sleep. Interestingly, sleep typically occurs in 90-120 minute cycles, with transitions from the N-stages of sleep in the first part of the night to REM sleep in the latter.

Age plays a huge factor in normal sleeping patterns. Newborns need between sixteen to eighteen hours of sleep a day, preschoolers need ten to twelve hours, and school age children and teenagers need nine or more hours. Because deeper N3 and REM sleep states diminish as individuals age, older adults experience more difficulty getting to sleep and staying asleep. At a time when individuals tend to need more reparative and restorative sleep, they actually receive less.

Some of the most common sleep disorders include insomnia (difficulty getting to sleep and staying asleep), sleep apnea (where breathing may stop or be blocked for brief periods during sleep), sleep deprivation (not getting enough sleep), restless leg syndrome (an uncontrollable need to move legs at night, at times accompanied by tingling or other discomfort), narcolepsy (a central nervous system disease that results in daytime sleepiness and other issues, including loss of muscle tone and more), and problem sleepiness (when daytime sleepiness interferes with regular responsibilities, such as working or studying).

In addition to sleeping disorders, lack of necessary sleep can cause a myriad of other physical and emotional problems. It contributes to adrenal fatigue, poor digestion, weight gain and/or obesity, grogginess, decreased focus and concentration, memory problems, increased irritability and frustration levels and other mood challenges, heart disease, a compromised immune system, and a higher likelihood of chronic or autoimmune conditions.

When children don't get the sleep they need, both physical and emotional development can be negatively affected. The necessity for regular, healthy sleeping patterns is apparent when one considers the serious difficulties and disorders caused by lack of sleep.

Countless individuals have turned to natural remedies to promote ease in falling asleep, staying asleep, and reaching the deeper levels of sleep. There are supplements and essential oils that work together to reduce symptoms of the more serious sleeping disorders and should be considered as a viable addition or alternative to sleep treatments as advised by medical professionals. The benefits of using essential oils such as lavender to promote healthy sleep are numerous and astounding, and the results can be life-altering for the chronically sleep deprived.

TOP SOLUTIONS

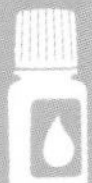

SINGLE OILS

Lavender - calms, relaxes, and sedates; supports parasympathetic system (pg. 108)

Vetiver - grounds and promotes tranquility (pg. 134)

Roman chamomile - balances hormones; sedates, calms, and relaxes (pg. 125)

By Related Properties

For definitions of the properties listed below and more oil options, see Oil Properties Glossary (pg. 435) and Oil Properties (pg. 436).

Analgesic - arborvitae, basil, bergamot, birch, black pepper, cassia, cinnamon, clary sage, clove, coriander, cypress, eucalyptus, fennel, frankincense, ginger, helichrysum, jasmine, juniper berry, lavender, lemongrass, marjoram, melaleuca, oregano, peppermint, ravensara, rosemary, white fir, wild orange, wintergreen

Antidepressant - clary sage, coriander, frankincense, geranium, jasmine, lavender, lemongrass, melissa, oregano, patchouli, ravensara, rose, sandalwood, wild orange, ylang ylang

Calming - bergamot, birch, black pepper, cassia, clary sage, coriander, fennel, frankincense, geranium, jasmine, juniper berry, lavender, melissa, oregano, patchouli, roman chamomile, sandalwood, tangerine, vetiver, yarrow

Detoxifier - arborvitae, cassia, cilantro, cypress, geranium, juniper berry, lemon, lime, patchouli, rosemary, wild orange

Grounding - basil, cedarwood, clary sage, cypress, melaleuca, vetiver, ylang ylang

Relaxing - basil, cassia, cedarwood, clary sage, cypress, fennel, geranium, jasmine, lavender, marjoram, myrrh, ravensara, roman chamomile, white fir, ylang ylang

Restorative - basil, frankincense, lime, patchouli, rosemary, sandalwood, spearmint

Sedative - basil, bergamot, cedarwood, clary sage, coriander, frankincense, geranium, jasmine, juniper berry, lavender, lemongrass, marjoram, melissa, patchouli, roman chamomile, rose, sandalwood, spikenard, vetiver, ylang ylang

Related Ailments: Hypersomnia, Insomnia, Jet Lag, Narcolepsy, Periodic Limb Movement Disorder (PLMD), Sleep Apnea, Sleepwalking, Restless Leg Syndrome (RLS)

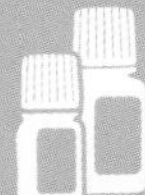

BLENDS

Calming blend - calms mind/emotions; promotes relaxation and restful sleep (pg. 142)

Grounding blend - promotes sense of well being and supports autonomic nervous system (pg. 150)

Focus blend - balances brain activity and calms overstimulation (pg. 149)

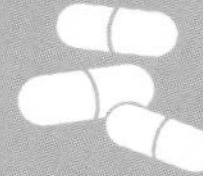

SUPPLEMENTS

Bone support complex (pg. 170), cellular vitality complex, defensive probiotic, **detoxification blend softgels (pg. 173)**, detoxification complex, energy & stamina, **essential oil omega complex (pg. 175)**, liquid omega-3 supplement, phytoestrogen multiplex, whole food nutrient supplement

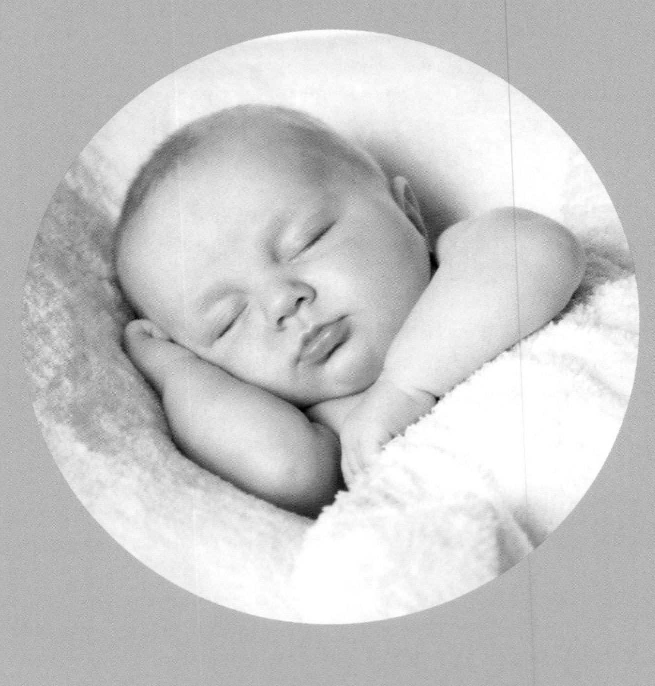

USAGE TIPS: To support optimal and restful sleep, inhalation and topical use of essential oils gives direct access to the brain through smell, relaxes tense muscles, and calms active minds.

- **Aromatic:** Diffuse selected oil(s) of choice, apply a few drops to clothing, bedding (e.g. pillow), or any other method that supports inhalation. Start exposure just before bedtime.
- **Topical:** Combine oils with soothing and relaxing massage techniques; apply oils on forehead, back, shoulders, under nose, and especially bottoms of feet from a pre-made or prepared roller bottle blend for ease. Applying oils on chest allows breathing in vapors. For chronic issues, use Oil Touch technique regularly.

Conditions

CONDITIONS (CONTRIBUTORS TO SLEEP ISSUES):

Alcohol, issues with - See *Addictions*
Anxiety - See *Mood & Behavior*
Bedtime, chronically late - See "Night owl" below
Brain injury - See *Brain*
Breathing issues - See *Respiratory*
Caffeine (avoid consuming within four to six hours of sleep) - See *Addictions*
Chronic pain - See *Pain & Inflammation*
CPAP machine, difficulties with - See *Respiratory*
Daytime napping - See *Energy & Vitality*
Depression - See *Mood & Behavior*
Dreaming, excessive - clary sage, geranium, frankincense, juniper berry, lavender, patchouli, roman chamomile, calming blend, grounding blend, tension blend
Drug abuse - See *Addictions*
Drug withdrawals - See *Addictions*
Emotional discomfort - bergamot, clary sage, geranium, juniper berry, melissa, ravensara, ylang ylang; see *Mood & Behavior*
Eating, excessive, late at night - See *Eating Disorders, Weight*
Cold extremities, poor circulation - cypress, coriander; see *Cardiovascular*
Fear (of sleeping, etc.) - bergamot, cardamom, coriander, patchouli, ravensara, roman chamomile, calming blend, grounding blend, soothing blend; see *Mood & Behavior*
Grief - See *Mood & Behavior*
Heart symptoms (i.e. rapid heart rate) - ylang ylang; see *Cardiovascular*
Hormone imbalances - clary sage; see *Men's Health* or *Women's Health*
Illness/chronic illness - See *Immune & Lymphatic*
Insomnia - See "Sleeplessness," "Sleeplessness, chronic" below
Insomnia, nervous tension - basil, lavender, marjoram, roman chamomile, rosemary, vetiver, calming blend, massage blend, tension blend, uplifting blend; see *Nervous*
Interferences in normal sleep schedule (i.e. jet lag, switching from day to night shift, up at night with a baby) - See "Jet lag ..." below
Jet lag, overly tired - arborvitae, basil, grapefruit, lemon, lemongrass, rosemary, tangerine, wild orange, focus blend, invigorating blend
Jet lag, can't go to sleep - lavender, patchouli, peppermint, wild orange; see "Sleeplessness" below
Melatonin levels low, irregular sleep cycles (REM) - black pepper, cedarwood, frankincense, ginger, lime, myrrh, rosemary (use during day), sandalwood, tangerine, ylang ylang, vetiver, calming blend, focus blend
Mental chatter/over-thinking - basil, cedarwood, rosemary, calming blend, cleansing, grounding blend
Muscle cramps/charley horses - See *Muscular*
Nervous tension - basil, bergamot, douglas fir, geranium, grapefruit, jasmine, lavender, melissa, roman chamomile, rose, sandalwood, vetiver, wild orange, ylang ylang, calming blend, grounding blend, invigorating blend, massage blend, tension blend; see *Mood & Behavior, Nervous*
Nicotine - See *Addictions*
Night eating syndrome - See *Eating Disorders, Weight*
Night owl - cedarwood, lavender, vetiver, wild orange, wintergreen, calming blend, grounding blend; see "Sleeplessness," "Sleeplessness, chronic" below
Night sweats - douglas fir, eucalyptus, ginger, lime, peppermint, cellular complex blend, detoxification blend, massage blend, women's blend, women's monthly blend; see *Endocrine (Thyroid), Immune & Lymphatic, Women's Health*
Nightmares - cinnamon, clary sage, cypress, eucalyptus, geranium, grapefruit, juniper berry, lavender, melissa, roman chamomile, white fir, wild orange, vetiver, calming blend, grounding blend
Over-excited/over-stimulated - lavender, patchouli, roman chamomile, sandalwood, wild orange; see *Mood & Behavior*
Pain or discomfort at night - soothing blend; see *Pain & Inflammation*
Periodic limb movement - marjoram, massage blend; see "Twitching" below
Psychiatric disorder - See *Mood & Behavior*
Restless legs - basil, cypress, geranium, ginger, grapefruit, lavender, patchouli, peppermint, roman chamomile, spearmint, wintergreen, calming blend, massage blend, soothing blend, tension blend
Restlessness - bergamot, black pepper, cedarwood, frankincense, lavender, patchouli, roman chamomile, wild orange, calming blend, grounding blend, joyful blend, massage blend, tension blend
Routine/schedule, poor - grounding blend; see "Melatonin levels low..." below
Serotonin levels low (precursor to melatonin) - bergamot, cedarwood, clary sage, grapefruit, melissa, patchouli, roman chamomile, ylang ylang; see *Mood & Behavior*
Sleep apnea - eucalyptus, lemongrass, peppermint, rosemary, thyme, wintergreen, cleansing blend, grounding blend, protective blend, respiratory blend, women's blend; see *Respiratory*
Sleep-walking - black pepper, geranium, lavender, vetiver, calming blend, cellular complex blend, grounding blend
Snoring - douglas fir, eucalyptus, geranium, patchouli, peppermint, rosemary, cleansing blend, detoxification blend, respiration blend, protective blend; see *Respiratory*
Stimulants, use of (medications, caffeine, energy drinks, supplements) - See *Addictions*
Stress - clary sage, frankincense, lavender, lime, vetiver, wild orange, calming blend, invigorating blend, joyful blend; see *Stress*
Teeth grinding - frankincense, geranium, lavender, marjoram, roman chamomile, wild orange, calming blend; see *Parasites*
Tranquility, lack of - cinnamon, clary sage, jasmine, melissa, roman chamomile, tension blend
Twitching/muscle spasms - basil, clary sage, coriander, cypress, eucalyptus, ginger, jasmine, lemongrass, marjoram, grounding blend, massage blend, soothing blend; see *Muscular*

CONDITIONS (RELATED TO, RESULT OF SLEEP ISSUES):

Adrenal fatigue - See *Endocrine (Adrenals)*

Alertness, lack of/poor daytime learning - bergamot; see *Focus & Concentration*

Depression - See "Serotonin levels low" above , *Mood & Behavior*

Difficulty controlling emotions - See *Mood & Behavior*

Driving, can't stay awake (pull over!) - basil, peppermint, rosemary, respiration blend

Drowsiness, daytime - basil, grapefruit, lemon, rosemary, wild orange, focus blend, invigorating blend; see *Energy & Vitality*

Focus, concentration compromised - See *Focus & Concentration*

Memory, poor/slow recall or response - bergamot, frankincense, rosemary; see *Focus & Concentration*

Narcolepsy - frankincense, lavender + wild orange, patchouli, sandalwood, vetiver, calming blend, focus blend; see *Brain*

Night eating syndrome - See *Eating Disorders, Mood & Behavior, Weight*

Physical discomfort/pain - frankincense, soothing blend; see *Pain & Inflammation*

Sleep, lack of/deprivation - geranium, lavender, patchouli, cellular complex blend, detoxification blend, tension blend; see *Energy & Vitality*

Sleep, poor - lavender, marjoram, roman chamomile, sandalwood, vetiver, calming blend

Sleeplessness - basil, cedarwood, clary sage, frankincense, geranium, lavender, patchouli, roman chamomile, sandalwood, vetiver, wild orange, calming blend, comforting blend, grounding blend, inspiring blend, renewing blend

Sleeplessness, chronic - bergamot, cedarwood, cypress, jasmine, lavender, melissa, peppermint, roman chamomile, sandalwood, tangerine, thyme, vetiver, wild orange, ylang ylang, calming blend, comforting blend, grounding blend, inspiring blend, renewing blend, uplifting blend

Weakened immunity - See *Immune & Lymphatic*

Weight gain - See *Weight*

Remedies

Avoid using essential oils which stimulate at night, for example rosemary and peppermint. Instead opt for oils which relax, such as vetiver and roman chamomile.

SLEEP-PROMOTING BATH RECIPES

- To help fall asleep: Add a few drops lavender to 1 cup Epsom salts; dissolve in hot bath (Epsom salts offer a good source of magnesium, which supports relaxation)
- Sleep tonight; sleep in tomorrow: Mix 5 drops patchouli oil, 2 drops wild orange oil, and 1 drop frankincense oil with Epsom salts; soak fifteen to twenty minutes.

SLEEP

STOP SNORING BLEND

18 drops marjoram
12 drops geranium
12 drops lavender
8 drops eucalyptus
5 drops cedarwood
Combine in spray bottle. Mist room generously, lightly spray pillow, apply to throat, inhale.

ROLLER BOTTLE REMEDIES FOR SLEEP & ANXIETY ISSUES

For all recipes use a 10ml roller bottle; after placing essential oils in bottle, fill remainder with fractionated coconut oil; use on feet, back of neck

- Recipe #1: 20 drops calming blend, 10 drops vetiver, and 10 drops wild orange
- Recipe #2: 3 drops each of cedarwood, patchouli, grounding blend, vetiver, roman chamomile
- Recipe #3: 3 drops each of juniper berry, grounding blend, vetiver, patchouli, ylang ylang
- Recipe #4: 7 drops each of bergamot, calming blend, roman chamomile, vetiver, ylang ylang, and 3 drops patchouli

SLEEPY-TIME MASSAGE RUB (Yield: ½ cup)

¼ cup cocoa butter
¼ cup coconut oil
20 drops of lavender
6 drops of white fir
6 drops cedarwood
10 drops of frankincense

- Substitutions: Replace any of above oils with ylang ylang, roman chamomile, vetiver, cedarwood, or clary sage as desired to promote relaxation and restful night's sleep.
- Instructions: Warm coconut oil and cocoa butter in a small pan until melted. Let rest on counter for ten minutes. Once cooled, add essential oils to mixture, then cool it in fridge for 1 hour. Desired texture is firm, not hard. Whip on high with electric mixer until softened and forms peaks. Apply a small, pea-sized amount and massage into feet before bed. Save remainder for additional treatments. Store in a cool place.

DIFFUSE TO ASSIST WITH GOING TO & STAYING ASLEEP:

Place essential oils in diffuser (add water when required); diffuse

- 1 drop each of cedarwood, patchouli, grounding blend, vetiver, roman chamomile
- 8 drops calming blend,
  3 drops wild orange

BEDTIME "TEA" FOR RELAXATION

Steep chamomile tea and add 2 drops lavender oil (make sure you have pjs on before finishing tea; it works great!)

QUIET THE MIND & BODY

- Stop the mind chatter: 1-3 drops each of grounding blend, and calming blend layered on bottoms of feet, back of neck at night; also breath in.
- For more restful sleep: 3 drops cellular complex blend on bottoms feet at night
- Kids' lights out: Layer vetiver, cedarwood, patchouli, calming blend, ylang ylang

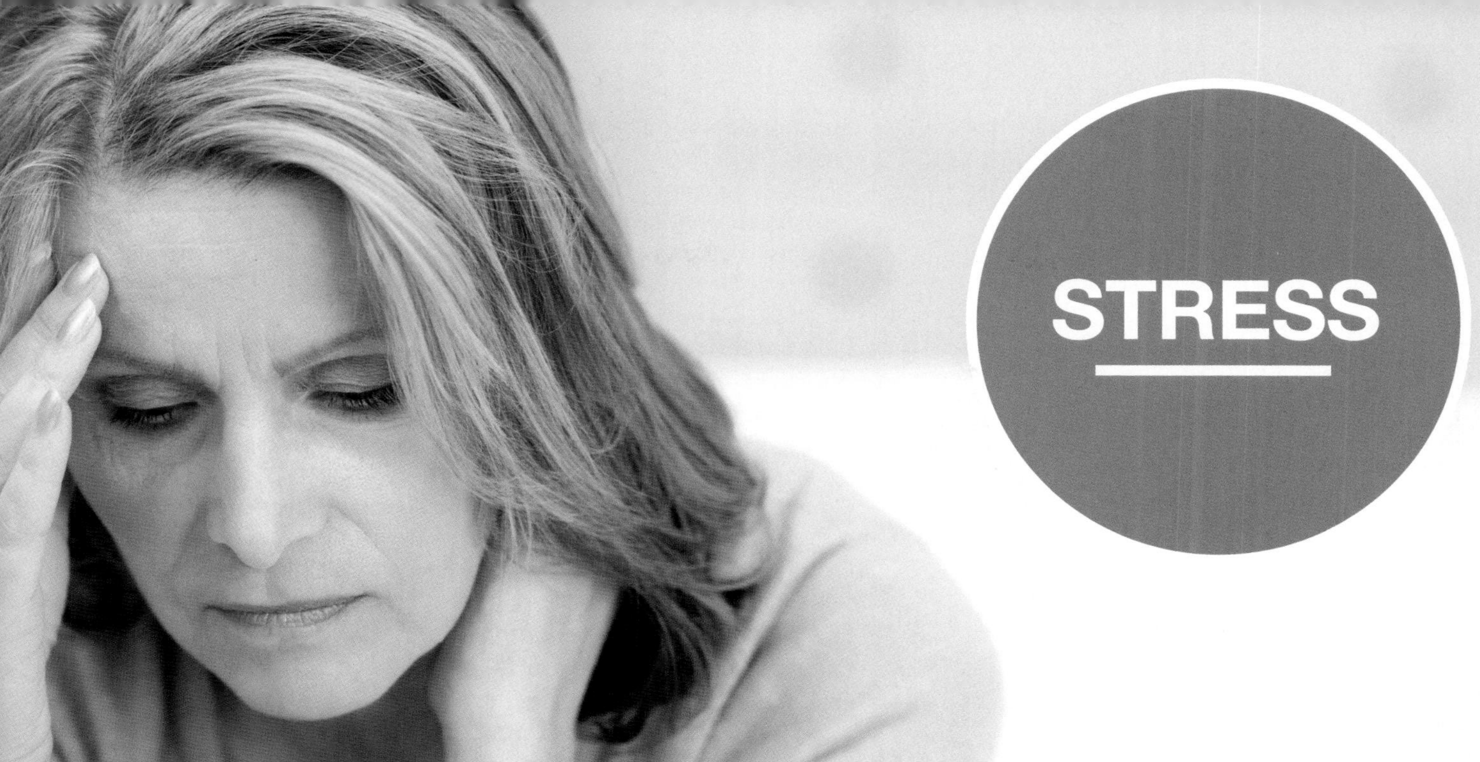

STRESS

UNDER NORMAL conditions, individuals are able to maintain homeostasis, a state where one is healthy, alert, and effective, and where body systems are operating as they should. Conversely, stress is the body's physiological response to overwhelming stimuli, a condition that directly challenges the body's ability to maintain homeostasis. When a stressful event or condition is perceived, the sympathetic nervous system is activated, which causes a fight-or-flight response in the body.

The fight-or-flight response initiates a chain reaction of activity in the body, starting with the central nervous system. Various parts of the brain, adrenal glands, peripheral nervous system (PNS), and other body systems work together to secrete hormones, such as adrenaline and cortisol, into the bloodstream. These hormones send messages instructing the immediate suspension of uncritical activities, such as those of the digestive, reproductive, and immune systems. All bodily energy and resources are directed to supporting heart and brain function.

Once the body's response to stress has been activated, a number of physical changes immediately occur. Stress reduces the blood-brain barrier's ability to block hormones and chemicals from entering the brain, thereby allowing corticosteroids to speed up the brain's ability to process information and make a decision. Cortisol deactivates the immune system, which does not cause serious problems as long as it is only a temporary, acute, response to stress.

When stress becomes chronic, however, some extremely serious situations can result. Over time, neuroplasticity of the brain is compromised, which results in the atrophy and destruction of neuron dendrites, and the brain loses the ability to form new connections or even process new sensory information (both being vital brain functions). When the immune system is repressed for an extended period of time, the body pays a significant toll. Risk of heart attack and stroke increases, anxiety and depression are more likely, and infertility can result, as well as a number of other chronic conditions including asthma, back pain, fatigue, headaches, serious digestive issues, and more.

It stands to reason that individual interpretation of relationships and other stimuli directly impact the level of stress experienced. When an individual can honestly assess a situation and choose to interpret it differently, this simple change in thinking can help reprogram an individual's stress response.

Essential oils are excellent support for effectively reprogramming the stress response on a chemical level. For example, when the cell membrane is hardened, cells suspend activity, rich nutrients and oxygen from the blood are not able to enter the cell, and toxic waste inside the cell is unable to escape. The chemical compounds in citrus oils, when inhaled, help cells to return to their normal state, thus allowing the interchange of nutrients and release of toxins to resume. On a physiological cellular level, the body's descent into fight-or-flight is interrupted, and the body is quickly able to shift towards homeostasis. There are numerous viable essential oils solutions that can interrupt unhealthy stress responses and prevent additional negative results.

TOP SOLUTIONS

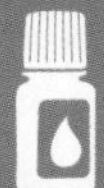

SINGLE OILS

Lavender - calms and relieves stress (pg. 108)
Roman chamomile - calms reduces stress (pg. 125)
Wild orange - energizes while reducing anxiety and depression (pg. 136)
Frankincense - reduces depression, trauma, and tension (pg. 100)
Vetiver - improves focus and sedates (pg. 134)

By Related Properties

For definitions of the properties listed below and more oil options, see Oil Properties Glossary (pg. 435) and Oil Properties (pg. 436).

Calming - bergamot, birch, black pepper, cassia, clary sage, coriander, fennel, frankincense, geranium, jasmine, juniper berry, lavender, melissa, oregano, patchouli, roman chamomile, sandalwood, tangerine, vetiver, yarrow
Energizing - basil, bergamot, clove, cypress, grapefruit, lemon, lemongrass, lime, rosemary, tangerine, white fir, wild orange
Grounding - basil, cedarwood, clary sage, cypress, melaleuca, vetiver, ylang ylang
Refreshing - cypress, geranium, grapefruit, lemon, lime, melaleuca, peppermint, wild orange, wintergreen
Relaxing - basil, cassia, cedarwood, clary sage, cypress, fennel, geranium, jasmine, lavender, marjoram, myrrh, ravensara, roman chamomile, white fir, ylang ylang
Uplifting - bergamot, cardamom, cedarwood, clary sage, cypress, grapefruit, lemon, lime, melissa, sandalwood, tangerine, wild orange, ylang ylang

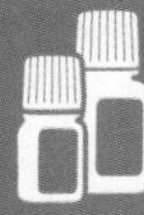

BLENDS

Invigorating blend - energizes while reducing anxiety and depression (pg. 153)
Grounding blend - balances mood while reducing stress and trauma (pg. 150)
Calming blend - reduces anxiety and stress (pg. 142)
Tension blend - relieves tension and stress (pg. 165)
Women's blend - balances hormones and calms anxiety (pg. 168)

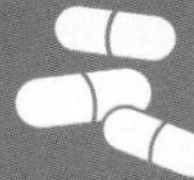

SUPPLEMENTS

Bone support complex (pg. 170), cellular vitality complex, digestion blend softgels, **energy & stamina complex (pg. 174)**, **essential oil omega complex (pg. 175)**, liquid omega-3 supplement, phytoestrogen multiplex, **whole food nutrient supplement (pg. 177)**

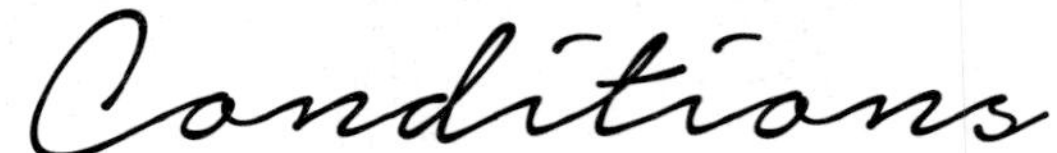

Conditions

For more emotions associated with stress (i.e. anxiety, depression) - see *Mood & Behavior*
Accelerated aging - frankincense, jasmine, sandalwood, ylang ylang, anti-aging blend, metabolic blend
Anxiety - bergamot, clary sage, frankincense, lavender, vetiver, wild orange, calming blend, focus blend, grounding blend, inspiring blend, invigorating blend, renewing blend; see *Mood & Behavior*
Behavioral stress - See *Addictions, Eating Disorders, Weight*
Busy-ness - juniper berry, calming blend, grounding blend
Chest pain - basil, cypress, lavender, marjoram, rosemary, sandalwood, thyme, wild orange, cellular complex blend, protective blend, soothing blend; see *Cardiovascular*
Constricted breathing - bergamot, frankincense, lavender, roman chamomile, grounding blend, inspiring blend, invigorating blend; see *Respiratory*
Depression - bergamot, frankincense, wild orange, ylang ylang, calming blend, invigorating blend, joyful blend, women's monthly blend; see *Mood & Behavior*
Energy, lack of stress - See *Energy & Vitality*
Endure stress and avoid illness - vetiver; see *Immune & Lymphatic*
Environmental stress - cinnamon, frankincense, geranium, juniper berry, sandalwood, wild orange, invigorating blend, grounding blend, renewing blend
Fainting - basil, bergamot, cinnamon, cypress, frankincense, lavender, peppermint, rosemary, sandalwood, wild orange; see *Cardiovascular*
Fatigue/exhaustion - basil, bergamot, cinnamon, lemon, lime, cellular complex blend, detoxification blend, grounding blend, encouraging blend, joyful blend, metabolic blend; see *Energy & Vitality*
Headache and migraine - frankincense, lavender, peppermint, wintergreen, soothing blend, tension blend; see *Pain & Inflammation*
Heart disease - geranium, lime, ylang ylang; see *Cardiovascular*
Illness, stress related - bergamot, lemon, rosemary; see *Immune & Lymphatic*
Insomnia - lavender, roman chamomile, marjoram, vetiver, calming blend, grounding blend, inspiring blend; see *Sleep*
Mind/thought-related/poor memory stress - See *Brain, Focus & Concentration*
Mood-related, moodiness driven stress - See *Mood & Behavior*
Muscle tension or pain - lavender, marjoram, peppermint, wintergreen, massage blend, soothing blend, tension blend; see *Muscular, Skeletal, Pain & Inflammation*
Nervous tension - calming blend, douglas fir, focus blend; see *Mood & Behavior, Nervous*
Obesity/overeating - bergamot, cinnamon, clary sage, geranium, ginger, grapefruit, jasmine, sandalwood, ylang ylang, invigorating blend, metabolic blend, women's blend; see *Weight, Eating Disorders*
Physical stress - geranium, lavender, invigorating blend, reassuring blend; see *Athletes*
Sex drive, change in - rose, ylang ylang, women's blend, joyful blend; see *Intimacy*
Shock - bergamot, frankincense, geranium, helichrysum, melaleuca, peppermint, roman chamomile, encouraging blend, focus blend, joyful blend; see *First Aid*
Sleep problems - lavender, wild orange, calming blend, grounding blend; see *Sleep*
Stomach, upset - peppermint, digestion blend; see *Digestive & Intestinal*
Stress, lack of management - coriander, wintergreen
Teeth grinding - frankincense, geranium, lavender, marjoram, roman chamomile, wild orange, calming blend; see *Parasites*
Tension - cedarwood, ginger, lavender, lemongrass, peppermint, wintergreen, calming blend, tension blend; see *Muscular*
Trauma stress, intense - cedarwood, frankincense, jasmine, lavender, melissa, roman chamomile, vetiver, ylang ylang, calming blend, grounding blend, focus blend; see *Limbic, Mood & Behavior*

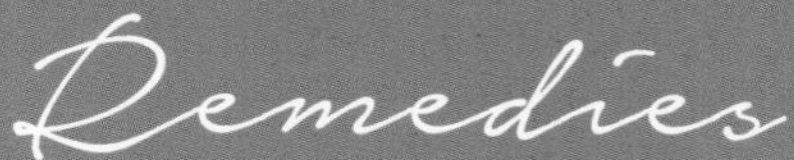

ROLLER BOTTLE REMEDIES

LIFT AND CALM BLEND
10 drops frankincense
12 drops invigorating blend
8 drops lavender
4 drops peppermint
Combine oils into a roller bottle and fill remainder with fractionated coconut oil. Apply to pulse points and behind the ears.

EXHAUSTION BLEND
10 drops eucalyptus
8 drops rosemary
7 drops bergamot
7 drops grapefruit
Combine oils into a roller bottle and fill remainder of bottle with fractionated coconut oil. Apply to pulse points and behind the ears to help when feeling exhausted.

MOTIVATION BLEND
10 drops lime
10 drops wild orange
5 drops frankincense
5 drops black pepper
Combine oils into a roller bottle and fill remainder with fractionated coconut oil. Apply to pulse points and behind the ears.

ANXIETY BLEND
10 drops bergamot
10 drops lemon
10 drops invigorating blend
10 drops lime
10 drops lavender
5 drops grounding blend
5 drops calming blend
Combine oils into a roller bottle and fill remainder with fractionated coconut oil. Apply to pulse points and behind the ears to help reduce feelings of anxiety.

MENTAL CLARITY BLEND
12 drops lemon
8 drops rosemary
4 drops cypress
2 drops peppermint
Combine oils into a roller bottle and fill remainder with fractionated coconut oil. Apply to pulse points and behind the ears to help increase mental clarity.

CHILL PILL BLEND
10 drops clary sage
15 drops bergamot
20 drops grapefruit
25 drops wild orange
15 drops frankincense
10 drops lemon
Combine oils into a roller bottle and fill remainder with fractionated coconut oil. Apply to pulse points and behind the ears.

BATH REMEDIES

The Basic De-Stress Bath
1 cup Epsom salts or sea salt
1/ 2 cup baking soda
10 drops lavender
Drop oil onto dry mixture of salt and baking soda, stir. Soak in tub as desired. Repeat throughout the week as necessary. This is a basic recipe. To individualize and cater to each unique stressful situation, select appropriate oils from Conditions list above. Then simply add 10-15 drops to bath. Combining a few oils or using an existing blend is an excellent way to enjoy the benefits of multiple oils at once.

Here are some favorites to choose from:

Bliss Bath - 7 drops calming blend and 7 drops roman chamomile

Calming Bath - 10 drops calming blend

De-Stress & Focus Bath - 5 drops calming blend and 5 drops frankincense

Energizing & Calming Bath - 7 drops wild orange oil and 8 drops lavender oil or calming blend

Get-My-Heart-Back-in-the-Project - 2 ylang ylang and 6 wild orange

Grounding Bath - 10 drops grounding blend

Quiet-the-Mind Bath - 9 drops sandalwood oil , 5 drops lavender oil and 1 drop cedarwood oil

Reviving & Relaxing Bath - 10 drops invigorating blend

Soothing Bath - 10 drops soothing blend

Take Out Tantrums Bath - 4 drops calming blend, 3 drops lavender and 2 drops tension blend

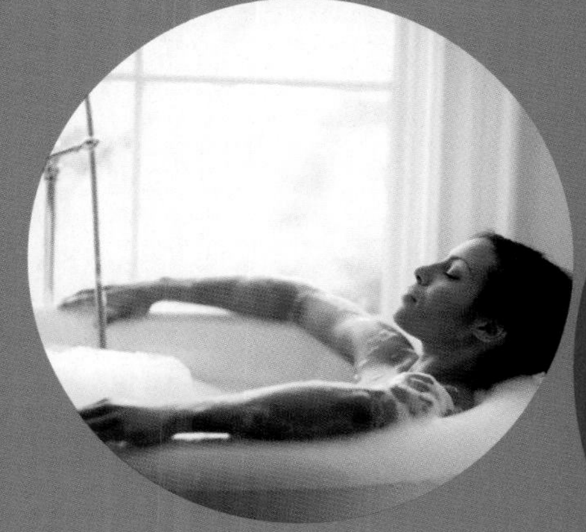

Tension Tamer Bath - 4 drops calming blend and 4 drops tension blend

Warm, Relax, Revive the Weary and Painful Bath - 4 drops ginger, 6 drops wild orange, 6 drops clove and 2 drops lavender

STRESS

USAGE TIPS: Managing and eliminating stress. Essential oils are extremely effective for stress reduction. Any method of application can be successful. Here are some primary methods:

- **Aromatic:** Get/create exposure to an aroma as a first step to success for an immediate invitation to relax, calm down, get focused or whatever is needed at the time. Diffuse favorite oils, inhale from bottle or hands, apply a few drops to clothing, or apply under nose.
- **Topical:** Apply to tense or tired muscles on back, shoulders, neck, legs, or anywhere the stress is affecting the body. This topical use also allows for an aromatic experience. Consider use on the chest, gland locations, base of skull (especially in suboccipital triangles), behind ears, or across forehead, and perfume points.
- **Internal:** Stress often affects internal activity such as digestion; choose and use oils according to needs.

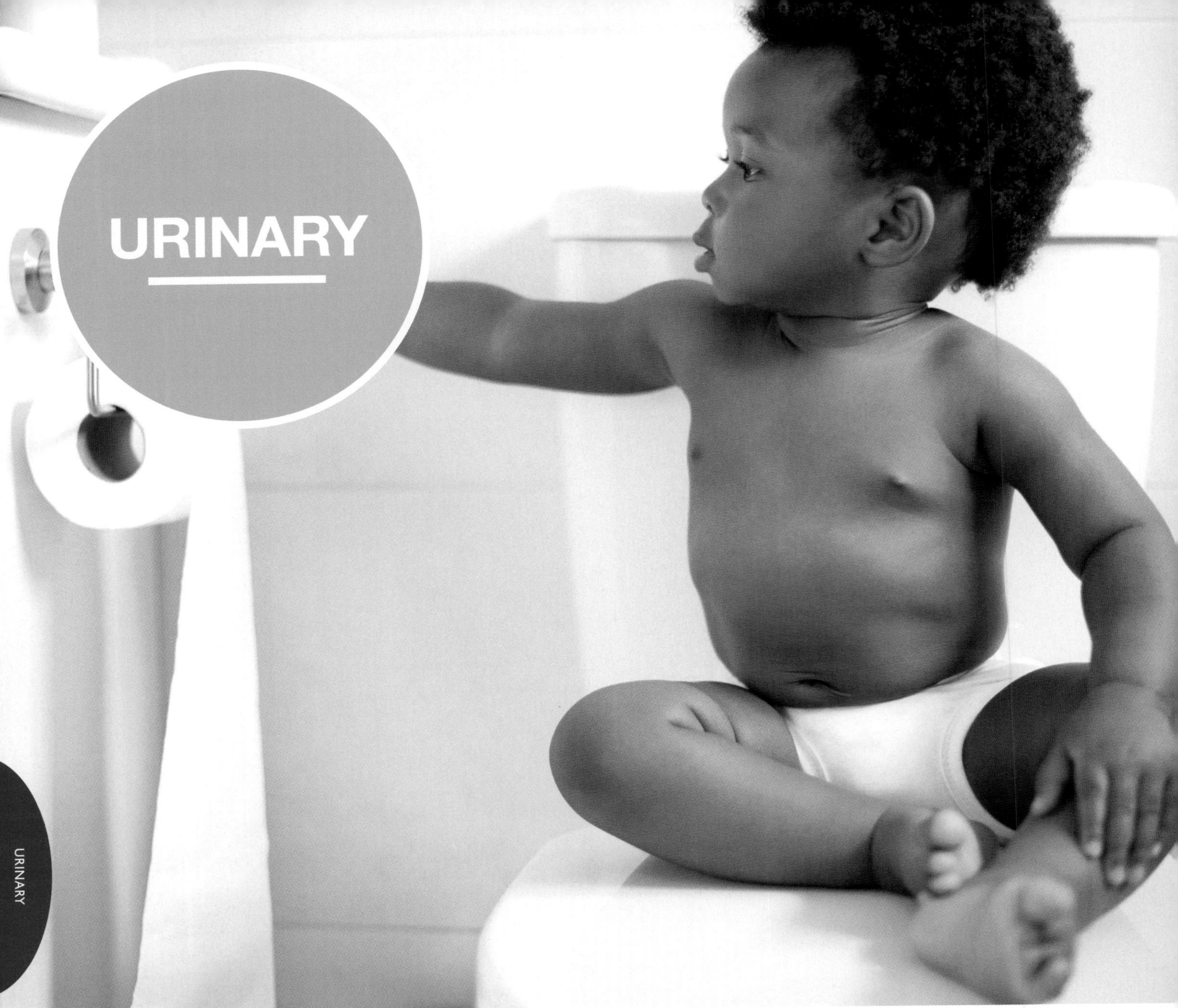

THE URINARY TRACT consists of the kidneys, ureters, bladder, and urethra. The principal function of the urinary system is to maintain the volume and composition of body fluids within normal limits. One aspect of this function is to rid the body of waste products that accumulate as a result of cellular metabolism and, because of this, it is sometimes referred to as the excretory system. While it plays a major role in excretion, however, it relies on other organs to support this function.

The urinary system maintains appropriate fluid volumes, pH and chemical balances, and electrolyte levels through complex processes in the kidneys and by regulating the amount of water that is excreted in the urine. Urine is formed in the kidneys through a blood filtration process and carries waste products and excess fluid to the ureters, tubes made of smooth muscle fibers that propel urine toward the urinary bladder, where it is stored until it is expelled from the body. The moving of urine from the bladder through the urethra and out of the body is called urination, or voiding.

The kidneys are also responsible for regulating sodium and potassium levels. No less important is the kidneys' ability to remove drugs from the body, release hormones that regulate blood pressure, produce an active form of vitamin D, which promotes strong, healthy bones, and control the production of red blood cells.

Most individuals operate in a constant state of dehydration, which takes its toll on overall health, but particularly impacts kidney health. In addition to adequate water intake, there are some essential oils that are extremely effective in supporting kidney health and helping the body to quickly rid itself of UTI discomfort and infections and even stones. While it is of utmost importance to utilize the services of medical professionals in the case of a prolonged or serious condition, essential oils can serve as a powerful first line of defense.

TOP SOLUTIONS

SINGLE OILS

Lemon - helps dissolve stones and acts as diuretic (pg. 110)
Juniper berry - acts as diuretic; tonifies bladder and supports urinary system (pg. 107)
Lemongrass - decongests urinary tract and fights urinary infections (pg. 112)
Cypress - resolves incontinence and excessive water/fluid retention (pg. 93)
Thyme - supports healthy prostate and circulation; fights urinary infections (pg. 133)
Eucalyptus - relieves infection, stones (pg. 97)
Cardamom - antioxidant and combats infection

By Related Properties

For definitions of the properties listed below and more oil options, see Oil Properties Glossary (pg. 435) and Oil Properties (pg. 436).

Anti-infectious - arborvitae, basil, bergamot, cardamom, cedarwood, cinnamon, clove, cypress, eucalyptus, frankincense, geranium, lavender, marjoram, melaleuca, patchouli, roman chamomile, rose, rosemary
Anti-inflammatory - arborvitae, basil, bergamot, birch, black pepper, cardamom, cassia, cedarwood, cinnamon, cypress, dill, eucalyptus, fennel, frankincense, geranium, ginger, helichrysum, lavender, lemongrass, lime, melaleuca, melissa, myrrh, oregano, patchouli, peppermint, rosemary, sandalwood, spearmint, spikenard, wild orange, wintergreen, yarrow
Cleanser - arborvitae, cilantro, eucalyptus, grapefruit, juniper berry, lemon, thyme, wild orange
Detoxifier - arborvitae, cassia, cilantro, cypress, geranium, juniper berry, lemon, lime, patchouli, rosemary, wild orange
Diuretic - arborvitae, basil, bergamot, birch, cardamom, cedarwood, cypress, eucalyptus, fennel, frankincense, geranium, grapefruit, helichrysum, juniper berry, lavender, lemon, lime, marjoram, patchouli, ravensara, rosemary, sandalwood, thyme, white fir, wild orange, wintergreen
Purifier - arborvitae, cinnamon, eucalyptus, grapefruit, lemon, lemongrass, lime, marjoram, melaleuca, oregano, wild orange

Related Ailments: Bed-Wetting, Berger's Disease, Incontinence, Kidney Infection, Kidney Stones, Overactive Poor Urine Flow, Ureter Infection, Urinary Tract Infection (UTI), Urination (Painful/Frequent)

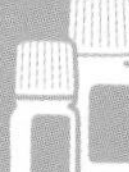

BLENDS

Cellular complex blend - antioxidant; cleanses and disinfects urinary tract (pg. 143)
Detoxification blend - supports proper liver and kidney function (pg. 146)
Metabolic blend - acts as diuretic and detoxifies (pg. 157)
Protective blend - promotes blood flow and elimination of waste (pg. 158)

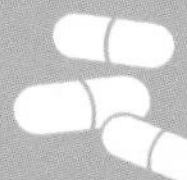

SUPPLEMENTS

Cellular vitality complex, **detoxification blend softgels (pg. 173), detoxification complex (pg. 172), essential oil cellular complex (pg. 174)**, metabolic blend softgels, **protective blend softgels (pg. 182)**, whole food nutrient supplement

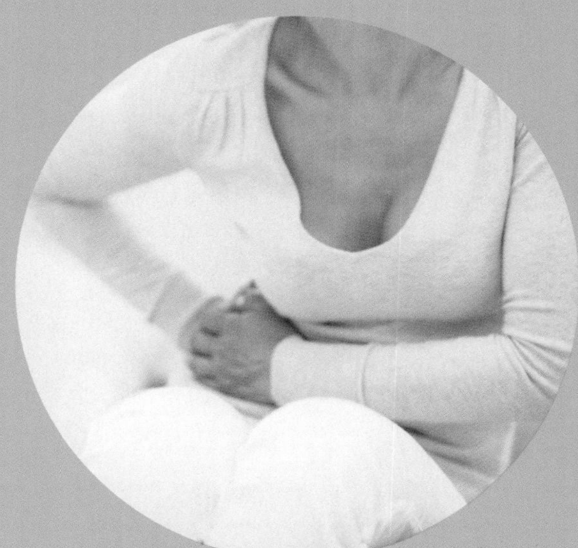

URINARY

USAGE TIPS: For best success in supporting urinary conditions

- **Internal:** Use softgels or place drops of oil(s) in a capsule and consume every few hours for acute situations; or under tongue or in water.
- **Topical:** Place over urinary areas of bladder/kidneys. Use carrier oil as needed to prevent sensitivity; spine, bottoms of feet also excellent locations.
- **Aromatic:** Diffuse oils through night for nighttime concerns such as bed-wetting.

Conditions

Abdominal pain - coriander, grapefruit, ginger, lavender, oregano, rosemary, cleansing blend; see *Digestive & Intestinal*

Bed-wetting - black pepper, cypress, frankincense, juniper berry, thyme, massage blend

Disorders - basil, bergamot, birch, cypress, juniper berry, lavender, lemongrass, lime, rosemary, sandalwood, thyme, wintergreen, cellular complex blend, digestion blend

Dribbling/minor leaks - cypress, marjoram, thyme, cellular complex blend

Edema - See "Water Retention" below

Excrete uric acid/toxins - cardamom, juniper berry, lemon, rosemary, cleansing blend, grounding blend

Hesitancy, urine flow - basil, ginger, thyme, metabolic blend

Incontinence - cypress, spearmint, renewing blend

Incontinence, emotional (repression of emotions) - black pepper, lavender, vetiver; see *Mood & Behavior*

Infections, bladder - arborvitae, birch, bergamot, cedarwood, cinnamon, clove, eucalyptus, fennel, juniper berry, lemon, lemongrass, rosemary, sandalwood, spearmint, thyme, white fir, wintergreen, cleansing blend, comforting blend, protective blend

Infections, kidney - bergamot, cardamom, cinnamon, coriander, fennel, juniper berry, lemon, lemongrass, rosemary, sandalwood, spearmint, thyme, cellular complex blend, cleansing blend, inspiring blend, protective blend

Infections, urinary - bergamot, cedarwood, cinnamon, fennel, lemon, lemongrass, geranium, juniper berry, rosemary, sandalwood, thyme, white fir, cellular complex blend, cleansing blend, inspiring blend, protective blend

Ketones in urine - coriander, fennel, juniper berry, rosemary, thyme

Kidney, circulation - basil, coriander, juniper berry

Kidney, lack of tone/weak - geranium, helichrysum, juniper berry, lemongrass, rosemary

Kidney stones - birch, cinnamon, clary sage, eucalyptus, fennel, geranium, juniper berry, lemon, sandalwood, spearmint, wild orange, wintergreen, renewing blend

Kidney, toxic - bergamot, cardamom, coriander, grapefruit, juniper berry, lemon, lemongrass, cleansing blend, detoxification blend, metabolic blend

Low-force/volume urine stream - cardamom, cinnamon, lemon, juniper berry, marjoram, thyme, comforting blend, massage blend, metabolic blend

Nausea/vomiting - bergamot, clove, fennel, ginger, lemon; see *Digestive & Intestinal*

Pelvic pressure - basil, cypress, clary sage, ginger, lavender, peppermint, metabolic blend

Perspiration, lack of - cardamom, cilantro, ginger, juniper berry, lemongrass, oregano, cleansing blend

Pus or blood in urine - basil, cardamom, frankincense, lemon, melaleuca, oregano, sandalwood, cellular complex blend, cleansing blend, detoxification blend, invigorating blend, protective blend; see suggestions for various urinary infections; see *Immune & Lymphatic*

Sharp/spastic pains in kidneys or bladder when urinating - basil, cardamom, cilantro, clary sage, cypress, grapefruit, juniper berry, lavender, lemon, marjoram, roman chamomile, thyme, white fir, tension blend

Swollen ankles, toes, fingers - basil, cypress, frankincense, grapefruit, lemon, marjoram, patchouli, massage blend

Urination, painful/burning/frequent - basil, birch, cinnamon, juniper berry, lemongrass, sandalwood, detoxification blend, massage blend, protective blend

Urgency of urination - cypress, frankincense, oregano, digestion blend, grounding blend, soothing blend

Water retention (edema) - cardamom, cedarwood, cinnamon, cypress, douglas fir, eucalyptus, fennel, frankincense, geranium, grapefruit, juniper berry, lavender, lemon, rosemary, tangerine, thyme, white fir, wild orange, wintergreen, comforting blend, detoxification blend, inspiring blend, massage blend, metabolic blend, renewing blend

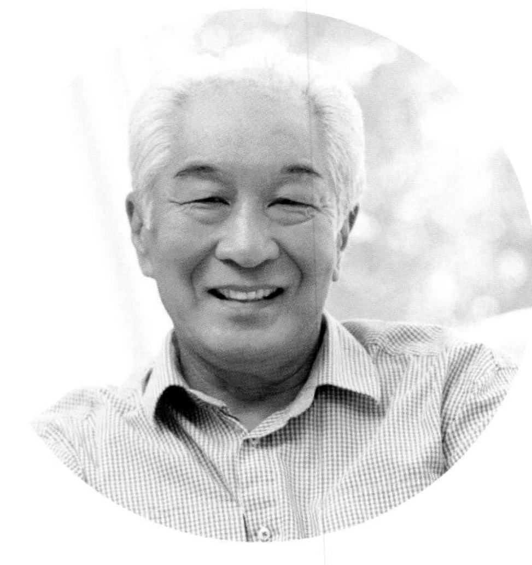

Remedies

ROCKIN RELIEF (for kidney stones)
4 drops helichrysum
4 drops juniper berry
5 drops grapefruit
5 drops lemon
Combine in a 15ml bottle, fill remainder with carrier oil. Apply over lower back every twenty minutes and cover with hot, moist compress. Note: avoid alcohol, sugars, refined foods, and drink ample amounts of water.

FIRE EXTINGUISHER (supports resolving urinary burning/infection)
2 drops sandalwood
6 drop cleansing blend
4 drops juniper berry
5 drop lemongrass
Combine in a 5ml roller bottle, fill remainder with carrier oil. Apply topically on lower abdomen over bladder and on lower back over kidneys every twenty minutes during daytime hours until pain no longer reoccurs. 1 drop protective blend in a glass of water internally morning and evening. Continue bladder blend three times daily. Take protective blend in water for three days after pain subsides.
Note: avoid alcohol, sugars, refined foods, drink ample amounts of water.

IN CONTROL (bladder control - for incontinence/bed-wetting)
1 drop juniper berry
1 drop of cypress
Combine in palm and apply topically across lower abdomen, use for occasional inconvenient urges, or three-plus times a day for chronic control issues.

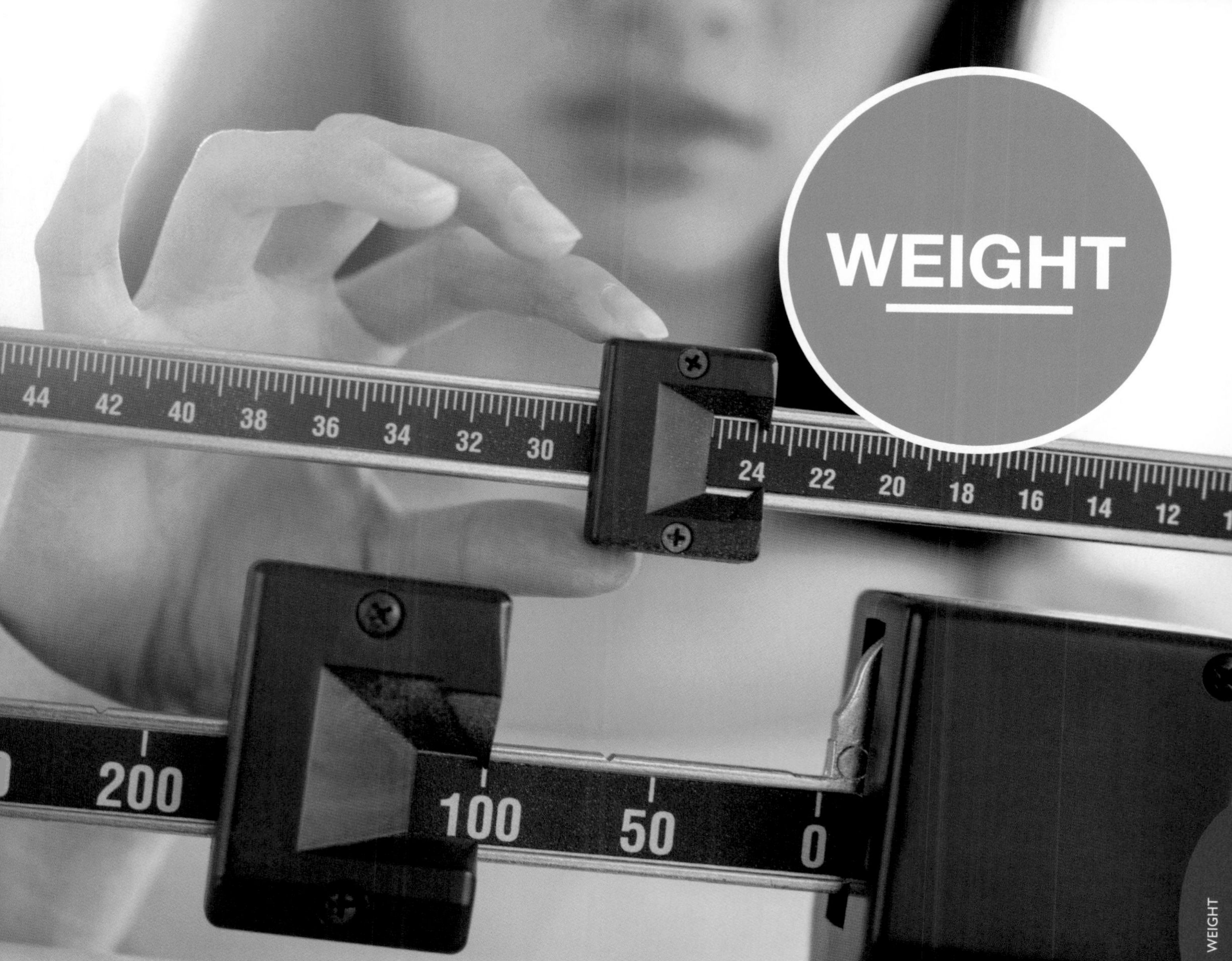

WEIGHT GAIN can result from an increase in muscle mass, fat deposits, or excess fluids such as water. The most common causes of weight gain are from excessive eating and poor nutrition. Food is made up of calories, or units of energy. Physical activity and normal body metabolism burn calories. When a person takes in more calories than the body uses, the extra calories are stored as fat subsequently enlarging or decreasing the "size" of fat cells depending on the balance of energy in the body. When fat cells build up or accumulate, it causes increased fat or obesity.

Other factors that may cause weight gain include medication, lack of lean muscle mass, inactivity, hypothyroidism, menopause, pregnancy, or slow metabolism. Sometimes toxicity levels within the body can encourage the body to hold onto fat; when there are too many toxins for the body to handle, the fats are diverted into fat cells – the only place in the body where natural insulation provides protection for vital body organs. Later, when individuals try to lose weight, despite effort it seems to prove to be next to impossible. These protective fat cells are programmed to guard the vital organs at all costs; therefore they cannot let go of their cargo.

Being overweight can bring about undesirable emotional effects such as depression, anxiety, and mood swings. Excess weight or obesity can cause exhaustion or fatigue and challenge individuals participating in various activities, a scenario especially difficult for overweight parents with active children. It causes undue stress on joints, bones, and muscles. Carrying excess fat can also dramatically increase the risk of developing deadly and debilitating diseases.

Essential oils and whole-food supplementation can be powerful allies in the process of maintaining a healthy weight and losing excess weight. Essential oils have the ability to coax toxic fat cells into releasing their contents, help break down the toxins, and, with proper hydration, flush them out of the body. Oils can also support the body's insulin response, reduce cravings, and provide a feeling of satiety. Supplements can give the cells the energy they need to carry out proper body function, including extra fuel for working out. Digestive enzymes help the body break down and utilize nutrients for maximum support.

TOP SOLUTIONS

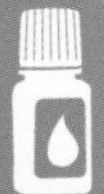

SINGLE OILS

Grapefruit - curbs cravings, reduces appetite, and induces fat burning (pg. 104)

Cinnamon - inhibits formation of new fat cells; balances blood sugar (pg. 86)

Peppermint - enhances sense of fullness; reduces cravings and appetite (pg. 122)

Ginger - encourages fat burning and promotes satiation (pg. 103)

By Related Properties

For definitions of the properties listed below and more oil options, see Oil Properties Glossary (pg. 435) and Oil Properties (pg. 436).

Analgesic - arborvitae, bergamot, black pepper, cassia, cinnamon, clary sage, clove, coriander, cypress, eucalyptus, frankincense, helichrysum, jasmine, juniper berry, lavender, lemongrass, marjoram, oregano, peppermint, ravensara, rosemary, white fir, wild orange, wintergreen

Antidepressant - basil, bergamot, clary sage, coriander, dill, frankincense, geranium, grapefruit, jasmine, lavender, lemon, lemongrass, melissa, oregano, patchouli, ravensara, rose, wild orange

Calming - bergamot, birch, black pepper, cassia, clary sage, coriander, fennel, frankincense, geranium, jasmine, juniper berry, lavender, oregano, patchouli, roman chamomile, sandalwood

Detoxifier - arborvitae, cassia, cilantro, cypress, geranium, juniper berry, lemon, lime, patchouli, rosemary, wild orange

Energizing - basil, clove, cypress, grapefruit, lemongrass, rosemary, white fir, wild orange

Steroidal - basil, birch, cedarwood, clove, fennel, patchouli, rosemary, thyme

Stimulant - arborvitae, basil, bergamot, birch, black pepper, cardamom, cedarwood, cinnamon, clove, coriander, cypress, dill, eucalyptus, fennel, ginger, grapefruit, juniper berry, lime, melaleuca, myrrh, patchouli, rosemary, spearmint, thyme, vetiver, white fir, wintergreen, ylang ylang

Stomachic - basil, cardamom, cinnamon, clary sage, coriander, fennel, ginger, juniper berry, marjoram, melissa, peppermint, rose, rosemary, tangerine, wild orange, yarrow

Uplifting - bergamot, cardamom, cedarwood, clary sage, cypress, grapefruit, lemon, lime, melissa, sandalwood, tangerine, wild orange, ylang ylang

Related Ailments: Excessive Appetite, Autointoxication, Cellulite, Loss of Appetite, Obesity, Overeating

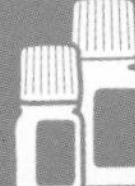

BLENDS

Metabolic blend - balances metabolism, eliminates cravings, and lifts mood; acts as diuretic (pg. 157)

Detoxification blend - support body's ability to remove toxins and waste effectively (pg. 146)

Cellular complex blend - improves function of the endocrine system and thyroid (pg. 143)

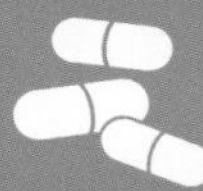

SUPPLEMENTS

Cellular vitality complex, defensive probiotic, **detoxification complex (pg. 173)**, digestion blend softgels, essential oil omega complex, fruit & vegetable supplement powder, **meal replacement shake (pg. 179)**, **metabolic blend softgels (pg. 180)**, phytoestrogen multiplex, whole food nutrient supplement

USAGE TIPS: For weight management, the focus is primarily on what and how much food is consumed (appetite) and how well it is utilized as fuel by the body (metabolism). Additionally, balancing other processes such as elimination, blood sugar, and hormones is often necessary for long-lasting results. See suggested programs in "Remedies" below. With that in mind:

- **Internal:** Ingesting oils for support with appetite, cravings and metabolism, including the ability to burn fat and release it along with toxins is very effective. Place drops of oils in a capsule for systemic or on-going support. Drink oils in water; drop on tongue. Be generous with usage for this purpose.
- **Topical:** Use to assist the body to detox and target specific zones. Consider applying blends of oils to areas like the abdomen, thighs, and arms as a treatment. Use a carrier oil if necessary to prevent sensitivity especially with oils like cinnamon.
- **Aromatic:** Excellent for supporting appetite control. Inhale as needed.

Conditions

Anorexia - See *Eating Disorders*

Appetite, excess - bergamot, ginger, grapefruit, juniper berry, lemon, peppermint, metabolic blend, renewing blend; if due to nutritional deficiencies see *Weight* - "Supplements"

Appetite, imbalanced - grapefruit, wild orange, metabolic blend

Appetite, loss of - bergamot, black pepper, cardamom, coriander, fennel, ginger, grapefruit, lemon, patchouli, spearmint, thyme, cleansing blend, digestion blend, inspiring blend, metabolic blend, tension blend

Blood sugar imbalance - cassia, cinnamon, coriander, fennel, rosemary, metabolic blend, protective blend, uplifting blend; see *Blood Sugar*

Cellulite - birch, cypress, eucalyptus, geranium, ginger, grapefruit, lemongrass, lemon, lime, rosemary, tangerine, white fir, wild orange, wintergreen, metabolic blend; see *Detoxification*

Cravings - ginger, grapefruit, peppermint, metabolic blend

Cravings, sugar - cassia, cinnamon, clove, grapefruit, metabolic blend

Eating, over/binging/compulsive - bergamot, black pepper, cedarwood, cinnamon, ginger, grapefruit, juniper berry, lemon, oregano, patchouli, peppermint, joyful blend, metabolic blend

Edema/swelling/water retention - basil, cypress, ginger, juniper berry, lemon, lemongrass, patchouli, rosemary, tangerine, metabolic blend; see *Urinary*

Emotional/stress-induced eating - bergamot, grapefruit, metabolic blend; see *Eating Disorders, Mood & Behavior*

Energy, low/fatigue/exhaustion - basil, lime, peppermint, rosemary, jasmine; see *Energy & Vitality*

Excessive weight/obese - birch, cinnamon, fennel, ginger, grapefruit, juniper berry, lemon, oregano, tangerine, wild orange, wintergreen, metabolic blend

Fat, breakdown/dissolve - grapefruit, lemon, spearmint, tangerine, metabolic blend

Food addiction - basil, black pepper, cardamom, ginger, grapefruit, metabolic blend; see *Addictions*

Hunger pains - fennel, myrrh, oregano, peppermint, focus blend; see *Digestion & Intestinal*

Inability to lose weight - cinnamon, coriander, spearmint, detoxification blend, metabolic blend; see *Candida, Detoxification*

Metabolism, slow - cassia, clove, ginger, lemongrass, spearmint, metabolic blend

Metabolism, too fast - ginger, metabolic blend, myrrh, respiration blend drops

Overindulgence of food - grapefruit, juniper berry, peppermint, metabolic blend

Pancreas, inflamed - dill, fennel; see *Endocrine (Pancreas)*

Satiety/satiation, lack of - bergamot, dill, fennel, ginger, grapefruit, peppermint

Sagging skin - helichrysum, grapefruit, anti-aging blend, massage blend; see *Integumentary*

Sense of self, poor/self worth, lack of - bergamot, grapefruit, jasmine, joyful blend; see *Mood & Behavior*

Stretch marks - frankincense, geranium, lavender, sandalwood, tangerine, anti-aging blend; see *Integumentary*

Thyroid imbalances - coriander, frankincense, clove, ginger, rosemary, anti-aging blend; see *Endocrine (Thyroid, Adrenal)*

Toxicity - lemon, grapefruit, rosemary, detoxification blend, metabolic blend; see *Detoxification*

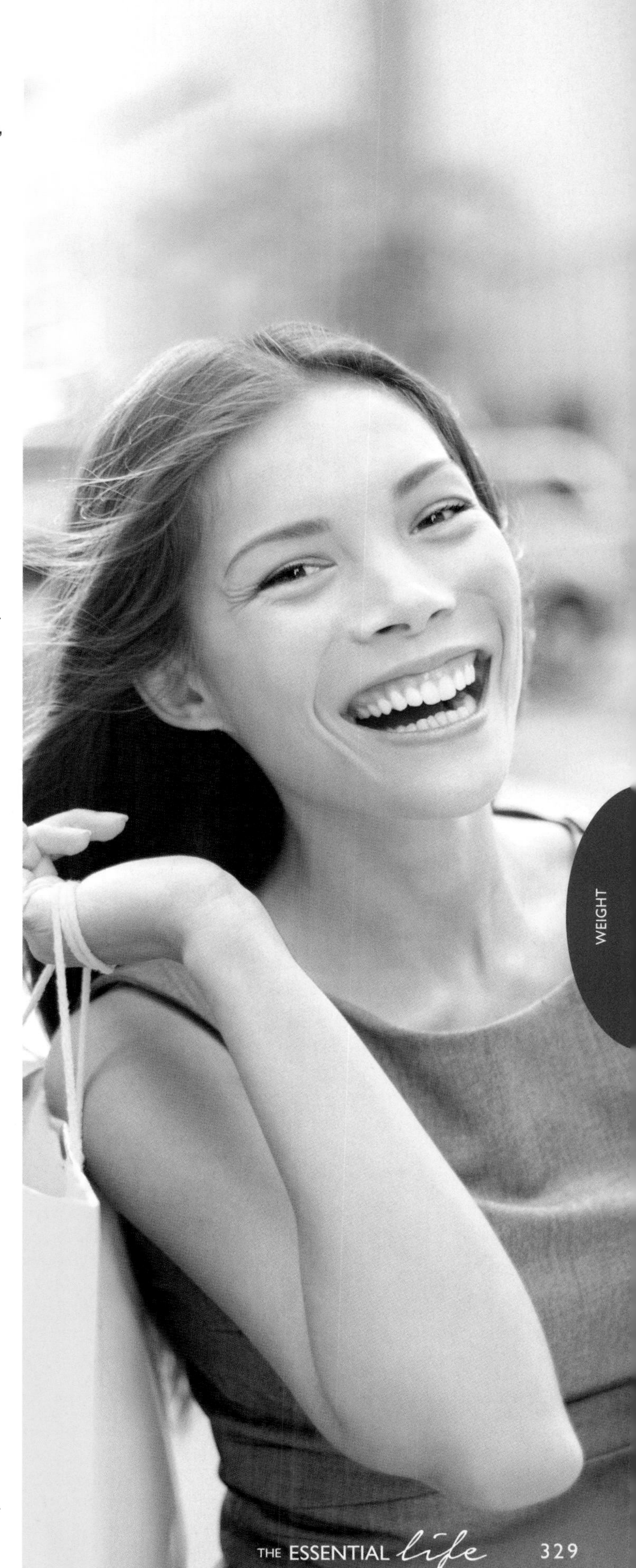

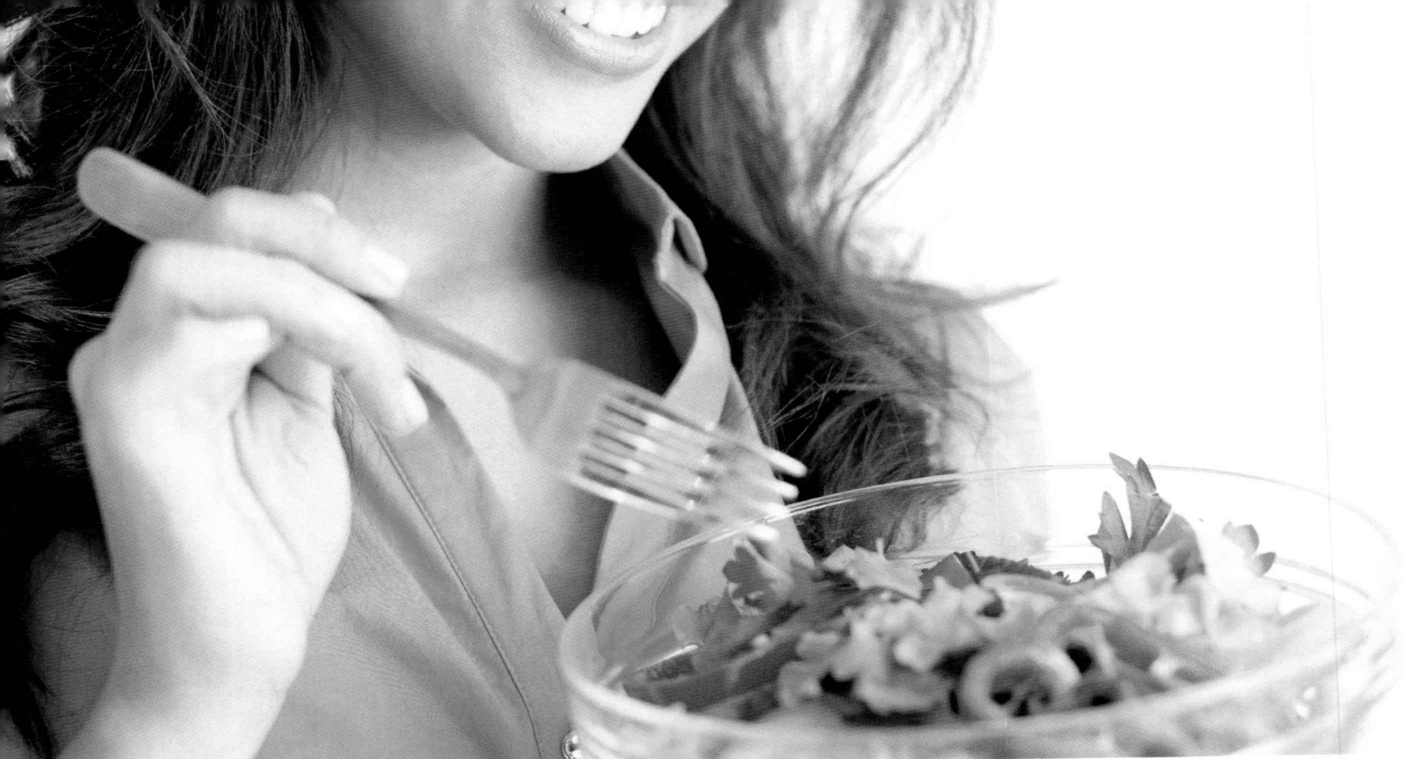

Weight Loss Program

	10-30 days (Pre-Cleanse)	10 days (Cleanse)	20 days (Restore)	30 days (Maintain)
UPON RISING	metabolic blend in or with water			
MORNING MEAL	- meal replacement shake - whole food nutrient supplement - essential oil omega complex - detoxification complex - food enzymes ***	- meal replacement shake - whole food nutrient supplement Essential oil omega complex - GI cleansing softgels * - detoxification blend	- meal replacement shake - whole food nutrient supplement - essential oil omega complex - food enzymes *** - defensive probiotic **	- meal replacement shake - whole food nutrient supplement - essential oil omega complex [optional: food enzymes ***]
BETWEEN MEALS	metabolic blend in or with water			
NOON MEAL	- meal replacement shake - food enzymes ***	- meal replacement shake - GI cleansing softgels *	- Healthy Meal or meal replacement shake - food enzymes ***	- Healthy Meal or meal replacement shake [optional: food enzymes ***]
BETWEEN MEALS	metabolic blend in or with water			
MORNING MEAL	- Healthy Meal - whole food nutrient supplement - essential oil omega complex - detoxification complex - food enzymes ***	- Healthy Meal - whole food nutrient supplement - essential oil omega complex - food enzymes *** - GI cleansing softgels * - detoxification blend	- Healthy Meal - whole food nutrient supplement - essential oil omega complex - food enzymes *** - defensive probiotic **	- Healthy Meal - whole food nutrient supplement - essential oil omega complex [optional: food enzymes ***]
BETWEEN MEALS	metabolic blend in or with water			
EXERCISE	Aerobic (20+ minutes 3X per week) Resistance (10+ minutes 3X per week) Flexibility (5-20 minutes daily)			

* GI cleansing softgels- start with 1 softgel a day, increasing to 3 a day as comfortable.
**Defensive probiotic will last for 15 days (2 capsules per day for 15 days in a 30-count bottle)
*** Food enzymes - take 1-2 per meal

NOTE: Metabolic blend should be taken 5 drops 5X daily (only mentioned 4X above) fit the 5th in during the day (there are 5 drops per softgel)
CAUTION: Always follow common sense, and the advice of your health care professional***

Remedies

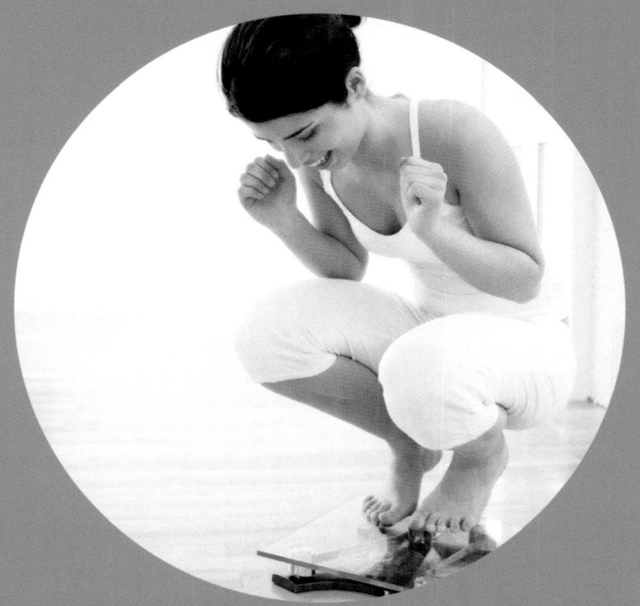

WEIGHT LOSS DETOX AND METABOLISM BOOST

- Take 5 drops metabolic blend in capsule or water two to five times per day.
- Take 3 drops detoxification blend in capsule two times a day. Can combine oils.
- Take 1-2 capsules of food enzymes with every meal.
- Apply grapefruit topically to troubled areas. Dilute as needed or desired.
- Address thyroid - see Endocrine (Thyroid).
- Rub 1-2 drops of grounding blend on bottoms of feet morning and evening.
- As a morning meal, use meal replacement shake. Add cinnamon, cassia, or citrus oil to enhance flavor and benefits.

BODY SLIMMING WRAP

30 drops metabolic blend
15 drops eucalyptus
15 drops peppermint
10 drops grapefruit
10 drops lavender
10 drops women's monthly blend
5 drops wintergreen

Use a 4 ounce glass bottle with a sprayer top for ease of use. Mix oils in bottle. Swirl. Fill remainder with fractionated coconut oil. Optional: add oils to approximately 4 ounces of non-scented natural lotion as an alternative.

Instructions for use:

- Step 1: Measure the areas to be addressed prior to use.
- Step 2: Spray or apply mixture to areas of concern.
- Step 3: Place and wrap around body cotton fabric (e.g. muslin) or paper towel as a barrier between skin and plastic wrap so as not to absorb toxins from plastic (oils breakdown some plastics).
- Step 4: Using plastic wrap, wrap around about 3-4 layers
- Step 5: Leave on for anywhere from a few hours to overnight as desired and then remove.
- Step 6: Measure treated areas again and record difference.

NOTE: Drink plenty of water with lemon oil (4 drops per 16 ounces) before and after treatment. It is an excellent diuretic and helps release toxins from fat.

WEIGHT LOSS TUMMY RUB

8 drops fennel
5 drops grapefruit
4 drops patchouli
2 ounces fractionated coconut oil

Blend and store in glass bottle. Recipe can be doubled as desired. Apply to tummy. Enhance the effects by adding metabolic blend to your water all day long.

CELLULITE/WEIGHT LOSS/DETOX BATH

2 cups Epsom salt
1 cups baking soda
10 drops metabolic blend

Mix ingredients and use desired quantity in the bath. Soak twenty minutes or longer two to three times a week. Drink lots of water during and/or after. Add 5 drops metabolic blend per 16 ounces drinking water for enhanced results and as a daily habit.

AROMATHERAPY APPETITE CONTROL INHALER BLENDS

Pick a blend below and place into inhaler. Breathe in scent of blend with three long deep breaths through nostrils. Use inhaler prior to eating and when appetite is triggered.

- **Sexy Citrus**
  30 drops grapefruit
  4 drops lemon
  1 drop ylang ylang

- **Marvelous Mint**
  20 drops peppermint
  10 drops bergamot
  4 drops spearmint
  1 drop ylang ylang

- **Herbal Mix**
  15 drops basil
  15 drops marjoram
  1 drop oregano
  1 drop thyme

CRAVE AWAY

Place 1-3 drops of grapefruit into palms, rub hands together vigorously; cup hands together and slowly inhale. May augment with a drop of patchouli.

"TONE" UP YOUR MUSCLES

Combine 4 drops basil, 3 drops cypress, 3 drops rosemary, 3 drops lavender with 1 teaspoon of carrier oil. Rub into muscles before workout. Enhances muscle tone, prevents sore muscles.

LOVE YOURSELF

Apply 1-2 drops grapefruit topically to chest or diffuse to encourage positive relationships with physical self.

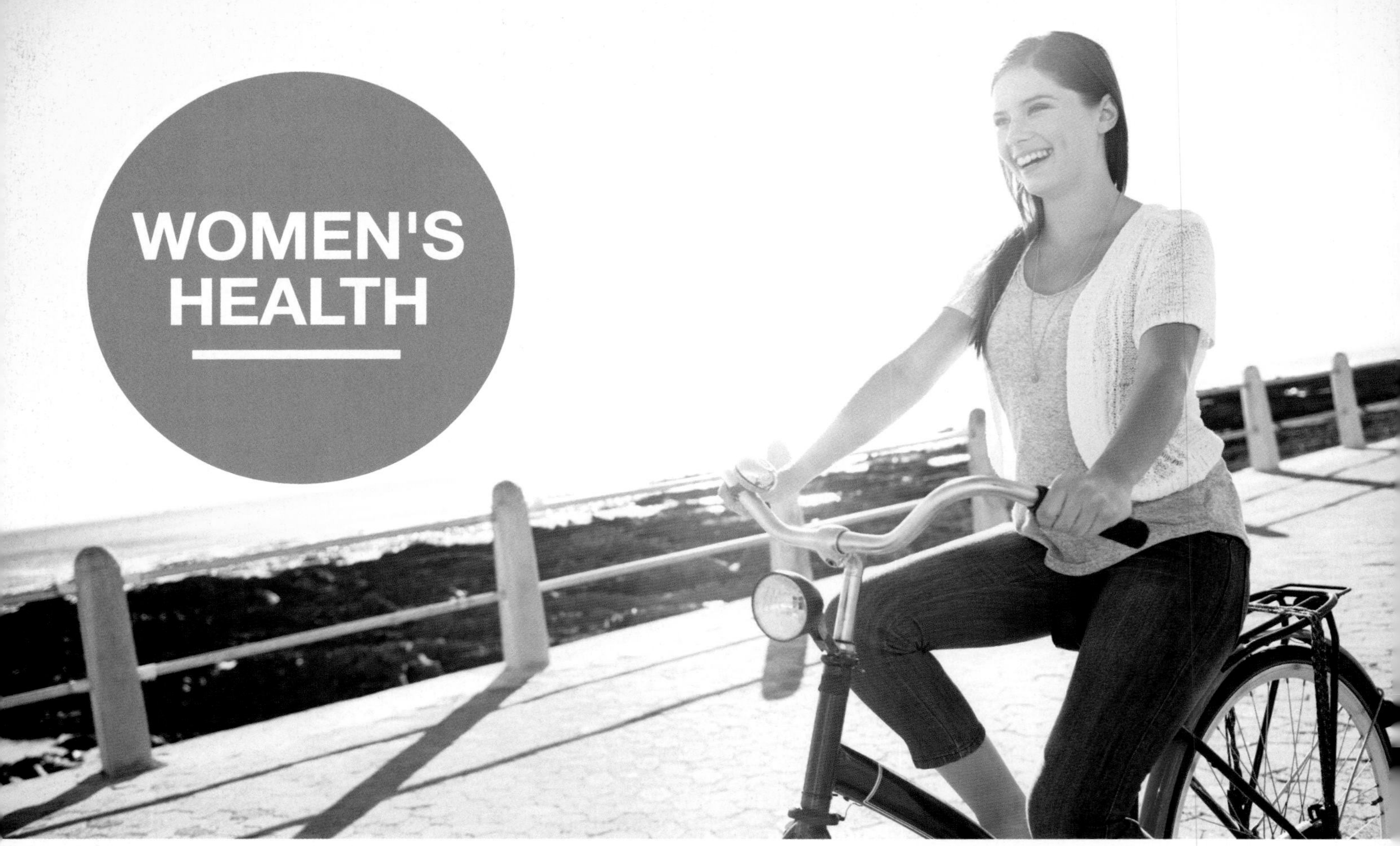

WOMEN'S HEALTH

WOMEN face health challenges specific to their gender including, but not limited to, the reproductive system, brain, heart, skeleton, and hormone issues. Many women suffer from high cortisol levels, which lead to fatigue, weight changes, depression, anxiety, and digestive problems. At all stages of life, most women do their best to maintain homeostasis while multitasking. Physical and emotional stress can be a cause and symptom of many women's issues.

The female reproductive system works closely with other systems, specifically the endocrine system. The female reproductive system includes the ovaries, fallopian tubes, uterus, cervix, external genitalia, and breasts. The ovaries are responsible for producing egg cells as well as secreting the hormones estrogen and progesterone. These hormones are vital to reproductive health and fertility, but they also play a role in the balance of a woman's emotional and physical health. They influence other body tissue and even bone mass. Hydration and nutrition can directly impact the production of these hormones. Women with lower body fat sometimes do not produce enough of the sex hormones and can encounter amenorrhea (an abnormal absence of menstruation) and decreased bone density.

For approximately forty years of their lives women experience the menstruation cycle. This monthly cycle (26-35 days) involves egg development and release from the ovaries, the uterus preparing to receive a fertilized egg, and the shedding of the uterine lining if an egg is not fertilized. Many women experience difficulty during the second half of this cycle in the form of premenstrual syndrome and menstrual cramps. Irritability, anxiousness, bloating, headaches, and even migraines can be common at this time. The cycle is maintained through the secretion of the sex hormones. An imbalance of sex hormones can lead to a lack of period as well as irregular and/or extended bleeding. This can be linked to polycystic ovary syndrome or endometriosis.

As a woman ages, the sex hormones begin to diminish. Menopause refers to the time when menstruation no longer occurs due to diminished sex hormones, specifically after a lack of twelve periods. This change leads to periodic instability of functions in the body, and side effects such as hot flashes, mood swings, vaginal dryness, fluctuations in sexual desire, fatigue, forgetfulness, and urinary incontinence can occur.

Nutrition and hydration are important keys to a woman's health. Daily supplements that include a whole food nutrient supplement, essential oil omega complex, bone supplement complex, and phytoestrogen multiplex will help a woman's body be able to regulate hormones properly. The phytoestrogen multiplex is a natural form of estrogen-like therapy, assisting to balance not only a deficiency, but also any excess of the wrong kind and harmful estrogen metabolites. The woman's monthly blend can be applied to the wrists, ankles, and directly over the abdomen when symptoms of PMS and menopause are occurring. Grapefruit and thyme oils support healthy progesterone levels, the counterbalance hormone to estrogen. Also, mood-enhancing oils, including joyful blend, calming blend, invigorating blend, and grounding blend, can help with depression and other emotions that may be prevalent for women.

TOP SOLUTIONS

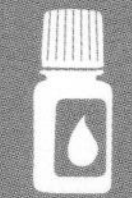

SINGLE OILS

Rose - helps overcome frigidity and infertility; promotes healthy menstruation (pg. 126)
Geranium - supports hormone, emotional balance, and fertility (pg. 102)
Ylang ylang - promotes healthy libido; relaxes (pg. 139)
Clary sage - enhances endocrine system function and balances hormones (pg. 88)
Grapefruit - supports healthy progesterone levels and breast health (pg. 104)
Jasmine - promotes a healthy uterus, libido (pg. 106)
Ginger - promotes healthy menstruation and libido; relieves cramps (pg. 103)
Fennel - supports healthy estrogen levels and supports healthy ovaries (pg. 98)
Thyme and oregano - supports healthy progesterone levels (pg. 133) (pg. 120)

By Related Properties

For definitions of the properties listed below and more oil options, see Oil Properties Glossary (pg. 435) and Oil Properties (pg. 436).

Analgesic - arborvitae, basil, bergamot, birch, black pepper, cassia, cinnamon, clary sage, clove, coriander, cypress, fennel, frankincense, ginger, helichrysum, jasmine, juniper berry, lavender, lemongrass, marjoram, melaleuca, oregano, peppermint, rosemary, white fir, wild orange, wintergreen
Antidepressant - basil, bergamot, cinnamon, clary sage, coriander, dill, frankincense, geranium, grapefruit, jasmine, lemon, lemongrass, melissa, oregano, patchouli, ravensara, rose, sandalwood, wild orange, ylang ylang
Antihemorrhagic - geranium, helichrysum
Aphrodisiac - black pepper, cardamom, cinnamon, clary sage, clove, coriander, ginger, jasmine, juniper berry, patchouli, peppermint, ravensara, rose, rosemary, sandalwood, spearmint, thyme, vetiver, wild orange, ylang ylang
Detoxifier - arborvitae, cassia, cilantro, cypress, geranium, juniper berry, lemon, lime, patchouli, rosemary, wild orange
Emmenagogue - arborvitae, basil, cassia, cedarwood, cinnamon, clary sage, dill, fennel, ginger, jasmine, juniper berry, lavender, marjoram, myrrh, oregano, peppermint, roman chamomile, rose, rosemary, spearmint, thyme, wintergreen
Galactagogue - basil, clary sage, dill, fennel, jasmine, lemongrass, wintergreen

Related Ailments: Amenorrhea, Dysmenorrhea, Endometriosis, Estrogen Imbalance [Detoxification], Excessive Menstrual Bleeding, Female Hormonal Imbalance [Detoxification], Fibrocystic Breasts [Endocrine], Fibroids [Cellular Health], Hot Flashes, Infertility, Irregular Menstrual Cycle, Lack Of Ovulation, Libido (low) for Women, Menopause, Menorrhagia, Menstrual Pain, Ovarian Cyst, Pelvic Pain Syndrome, Perimenopause, PMS, Polycystic Ovary Syndrome (PCOS), Scanty Menstruation, Vaginal Yeast Infections [Candida], Vaginitis

BLENDS

Women's blend - stabilizes mood and supports proper endocrine function (pg. 168)
Women's monthly blend - supports monthly cycle (pg. 167)
Encouraging blend - supports healthy reproductive function (pg. 148)

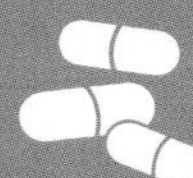

SUPPLEMENTS

Bone support complex (pg. 170), cellular vitality complex, essential oil cellular complex, **essential oil omega complex (pg. 175)**, liquid omega-3 supplement, **phytoestrogen multiplex (pg. 181)**, **whole food nutrient supplement (pg. 183)**

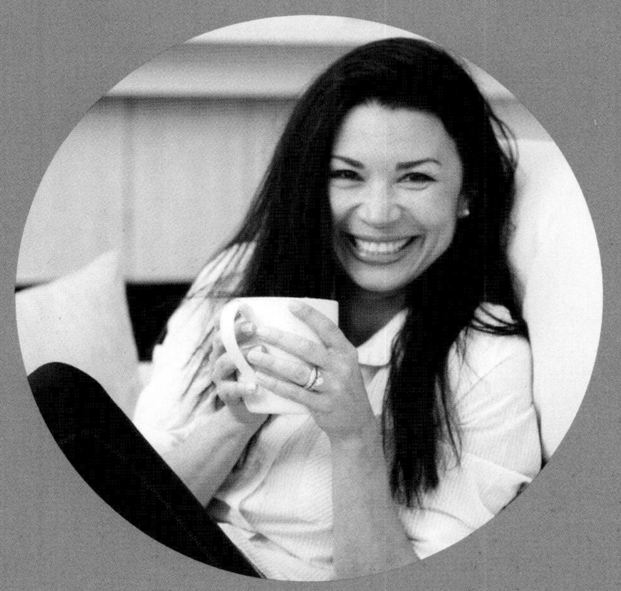

USAGE TIPS: For best results for women's health

- **Aromatic:** Women are very sensitive and emotionally responsive to aromas. Consider regular use for promoting emotional stability. Diffuse selected oils that derive desired results. Additionally, use favorite oils to wear as perfume; apply to wrists and neck. Smell wrists throughout the day. Reapply as needed.
- **Topical:** Apply selected oils to back of neck and shoulders or other areas of need (e.g. back, for menstrual cramps) to reduce tension, soothe sore muscles, reduce spasms.

Remedies

COOL YOUR HOT MESS (for PMS)
12 drops wild orange
9 drops clary sage
6 drops geranium
6 drops roman chamomile
Combine in a 5ml bottle/roller bottle, fill remainder with carrier oil. Apply to pulse points, cup hands together over nose and mouth and inhale.

HE'LL NEVER KNOW (for symptoms of PMS/menopause)
12 drops geranium
6 drops ylang ylang
4 drops clary sage
Combine in a 5ml bottle/roller bottle, fill remainder with carrier oil. Apply over lower abdomen and lower back (female organs are in between), use on wrists for emotional support, cup hands together over nose and mouth and inhale. Or apply women's monthly blend in same manner.

MENORRHAGIA (HEAVY FLOW)
6 drops roman chamomile
4 drops geranium
3 drops lemon
2 drops cypress
Combine in 15 ml bottle/roller bottle, fill remainder with carrier oil. Massage onto abdomen and pelvic area (above uterus) several times daily, starting the week before menstruation.

FIXUS (PILARIS KERATOSIS)
15 drops lavender
15 drops geranium
15 drops melaleuca
15 drops myrrh
15 drops oregano
Combine in 2-ounce spray bottle, fill remainder with carrier oil. Apply three to five times a day to affected area, shaking lightly before each use.

BREAST ENHANCER
Apply 1 drop of vetiver across top of breasts two times per day until desired results are achieved (generally a couple months). Can add complimentary oils to change aroma. NOTE: This suggestion is suited for women who have lost or never had breast mass due to intense exercise levels [i.e. runners] or breastfeeding, etc. Vetiver will not have a negative impact on women with larger breasts so its unnecessary to avoid usage for other purposes.

BREAST DETOX
- Apply 4 drops frankincense oil to each breast twice daily for thirty days. Do detox two to four times per year. Use a carrier oil for easier distribution.
- Eucalyptus and grapefruit are also excellent for breast health, applied topically with a carrier oil. Apply for discomfort or concern.

FERTILITY BLEND
12 drops clary sage
10 drops fennel
7 drops geranium
8 drops lavender
8 drops bergamot
Bonus: add 3 drops rose if available
Combine oils in 10ml roller bottle; fill remainder with fractionated coconut oil. Apply to lower abdomen twice daily, targeting ovary and uterus areas.

FERTILITY PROTOCOL
- **Diet:** See *Candida*
- **Supplementation:** (See *Candida* for a more in-depth program):
  - › Cellular vitality complex, whole food nutrient complex, essential oil omega complex - take as directed
  - › Defensive probiotic - take 1 capsule three times on days 11-15 of monthly cycle; then take one per day on day 16 until end of monthly cycle (onset of menstruation). Repeat monthly until desired results are achieved.
  - › GI cleansing softgels - take first ten days of monthly cycle, 1-3 capsules three times a day
  - › Phytoestrogen multiplex - take 1 capsule every day to eliminate harmful estrogen metabolites and maintain healthy estrogen levels.
- **Essential oil use:**
  - › Geranium - apply two times a day over liver, adrenal glands, kidneys areas to support healthy production of progesterone.
  - › Grapefruit - take 16 drops under tongue or in a capsule every morning to support healthy progesterone levels.
  - › Women's monthly blend - apply to sides of feet under ankle bones, abdomen, and wrists for hormone and mood balancing

Follow program until becoming pregnant. Then discontinue GI cleansing softgels, phytoestrogen multiplex, women's monthly blend. Continue everything else throughout pregnancy. Reduce defensive probiotic consumption to 1-2 per day to maintain healthy terrain.

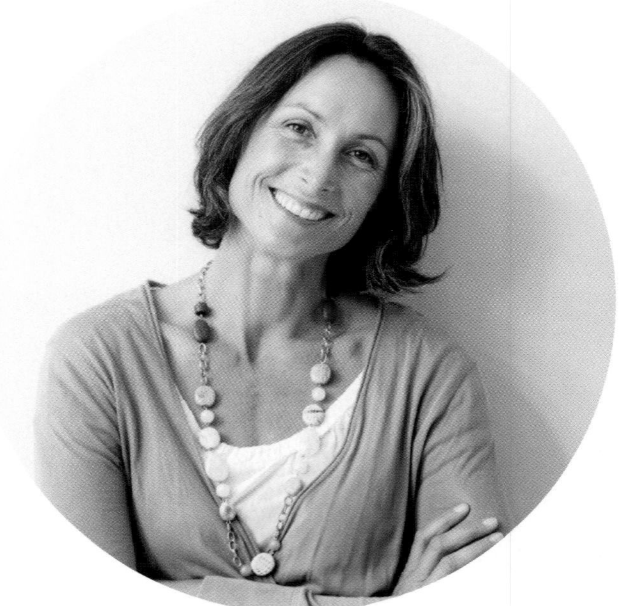

Conditions

Breast, cellular health - eucalyptus, frankincense, grapefruit, cellular complex blend

Breast size, too small (want to enlarge) - black pepper, clary sage, fennel, geranium, myrrh, vetiver, yarrow, anti-aging blend, cellular complex blend, invigorating blend, reassuring blend, women's blend, women's monthly blend (these oils will not cause already larger breasts to enlarge further)

Breasts, tender - clary sage, fennel, geranium, helichrysum, lavender, lemon, myrrh, roman chamomile, yarrow, cellular complex blend, detoxification blend, invigorating blend, women's blend, women's monthly blend

Candida - See *Candida*

Cysts, ovarian - basil, clary sage, cypress, fennel, frankincense, geranium, grapefruit, lemon, rosemary, thyme, cellular complex blend, cleansing blend, detoxification blend, metabolic blend, women's blend, women's monthly blend; see *Blood Sugar*

Endometriosis - arborvitae, basil, bergamot, black pepper, clary sage, cypress, eucalyptus, frankincense, geranium, ginger, lemon, lemongrass, rosemary, sandalwood, anti-aging blend, cellular complex blend, cleansing blend, ylang ylang, detoxification blend, invigorating blend, joyful blend, protective blend, reassuring blend, women's blend, women's monthly blend

Estrogen dominance - basil, clove, lemongrass, thyme, cleansing blend, detoxification blend, renewing blend

Estrogen, false/xenoestrogens - clary sage, oregano, thyme, cleansing blend, detoxification blend; see *Candida, Detoxification*

Estrogen, imbalanced/low - basil, clary sage, coriander, cypress, lavender

Female organs, tone - fennel, lemongrass, sandalwood, women's blend, women's monthly blend

Fibroids - basil, clary sage, eucalyptus, frankincense, helichrysum, lemon, lemongrass, melaleuca, sandalwood, thyme, cellular complex blend, reassuring blend

Frigidity - jasmine, rose, ylang, ylang, inspiring blend, massage blend, reassuring blend, women's blend; see "Aphrodisiacs" property, *Intimacy*

Genital warts - arborvitae, frankincense, lemongrass, melissa, thyme, detoxification blend

Headache, migraine/cyclical - basil, clary sage, fennel, geranium, lavender, melissa, peppermint, rosemary, roman chamomile, cellular complex blend, tension blend, women's monthly blend, women's blend

Hemorrhoids - cypress, helichrysum, myrrh, roman chamomile, sandalwood, detoxification blend, digestion blend, massage blend; see *Cardiovascular*

Hormones, imbalanced (general) - jasmine, geranium, ylang ylang, encouraging blend, renewing blend, women's blend, women's monthly blend

Hot flashes - clary sage, eucalyptus, lemon, peppermint, women's blend, women's monthly blend; see *Endocrine (Thyroid)*

Infertility - basil, clary sage, cypress, fennel, frankincense, jasmine, melissa, roman chamomile, rose, rosemary, thyme, ylang ylang, cellular complex blend, inspiring blend; see *Candida, Blood Sugar*, "Progesterone, low" below

Low libido - black pepper, cardamom, cinnamon, clary sage, clove, coriander, ginger, jasmine, juniper berry, patchouli, peppermint, ravensara, rose, rosemary, sandalwood, spearmint, thyme, vetiver, wild orange, ylang ylang, invigorating blend; see "Aphrodisiacs" property, *Intimacy*

Mammary gland support - clary sage, geranium, grapefruit, cellular complex blend, invigorating blend, women's blend; see "Breast Detox" recipe below

Menopause problems - basil, clary sage, cypress, fennel, geranium, lavender, roman chamomile, rosemary, thyme, wild orange, reassuring blend, women's blend, women's monthly blend

Menstruation (menses) cycle, irregular - cypress, fennel, jasmine, juniper berry, lavender, melissa, peppermint, rose, rosemary, thyme, cellular complex blend, renewing blend, soothing blend, tension blend, women's blend, uplifting blend, women's monthly blend

Menstruation (menses), heavy (menorrhagia) - clary sage, cypress, fennel, frankincense, geranium, spearmint, cellular complex blend, cleansing blend, detoxification blend, renewing blend, women's blend, women's monthly blend

Menstruation (menses), lack of/absence (amenorrhea) - basil, cedarwood, dill, juniper berry, roman chamomile, cellular complex blend, detoxification blend, renewing blend, women's blend, women's monthly blend

Menstruation (menses), overly light - basil, cinnamon, ginger, rosemary, cellular complex blend, cleansing blend, detoxification blend, invigorating blend, women's blend, women's monthly blend

Menstruation (menses), painful (dysmenorrhea) - basil, cardamom, cinnamon, clary sage, coriander, cypress, dill, frankincense, ginger, lemongrass, jasmine, peppermint, complex blend, cleansing blend, detoxification blend, women's blend, uplifting blend, women's monthly blend

Menstruation (menses), prolonged - frankincense, geranium, cellular complex blend, women's blend, women's monthly blend

Miscarriages (multiple) - clary sage, frankincense, grapefruit, lemon, oregano, thyme, cellular complex blend, cleansing blend, detoxification blend, invigorating blend, women's blend, women's monthly blend

Night sweats - clary sage, eucalyptus, ginger, lemon, lime, peppermint, cellular complex blend, detoxification blend, massage blend, tension blend, women's blend, women's monthly blend; see *Endocrine (Thyroid), Immune & Lymphatic*

Ovaries - clary sage, frankincense, geranium, rosemary, cellular complex blend, detoxification blend, women's monthly blend

Ovulation, irregular - melissa, rose

Pelvic pain - coriander, cypress, geranium, ginger, tension blend, women's monthly blend

Perimenopause - cardamom, clary sage, cypress, fennel, lavender, roman chamomile, rosemary, cellular complex blend, detoxification blend, reassuring blend, women's blend, women's monthly blend

PMS - bergamot, clary sage, cypress, fennel, geranium, grapefruit, jasmine, lavender, roman chamomile, reassuring blend, women's monthly blend

Postpartum depression - See *Pregnancy, Labor & Nursing*

Progesterone, low - clove, geranium, grapefruit, oregano, thyme, detoxification blend, women's blend, women's monthly blend

Rhythm method, use of (to regulate cycle) - melissa, rose

Sterility - geranium, cleansing blend, detoxification blend, women's blend, women's monthly blend; see "Infertility" above

Uterus, cleansing and purifying - clary sage, geranium, lemon, melaleuca, rose, cleansing blend, detoxification blend, invigorating blend, women's blend, women's monthly blend

Uterus, cramping - black pepper, cypress, jasmine, juniper berry, women's blend, women's monthly blend

Uterus, damaged/degenerated - frankincense, geranium, lemongrass, sandalwood, cellular complex blend, women's blend

Uterus lining, unhealthy - frankincense, geranium, grapefruit, jasmine, cellular complex blend, women's blend

Uterus, prolapsed/lack of tone - fennel, frankincense, juniper berry (stimulates uterine muscles), melissa, rose, wild orange, women's blend, women's monthly blend

Vaginal, candida/thrush - melaleuca, myrrh, oregano, thyme, cleansing blend, detoxification blend, metabolic blend, protective blend; see *Candida*

Vaginal discharge - clary sage, frankincense, lavender (thick, yellow), cellular complex blend, cleansing blend, detoxification blend, protective blend, women's blend; see *Candida*

Vaginal dryness - clary sage, grounding blend; see *Integumentary*

Vaginal infection/inflammation - clary sage, eucalyptus, frankincense, rosemary, spearmint, cellular complex blend, detoxification blend, protective blend, reassuring blend, women's blend

Emotional Well-Being

There is a significant connection between emotional and physical health. The body releases various chemicals in response to emotions. For example, the body's release of serotonin, dopamine, or oxytocin results in an uplifting emotion and positive sensation in the body. An experience of stress causes the brain to instruct the release of cortisol, and the body's response will be one of urgency and perhaps even fear.

Emotional stress, whether acute or chronic, can have profound effects on the body. A range of illnesses, from headaches to digestive issues, lack of sleep, and heart disease, can be the result of emotions such as grief, anxiety, and depression taking a toll on the immune system and other cells, tissues, and organs of the entire body.

Examining activity at a cellular level can assist in the understanding of how emotions can affect body functions. Embedded in the surface of the cell membrane are protein molecules known as receptors. These receptors face outward and continuously scan for, communicate with, and solicit needed chemicals that exist outside the cell.

These solicited chemicals attach to receptors, distribute information, and produce biochemical responses within the cell to adapt to environment and stimuli. In this way the receptors play a unique and important role in cellular communication. The binding chemical, called a ligand, is classified as a "messenger molecule," because it sends information to cells that will influence the cell's development and function. A ligand can be a neurotransmitter, hormone, pharmaceutical drug, toxin, parts of a virus, or a neuropeptide used by neurons to communicate with each other.

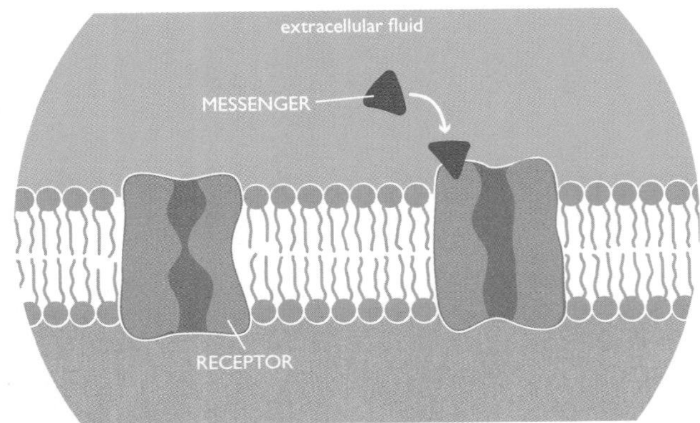

While numerous receptors are found in most cells, each receptor will only bind with ligands of a particular structure, much like how a lock will only accept a specifically shaped key. When a ligand binds to its corresponding receptor, it activates or inhibits the receptor's associated biochemical pathway.

There are two types of ligands: endogenous and exogenous. Endogenous ligands, such as serotonin, are produced in the body and can have an impact on emotions. Exogenous ligands are substances that are introduced into the body and have a similar effect. They, too, are messenger molecules and can come from a variety of sources such as medications or essential oils.

The Messages of Emotions

The hypothalamus – the "control and command center" of the brain – converts mental thoughts and emotions into hundreds of different types of ligands, specifically neuropeptides. The emotions triggered by a perceived threat, for example, are powerful and initiate the release of specific messenger molecule chemicals which, as indicated above, attach to certain receptor sites of cells and affect cell function. What the hypothalamus "believes to be true" determines what the "factory" produces, and chemical production ensues. Neuropeptides affect our chemistry, and our chemistry affects our biology. Bottom line: emotions trigger cell activity!

The Scent Alarm

The sense of smell is our most primal, and it exerts a powerful influence over our thoughts, emotions, moods, memories, and behaviors. A healthy human nose can distinguish over one trillion different aromas through hundreds of distinct classes of smell receptors. By way of comparison, we only have three types of photoreceptors used to recognize visual stimuli. Olfaction is far more complex than sight, and we are ten thousand times more capable of smelling than tasting.

It's accurate to say we "smell" danger. Our sense of smell is inextricably connected to our survival, and it plays a major role in remembering what is and isn't safe and what is pleasurable. Why remember danger, stress, trauma, and pleasure? To learn from experience so we can protect ourselves, survive, and procreate. If it wasn't safe this time, we can avoid it the next time; or if it was pleasurable (e.g. food, physical intimacy), we want to participate again. People, environments, food: smelling them is part of everyday life.

OLFACTORY SYSTEM

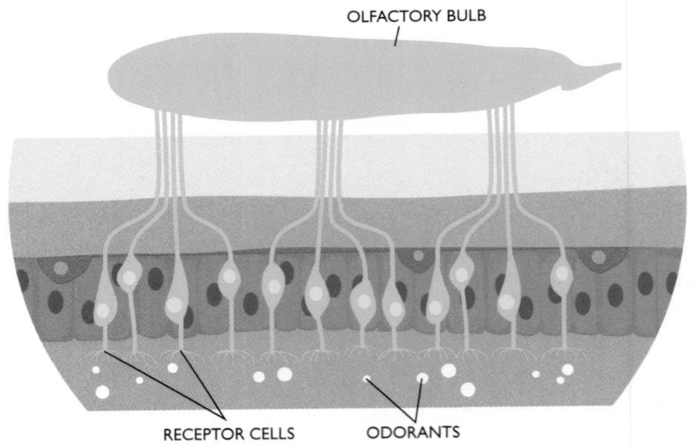

Aromas serve as exogenous ligands. They are received via olfactory receptors, which are highly concentrated in the limbic system, the primitive part of the brain and seat of emotion. In the center lies the amygdala, which instantly receives the incoming scent information before other higher brain centers. By the time the information reaches our "thinking" and decision-making cortex and we actually figure out what we smelled, the scent has already triggered emotional and body chemistry responses.

The amygdala is the storehouse of traumas and contains the densest concentration of neuropeptides, affecting cellular memory. Smell is the primary sense that unconsciously activates and affects traumatic memories stored there. Acting as the watchdog, the amygdala is constantly on the lookout for danger or threats. As it belongs to the more primitive part of our brain it doesn't have the intelligence to discern between real threats versus perceived threats (e.g. a saber-toothed tiger versus a missed bus stop or being late to work and an angry boss). It passes on its concerns and notifies the hypothalamus when safety and security are at risk, which then in turn notifies the pituitary, which alerts the adrenal glands, which sets off the alarm for fight-or-flight stress response and releases cortisol and adrenaline. Bottom line: The emotional stress triggered the release of the stress hormones.

Many researchers agree that physical illnesses are often the result of an emotional inflammatory response to trauma or negative experiences. What can begin as "emotional inflammation" can later become physical issues and disease. Although medical technology is not advanced enough to see them, memories, trauma, and painful emotions are stored in the body and eventually manifest as physical inflammation when the body's tissues follow suit.

FOOD & MOOD

What you put in your mouth has a direct impact on emotions. Nutritional deficiencies, food sensitivities, blood sugar imbalances, substance abuse, and stimulants (like caffeine) affect biochemistry and contribute to mood fluctuations and compromised emotional states.

Additives in processed foods generate adverse chemical reactions within the body and drastically affect mood and behavior in many children and adults. Some of these synthetic substances are labeled "excitotoxins" by nutritionists and wellness experts. These include additives such as high fructose corn syrup, trans-fats, artificial flavors, artificial colors, artificial sweeteners, MSG, and other preservatives. These chemicals deliver messages to the brain and cells of the body just like any exogenous ligand. More than one specific ligand can "fit" into a receptor. As heroin fits in the same opiate site as endorphins, so can these toxic food chemicals unlock receptor sites in our brain and transmit influences that, if we knew, we would never let in.

So once again, we have a choice on what chemical soup we want to ingest. The old adage, "we are what we eat," could not ring more true. Or perhaps it gets rewritten here: We emote or express emotionally what we eat.

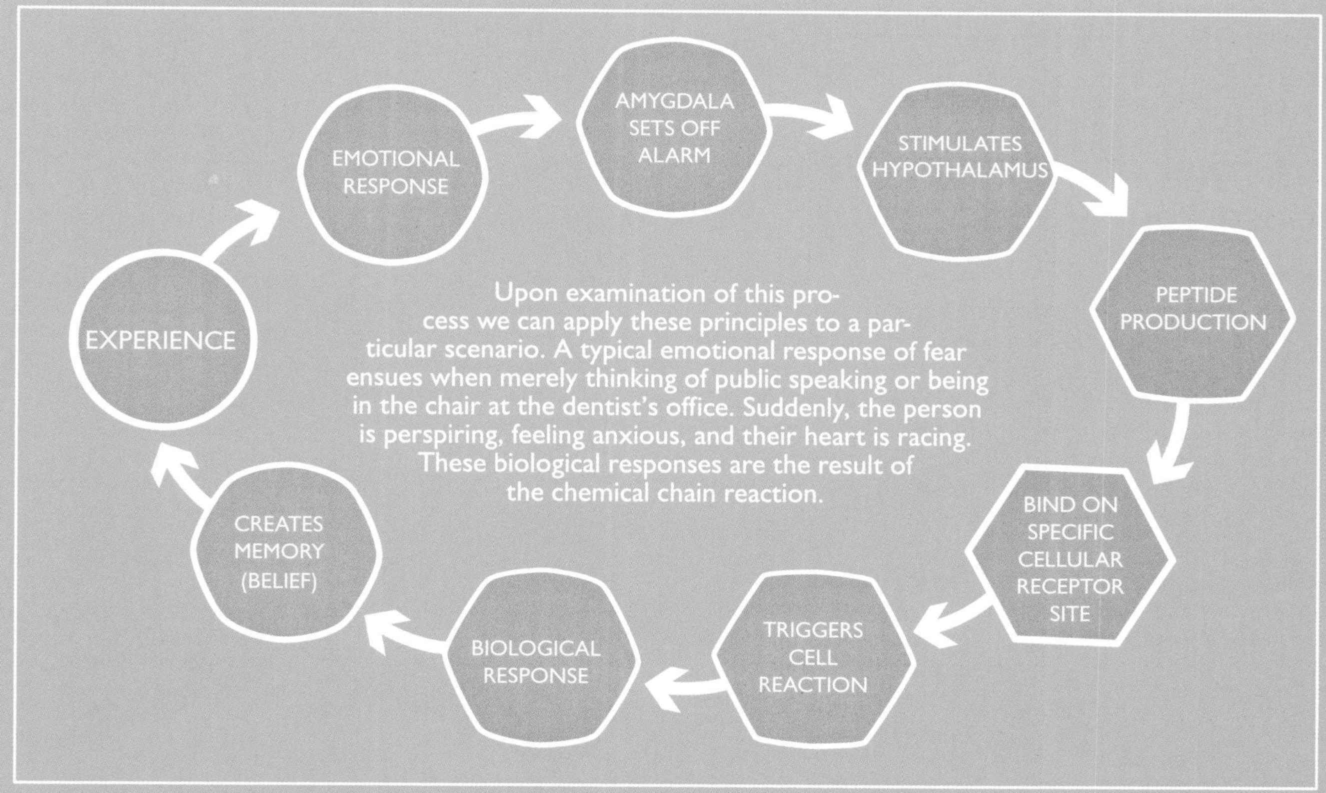

The Importance of the Sense of Smell

Smell can be used beneficially in healing efforts as well. Scents are experienced long before words. Whether for relieving stress, stabilizing mood, improving sleep, eliminating pain, relieving nausea, or improving memory and energy levels, scents can actually change nervous system biochemistry.

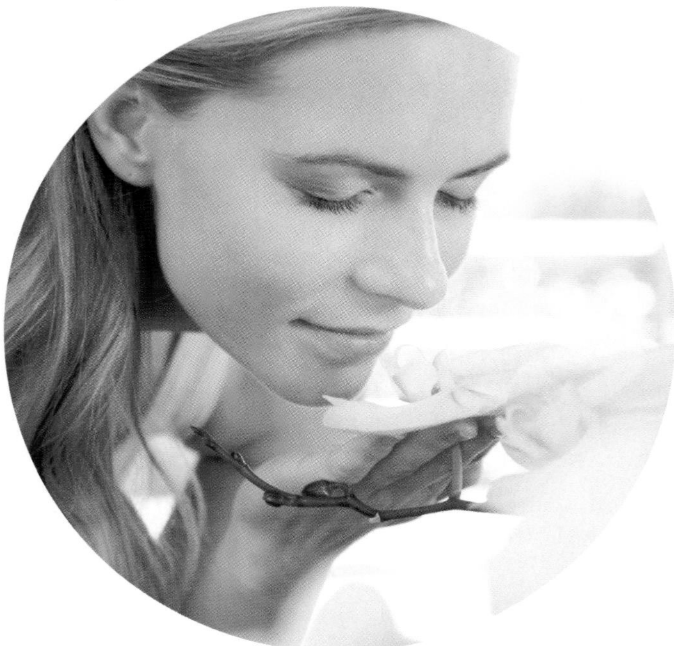

Essential oils can facilitate a rapid emotional response in the brain and the body to facilitate such a release. Essential oils are powerful biochemical agents for emotional balance, wellness, and toxic release, which can be paired or partnered with any holistic or medically-derived program to create a successful approach to mental and emotional wellness.

The Power of Essential Oils Choose Your Mood

Moods are often perceived as having chosen us, as if they are happening *to* us. Rather, the chemical impact of our emotions and other exogenous ligands is the real chooser of moods. That's why we reach for certain foods, sugar, caffeine, or a drug of choice (see "Food & Mood" for more information), interact with certain people, do certain things, and act out certain behaviors because of how it makes us feel and to get a "chemical" hit.

What if we could use this knowledge to choose the mood we want to feel and then actually feel it - without harmful substances or recreational drugs? What if we could think of a desired mood and then choose to use a healthful exogenous ligand that is capable of creating it? With essential oils, we have the ability to direct our own emotional traffic!

OUR SECOND BRAIN

Digestive issues and disorders are growing rampant, in part because of the refined and processed foods that are prevalent in today's diets. The gut is considered the body's "second brain" because of its impact on mood states. In recent years, scientists have discovered that there are more neurotransmitters (a type of ligand) in the gut than there are in the brain, and, among other things, healthy mood management depends on how well these neurotransmitters relay messages to each other.

Serotonin is a chemical responsible for maintaining mood balance, social behavior, appetite and digestion, sleep, memory, and sexual desire and function. The majority of the body's serotonin, between 80-90 percent, can be found in the gastrointestinal tract. Gut health, then, promotes emotional health and mood stabilization. How can an individual hope to experience healthy moods if their cells are depleted of nutrition and if their neurotransmitters reside in an area with blockages and inflammation? How can the over one hundred million neurons embedded in the gut influence healthy emotions when inflammation, blockages, candida, and other harmful bacteria are overpopulated and system imbalances are standard?

Detoxifying the body can improve emotional health. Toxicity symptoms in the body can directly mirror many depressive symptoms and may include insomnia, foggy thinking, low energy, digestive issues, dampened immune function, and allergies. New studies even suggest that depression may be a type of "allergic reaction" to inflammation.

Chemical compounds found in essential oils stimulate a range of gentle to more intense detoxification effects (depending on use) and promote a natural cleanse for the digestive, endocrine, immune, and lymphatic and other detoxification systems and channels of the body. This, in turn, boosts mood and restores mental and physical energy.

Blood sugar imbalances can also trigger depressive symptoms. Certain essential oils, like cinnamon, coriander, and fennel, support metabolic function and assist in moderating blood sugar levels. Omega 3-fatty acids, food enzymes, chelated minerals and B and D vitamins found in a whole food nutrient supplement, antioxidants, and polyphenol supplements also help to regulate blood sugar levels, as well as reduce inflammation, boost energy, and support the gut with the right combination of good fats and other nourishing components.

Rather than feeling victimized by our emotional states, what if we had our own apothecary of essential oils in the home? Such a collection offers a cornucopia of emotional states for ready access. Like an eager child opening a box of candy, relishing the array of colors and designs and imagining the flavors waiting to tantalize her tongue and brighten her spirit, we, too, can delight in selecting and generating moods with the use of essential oils.

As natural exogenous ligands, essential oils can powerfully influence our emotions, much like mood-altering drugs like morphine, but with healthful results. Unlike synthetic medications or drugs that are designed to alter behavior, their complex molecular structure allows them to intelligently bind to the receptor sites of cells in our body and support a desired effect to restore balance and healthy function.

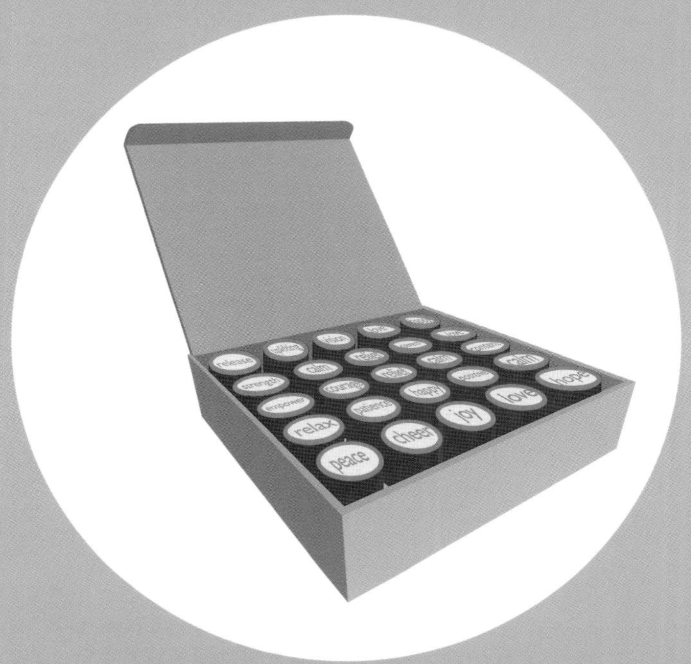

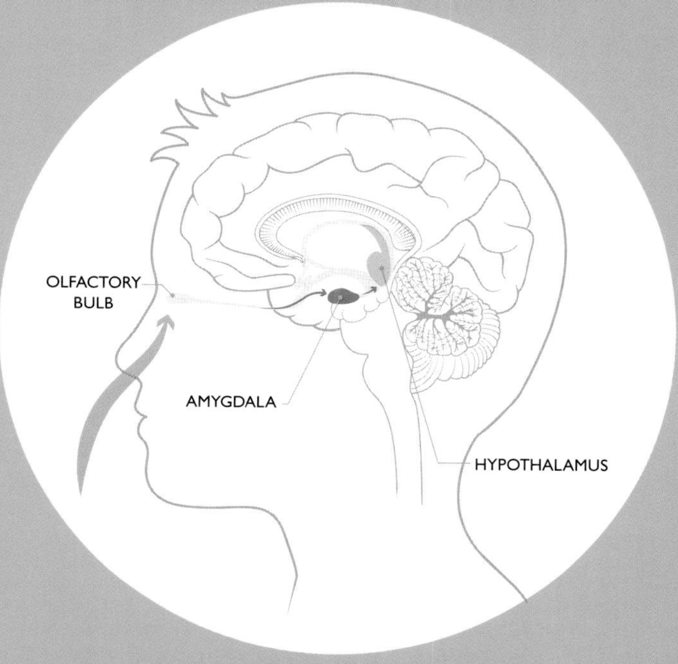

Taking It to the Next Level

Emotional healing and rebalancing of moods is accomplished when a new stimulus is introduced to the same chain of command in the brain. As we've already discussed, an aroma (stimulus) enters the olfactory system, and in turn the limbic system and amygdala, hypothalamus, and other parts of the brain and body. Depending on what aroma is introduced and the information it conveys determines the brain's response. Traumatic memories stored in the amygdala can be released by utilizing the sense of smell and essential oils. If the significance an individual attaches to a past experience can be shifted, the amygdala can release the trauma of the memory. This is what makes aromatherapy a wonderful means for emotional healing and rebalancing moods. Here is an example:

If an individual is deficient in serotonin for an extended period of time, their habitual response to life's situations might be more anxious or angry, more hopeless, more sad, more phobic, more thoughts of "what-if?". If he begins using wild orange, for example, a known antidepressant oil due to its capacity to uplift, detoxify, and calm, he would find himself irresistibly more happy and with a plausible capacity to be more hopeful, trusting, less reactive, and more calm. He also, therefore, has a potential to react to experiences and respond to memories differently.

Here's another example. A young child experiences a high level of trauma, such as a parent suffering with cancer who subsequently passes away. The child's body experiences tremendous chemical expenditures to support the experiences of stress, trauma, and grief. And then, if more trauma occurs, say the deceased parent is replaced and the surviving parent remarries, additional chemicals are released to cope with a new stepparent and stepsiblings.

If, during, or after traumatic seasons of this child's life, her chemical reserves are not replenished, her coping capacity is literally chemically diminished. She might find herself crying more, experiencing meltdowns more easily, perhaps being teased for being a crybaby, or simply coping less effectively with everyday life. A missed homework deadline, low grade, or athletic performance failure may seem a crushing blow. The same exact events could happen to another person with full reserves who moves through it gracefully. What's the difference?

One of the most important chemicals we have to work in these kinds of situations is endorphins. The name itself reveals it to be an endogenous ligand: "endo-morphine," self-made morphine or *endorphin*. When endorphins are lacking, coping challenges arise. Endorphins serve us not only in our ability to experience pleasure, but also to appropriately buffer us from pain, both physical and emotional. The craving for its benefits will drive any number of behaviors when levels are low.

Typically two types of addictions may arise. One is generally met by abnormally intense levels of thrill or pleasure, as intensity is required in order to get the chemical "hit." The endogenous ligand, endorphins, is the body's "drug" of choice, received on an opiate receptor site. Activities of greater and greater intensity may be pursued to increase the production of endorphins. Bungee jumping, pornography use, playing intense video games, exaggerated sexual activity, gambling, overconsumption of comfort foods, or other behaviors known to generate endorphins become appealing in an attempt to fill a need.

The second addiction is usually focused on exogenous ligands in the form of pain-numbing opiate drugs, including opium, heroin, vicodin, oxycodone, and other prescription pain medications. Opiate drugs are received on the same opiate receptor sites. Either addiction, is powerful as chemical needs remain unmet.

Returning to the story of the child who lost her parent, one of the main chemicals likely low, based on circumstances described, is endorphins. If those diminished reserves of endorphins were never replenished, she would potentially grow into an adult continually experiencing the inability to cope with life or fully experience pleasure, never fully recovering from the trauma, ever searching for ways to numb the pain and meet her emotional needs. Her body is simply lacking the chemical capacity to fully heal. The body needs to increase its reserves and ability to manufacture the chemicals needed.

Now to explore a potential solution, the essential oil of helichrysum. Helichrysum has powerful analgesic and pain-relieving therapeutic benefits. It is high in many chemical constituents, one known as ketones; a compound with powerful, regenerative benefits. As the child-turned-adult uses this oil and her body experiences this chemistry, she is exposed to generous amounts of healthy pain-killing/numbing chemicals. What science has yet to identify is what happens in the body from here.

Whether a chemical need is met or a pathway of reception is opened up is not known. What is happening potentially for the woman, however, is she finally feels relief from "pain." Her coping capacity is increased. She handles life better. With natural, healing chemicals on board in rich supply she finally experiences healing.

The diverse and concentrated chemical constituents in essential oils work to cleanse, ground, lift, balance, and calm the central nervous system and the emotional body. Some essential oils – like frankincense, patchouli and sandalwood – have high concentrations of sesquiterpene molecules that have been clinically demonstrated to cross the blood-brain barrier. These molecules have significant oxygen supporting effects on the brain and, when combined with aromatic stimulation, can assist the amygdala in releasing the effects of stored memories.

Here are some additional demonstrated mental and emotional benefits:

- Cleanse negative memories
- Reduce stress, anxiety, and tension
- Offset mental fatigue
- Uplift mood
- Calm the central nervous system
- Relax muscular tension
- Induce restful sleep
- Invigorate the senses
- Increase feelings of courage and determination
- Promote a cathartic effect (facilitating the release of stuck emotions)
- Support DNA correction and expression

In conclusion, aromatherapy offers many practical healing advantages, but perhaps one of the most fascinating is the relationship it has with emotional well being. Inhalation of essential oils with the resulting aromatic exposure is the most effective method of impacting the brain for emotional wellness. Some studies demonstrate that essential oils have the highest bio-frequency of any consumable natural substance.

Essential oils offer a fresh, effective support tool to aid in the emotional healing process and to shift out of old habits and ineffective coping patterns. Aromatherapy allows the individual to harness the olfactory power of plants for healing, or simply to enhance a state of well being using scents to create a powerful influence over how one thinks, feels, and behaves.

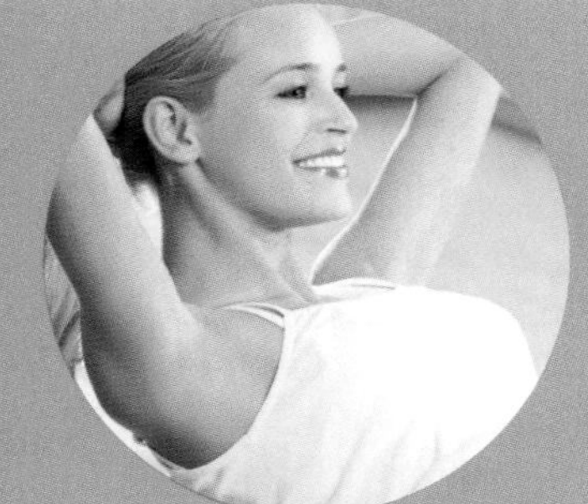

MOVE IT, MOVE IT

Studies indicate that moderate exercise of thirty minutes a day for three days a week has an antidepressant effect on a large percentage of depressed subjects. But many who are anxious or depressed lack the energy or sensory motivation to begin an exercise regime. Essential oils like peppermint, cypress, and wintergreen support the flow of blood and oxygen and the sensory "oomph" to engage in physical activity. Other oils aid in relieving muscle tension and assisting with muscle recovery. Helichrysum, for example, contains natural chemical components that have a regenerative effect both physically and emotionally.

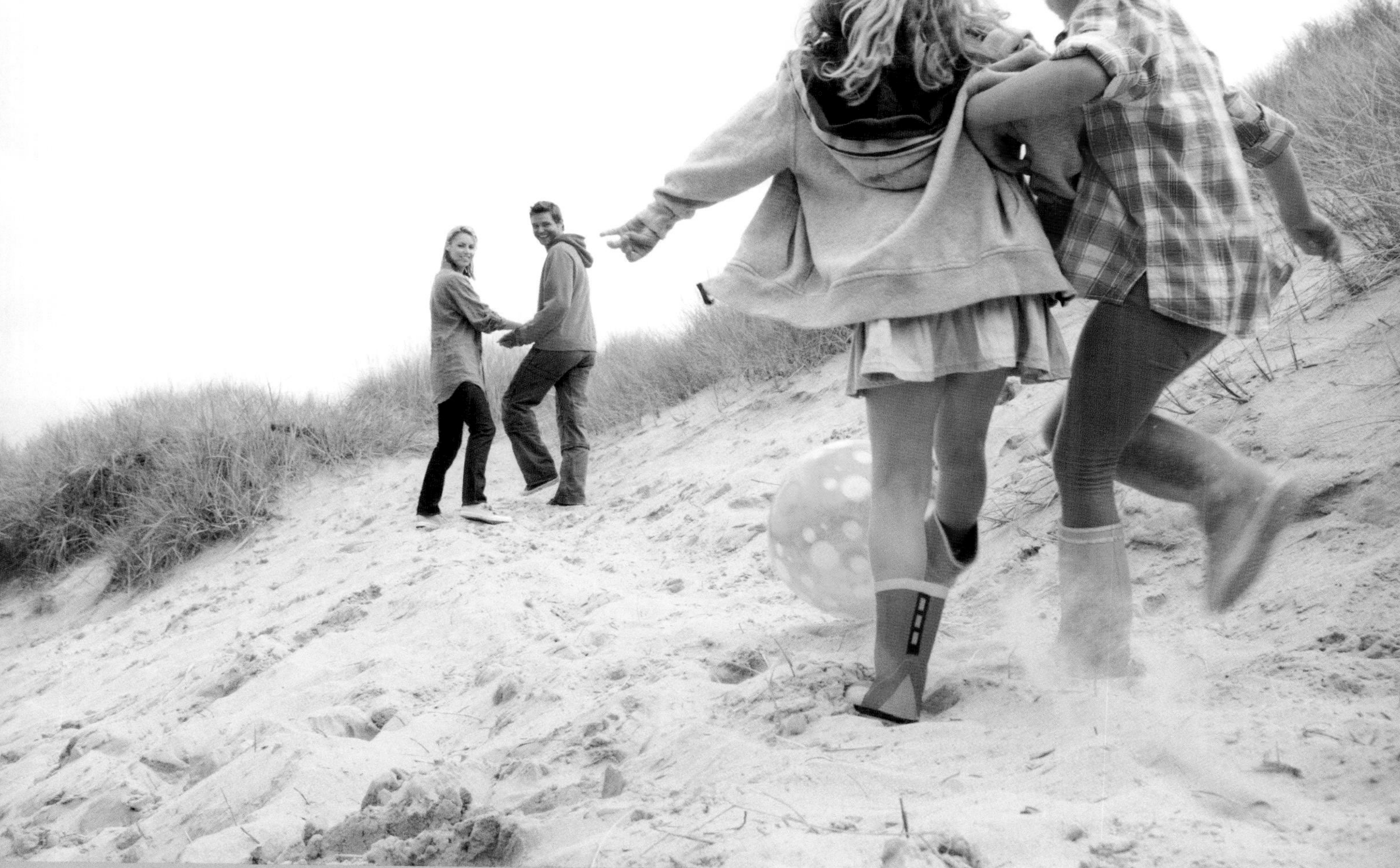

Practical Application

As essential oils are used topically, aromatically, and internally, the body's vibration is raised and its emotional frequencies are impacted, as is the capacity for emotional well being. Each individual oil with its diverse chemistry has the ability to be a tremendous multi-tasker and work in multiple areas of interest simultaneously. Additional benefits to essential oil use comes from combining oils to create synergistic blends. See Application Methods in this book to learn more.

Application methods also impact the body's response to aromatherapy in emotional health and healing:

- Aromatic use is the fastest way to access the mood center of the brain and invite the release of negative stored emotions. It is also helpful to use the oils aromatically when resetting new, healthy belief patterns.
- Topical use assists the body in moving from a stress response to a repair or restore response necessary to create an environment where emotional healing can take place.
- Internal use of essential oils supports healthy chemical reactions in the body, nourishment of cells, and release of toxins. This internal support fosters a healthy and balanced emotional environment. Cleansing the internal environment allows emotions to be recognized and processed more readily.

SWEET DREAMS

Adequate sleep is crucial to mental health and brain function. Insomnia and restless sleep are a problem for many who experience depressed or anxious mood states. Pairing a resin or tree essential oil like vetiver, cedarwood, sandalwood, or frankincense with a citrus oil like wild orange, lime, lemon, or bergamot has been found to stabilize mood fluctuations, ground the body, and promote a relaxation response in preparation for sleep. Flower oils like lavender, roman chamomile, clary sage, geranium, and ylang ylang aid in quieting mental chatter and calming the nervous system.

Similarly, many studies have been conducted on the powerful mental, physical, and emotional benefits of meditation. Meditation is a practice that seeks to achieve a focused state of relaxation. The essential oils listed above can help to still the mind, open air pathways, and calm the mind and heart.

Emotional Index

Essential oils are some of nature's most powerful remedies for emotional health. Below are lists designed to introduce the concept of associating an oil to an emotion or vice versa as well as serve as an ongoing resource. Select specific targeted emotional states to address and then identify corresponding oils. **If you want to research specific mood conditions, refer to *Focus & Attention* and *Mood & Behavior* sections of this book.**

ESSENTIAL OIL	UN-BALANCED EMOTION	BALANCED EMOTION
Arborvitae	Overzealous	Composed
Basil	Inundated	Relieved
Bergamot	Inadequate	Worthy
Birch	Cowardly	Courageous
Black Pepper	Repressed	Honest
Cardamom	Self-centered	Charitable
Cassia	Uncertain	Bold
Cedarwood	Alone	Connected
Cilantro	Obsessed	Expansive
Cinnamon Bark	Denied	Receptive
Clary Sage	Limited	Enlightened
Clove	Dominated	Supported
Coriander	Apprehensive	Participating
Cypress	Stalled	Progressing
Dill	Avoiding	Intentional
Douglas Fir	Upset	Renewed
Eucalyptus	Congested	Stimulated
Fennel	Unproductive	Flourishing
Frankincense	Separated	Unified
Geranium	Neglected	Mended
Ginger	Apathetic	Activated
Grapefruit	Divided	Validated
Helichrysum	Wounded	Reassured
Jasmine	Hampered	Liberated
Juniper Berry	Denying	Insightful
Lavender	Unheard	Expressed
Lemon	Mindless	Energized
Lemongrass	Obstructed	Flowing
Lime	Faint	Enlivened
Marjoram	Doubtful	Trusting
Melaleuca	Unsure	Collected
Melissa	Depressed	Light-filled
Myrrh	Disconnected	Nurtured
Oregano	Obstinate	Unattached
Patchouli	Degraded	Enhanced
Peppermint	Hindered	Invigorated
Ravensara	Uncommitted	Resolute
Roman Chamomile	Frustrated	Purposeful
Rose	Isolated	Loved
Rosemary	Confused	Open-minded
Sandalwood	Uninspired	Devoted
Spearmint	Weary	Refreshed
Spikenard	Agitated	Tranquil
Tangerine	Oppressed	Restored
Thyme	Unyielding	Yielding
Vetiver	Ungrounded	Rooted
White Fir	Blocked	Receiving
Wild Orange	Drained	Productive
Wintergreen	Stubborn	Accepting
Yarrow	Erratic	Balanced

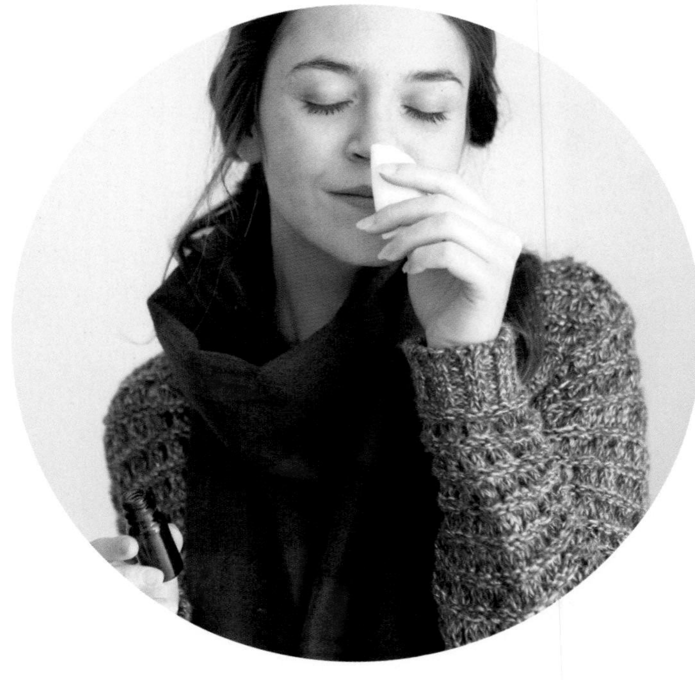

EMOTIONS

If you want to feel the positive emotion listed, use the associated oil.

Accepting	wintergreen	**Flourishing**	fennel	**Receiving**	white fir
Activated	ginger	**Flowing**	lemongrass	**Receptive**	cinnamon bark
Balanced	yarrow	**Honest**	black pepper	**Refreshed**	spearmint
Bold	cassia	**Insightful**	juniper berry	**Relieved**	basil
Charitable	cardamom	**Intentional**	dill	**Renewed**	douglas fir
Collected	melaleuca	**Invigorated**	peppermint	**Resolute**	ravensara
Composed	arborvitae	**Liberated**	jasmine	**Restored**	tangerine
Connected	cedarwood	**Light-filled**	melissa	**Rooted**	vetiver
Courageous	birch	**Loved**	rose	**Stimulated**	eucalyptus
Devoted	sandalwood	**Mended**	geranium	**Supported**	clove
Energized	lemon	**Nurtured**	myrrh	**Tranquil**	spikenard
Enhanced	patchouli	**Open-minded**	rosemary	**Trusting**	marjoram
Enlightened	clary sage	**Participating**	coriander	**Unattached**	oregano
Enlivened	lime	**Productive**	wild orange	**Unified**	frankincense
Expansive	cilantro	**Progressing**	cypress	**Validated**	grapefruit
Expressed	lavender	**Purposeful**	roman chamomile	**Worthy**	bergamot
Exuberant	ylang ylang	**Reassured**	helichrysum	**Yielding**	thyme

If you are feeling the negative emotion listed, use the associated oil.

Agitated	spikenard	**Doubtful**	marjoram	**Overzealous**	arborvitae
Alone	cedarwood	**Drained**	wild orange	**Repressed**	black pepper
Apathetic	ginger	**Erratic**	yarrow	**Self-centered**	cardamom
Apprehensive	coriander	**Faint**	lime	**Separated**	frankincense
Avoiding	dill	**Frustrated**	roman chamomile	**Stalled**	cypress
Blocked	white fir	**Hampered**	jasmine	**Stubborn**	wintergreen
Burdened	ylang ylang	**Hindered**	peppermint	**Uncertain**	cassia
Confused	rosemary	**Inadequate**	bergamot	**Uncommitted**	ravensara
Congested	eucalyptus	**Inundated**	basil	**Ungrounded**	vetiver
Cowardly	birch	**Isolated**	rose	**Unheard**	lavender
Degraded	patchouli	**Limited**	clary sage	**Uninspired**	sandalwood
Denied	cinnamon bark	**Mindless**	lemon	**Unproductive**	fennel
Denying	juniper berry	**Neglected**	geranium	**Unsure**	melaleuca
Depressed	melissa	**Obsessed**	cilantro	**Unyielding**	thyme
Disconnected	myrrh	**Obstinate**	oregano	**Upset**	douglas fir
Divided	grapefruit	**Obstructed**	lemongrass	**Weary**	spearmint
Dominated	clove	**Oppressed**	tangerine	**Wounded**	helichrysum

SECTION 5

NATURAL LIVING RECIPES

The Natural Living Recipes section takes living the ESSENTIAL LIFE to the next level. The recipes and tips here show how essential oils can enhance every area of life. They are the go-to tool of choice because they contribute to most every part of a great lifestyle.

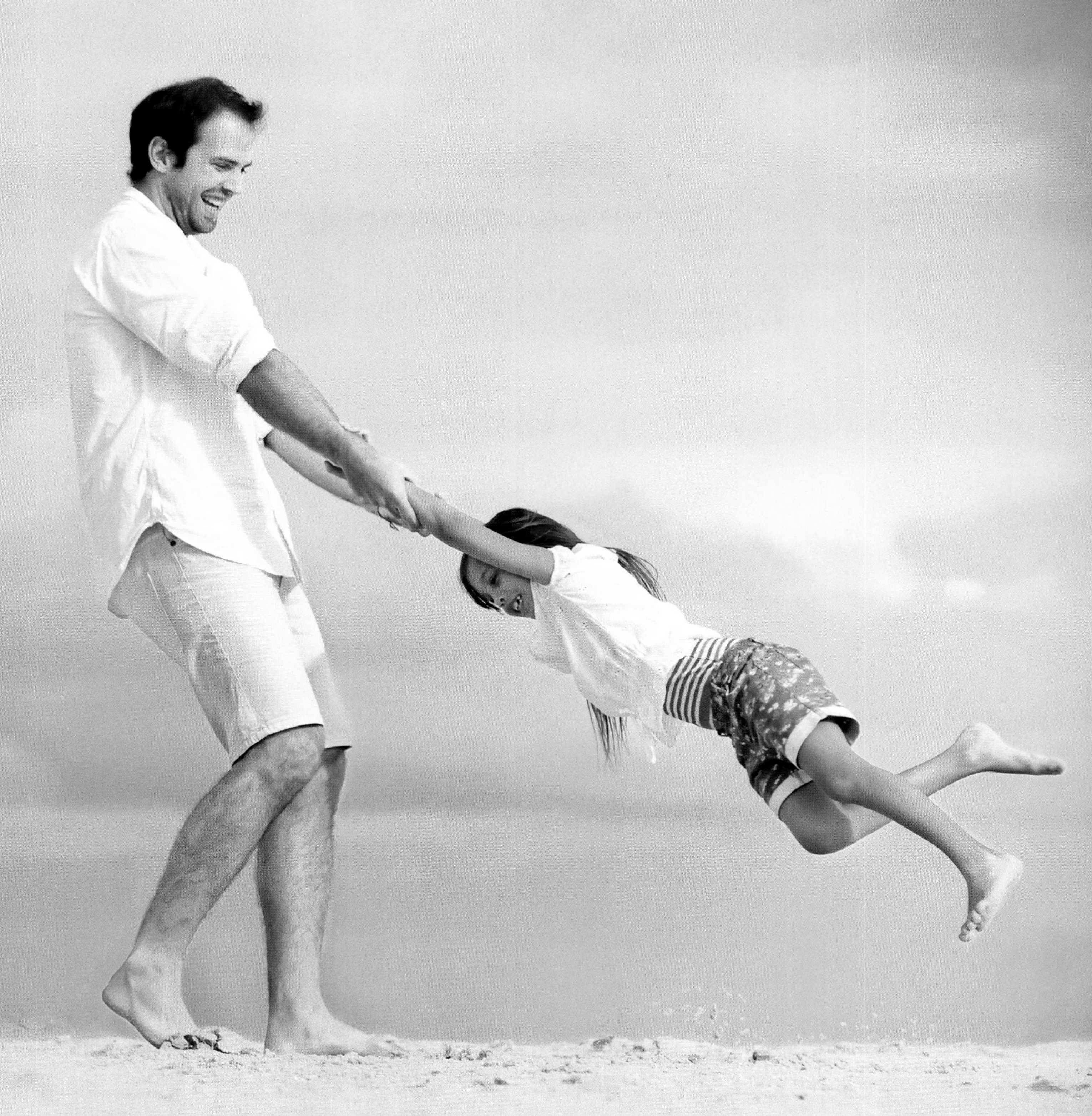

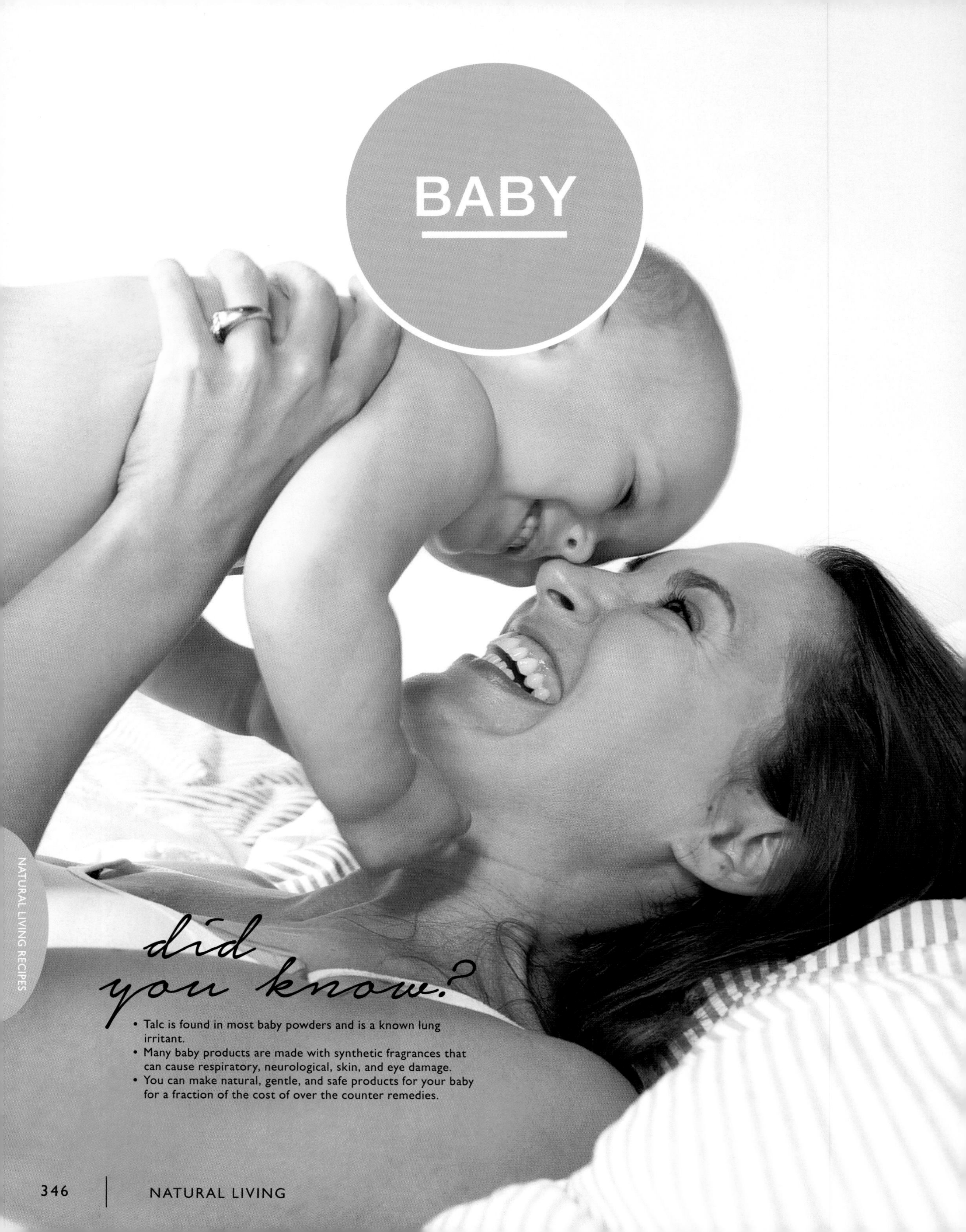

BABY

did you know?

- Talc is found in most baby powders and is a known lung irritant.
- Many baby products are made with synthetic fragrances that can cause respiratory, neurological, skin, and eye damage.
- You can make natural, gentle, and safe products for your baby for a fraction of the cost of over the counter remedies.

Diaper Rash Relief

½ cup coconut oil
15 drops melaleuca essential oil
15 drops lavender essential oil
15 drops frankincense essential oil

In a small glass spray bottle mix oils together. Spray a thin layer directly onto rash area and reapply as needed.

Calming Colic Blend

3 drops digestion blend essential oil
2 drops ginger essential oil
1 teaspoon coconut oil

Mix together and massage ointment over baby's tummy and lower back. Repeat 3 to 5 times daily.

Cradle Cap Moisturizer

1 teaspoon coconut oil
3 drops lavender essential oil

Mix together in palms and rub on the baby's scalp. Add cocoa butter if additional softening as needed.

Winter Cheeks Balm

¼ cup coconut oil
¼ cup olive oil
2 tablespoon beeswax
20 drops lavender essential oil

In a small mason jar mix ingredients together, and lower the jar into a warm saucepan partially filled with water. On low heat melt beeswax, coconut oil, and olive oil together, stirring every few minutes. After wax is completely melted remove from heat and add lavender. Mix together and cool until hardened. Rub balm over reddened cheeks to ease and protect.

Baby Stain Remover Spray

8 ounces water
2 tablespoons borax
20 drops lemon essential oil

Add borax and oils to a spray bottle. Add water and shake thoroughly. Spray directly on stain and wash.

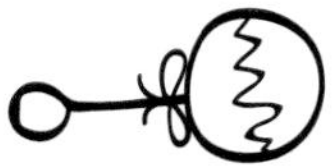

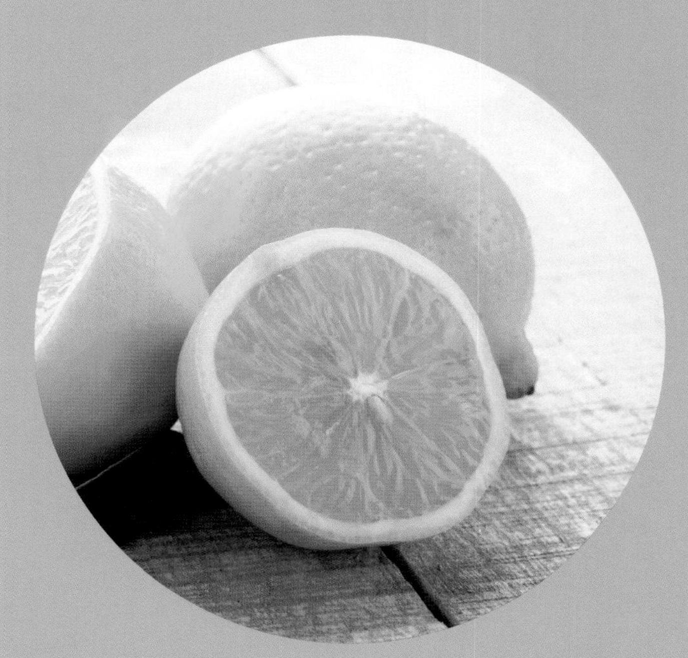

tips

- To clean baby's toys combine 2 drops lemon with 4 ounces of white vinegar in a glass spray bottle. Fill remaining with water and spray.
- To ease colic, apply 1-2 drops of digestion blend on baby's feet.
- To calm a crying or overtired baby put 1 drop lavender or calming blend under baby's nose and forehead.
- Scent children's drawers with their favorite essential oils applied to cotton balls.
- To signal safety, comfort, or time for sleep, place 2 drops of lavender, calming, or grounding blend near breast or nearby during feedings.
- For a soothing bath, add 2-4 drops of roman chamomile or calming blend.
- To soothe sore gums mix 1-2 drops of roman chamomile, white fir, or clove essential oil with fractioned coconut oil and massage into baby's gums.

CLEANING

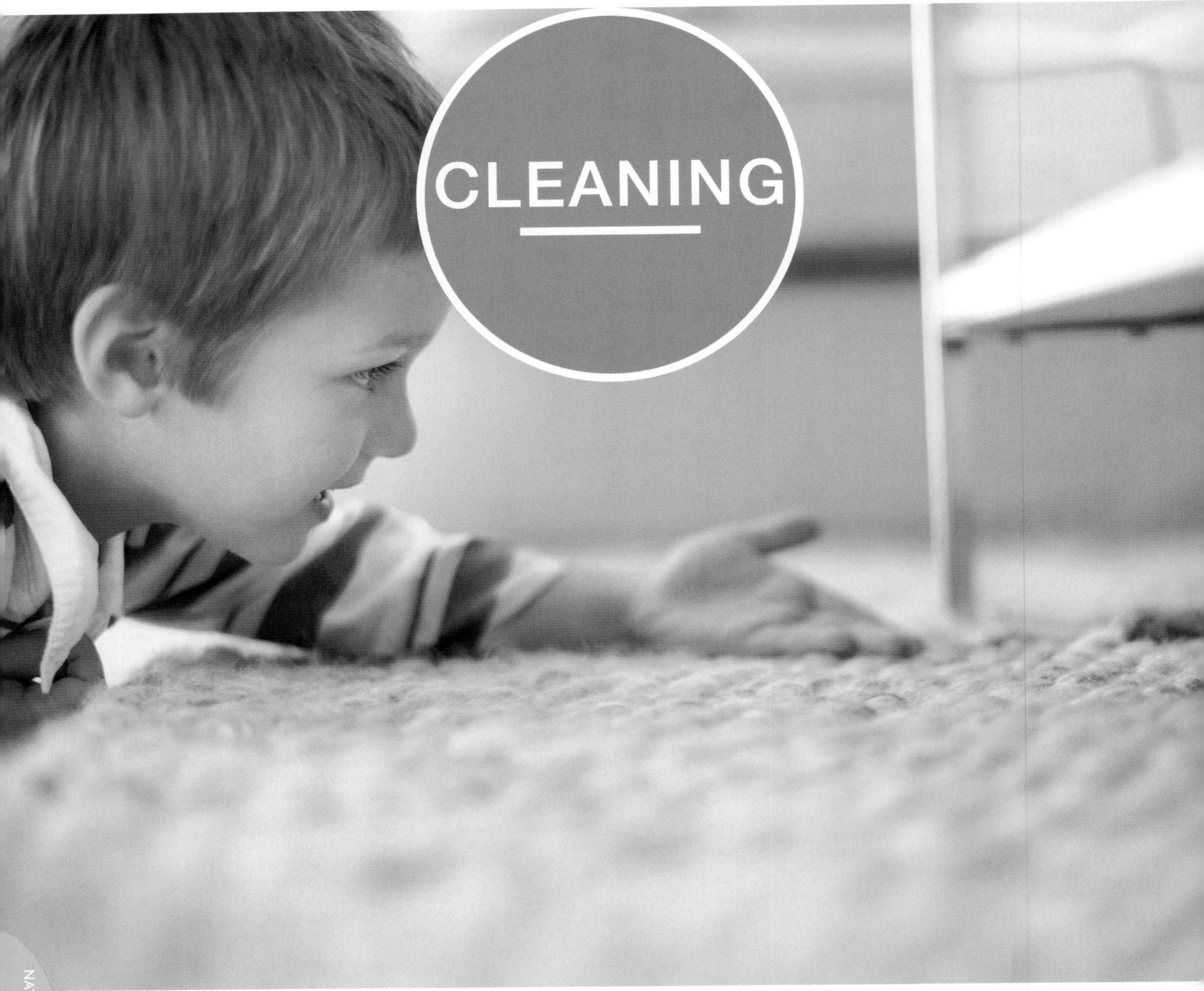

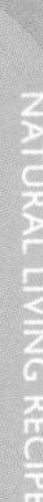

Fruit & Veggie Wash

It's important to wash any pesticides and germs off your fruits and vegetables. This solution removes all those residues and has germ-killing properties to boot.

½ cup apple cider vinegar
½ cup water
5 drops lemon essential oil
5 drops protective essential oil blend

Natural Scratch Remover

2 teaspoons lemon juice
1 teaspoons distilled white vinegar
3 drops lime essential oil

Mix ingredients in small bowl. Dip cloth into solution and rub onto wood surface. Rub on scratches until they disappear or on deeper scratches until they are managed. Buff away any residue with a dry cloth.

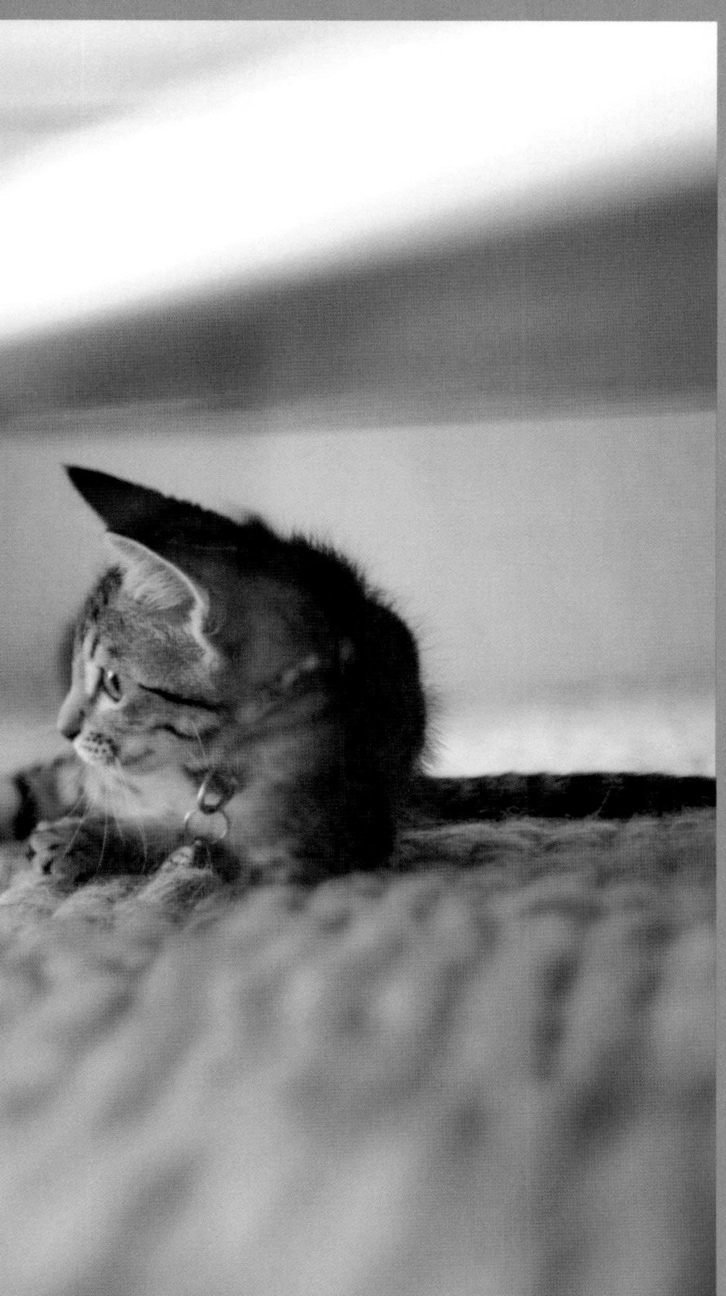

Upholstered Fabric Cleaner

¼ cup warm water
2 teaspoons castile soap
3 drops lime essential oil

Mix ingredients in a container. Dip cloth in the mixture and dab onto the stain for quick spot treatments on any fabric.

Carpet Freshener

2 cups baking soda
10 drops lemon essential oil
10 drops orange or grapefruit essential oil

Combine all ingredients in container. Sprinkle on carpet or rug and let sit for 15 minutes. Vacuum thoroughly.

Carpet Stain Remover

4 cups warm water, divided
½ teaspoon clear castile soap or dish soap
10 drops lemon essential oil

Mix 2 cups warm water, soap, and essential oil. Soak a rag in the mixture, wring out, and gently blot the stain. Use a clean rag soaked in the remaining 2 cups warm water to remove the residue. Alternate the soap solution with the fresh water until the stain is gone. Remember to blot, not rub, to remove a carpet stain as rubbing will ruin the carpet fibers.

Wood Cleaner & Polish

1 cup olive, almond, or fractionated coconut oil
½ cup water, distilled, or boiled and cooled
30 drops lemon essential oil
10 drops orange essential oil

Combine ingredients in a spray bottle or lidded container and shake well.
Spray or pour on a microfiber cloth and apply to surface to clean and polish any wood surface.

Hardwood Floor Cleaner

1 gallon warm water
½ cup distilled white vinegar
3 drops lemon or orange essential oil

Mix water, vinegar, and oil in a large bucket or container.
Mop with a dry mop or by hand with microfiber cloths.
Change solution as needed.

Leather Cleaner

¼ cup olive oil
½ cup regular vinegar
3 drops eucalyptus
A spray bottle

Mix the two ingredients together in your spray bottle and shake it well. Now you just have to spray the leather down and wipe it clean with a cotton cloth.
Please note that this recipe is perfectly safe for regular leather but is it not designed to be used on suede.

BATHROOM

CLEANING

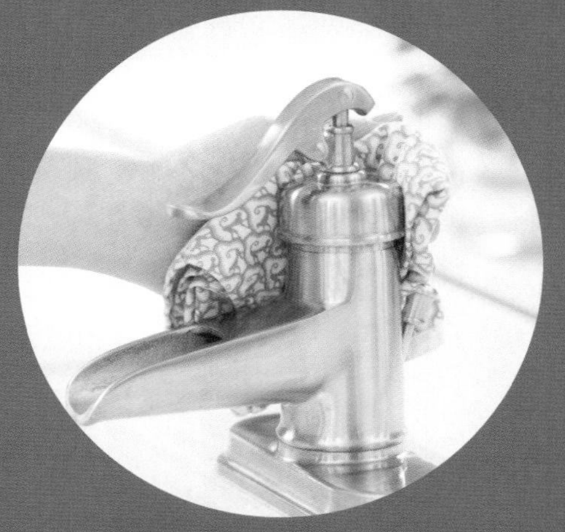

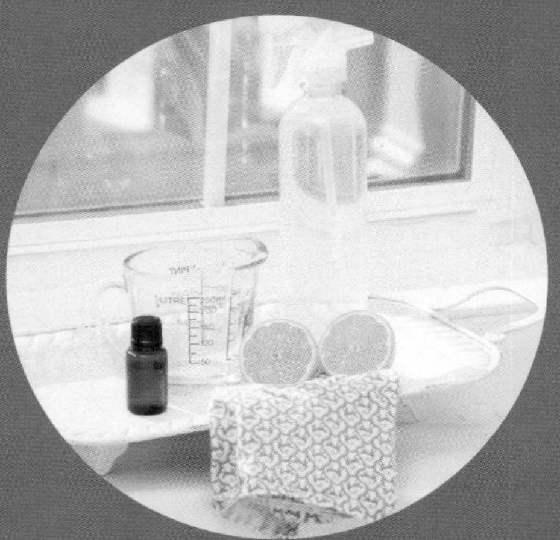

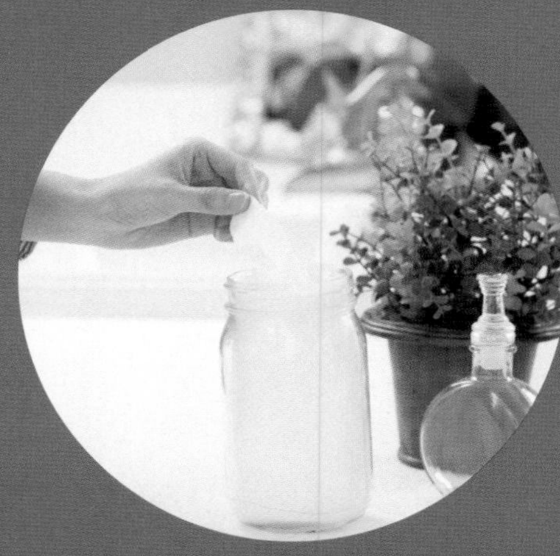

Soap Scum Remover

2 cups hot water
¼ - ½ cup borax
10 drops lemon essential oil

Add ingredients to a spray bottle and shake well. Spray windows or mirrors and wipe dry. Store in cool place for one to two months.

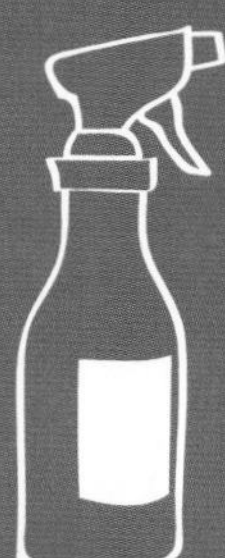

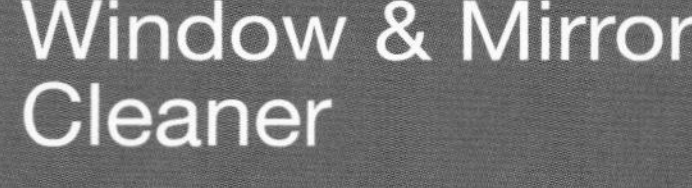

Window & Mirror Cleaner

2 cups water
2 tablespoons white vinegar
2 tablespoons rubbing alcohol
5 drops peppermint essential oil

Add ingredients to a spray bottle and shake well. Spray windows or mirrors and wipe dry. Store in cool place for for one to two months.

Disinfecting Cleaning Wipes

12 thick and durable paper towels
1 cup boiled and slightly cooled water
½ cup white vinegar
¼ cup rubbing alcohol
5 drops lavender essential oil
5 drops lemon essential oil

Cut paper towels in half and stack into a neat pile. Roll up and stuff into a quart size wide-mouth mason jar or large zip-lock bag. Mix ingredients and pour over paper towels. Put the lid on or zip and shake to moisten towels.

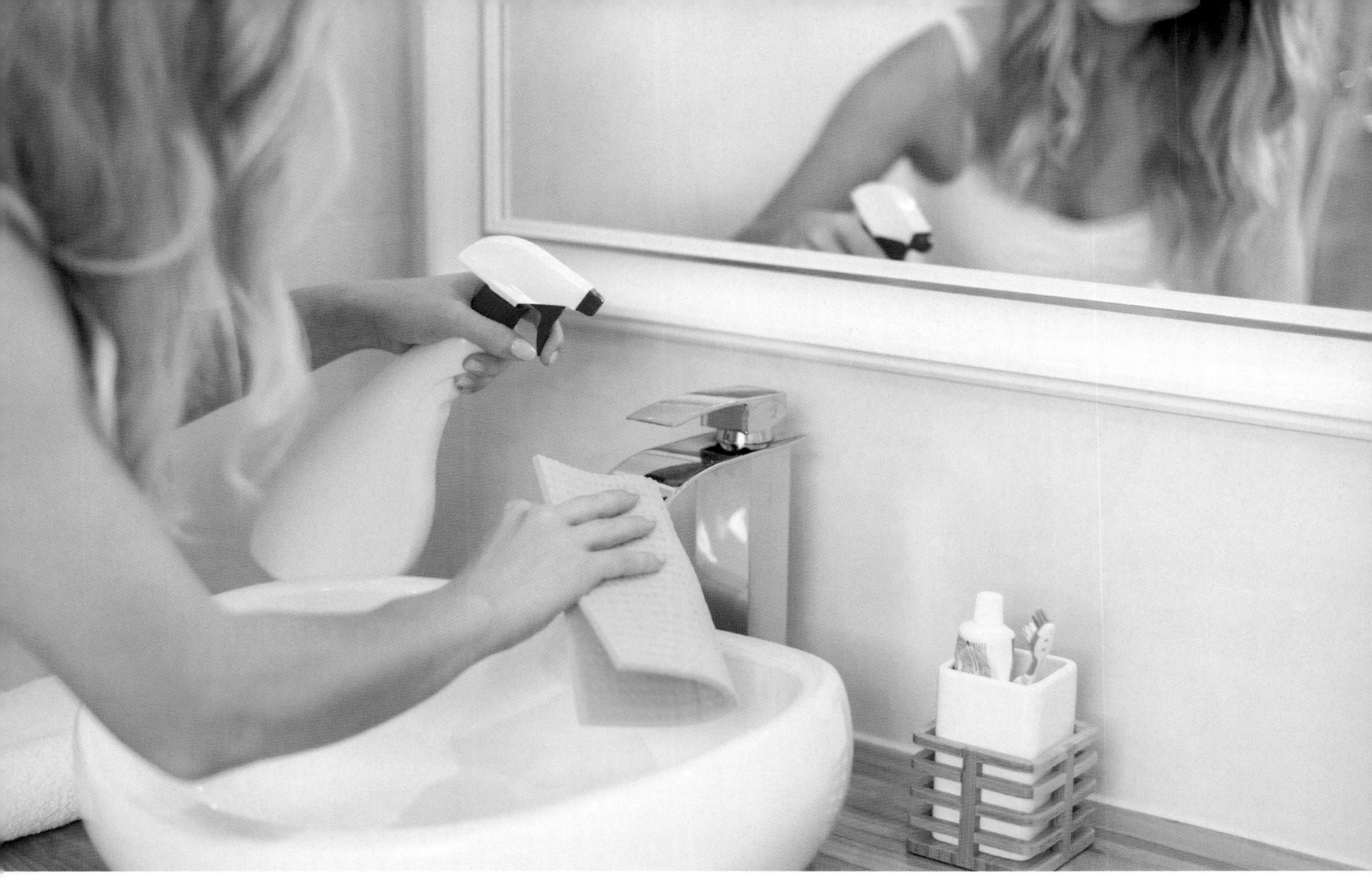

Mold & Mildew Preventer

2 cups water
30 drops melaleuca essential oil
10 drops peppermint essential oil

Add ingredients to a spray bottle and shake well. Spray directly on mold or mildew. Do not rinse. Repeat daily or weekly as needed.

Disinfecting Toilet Bowl Cleaner

½ cup baking soda
¼ cup white vinegar
10 drops melaleuca essential oil

Mix ingredients to dissolve baking soda. Add to toilet. Let sit for five to fifteen minutes. Scrub with a toilet brush and flush.

KITCHEN

CLEANING

Drain Cleaner

1/4 cup baking soda
1/4 cup distilled white vinegar
3 drops wild orange essential oil

Pour essential oil directly down drain, followed by baking soda, and then the vinegar. Allow to sit for fifteen minutes. Pour hot water down the drain, followed by cold water to unclog drains.

Sticker & Goo Remover

1 tablespoon baking soda
1 tablespoon almond or vegetable oil
2 drops lemon essential oil

Mix into a small glass bowl. Apply a small amount to the sticker or label and let sit for one to two minutes. Use a cloth or paper towel to remove. Apply again if needed.

Garbage Can Odor Tablets

2 cups baking soda
1 cup Epsom salts
1/4 cup water
10 drops lemon essential oil
5 drops peppermint essential oil
Ice cube tray

Combine dry ingredients. Slowly add water, then oils, and stir. Using a spoon, transfer mixture into the ice cube tray without overfilling the tray. Allow to dry overnight or until hardened. Place one to two tablets in the bottom of your garbage can and store the rest in an airtight container. Replace tablets as needed

Grill Cleaner

1/4 cup baking soda
2 tablespoons natural dish detergent
5 drops lemon essential oil
Distilled white vinegar

Combine the first three ingredients. Add vinegar until mixture has an olive-oil consistency. Brush mixture onto metal grill, and let sit for fifteen to thirty minutes. Use a damp scouring pad or grill brush to scrub surface clean. Rinse with water.

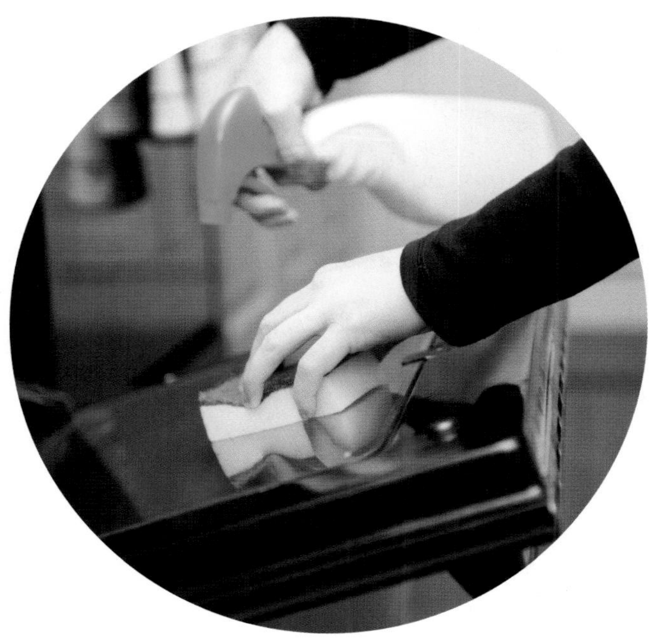

Oven Cleaner Spray

1 cup warm water
3 tablespoons baking soda
1 tablespoon castile soap
5 drops lemon essential oil
5 drops clove essential oil

Add all ingredients to a spray bottle and shake to combine. Spray liberally in the oven and let sit for fifteen minutes. Wipe clean with a sponge or cloth.

Oven Cleaner Paste

1 cup baking soda
1/2 cup water
1 tablespoon dish or castile soap
10 drops lemon essential oil

Combine ingredients in a bowl to form a paste. Apply with a sponge and let sit up to thirty minutes. Wipe off with clean cloth or sponge and water.

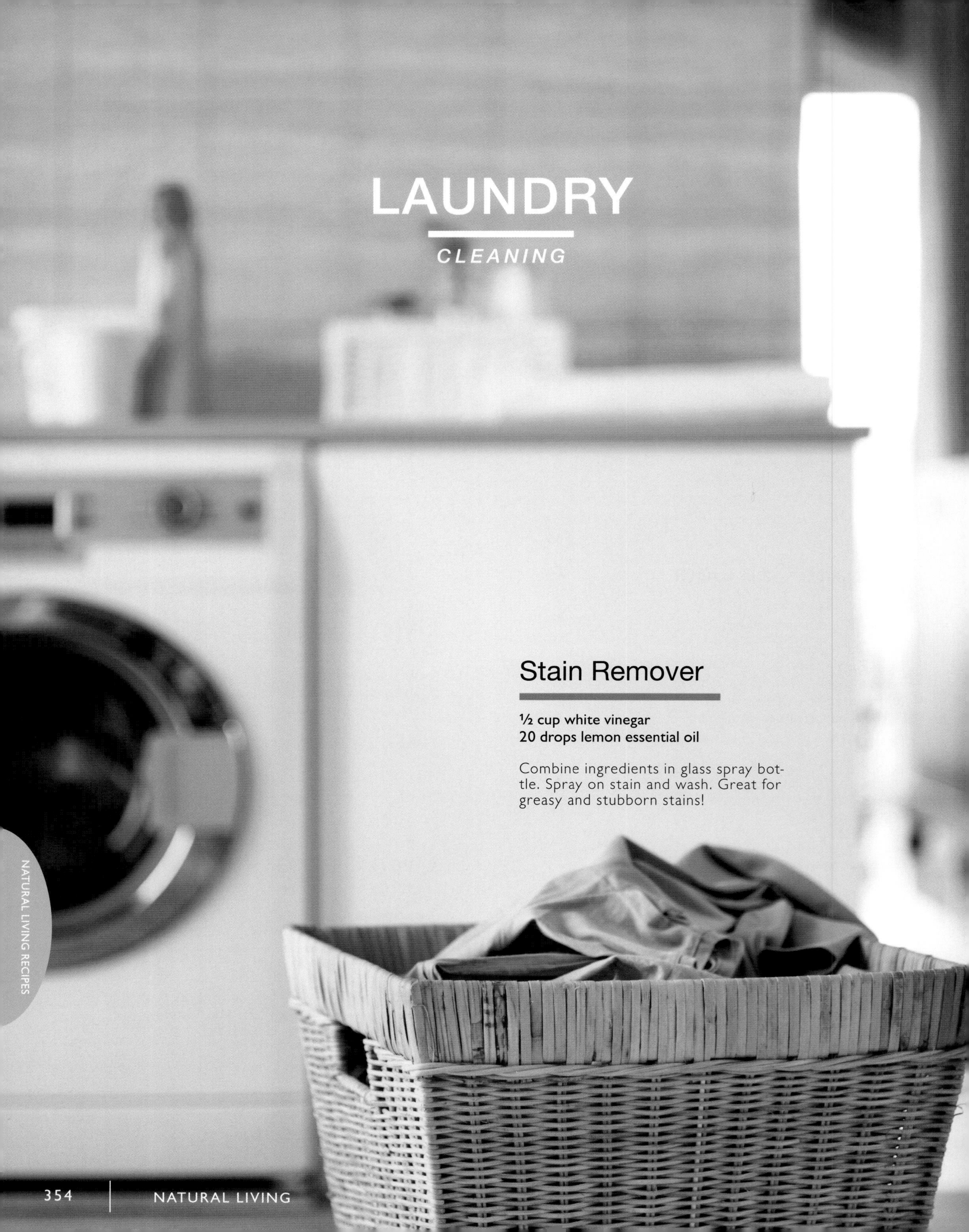

LAUNDRY

CLEANING

Stain Remover

½ cup white vinegar
20 drops lemon essential oil

Combine ingredients in glass spray bottle. Spray on stain and wash. Great for greasy and stubborn stains!

NATURAL LIVING RECIPES

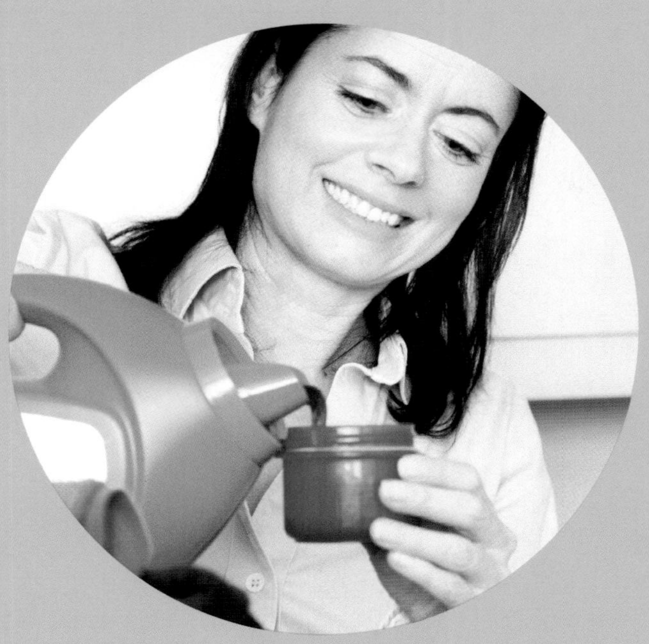

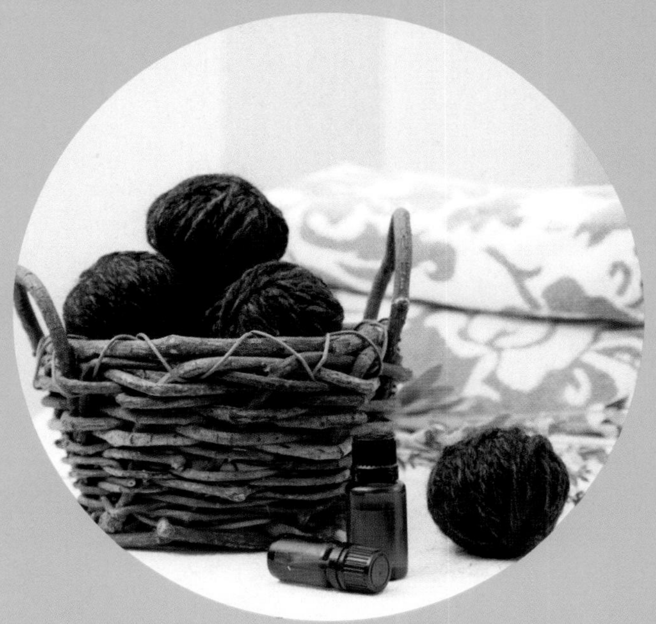

Liquid Fabric Softener

1 gallon distilled white vinegar
2 cups baking soda
20 drops clove essential oil
10 drops lemon essential oil

Combine ingredients in a large bowl or container and add ¼ to ½ cup per load. Your laundry will be softened and smell great.

Reusable Dryer Sheet

This is an easy and natural solution for a wonderfully scented dryer sheet.

1 6"x 6"piece of cotton or wool cloth (recycled T-shirts, sweaters, or socks, etc.)
2-4 drops orange or other essential oil

Place cloth in a container. Drop essential oil on fabric. Allow essential oil to dry thoroughly. Place dryer sheet on top of wet clothes in dryer and dry as usual. When sheet has lost its scent, simply add more oil.

Whitener & Brightener

2 ounces or ¼ cup hydrogen peroxide
10 drops lemon essential oil

Combine ingredients and pour into the bleach compartment of your washing machine or directly to the water. Launder as usual. Do not use on brights or colors. Hydrogen peroxide is a natural ingredient known for its bleaching properties.

Dryer Softener Balls

100% wool yarn or 100% animal yarn
Pantyhose (reuse pantyhose with runs in them)
4 to 6 drops of essential oil of choice

Take the end of the yarn and wrap it around your middle and index finger ten times. Remove it from the fingers and then wrap two or three times around the middle. (It should look like a bow.) Keep tightly wrapping the yarn around, making a round shape the size of a tennis ball. Cut the yarn and tuck the ends into the sides of the ball. Create four or more balls. Cut one leg off pantyhose. Place one yarn ball into the bottom and tie a knot above the ball. Repeat until all the balls have been added and secured. Once secured, felt (fusing together resulting in a ball) the yarn by washing and drying on the highest heat setting. When the balls are dry, remove the pantyhose and add 4-6 drops of your favorite essential oil. Toss in dryer with clothes.

Stain Stick

This is a quick recipe for spot treatments on any fabric.

½ 5-ounce bar castile soap
3 teaspoons water
4 drops melaleuca essential oil

Grate soap and place in microwave-safe bowl with water. Melt on low heat in microwave in thirty-second intervals for about a minute and a half. Once it has melted, let cool for five minutes and stir in essential oil. Pour into a stain stick container or deodorant container with a push-up bottom. Allow to cool to a solid state before using. Because melaleuca essential oil is a mild solvent, this stick will also help to remove set-in stains.

COOKING

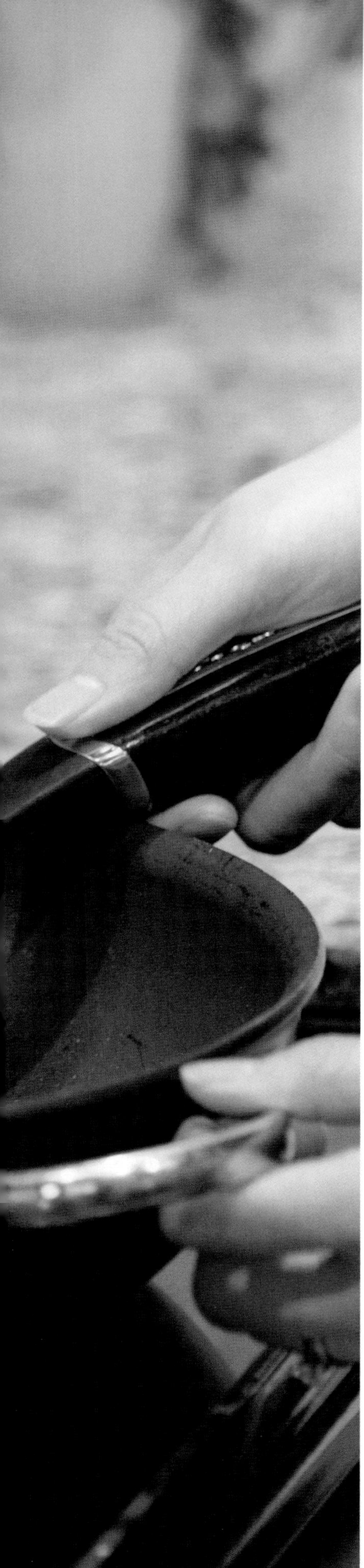

Tips for Cooking with Essential Oils

Adding essential oils to your favorite recipes makes it easy to incorporate their healthful benefits throughout the day. There are many variables with dealing with essential oils for cooking. If you have ever used fresh herbs instead of dried, you know the flavor and the quantity used is different. The same rule applies to essential oils for cooking. The oils are super-concentrated in flavor and aroma. You may find that some essential oil brands are more potent than others—this has to do with sourcing and purity. Essential oils can add a very subtle or very strong taste to your cooked dishes, depending on how much you use. We like to enjoy and identify as many flavors in our foods as possible, so use caution and know that less is best. Start with a tiny amount, then add more as you need it. If you get too much, the flavor will dominate and can spoil your dish.

The oils all have different viscosity as well, so some are thinner and some are thicker. The type of opening in the bottle you are using will affect the size of the drop. Using a dropper or syringe can help control what you are dispersing. Another good option is to drip onto a utensil first, then pull from that amount what you want to go into your dish or beverage.

You'll notice in the following recipes there are some interesting measurements that will help you add the right amount of essential oils to your cooking recipes. The best way to control quantity is to use the toothpick method.

1 toothpick dip = dip a toothpick into the essential oil and dip it once into the recipe
1 toothpick swirl = dip a toothpick into the essential oil and swirl it around in the recipe
1/2 drop = Drop an essential oil into a spoon, then use the tip of a sharp knife to obtain the desired amount of oil and add it to the recipe.

Be sure to use a fresh toothpick with each use so as not to contaminate your essential oil bottles.

Hot, savory, or spicy herbs are particularly hard to judge (for example, basil oil may be much more subtle in flavor than oregano), so the general rule should be: if it isn't citrus oil, use a toothpick until you test it or have a guaranteed recipe.

It's always best to mix your essential oils with an olive or other oil or liquid when cooking to more evenly disperse the flavor in your dish.

Baking typically requires more oil flavoring than cooking does. For example, where you might use 2 or 3 toothpick swirls of oregano in spaghetti sauce, you might use 2 or 3 drops when making artisan bread.

SUBSTITUTING OILS FOR HERBS

Substitute an oil for an herb to increase the health benefits and increase the flavor of any dish.

- **½ teaspoon dried herbs = 1½ teaspoons fresh herbs = 2-3 toothpick swirls essential oil**
- **1 teaspoon dried herbs = 1 tablespoon fresh herbs = 1 drop essential oil**

SUBSTITUTING OILS FOR CITRUS

- **1 teaspoon lemon extract = 1/8 teaspoon lemon essential oil = 16 drops**
- **1 tablespoon lemon zest = 1/16 teaspoon lemon essential oil = 8 drops**

BEVERAGES

COOKING

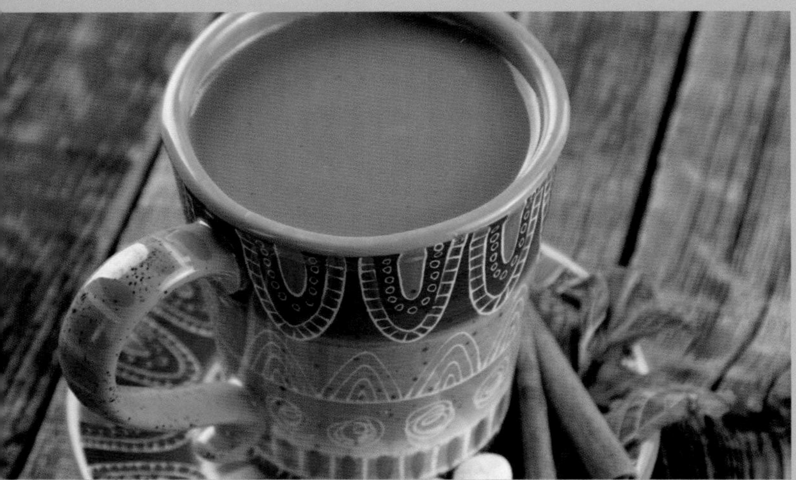

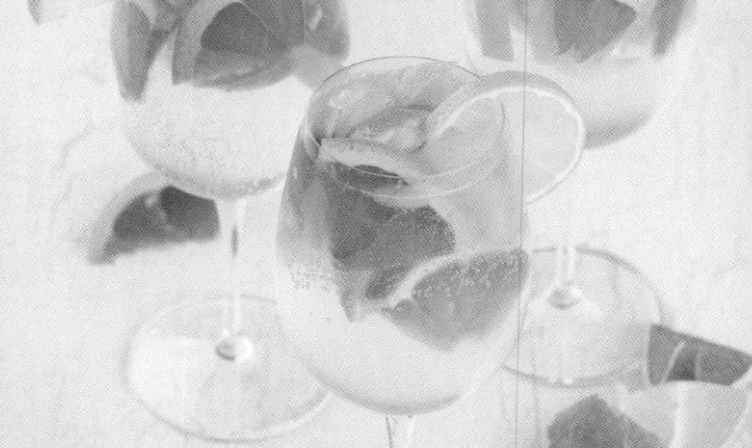

Hot Chocolate Bar

Hot chocolate, prepared.
Choose one or more of these essential oils:
• Peppermint • Cinnamon • Cassia • Cardamom • Orange
• Lemon • Pepper (gives a spicy kick)
Marshmallows, sprinkles, toffee bits, or candy canes for garnish

Prepare liquid hot chocolate as directed. Invite guests to dip toothpicks into their selection of essential oils and swirl into the chocolate. Garnish with candies if desired.

Overindulgence Tea

Hot water
Honey
10 drops wild orange essential oil
5 drops lemon essential oil
3 drops coriander essential oil
2 drops ginger essential oil
2 drops peppermint essential oil

Mix the essential oils In a small bottle. Dissolve one tablespoon honey into a cup of hot water. Stir in 2 drops of essential oil mixture. Sip until your tummy settles to help relieve the discomfort that is associated with overeating.

Frozen Blended Virgin Daiquiri

1+ cup frozen strawberries
1 teaspoon vanilla extract
1-2 drops lime essential oil
1 cup water
Stevia to sweeten

Mix all ingredients in blender. Add more sweetener or lime to taste. Add more water for a thinner consistency. For a creamy consistency, add a little plain yogurt.

Sparkling Citrus Drink

12 ounces selzer water
$1/8$-$1/4$ teaspoon stevia, to taste
6 drops grapefruit essential oil
6 drops lemon essential oil

Mix ingredients together and serve chilled or over ice. Garnish with a sprig of mint or a slice of lime, if desired. For a dash of color, add a tiny bit of red food coloring to create a pink color for the pink grapefruit.

tips

- Try adding these essential oils to still or sparkling water for a delicious flavor (and zero calories!)

- Peppermint
- Lemon
- Cardamom
- Protective blend
- Grapefruit
- Ginger
- Lime
- Grapefruit & cassia

- Add essential oil to ice cube trays. To distinguish the flavor and add to the presentation, you can include a drop of food coloring, zest of fruit, or leaf (e.g. peppermint or basil; dried citrus looks appealing as well).

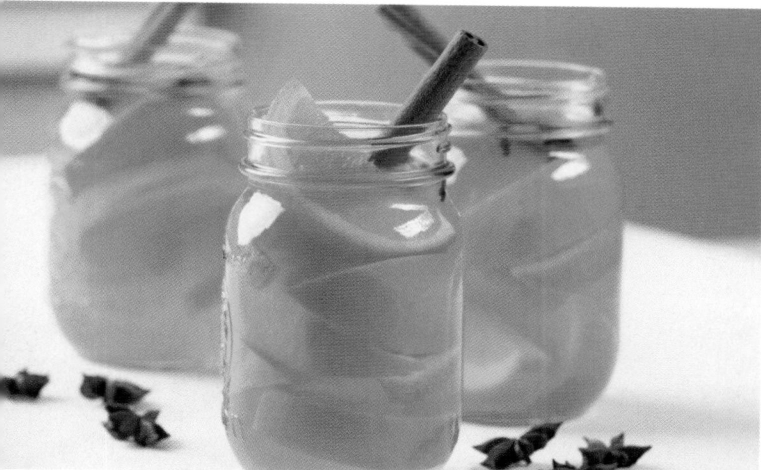

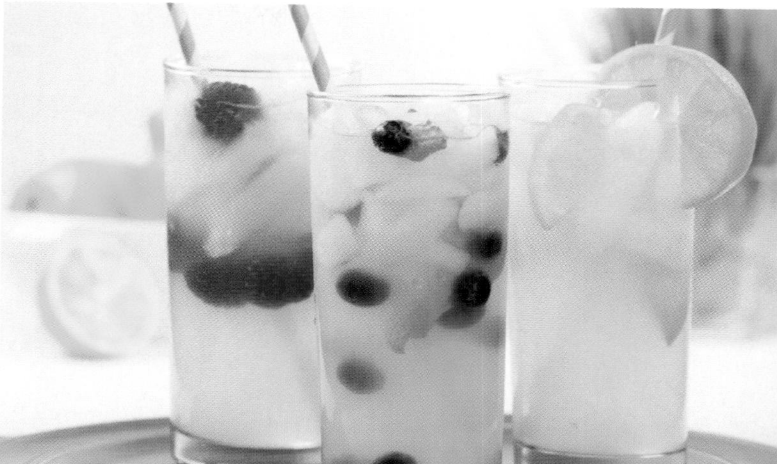

Hot Wassail

2 ½ cups apple cider
¾ cups cranberry juice
3 drops wild orange essential oil
1 drop lemon essential oil
2 toothpicks clove essential oil, swirled
2 toothpicks cinnamon essential oil, swirled
1 toothpick ginger essential oil (dip in and remove)

Combine juice, cider, and drops of wild orange and lemon essential oils in a saucepan. Bring to a simmer. Dip a toothpick into the remaining oils, then swirl or dip into the juice mixture. Pour into mugs and enjoy!

Green Berry Protein Shake

8 ounces almond milk (or milk of your choice)
3 scoops protein shake mix
1-2 cups fresh or frozen berries
2 scoops powdered greens mix or 1 large handful of fresh, washed spinach
2 drops ginger essential oil
2 drops grapefruit essential oil

Pour ingredients in blender, blend until smooth, and serve.

Lemonade Bar

Prepared lemonade of choice (8 ounces per person).
Various fresh fruits, like raspberries, strawberries, lemons, limes.
Toothpicks for flavoring with oils.

Choose one or more of these essential oils:
- Basil essential oil, 1 toothpick dip or to taste (great with raspberry lemonade)
- Lavender essential oil, 1 toothpick swirl or to taste
- Geranium essential oil, 1 toothpick swirl or to taste
- Ginger essential oil, 1 toothpick swirl or to taste
- Grapefruit essential oil, 3-4 toothpick swirls or to taste
- Lime essential oil, 2-3 toothpick swirls or to taste

Pour prepared lemonade into glasses, allowing your guests to add fruit and their choice of essential oils with the toothpicks. This is a fun crowd-pleaser!

Sweet Cassia & Grapefruit Water

Cassia essential oil provides an energy boost and fights infection in the body. Grapefruit essential oil is good for decreasing appetite and cleansing the body.

Add 10 drops of grapefruit and 2 drops cassia essential oils to a stainless steel or glass water bottle. Fill with chilled, filtered water and shake. Enjoy all day long!

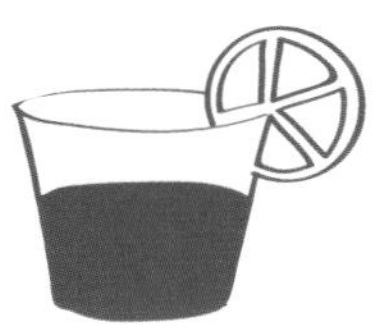

BREADS

COOKING

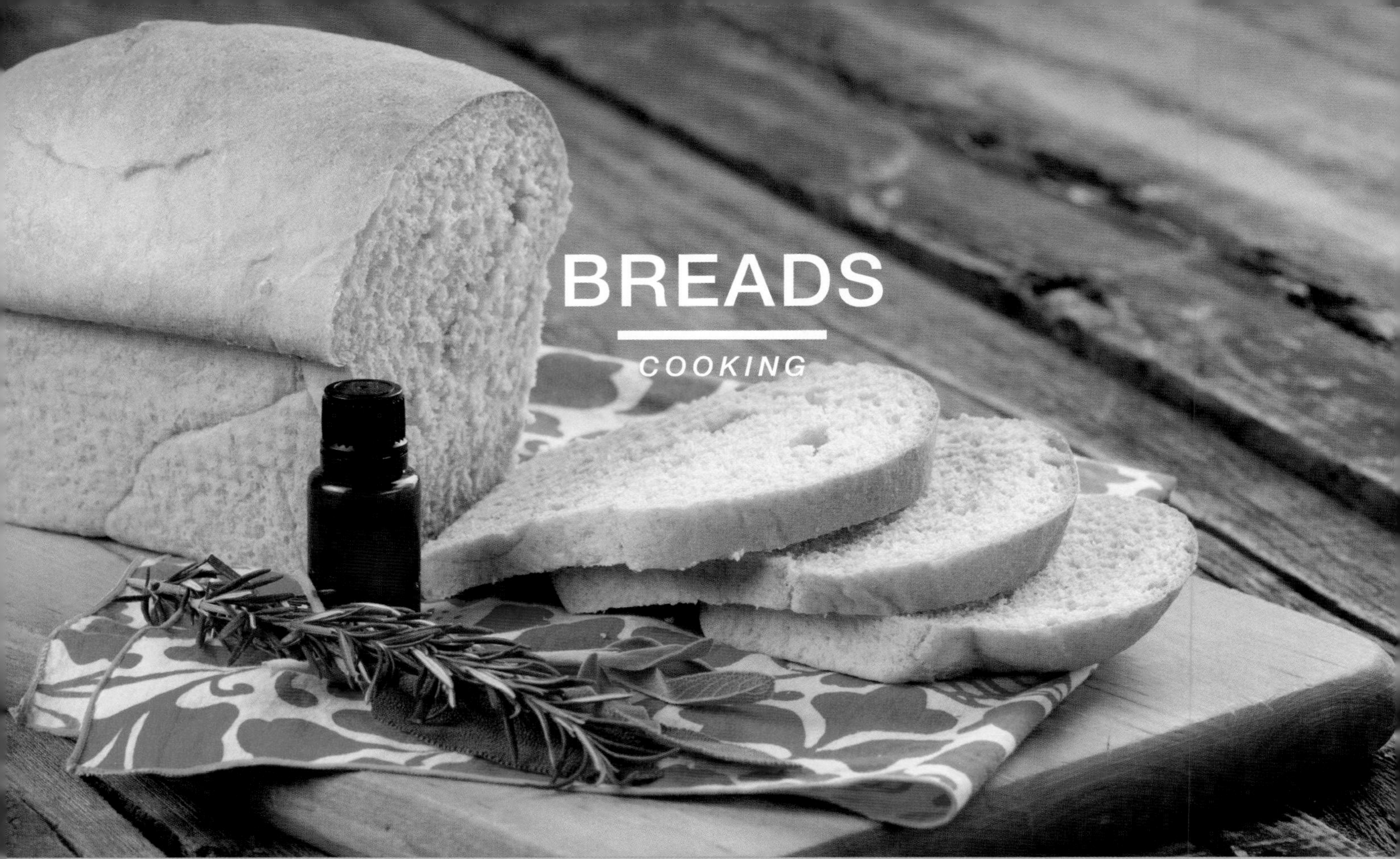

Wheat Herb Bread

2 drops thyme, sage, basil, rosemary, or oregano essential oil
1 ½ teaspoon honey (to taste)
1 ⅓ cups warm water
1 package or 2 ¼ teaspoons active dry yeast
1 ½ teaspoon sea salt
2 to 2 ¼ cups bread flour
1 ¾ cups whole wheat flour

Stir together essential oil drops and honey.
In a large bowl, combine water, yeast, and honey/essential oil mixture. Let stand for 5 minutes.
In a separate bowl, combine salt and flours. Stir flour mixture in gradually to water mixture until flour has been absorbed and the dough forms a ball.
In a mixer or by hand, knead dough until it is moderately stiff, smooth, and elastic.
Lightly spray a bowl with nonstick spray. Place dough in bowl, cover with a towel or plastic wrap (spray with nonstick spray), and let rise until doubled in size.
Remove dough from bowl, and punch down. Let rest for 10 minutes.
Spray an 8x4" bread loaf pan with nonstick spray. Shape dough to form a loaf and place in loaf pan. Let rise again until doubled in size, but not much higher than top of loaf pan. Put into a cold oven.
Bake in a 350 degrees oven for 25-30 minutes or more until golden on top and sides pull away from pan.

Tip: Great bread for dipping in your favorite olive oil (see Sauces recipes for ideas)

tips

Essential oils can flavor butters and oils for a savory, spicy, or sweet taste. For example, add cinnamon essential oil, stevia, and ground cinnamon to butter or oil for toast or biscuits. Add flavored butters or oil to the bread after it comes out of oven.

To your favorite bread recipes, add corresponding essential oils instead of herbs. You can also add orange essential oil-infused dried cranberries into sweet bread or muffin batters (see Snacks).

Make bread dips by flavoring olive oil with rosemary, thyme, and basil essential oils to taste. Mix balsamic vinegar with the flavored olive oil and serve with fresh bread chunks or slices.

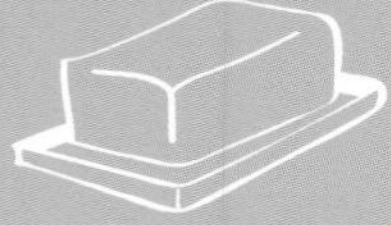

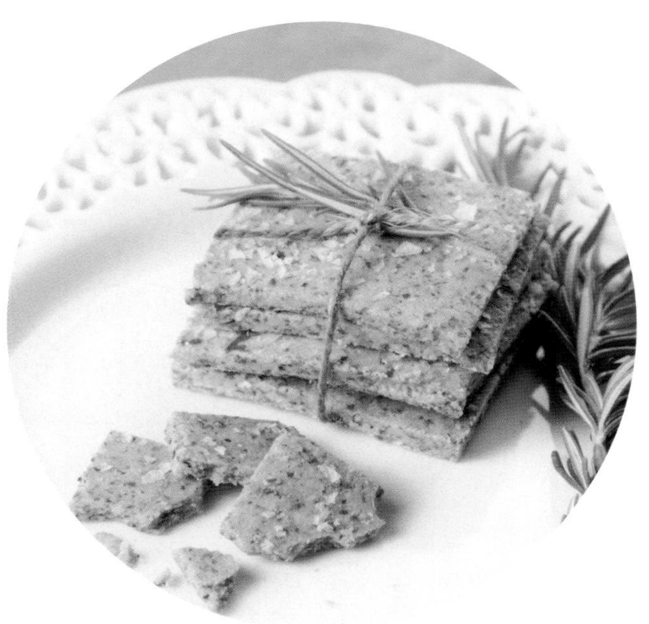

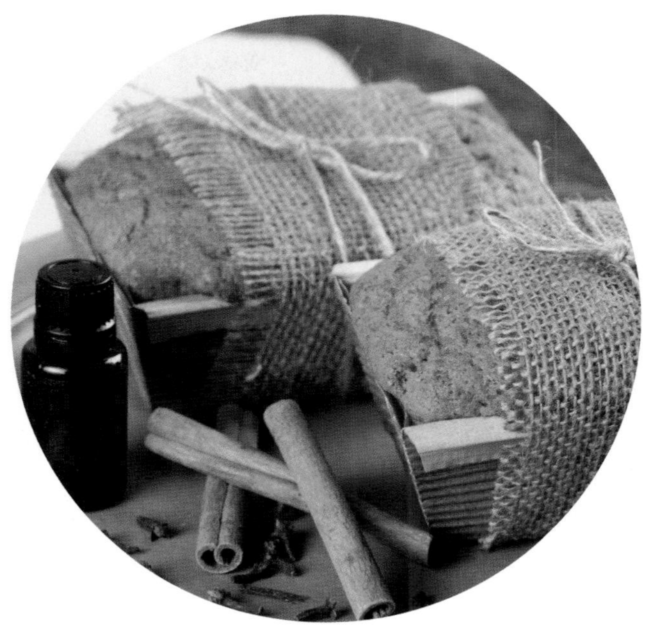

Herb Crackers

3 ½ cups blanched almond flour
½ teaspoon sea salt + ¼ reserved to sprinkle on top
2 tablespoon grapeseed or avocado oil
1 toothpick dip rosemary essential oil
1 toothpick dip thyme essential oil
1 toothpick dip black pepper essential oil
2 large eggs

Mix dry ingredients together. Mix oil, essential oils, and eggs in another bowl. Stir together dry and wet ingredients until thoroughly combined. Divide the dough into two parts. Prepare two baking sheets and three pieces of parchment paper.

Place one portion of the dough between two sheets of parchment paper and roll out till very thin. Remove top piece of parchment and set bottom layer of parchment and rolled-out cracker dough on baking sheet. Sprinkle kosher salt or sea salt over the cracker dough. Repeat process for the other half of the dough.

With pizza cutter or knife, cut squares into the dough. Bake for 12-15 minutes at 350 degrees. Let crackers cool completely on baking sheets before removing.

Zucchini Bread

3 eggs
2 cups sugar
1 cup canola oil
1 drop cinnamon essential oil
1 toothpick swirl clove essential oil
3 teaspoons vanilla
2 ¼ cups peeled, grated zucchini
3 cups flour
1 teaspoon baking soda
½ teaspoon salt
½ teaspoon baking powder
¼ teaspoons nutmeg
1 cup nuts, chopped

Beat eggs till light and fluffy.
Add sugar to eggs, mix well.
Add essential oils to canola oil, blend.
Mix oil, vanilla, and zucchini into eggs.
In a separate bowl, mix together flour, salt, soda, nutmeg, and baking powder. Add flour mixture to egg mixture; mix until blended. Stir in nuts. Spray 2 loaf pans with nonstick spray. Divide batter evenly between loaf pans. Bake 1 hour on a higher oven rack at 350 degrees or until done (toothpick or knife inserted into bread comes out clean). Oven temperatures vary greatly; check bread starting at 45 minutes cooking time.

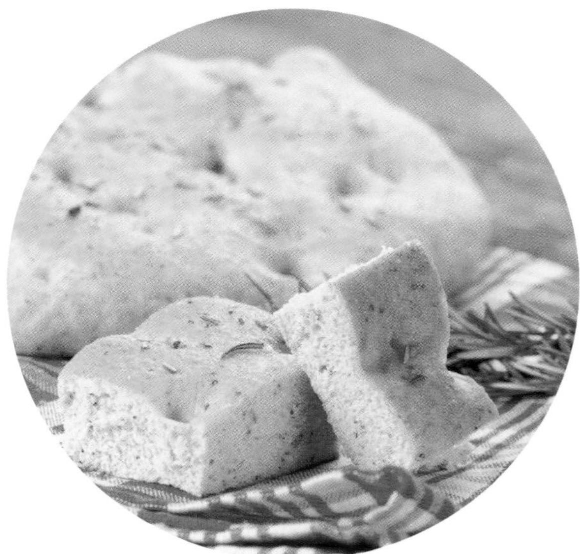

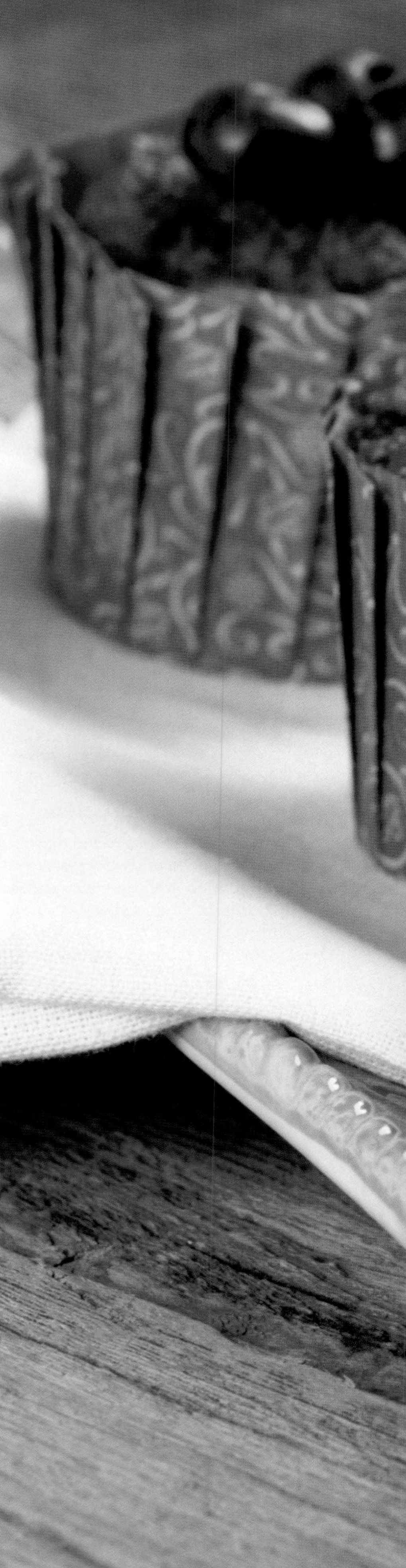

Herb Focaccia Bread

2 ¾ cups all-purpose flour (can use ½ whole wheat flour)
1 teaspoon salt
1 teaspoon sugar
2 ½ teaspoons instant yeast
1 large clove garlic, finely minced
¾ teaspoon dried rosemary or 1 tablespoon fresh rosemary, chopped
½ teaspoon dried thyme or ½ tablespoon fresh thyme, chopped
½ teaspoon dried oregano
½ teaspoon dried basil
1 tablespoon olive oil
1 cup warm water
Infuse olive oil with a toothpick of each oil: rosemary, thyme, oregano and basil

In a large bowl (or the bowl of a stand mixer), mix the flour, salt, sugar. Mix in the garlic and herbs. Pour in the water and olive oil and mix until the dough comes together, by hand or with a dough hook attachment, if using a stand mixer. Add in popped amaranth. Knead the dough until it has pulled away from the sides of the bowl (adding additional flour only if necessary - the dough will get less sticky as it kneads), about 4-6 minutes. The dough should be soft and pliable but not overly stiff. Likewise, it shouldn't leave a lot of sticky dough residue on your fingers. The goal is a soft, supple dough. Can add 2-3 tablespoons popped amaranth grain if desired.

Cover the bowl with lightly greased plastic wrap and let the dough rise for 30 minutes, until it is puffy. Deflate dough and allow to rest for 5 minutes.

Preheat the oven to 425 degrees. Lightly grease a large, rimmed baking sheet and with your hands, spread the dough out roughly an 8x10" rectangle. Use your knuckles or fingertips to make indentations over the dough, about every ½". Lightly brush dough's surface with olive oil and bake for 15 to 20 minutes, until golden brown.

Immediately after removing from the oven, stir together 1 tablespoon olive oil and ½ teaspoon salt and brush over the surface of the hot bread. Tear or slice into pieces and serve.

To pop amaranth - pop by placing in a pan that has been preheated at a high heat. Stir constantly until most of it has popped to white grain color.

Specialty Frostings/Glazes

Add 1-2 drops lemon or wild orange essential oil to glazes or frostings. If you make a lemon or citrus cake or pastry, you can try a toothpick dip of lavender essential oil with a drop of lemon essential oil in the glaze for a unique and delicious flavor combination.

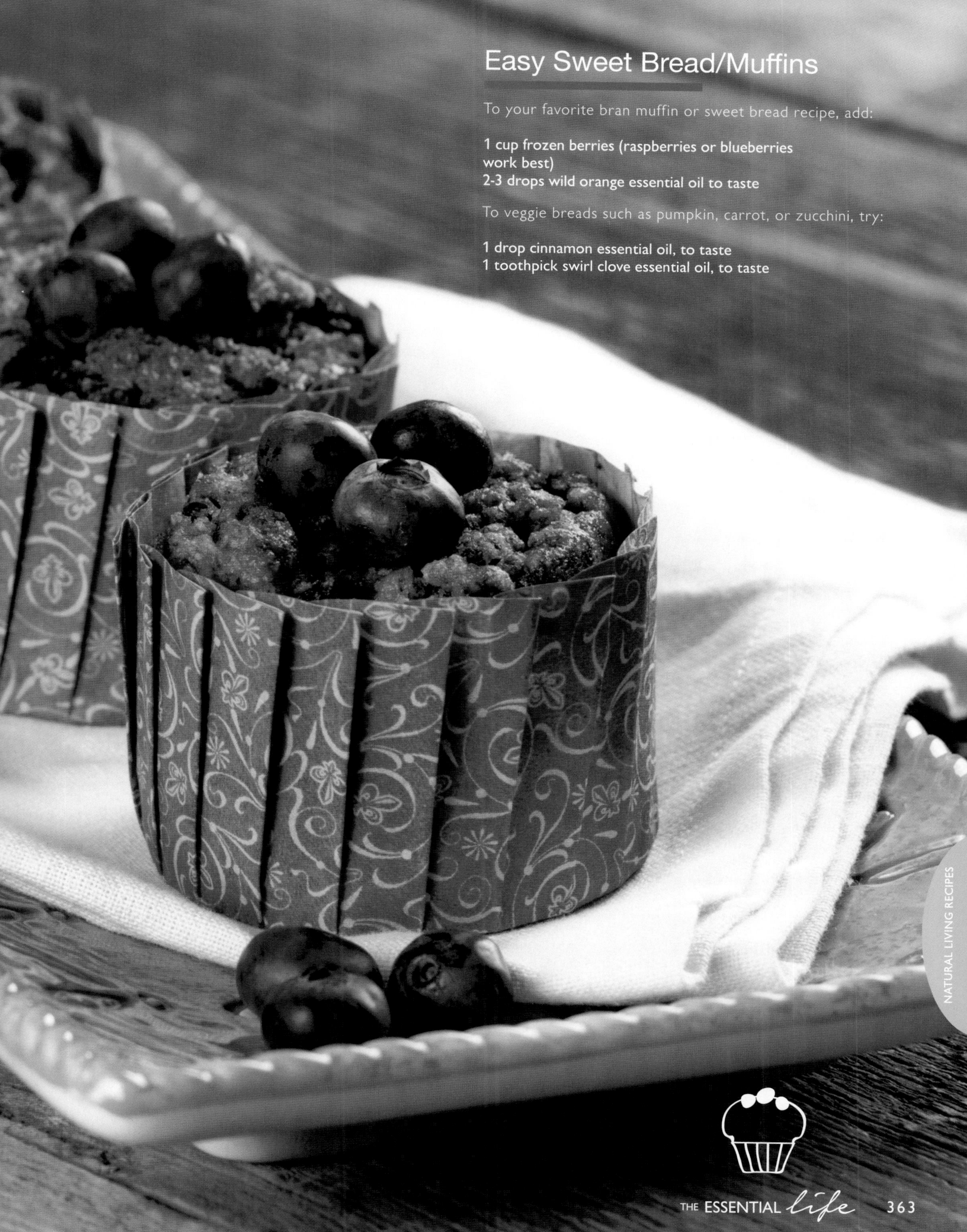

Easy Sweet Bread/Muffins

To your favorite bran muffin or sweet bread recipe, add:

1 cup frozen berries (raspberries or blueberries work best)
2-3 drops wild orange essential oil to taste

To veggie breads such as pumpkin, carrot, or zucchini, try:

1 drop cinnamon essential oil, to taste
1 toothpick swirl clove essential oil, to taste

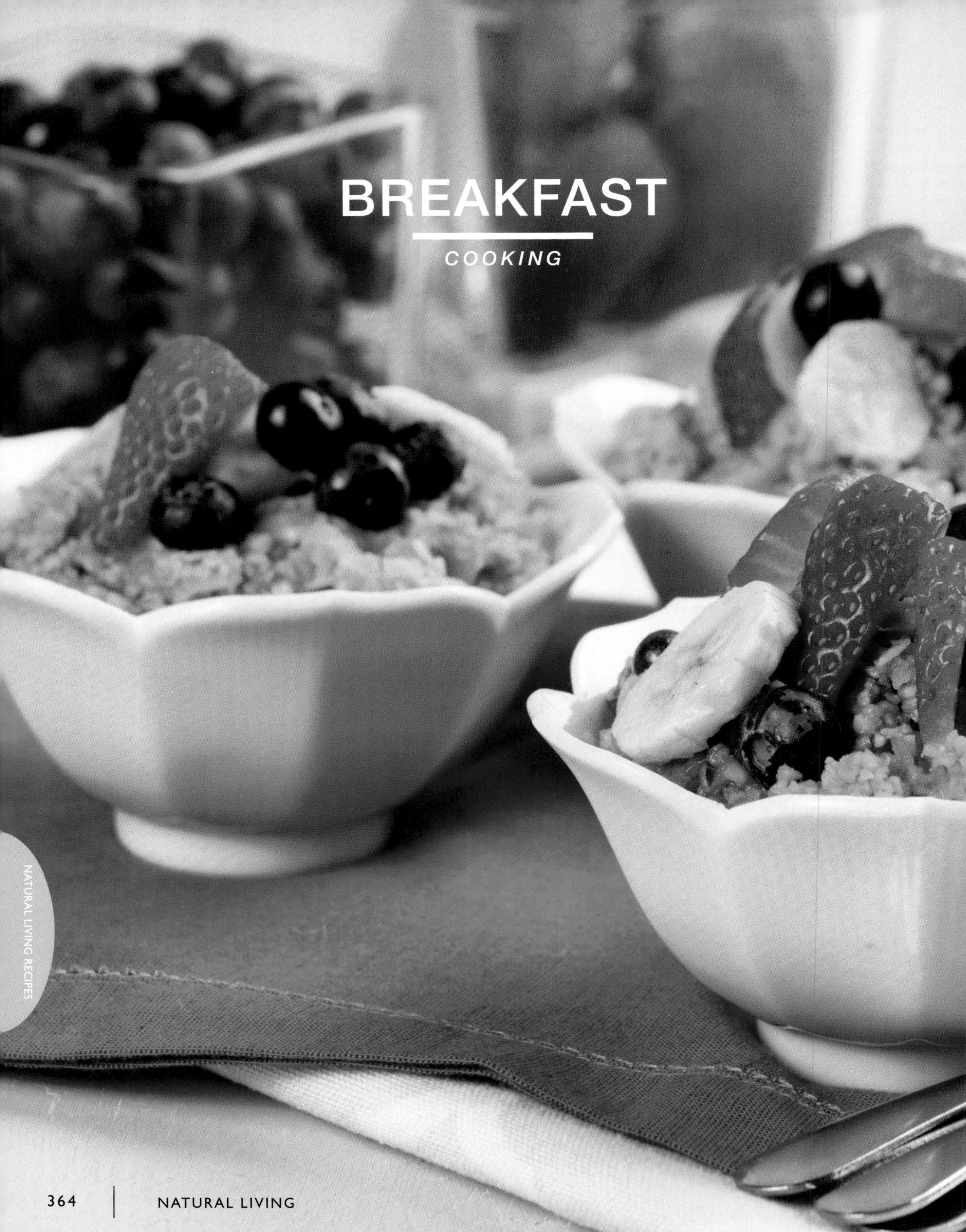

BREAKFAST

COOKING

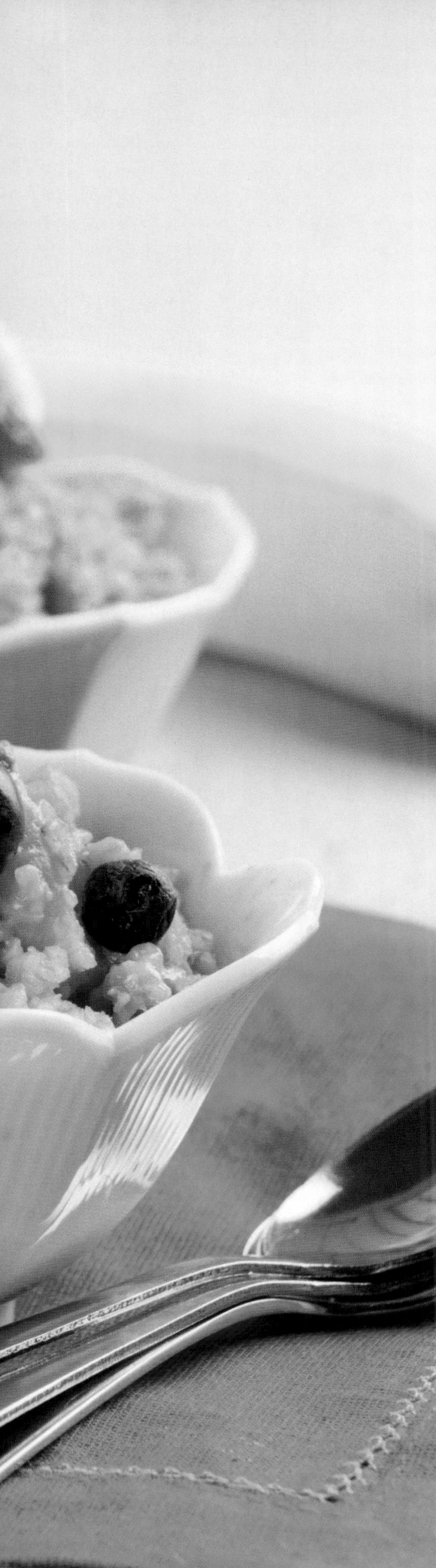

Baked Oatmeal

Dry ingredients:
2 cups rolled oats
½ cup brown sugar or raw coconut sugar
1 ¼ teaspoons baking powder
dash salt

Wet ingredients:
2 cups milk
1 drop cinnamon or protective blend essential oil
1 large egg
4 tablespoons melted butter
2 teaspoons vanilla extract

Variations that can be added:
*½ cup toasted chopped nuts
*½ cup plumped raisins
*2 bananas cut up and line bottom of pan with berries (cut sugar to ⅓ cup)
*1 ½ cups berries
*apple cinnamon—chop up 2 apples and simmer in the milk. Increase sugar to ½ cup and use cinnamon essential oil as noted above.

Mix dry ingredients in one bowl and wet ingredients in another. Butter an 8x8 baking pan or oven safe skillet. If using bananas, layer first. If not, spread dry ingredients evenly in pan. Pour the wet ingredients over the dry. Shake gently to distribute the liquid.

Bake at 375 degrees for 35-45 minutes until golden and set. Top with one of the following: sweet cream, cinnamon sugar or butter.

Makes 6 servings.

Easy Spiced Oatmeal

Use cinnamon, cassia, cardamom, or protective blend essential oils (to taste) to flavor plain oatmeal. To add essential oils to oatmeal, simply blend with your choice of milk (e.g. almond) and stir into oatmeal. Use honey or stevia to sweeten as desired.

Homemade Granola

3 ¼ cups rolled oats
4 tablespoons light brown sugar
¼ teaspoon kosher or sea salt
½ teaspoon nutmeg
½ cup honey
¼ cup vegetable oil
2 - 3 drops cinnamon or cassia essential oil (to taste)
1 teaspoon vanilla
1 - 1 ⅓ cups combined dried fruit, diced, seeds, or chopped nuts (raw or toasted) to your liking

Heat oven to 300 degrees, use middle rack. Combine oats, brown sugar, salt and nutmeg. Add essential oil to vegetable oil. In a different bowl, mix honey, oils, and vanilla to combine. Pour honey mixture over the oats. Mix thoroughly. Spread out on baking sheet and bake for 15 minutes, then stir. Stir every 5 minutes after that for at least 15 more minutes or until very light golden brown. Remove, let cool to room temperature. Add dried fruit, nuts and/or seeds to oats in a large bowl. If more chunky granola is desired, add sunflower seed kernels, wheat germ, oat bran, etc.

tips

Always use glass, ceramic, or metal bowls and spoons. Avoid plastic utensils and storage containers.

Make a yummy fruit dip as a side or topping by mixing 1 cup vanilla yogurt with 1/2 cup mashed berries and 1-2 drops lime essential oil.

You can add essential oils to your favorite breakfast drink or tea.

Ham & Cheese Crustless Quiche

2 cups Black Forest ham or crispy bacon, fully cooked and cubed or shredded
1 cup shredded cheese (good flavor) + 1/2 cup cheese to sprinkle on top
1/3 cup green onion, chopped, or 1/4 cup yellow onion
2 cups milk
5 large eggs
1 cup prepared dry biscuit mix
1/4 teaspoon sea salt
1 drop black pepper essential oil
1 toothpick cardamom or basil, dipped & swirled

Grease a pie pan or line with parchment paper sprayed with nonstick cooking spray. Place ham, cheese, and onions in bottom of pie pan. Beat remaining ingredients in bowl or blender and pour over the other ingredients. Bake at 400 degrees (bake on middle to higher rack) until light golden brown or until knife inserted in center comes out clean, approximately 30 minutes. Sprinkle reserved cheese on top and bake another 10 minutes until melted and bubbly.

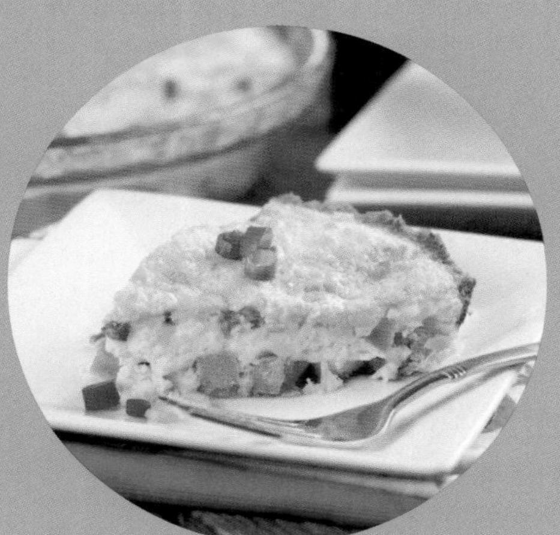

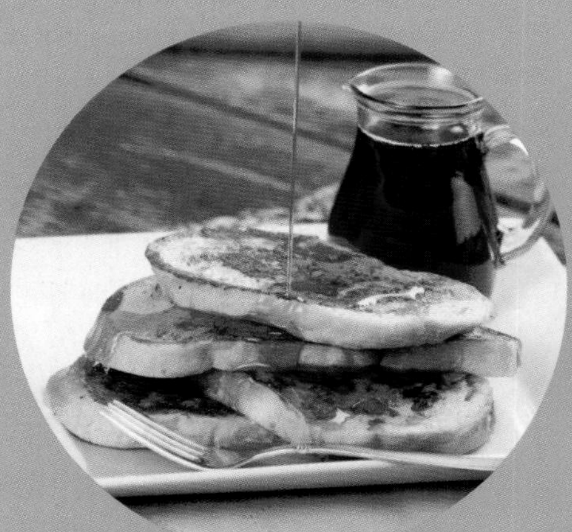

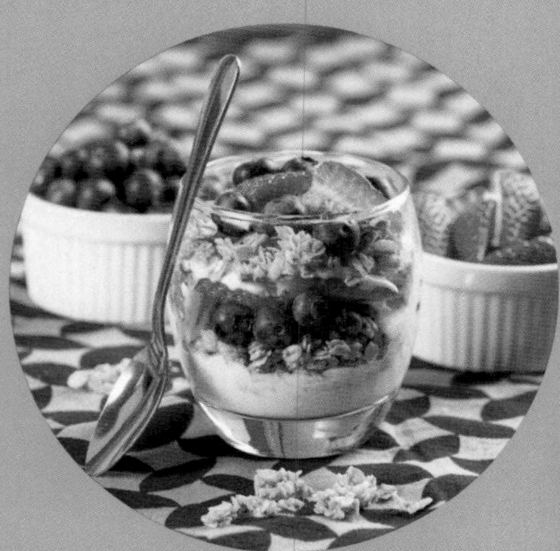

Spiced French Toast

3 large eggs
3/4 cup milk of your choice
1 teaspoon vanilla extract
1 drop cinnamon or protective blend essential oil
Dash of salt
Dash of pepper
6-8 slices bread of your choice

Whisk eggs until light and fluffy. Mix in remaining ingredients. Heat a skillet or griddle coated with coconut oil, butter, or a nonstick spray. Dip bread in batter, turning to coat, then place on griddle. Cook until golden, turn to cook the other side until golden. Top with butter and warm spiced syrup or spiced apple pie filling (see recipes). Note: Protective blend is great with white bread. Cinnamon is better for wheat bread.

Maple Syrup

1 bottle agave (approx. 18 ounces)
1/2 teaspoon maple extract
1/4 teaspoon vanilla extract
1 drop protective blend essential oil (for spicier syrup)

Mix, heat, and serve.

Yogurt Fruit Parfait

1/4 - 1/2 cup plain Greek yogurt
1 drop lime essential oil, or more to taste
Granola
1/4 cup blueberries

Blend lime with yogurt. Layer yogurt with granola and blueberries.

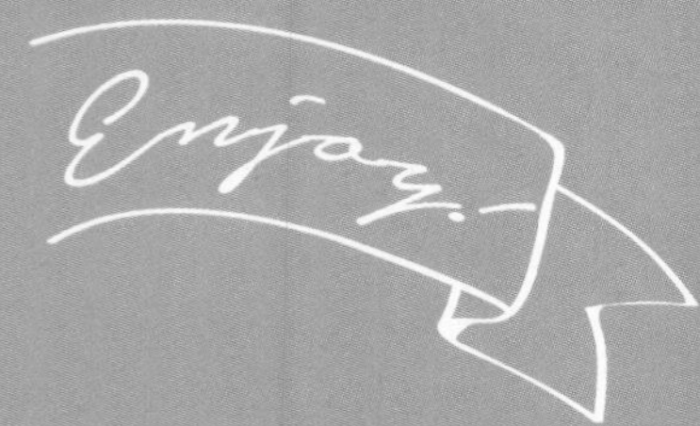

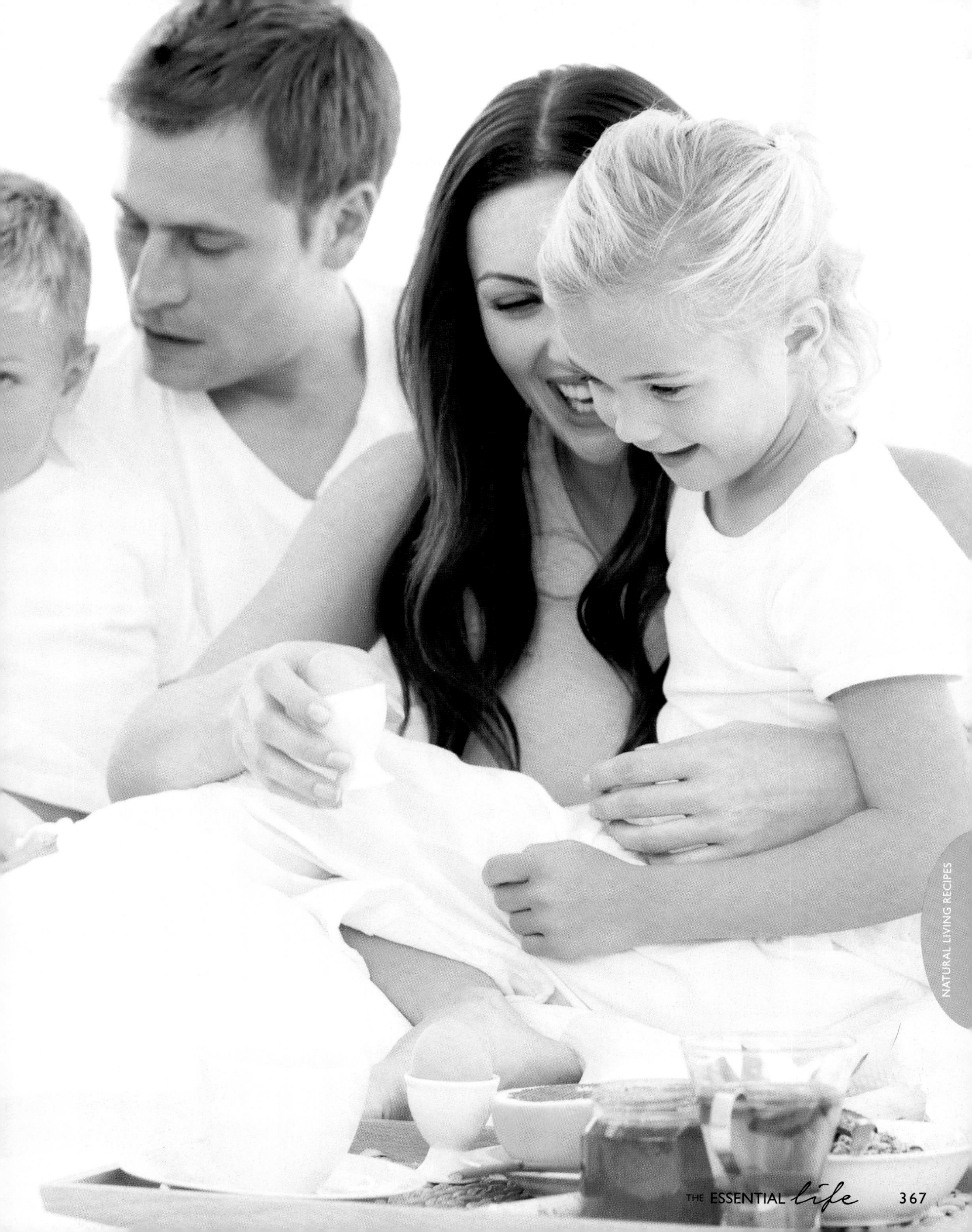

NATURAL LIVING RECIPES

DESSERTS

COOKING

Lemon Or Lime Bars

CRUST:
1 cup butter, softened (not melted)
2 cups flour
½ cup powdered sugar
¼ teaspoon sea salt

FILLING:
4 eggs
2 cups sugar
3 tablespoon lemon or lime juice
1 tablespoon water
¼ cup cornstarch
6 drops lemon or lime essential oil (or more to taste)

TOPPING (after baking):
⅓ - ½ cup powdered sugar
1 drop of lemon or lime essential oil

Mix butter, flour, ½ cup powdered sugar, and salt with pastry blender. Press into the bottom of 9x13" pan. (For nicer presentation, line pan with parchment paper so you can lift bars out of pan). Bake at 350 degrees for 15 minutes. While baking, mix eggs and sugar till light and fluffy. Add the lemon or lime juice, essential oil, water and cornstarch. Pour mixture over semi-cooked crust and bake at 350 degrees for 25-30 more minutes. Mix powdered sugar and citrus oil in baggie and shake it up. When lemon bars are done, sprinkle with citrus-infused powdered sugar on top by putting into metal strainer and shaking onto warm bars (let them cool a bit, but not completely).

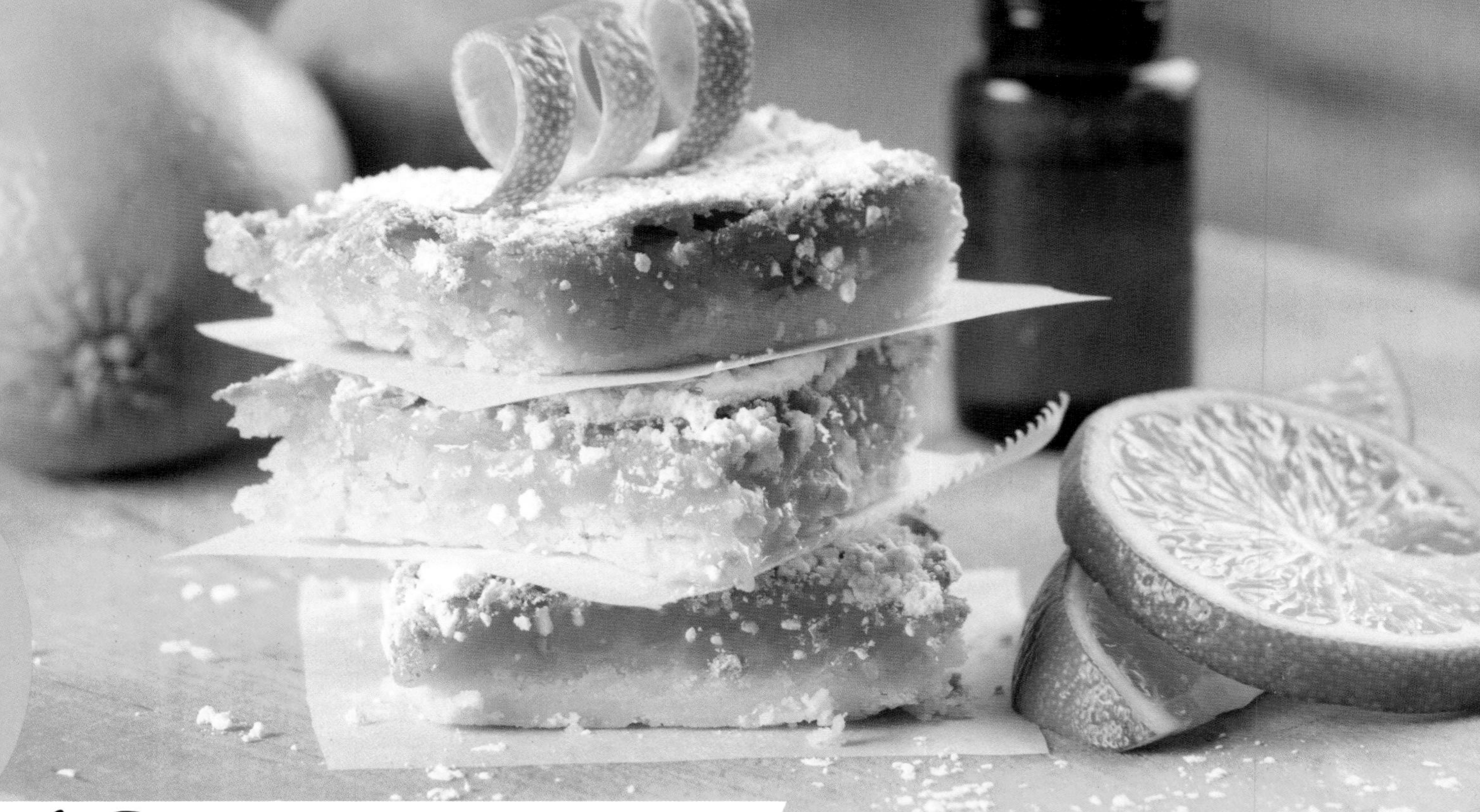

tips

Use pudding variations for making trifles, parfaits, and cream pies.

Flavor whipping cream and sugars (sprinkle on muffins or sugar cookies) with essential oils.

Strawberries Romanoff

Wash and rinse 1 quart strawberries and lay on paper towel to dry. Into sour cream or plain Greek yogurt, add 2 toothpick swirls lemon essential oil. Put brown sugar in a dish. Holding strawberry by the stem, dip into yogurt or sour cream essential oil mixture, then dab into brown sugar.

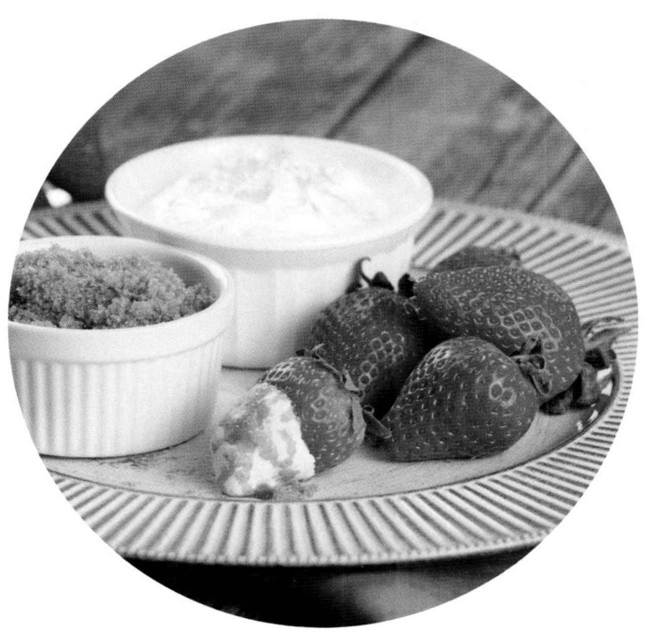

Ice Cream Log

Prepare desired cake recipe as directed. Instead of using a 9" x 13" pan, prepare a jelly roll pan with nonstick spray. Place parchment paper 2" larger than pan on all sides, and spray nonstick spray on parchment paper.
Spread cake batter thinly onto the paper.

Bake on a higher oven rack for 10-12 minutes at 350 degrees. Remove pan. Lift cake out of pan by holding all corners of parchment paper, let cool.

While cake is cooling, make ice cream mixture. Into 1 quart vanilla ice cream softened to the consistency of a thick milkshake, add your desired flavoring (e.g. peppermint, orange, lime, lemon, cinnamon, cardamom essential oils, chocolate chip pieces or sprinkles) to taste. Spread ice cream evenly on top of cooled cake mixture. Roll cake and ice cream using parchment paper, removing paper as you roll. Place roll onto a parchment-paper lined pan and freeze. Once frozen, you can wrap with plastic wrap to store in freezer. Slice and serve.

Pudding Variations

Use your favorite pudding recipe. Note: Don't add vanilla if using essential oils in pudding.

Citrus: Add 1 drop lemon, lime, grapefruit, or wild orange essential oils to hot pudding, after pudding has thickened. If you want to add more, add in "toothpick dip" increments.

Chocolate: In a microwavable dish, melt 1 cup chocolate chips and stir into hot pudding after pudding has thickened. Add 3 toothpick swirls peppermint essential oil to taste; 1 drop wild orange; 2 toothpick swirls cinnamon, cassia, or cardamom essential oils to taste.

Butterscotch: In a microwavable dish, melt 1 cup butterscotch chips and stir into hot pudding after pudding has thickened. Add 1 toothpick dip ginger essential oil to taste.

Banana: Chop a banana into small pieces; add to hot pudding. Add 1 toothpick swirl of invigorating blend essential oil or 1 swirl ginger essential oil.

Coconut: Add roasted coconut flakes to prepared pudding, add a dollop of whipped cream, and sprinkle shredded coconut on top.

Coconut lime: Add roasted coconut flakes to prepared pudding together with 2-3 toothpick swirls lime essential oil. Add a dollop of whipped cream and sprinkle shredded coconut on top.

Apple Pie Filling

5 cups apple slices, peeled
¼ cup water
¾ cup brown sugar
¼ cup flour
2 tablespoons granulated sugar
3 tablespoons butter
1 teaspoon vanilla
¾ teaspoon salt
½ teaspoon ground cinnamon
¼ - ½ teaspoon nutmeg
2 toothpick dips lemon essential oil
1 toothpick dip cinnamon essential oil
1 toothpick dip clove essential oil
1 toothpick dip ginger essential oil

Combine apples, brown sugar, and water. Cover and cook 8 minutes. Blend flour and granulated sugar together, stir into apple mixture. Cook on stovetop on medium heat, stirring constantly until thickened. Remove from heat. Add butter, vanilla, salt, cinnamon, nutmeg, and essential oils. Taste mixture and adjust flavors, if desired.

Add to prepared piecrust, bake with streusel on top, or use as a topping for pancakes or French toast.

DRESSINGS & MARINADES

COOKING

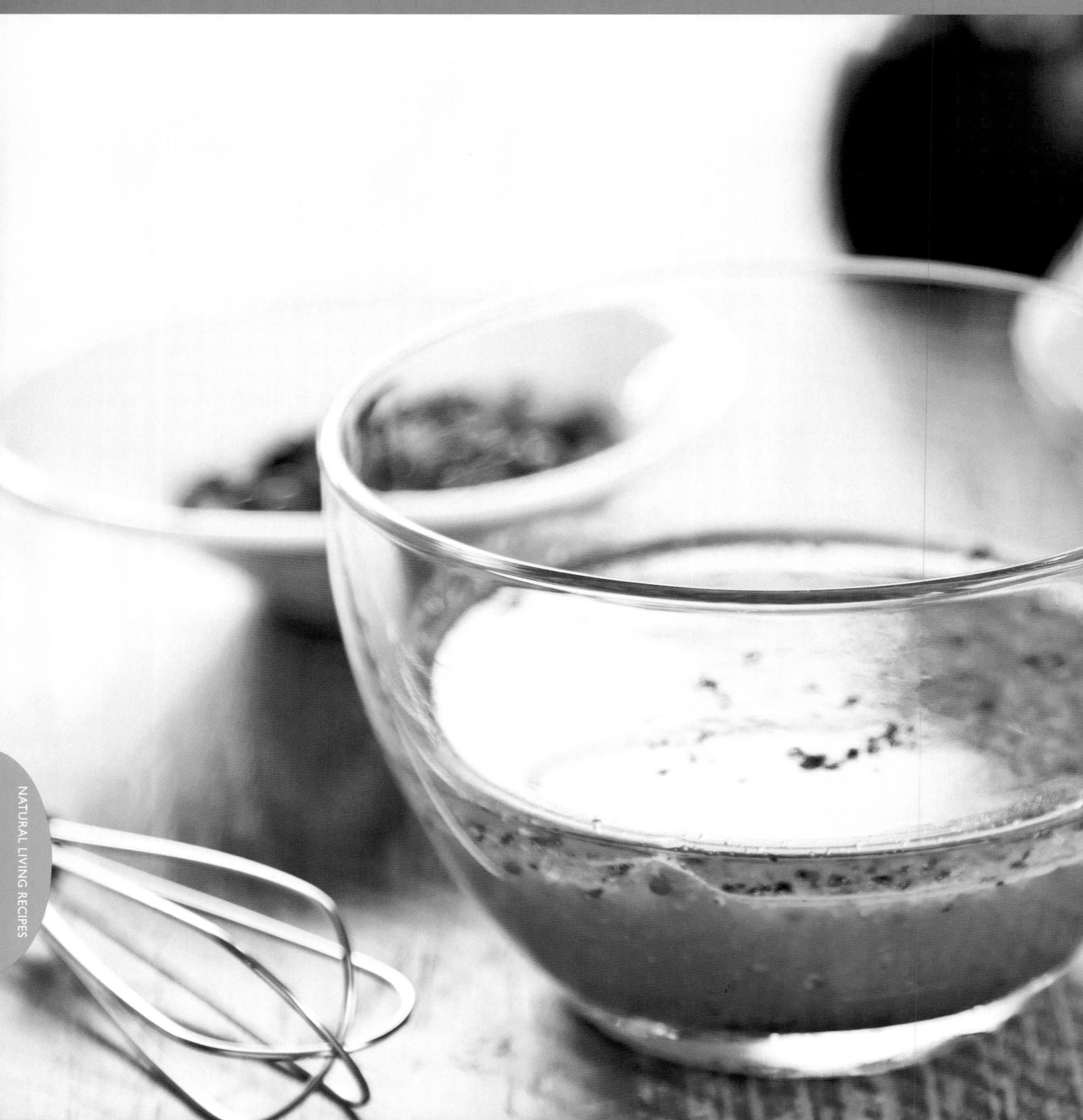

NATURAL LIVING RECIPES

Creamy Cilantro Dressing

½ cup buttermilk
½ cup mayonnaise
½ cup sour cream
1 package dry ranch buttermilk dressing mix
2 drops cilantro essential oil
6 stalks green onions, sliced
4 golden pepperoncini peppers
1 drop lime essential oil
1 teaspoon sugar

Combine all ingredients in blender and refrigerate. Serve on salads, tortillas, and as a focaccia/herb bread dip.

Basic Vinaigrette

⅔ cup olive oil
½ cup champagne or wine vinegar
2-3 teaspoons sugar or 1-2 drops stevia, to taste
1 teaspoon shallots or white onion, finely grated
1 teaspoon Dijon mustard
¼ teaspoon minced garlic
1-2 drops wild orange, grapefruit, or invigorating blend essential oils

Shake ingredients to mix well, and enjoy.

Strawberry Basil Dressing

6 frozen strawberries
1 ½ tablespoons water
2 toothpicks basil essential oil, swirled, to taste
1 toothpick dip of liquid stevia to sweeten, or more to taste Pinch of salt

Defrost strawberries just enough to soften them for easy blending. Coursely blend. In small bowl add basil essential oil and stevia to water and swirl. Add water mixture and salt to strawberries. Blend well to make one serving. Great on spinach salad in lieu of poppy seed dressing or sweet vinaigrette.

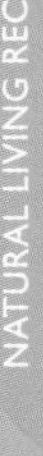

tips

- Essential oils absorb well into meats and make great marinades.
- When making vinegar dressings, pair ingredients. Balsamic or red wine vinegar (dark vinegars) pairs with raspberry or strawberry salads, beef, and lamb. White wine vinegar, rice, or champagne vinegars (light vinegars) go well with chicken, fish, pears, chunks of grapefruit, mango, or orange.
- Candied nuts and feta cheese go well with both dressings.

FERMENTED FOODS

COOKING

How To Make Wild Fermented Sauerkraut

Raw, unpasteurized sauerkraut delivers healthful probiotics to the digestive tract, increases body alkalinity, and increases nutrition absorption.

To make sauerkraut you will need a knife, cutting board, large mixing bowl, non-porous crock or Mason jar, and weighted jar.

Chop the cabbage into chunks of uniform size or shred into a bowl. Two heads of cabbage fill a ½ gallon jar nicely. Add any desired spices. Add coarse sea salt and mix throughout, using your hands to massage the mixture. The cabbage will begin to produce liquid (brine).

Using your fist or a wooden tamper, create an anaerobic environment by removing the air bubbles as you pack the vegetable mixture tightly into a crock or jar. Push until the brine starts to rise to the top of the veggies. Place a saucer or plate on top of the vegetables, covering them as closely to the edges as possible. Alternatively, use outer cabbage leaves to make a seal. Place a weight on top of the packed vegetables. A jar of water works well. Cover completely with a cloth and secure with a rubber band to keep bugs away.

During the first week, tamp the mixture down daily to help keep the veggies under the brine. Sometimes it takes a day or two to get the brine to stay above the veggies. This will help prevent mold from forming. Taste it after a week and see if you like it. You can let it ferment as long as you want, but most people prefer two to four weeks of fermentation in small batches. When it is too young, it will leave a carbonated feeling on your tongue, which disappears after about a week of fermentation.

The best temperature to ferment sauerkraut is 55-65 degrees. Put it in a pantry, root cellar, cupboard, or on your kitchen counter. A variation in this temperature is fine, but the best flavors develop within this range. When fermentation is complete, remove the weight, plate, or cabbage seal, scrape off the top layer, and enjoy the fresh healthy goodness below. Add essential oils after the sauerkraut is fermented.

Note: If mold forms, all is not lost. This is a test of your senses. Scrape off the mold and compost it. If the sauerkraut underneath smells okay, taste it. If it tastes "off," spit it out, and discard the batch!

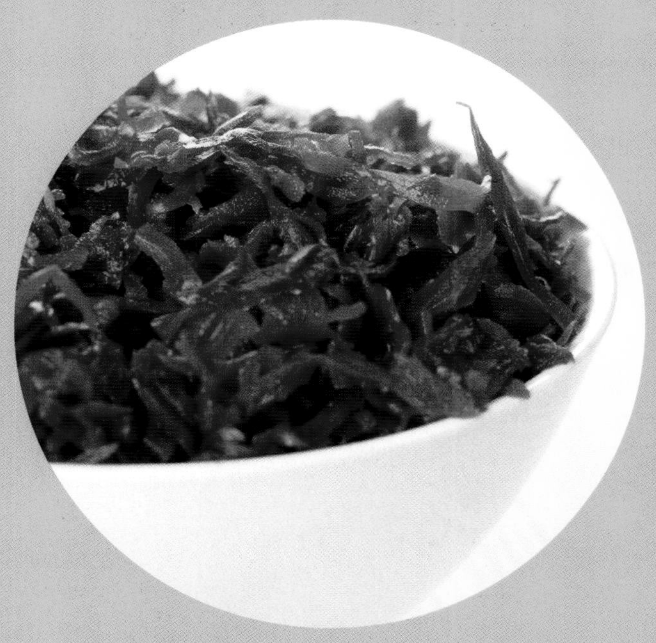

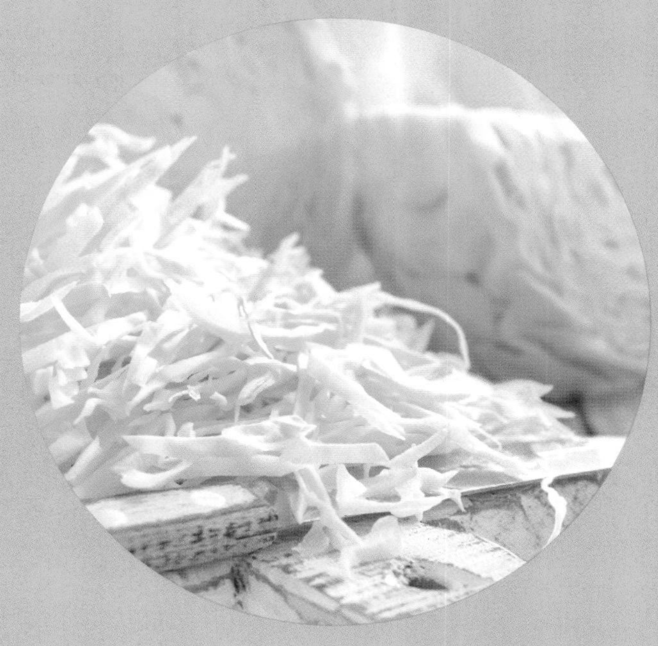

Basic Sauerkraut

1 to 1 ½ heads of cabbage
1 tablespoon sea salt per pound of cabbage
1 onion
2-3 tablespoons dill
2-3 tablespoons caraway seeds
2 drops of lemon essential oil to a pint size container of sauerkraut (after fermentation)

Red Cabbage & Apple Sauerkraut

1 to 1 ½ heads of red cabbage, finely shredded
2 Granny Smith apples, cored and shredded
¼ cup very thinly sliced red onion
1 tablespoon salt per pound of cabbage
5 whole peppercorns
3 whole cloves
1 cardamom pod
¼ teaspoon coriander seeds
⅛ teaspoon cinnamon

Combine cabbage, apple, and red onion. Sprinkle with salt and massage. Place the remaining ingredients in a small bowl. Crush with the back of a spoon or mortar and pestle. Add to cabbage mixture and follow basic recipe instructions.

Juniper Berry Sauerkraut

1 ½ to 2 heads red or green cabbage, shredded
1 to 1 ½ apples, peeled, cored, and coarsely chopped
1 tablespoon caraway seeds
1 ½ tablespoons juniper berries, crushed
1 tablespoon salt per pound of cabbage

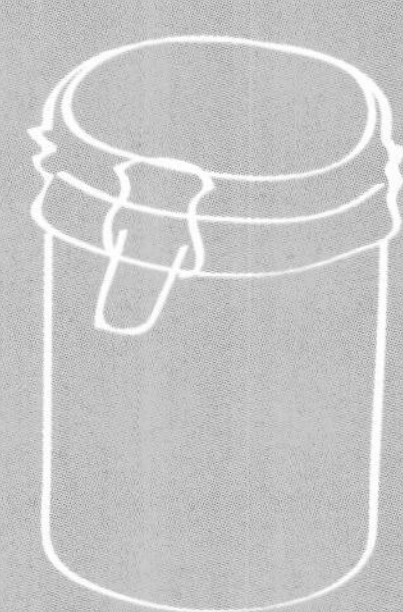

tip

You can use essential oils to flavor fermented foods after the fermenting process is completed. Simply add a toothpick-dip of your oil of choice to taste.

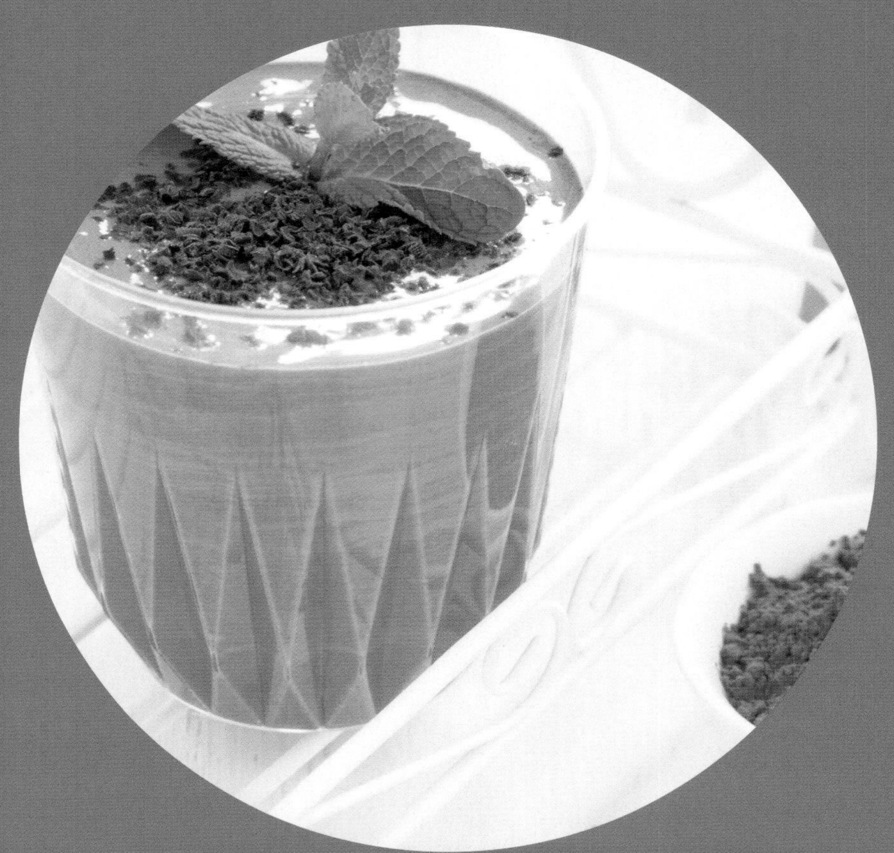

Organic Kefir with Blood Orange & Dark Chocolate

½ to 1 cup kefir
½ to 1 whole blood orange
A few squares of dark chocolate
2-4 drops citrus essential oil, optional
Mint leaves, optional

Pour the kefir in a bowl. Zest the orange, set aside. Peel the orange, cut into pieces, add to the kefir. Grate the dark chocolate over the kefir and oranges. Mix in the orange zest. Serve with a few mint leaves, if desired.

Kefir

Kefir is high in enzymes and probiotics and is alkalizing to the body. It stimulates mucosal immune response to protect from microbiological invasion of mucous membranes throughout the body. Kefir contains peptides that may restore normal immune function. Kefir is also good for lactose-intolerant people. The lactose found in milk is converted to lactic acid during the fermentation process.

1 tablespoon milk kefir grains
8-16 ounces goat or cow milk (raw, unpasteurized is the best choice)

Add 1 tablespoon kefir grains to 8-16 ounces of raw milk, place in a jar with a lid. Let it sit on the counter at room temperature for 24 to 72 hours, depending on how sour you like it and how warm your house is. Shake gently a couple times a day to redistribute the grains. When fermentation is complete, strain the milk and save the kefir grains to make a new batch. Put the strained kefir in a jar with a tight lid. Let it sit at room temperature for a few hours to increase fizziness. Then store in refrigerator.

Blueberry Kefir Smoothie

Blend together:
1 cup blueberries
1 cup kefir
2 large handfuls of greens
1 apple

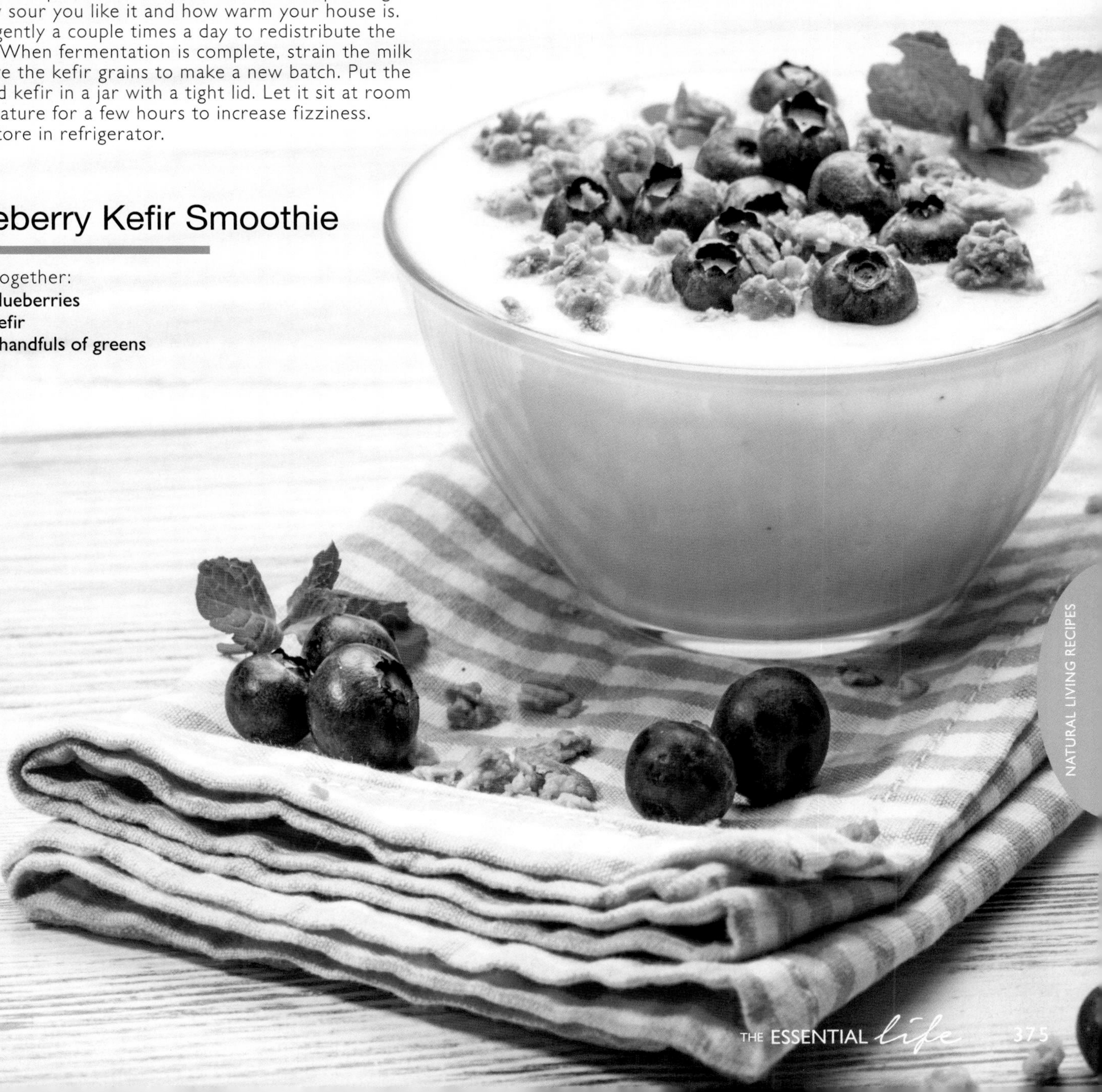

MAIN DISHES

COOKING

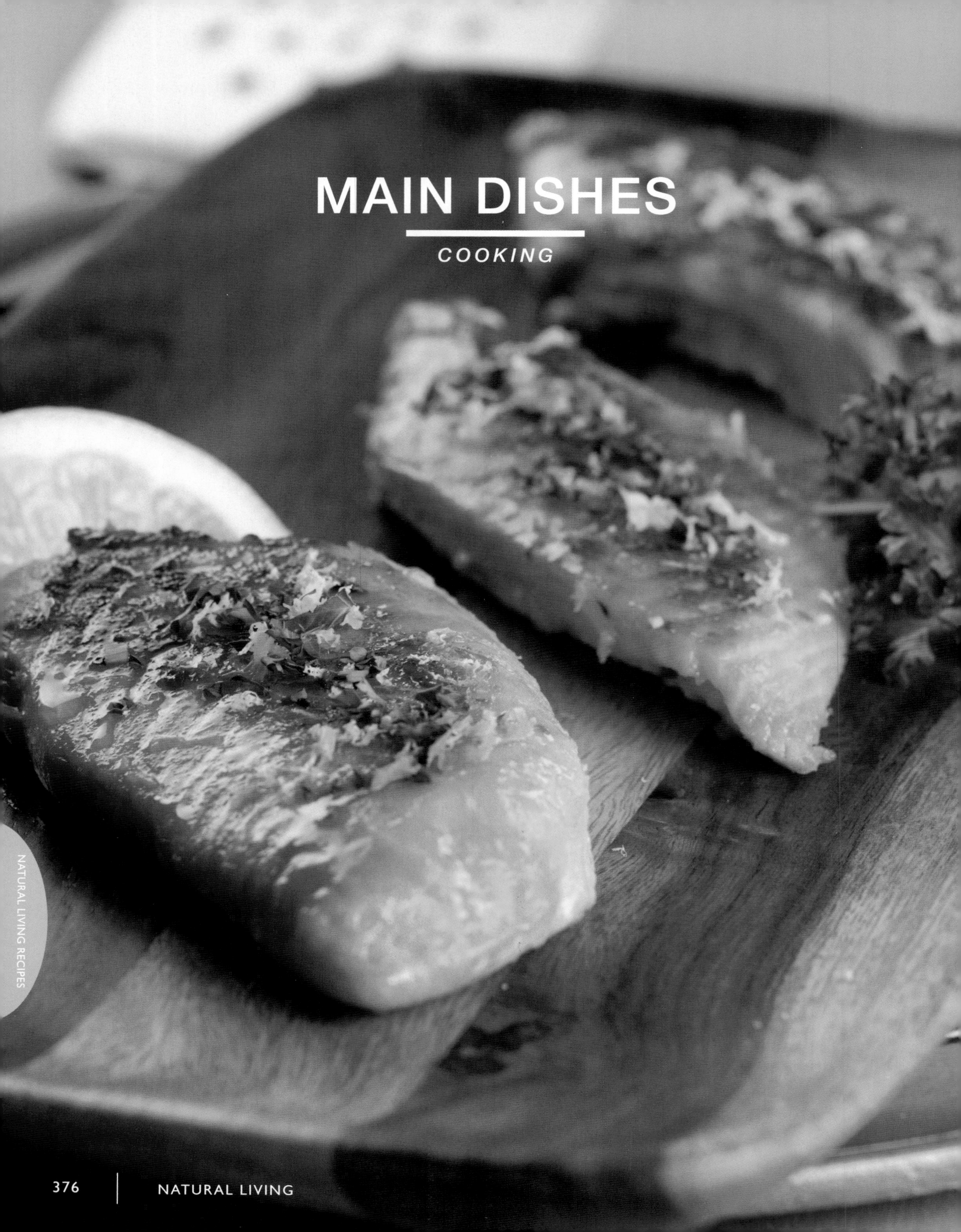

NATURAL LIVING RECIPES

Savory Brown Sugar Salmon

1 full filet salmon (½ salmon)

For marinade:
1 cup brown sugar
½ cup butter
¼ cup lemon juice
4 drops lemon essential oil

Put marinade ingredients in saucepan and warm over low heat, stirring until butter is melted and sugar is dissolved. Divide salmon fillet into two- to three-inch-wide steaks. Put marinade in a gallon zip-lock bag and add salmon pieces, flesh side down. Close bag tightly and marinate for at least 30 minutes.

Preheat broiler. Cover broiler pan with foil and place fish on pan, flesh side up. Broil until just flaky, drizzling marinade over fish while broiling. Turn and broil until skin starts to turn black. Remove pan from oven. Lift skin off fish with a fork and discard. Drizzle with marinade and broil for another minute or two. Turn again, pouring any remaining marinade over fish. Return to broiler and cook until fish is a light pink throughout. Place fish on a serving plate. Pour pan sauce over fish.

Lasagne Flavoring Ideas

To flavor your favorite lasagna recipes try:
Oregano essential oil (to taste)
Basil essential oil (to taste)
Rosemary essential oil (to taste)

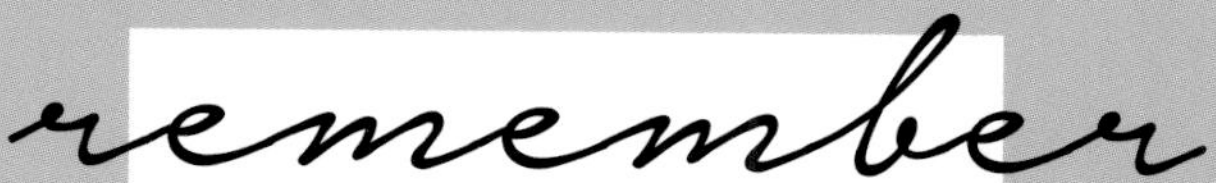

Certain essential oils go best with certain dishes.

- **Chicken:** basil, bergamot, black pepper, cassia, cilantro, cinnamon, ginger, grapefruit, lemon, lemongrass, lime, rosemary, tangerine sage, thyme, and wild orange.
- **Red meats**: basil, black pepper, cassia, cilantro, cinnamon, clove, coriander, fennel, ginger, grapefruit, lemongrass, lime, marjoram, oregano, wild orange, rosemary, tangerine, and thyme.
- **Vegetables:** basil, black pepper, cardamom, cilantro, fennel, ginger, grapefruit, lemon, lemongrass, and lime.

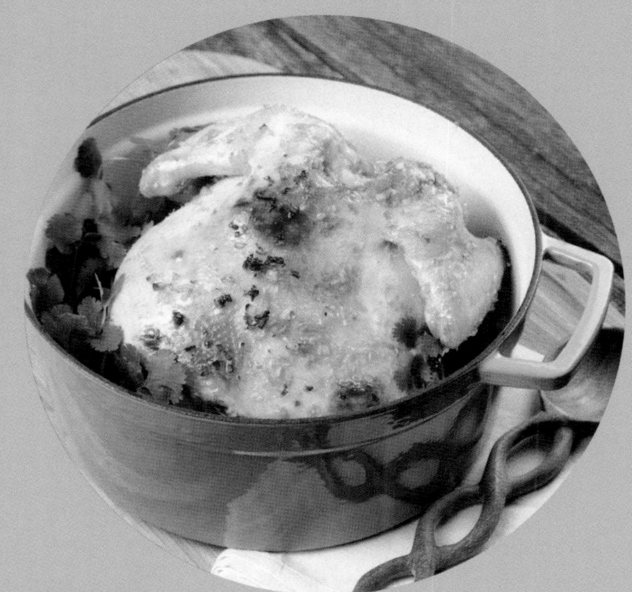

Thai Lemongrass Chicken

½ cup finely chopped lemongrass (3 or 4 stalks)
2 tablespoons finely chopped shallots
1 tablespoons finely chopped garlic
4 ½ teaspoons fish sauce
1 tablespoon soy sauce
1 pinch crushed red pepper flakes
1 ½ teaspoons kosher salt
2 tablespoons granulated sugar or 1 tablespoon agave
1 (3-4 pounds) whole chickens, rinsed and patted dry
2 tablespoons finely chopped fresh cilantro
1 tablespoon vegetable oil
3-4 drops lemongrass essential oil

In a nonreactive dish large enough to hold the chicken, combine all but 2 tablespoons of the lemongrass with all of the shallots, garlic, fish sauce, soy sauce, red pepper flakes, salt, and sugar. Add the chicken and turn it to coat, tucking some of the marinade underneath its skin. Pour any excess marinade into the bird's cavity. Marinate in the refrigerator for at least 3 hours, preferably overnight. Bring the chicken to room temperature before cooking it.

Heat the oven 350 degrees. Put the chicken, breast side down, on a rack in a roasting pan. Cook for 40 minutes. Turn the bird over and roast until the chicken is cooked and nicely browned, 20 to 30 minutes. The sugar in the marinade may cause the pan juices to burn, but this won't affect the chicken's flavor.

About 10 minutes before the chicken is done, combine the remaining 2 tablespoons of lemongrass with the cilantro and vegetable oil. Using a spoon, rub the mixture on the bird, spreading it evenly; continue roasting. The chicken is done when its juices run clear. Let the chicken sit for 10 minutes out of the oven before carving.

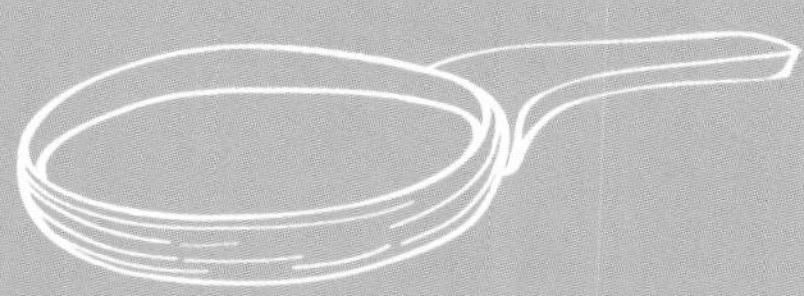

Herb-Marinated London Broil

1 London broil roast, pierced all over with a fork to absorb marinade
1 tablespoon white vinegar, sprinkled over roast and rubbed in to tenderize

For marinade:
1 cup red wine vinegar
½ cup olive oil
1 ½ tablespoons minced onion
2 teaspoons ground black pepper
1 drop black pepper essential oil
1 drop lemon essential oil
1 toothpick dip thyme essential oil
1 toothpick dip marjoram essential oil

Place London broil into baking dish to lay flat, cover with marinade. Let stand for at least 1 hour, turning every 15 minutes. Broil or grill to medium-rare or your preference. Let rest 10-15 minutes. Slice against the grain.

Oregano Parmesan Chicken

2 cups salad dressing
1 ½ cups fine grated Parmesan cheese
2-3 drops oregano essential oil (to taste, start with 2 drops)
4 boneless skinless chicken breasts

Mix salad dressing and Parmesan cheese. Add enough oregano essential oil to convey flavor, but not to overpower. Spoon over chicken. Bake at 350 degrees for approximately 45 minutes or until chicken is cooked to an internal temperature of 165 degrees. Serve with rice.

Enjoy!

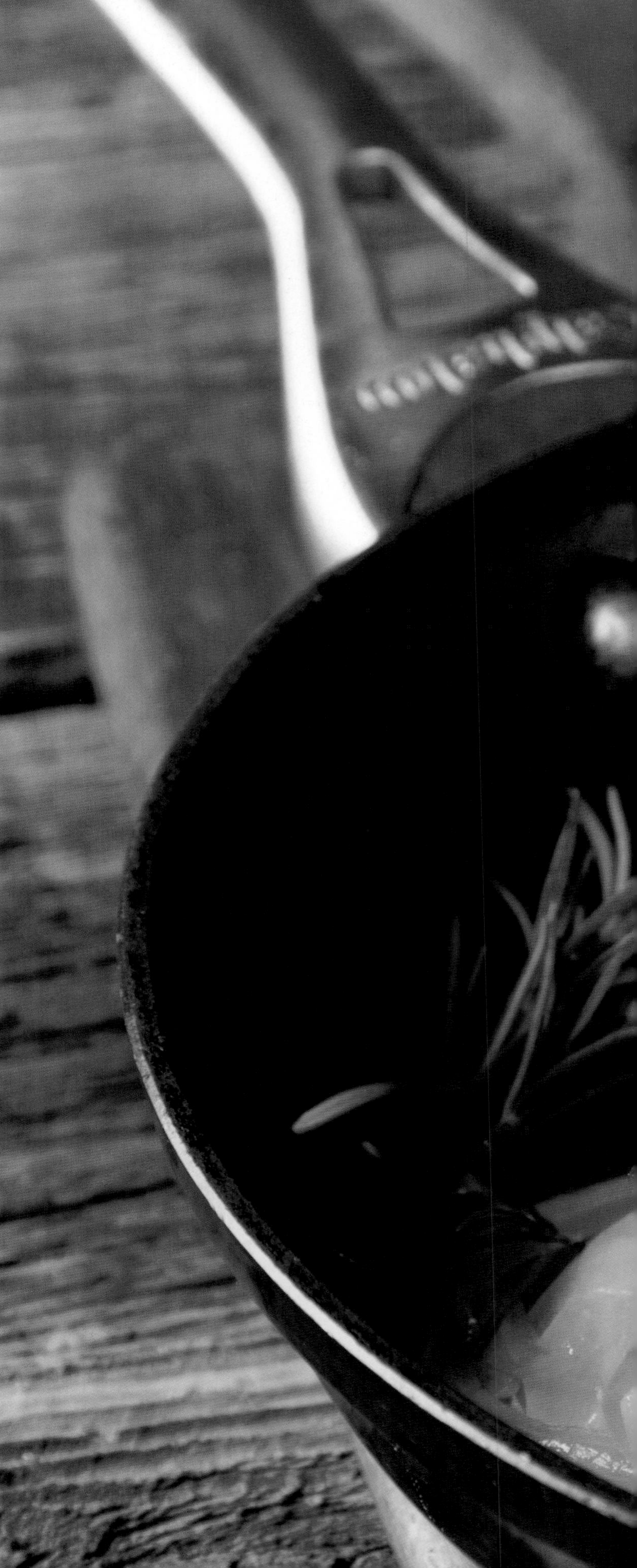

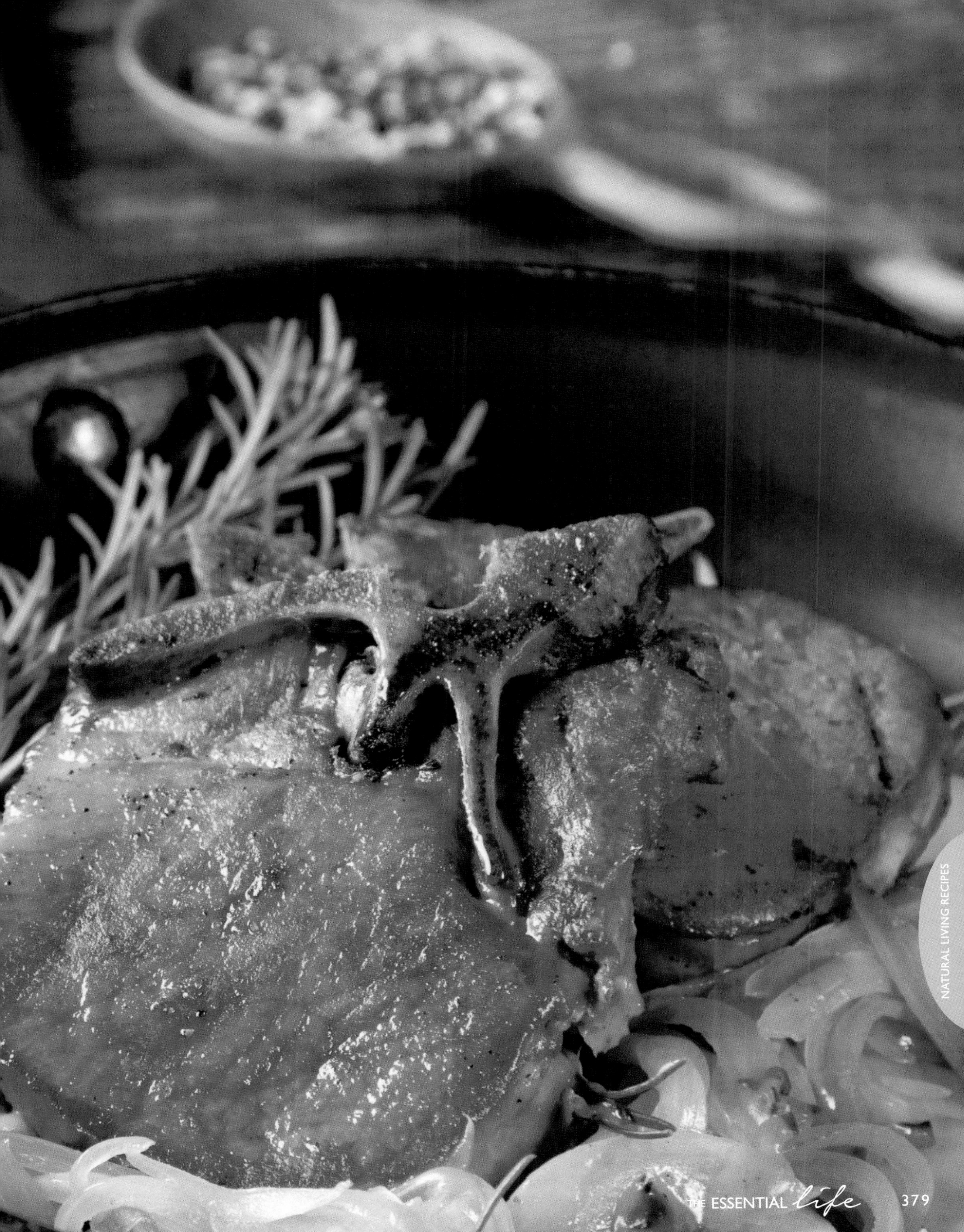

SALADS

COOKING

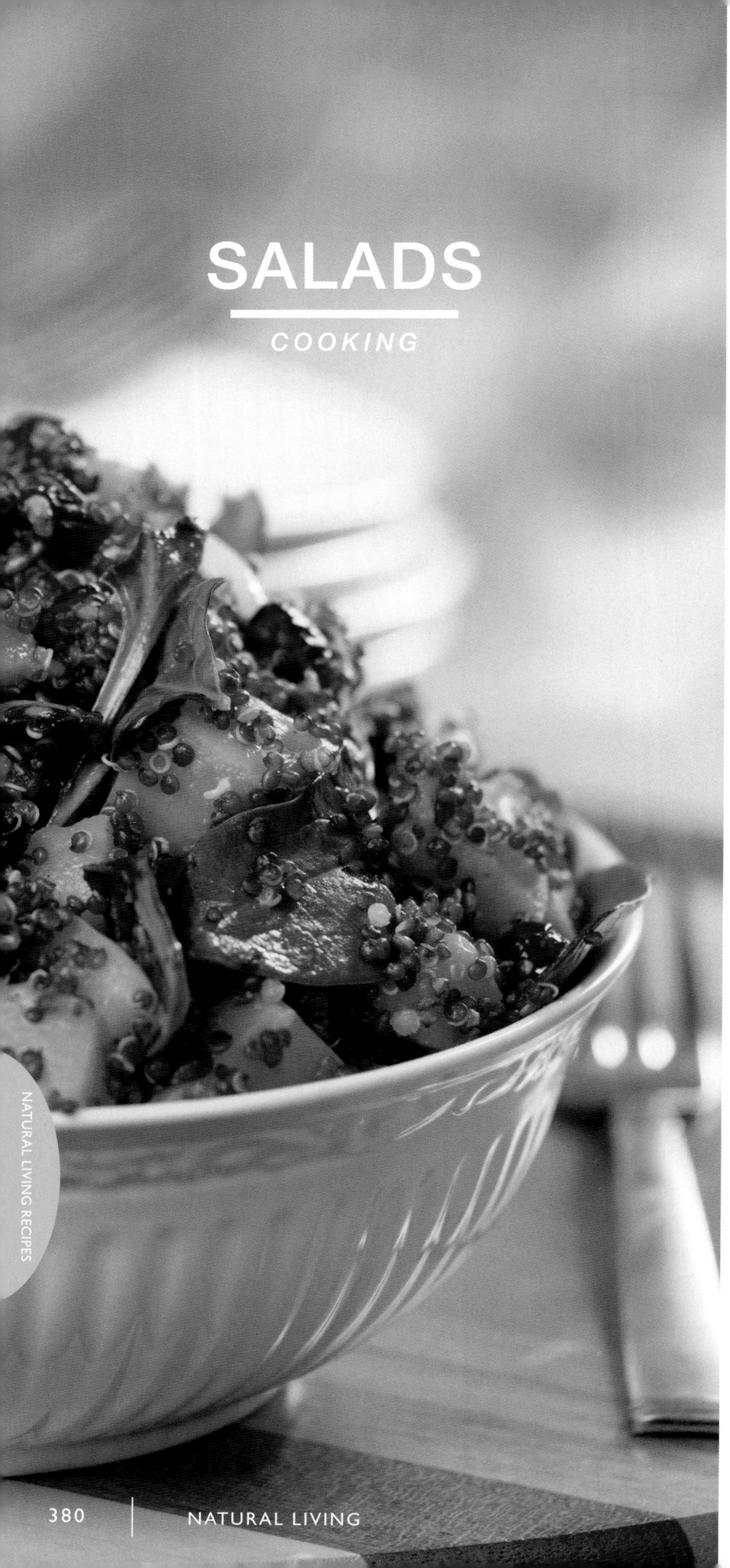

Warm Roasted Butternut Squash & Quinoa Salad

¾ cup dried cranberries
¾ cups baby spinach leaves
1 tablespoon fresh lemon juice
1 tablespoon raw honey
1 tablespoon olive oil
Large pinch of salt
1 toothpick black pepper essential oil
1 butternut squash, peeled and cut into a medium dice
½ teaspoon coarse salt
½ large sweet onion, thinly sliced
4 cups red quinoa, cooked and kept warm
1 ½ cup wheat berries, cooked kept warm

Place the spinach and dried cranberries in a large bowl. Cover and set aside.
Combine the lemon juice, honey, 1 tablespoon oilve oil, pinch of salt, and black pepper essential oil in a small bowl and whisk until combined. Set aside.
Preheat the oven to 425 degrees. Line a baking pan with tin foil.
Toss the diced butternut squash with 1 tablespoon olive oil and ½ teaspoon salt. Spread the squash out evenly on the tin foil lined baking sheet.
Roast the squash on the top rack of the oven for 15-20 minutes, or until squash is tender and turning golden brown on top. Remove from oven.
White the squash is roasting, place the ½ tablespoon olive oil in a small saute pan and heat to medium/high. Add the sweet onion and saute for 2 minutes. Reduce the heat to medium and continue to saute for another 5-6 minutes until the onion is lightly caramelized.
Add the hot butternut squash, hot onions, warm quinoa and wheat berries to the bowl of spinach and cranberries. Toss together to slightly wilt the spinach. Add the dressing and toss until well coated.
Serve warm.

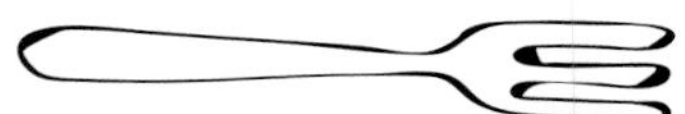

tips

- Use essential oils to infuse into olive oil and make seasoned croutons.
- See Spiced Almond recipe in Snacks to add crunch to your salads.
- See Dressings recipes as a companion to salad recipes.
- Essential oils are a fantastic addition to pasta salads.

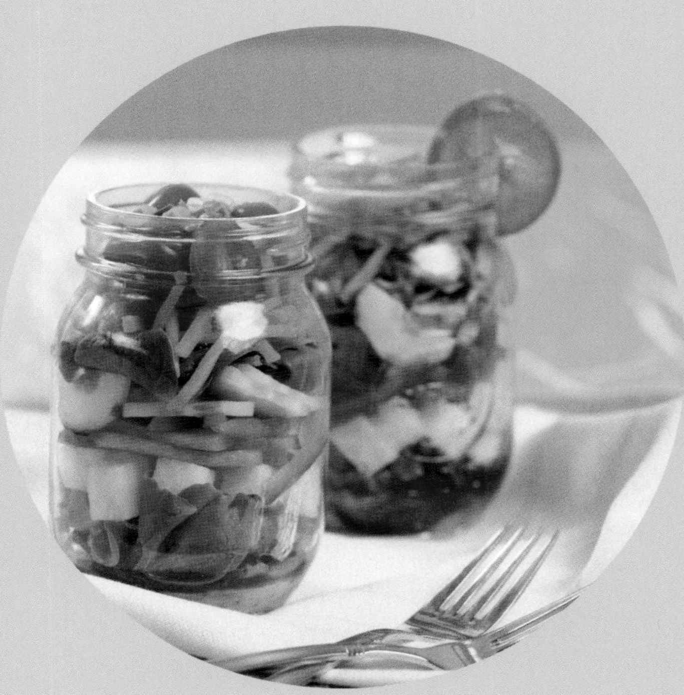

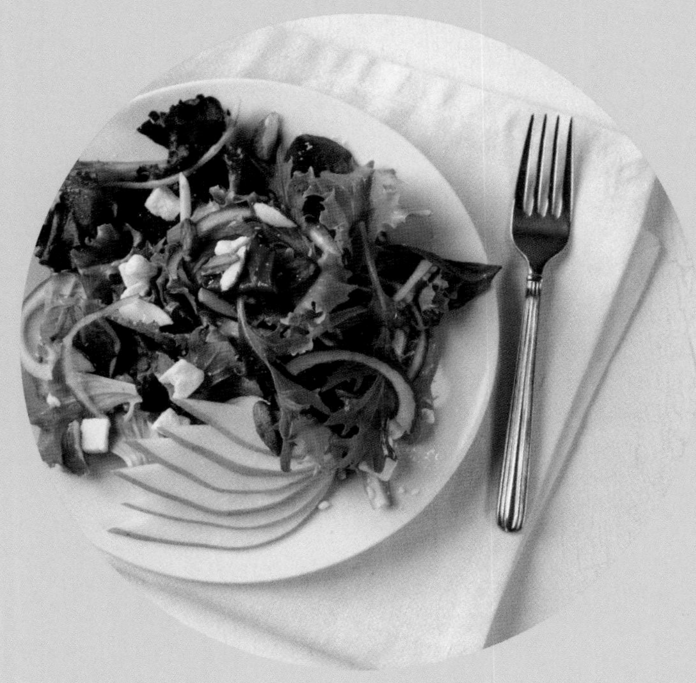

Salad in a Jar

½ lemon
1 toothpick swirl basil essential oil
Pinch salt
2 drops lemon or lime essential oil
1 tablespoon olive oil
Preferred salad vegetables

Into a quart-sized jar, squeeze ½ lemon and swirl in basil essential oil. Add salt, olive oil, and lemon or lime essential oil. Fill the jar with vegetables, adding the firmest vegetables first and placing salad greens at the top. Refrigerate. Salad lasts several days in the refrigerator. Before serving, turn jar upside down and shake to disperse dressing. Serve salad on large bowl or plate. If desired, add avocado, croutons, or other toppings.

Pear & Cheese Salad

4 cups mixed baby greens
⅓-½ cup crumbled goat, Gorgonzola, bleu, or feta cheese
1 pear, thinly sliced
¼-½ cup thinly sliced red onion
Crushed pecans or caramelized almonds
Pomegranate seeds, sprinkled on top (optional)

Top with Basic Vinaigrette dressing recipe (pg 371), using champagne vinegar and lemon essential oil for the citrus oil. Toss.

SAUCES & SEASONINGS

COOKING

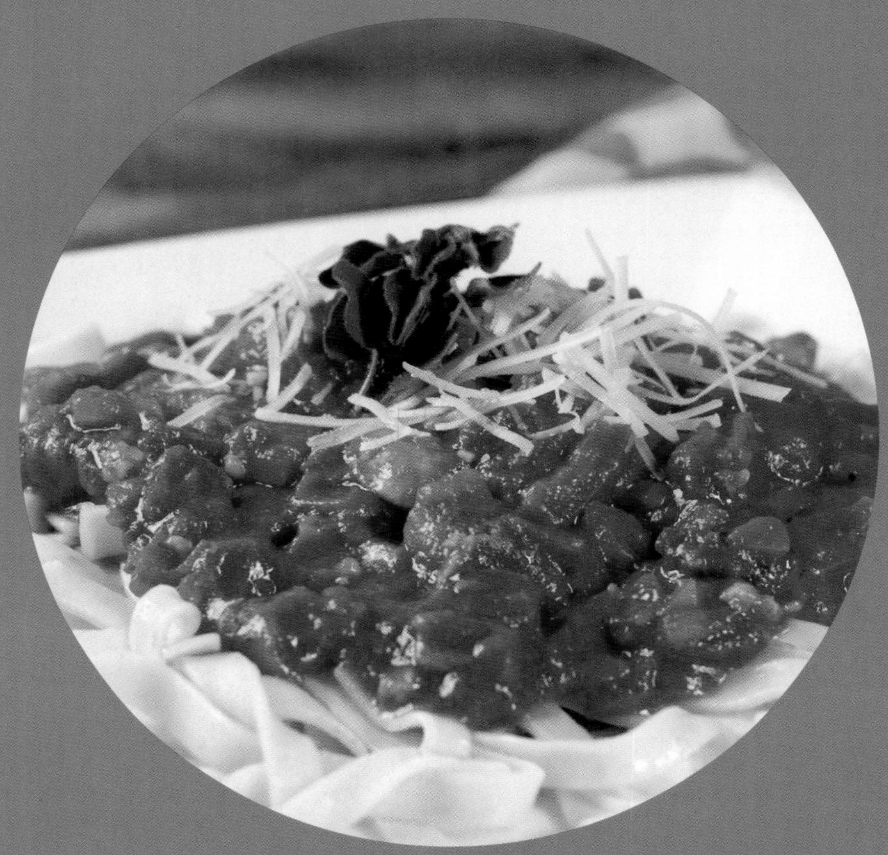

Fast & Easy Spaghetti Sauce

1 can diced or stewed tomatoes, drained
1 16 ounce can tomato sauce
1 4 ounce can tomato paste
4 ounces hot sausage or Italian sausage, pork or chicken is fine
4 to 6 ounces fresh mushrooms, sliced
1 medium onion, diced
1 medium bell pepper, diced

Garlic powder – start with 2 teaspoon and add to taste
Onion powder – start with 1 teaspoon
Basil essential oil – 1 toothpick dip and swirl into sauce, to start
Oregano essential oil – 1 toothpick dip and swirl into sauce, to start
Black pepper essential oil – 1 drop and more to taste

Cook onions until soft. Add sausage, cook until no longer pink. Add mushrooms and cook. Add tomatoes and cook for a few minutes. Add tomato paste and stir to combine. Add tomato sauce and stir to combine. Season with essential oils and spices, adding more to your taste. Once it's seasoned right, it's ready to serve.

Enjoy!

5 Star BBQ Sauce

2 cups ketchup
1 cups water
⅔ cup light brown sugar
½ cup apple cider vinegar
1 ¼ tablespoons Worcestershire sauce
½ tablespoon onion powder
½ tablespoon garlic, minced
½ tablespoon ground mustard
2 toothpick swirls liquid smoke
2 drops black pepper essential oil
1-2 drops lemon essential oil

Combine all ingredients except essential oils in saucepan, bring to boil. Reduce to low heat, add essential oils. Simmer, stirring often, 1 ½ hours.

Lemon-Parmesan Sauce for Fish

¾ cup mayonnaise (or vegan substitute)
⅔ cup grated Parmesan cheese
4-5 drops lemon essential oil
2 lemons, thinly sliced
Sliced fresh parsley

Mix ingredients well. Top each portion of cooked fish with sauce; broil 2-3 minutes until sauce puffs and turns golden brown. Garnish with sliced lemons and fresh parsley.

Salsa Flavoring Ideas

To flavor your favorite salsa recipe try adding:
Lime essential oil (to taste)
Toothpick dip cilantro essential oil (or to taste)
Toothpick dip black pepper essential oil (or to taste)

Pesto Flavoring Ideas

To your favorite pesto recipe, add one or all of the following:
1 toothpick dip black pepper essential oil (or to taste)
1 toothpick dip basil essential oil (or to taste)
1 toothpick dip lemon essential oil (or to taste)

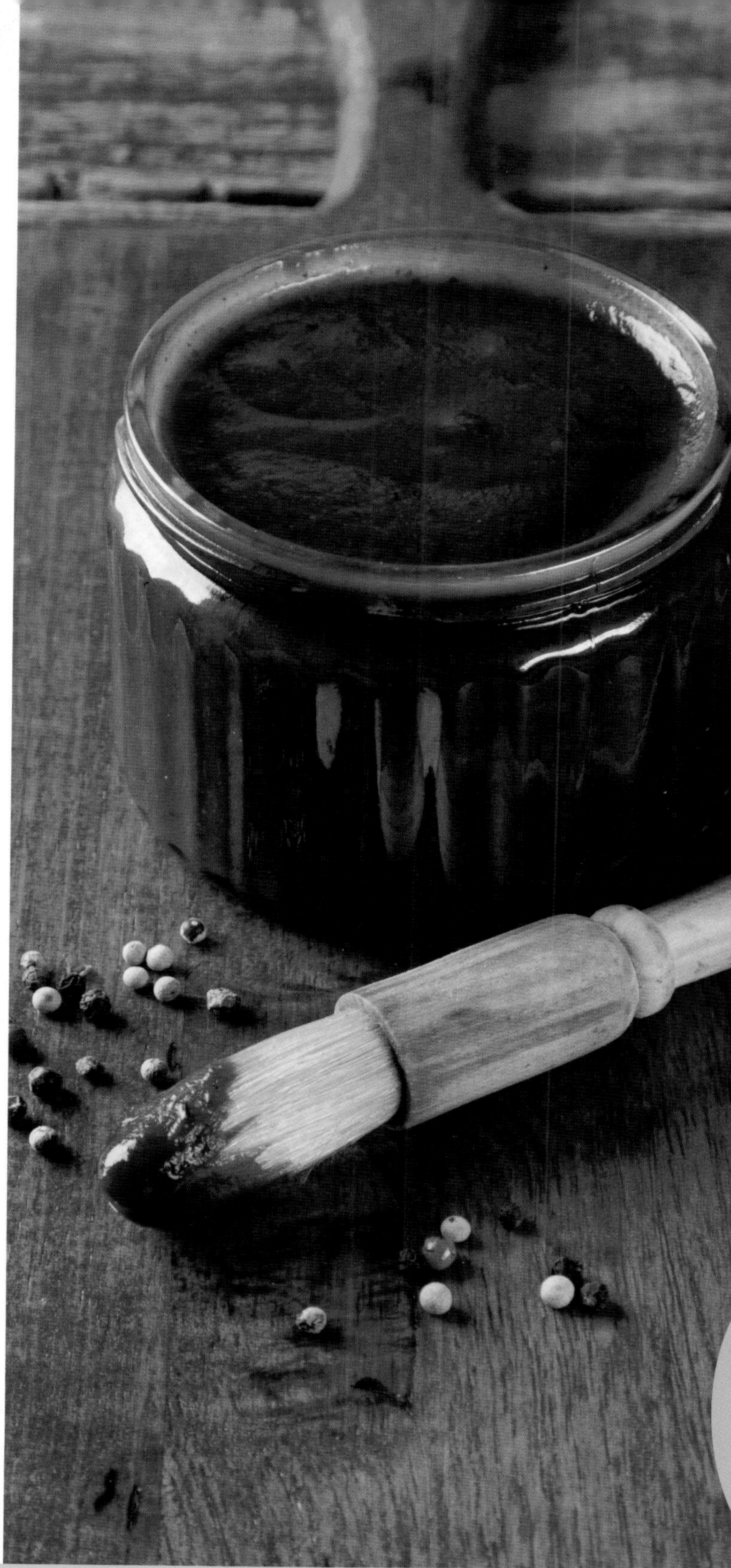

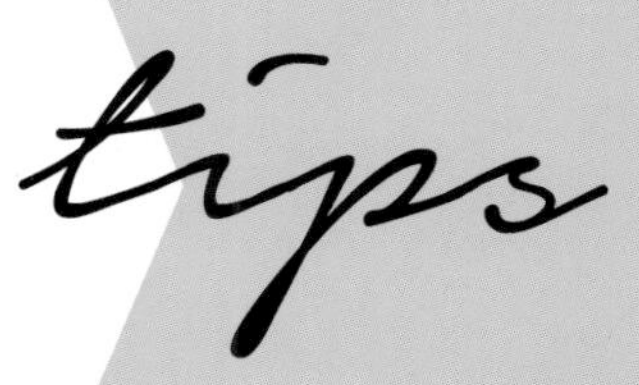

- Make a sweet glaze for chicken or fish by adding essential oils to honey and brushing on chicken or fish before baking.
- Add lemon essential oil to homemade hollandaise sauce.
- Use essential oils to make a honey dip for chicken wings.

Make herbed butters for steaks by adding favorite savory oils to whipped butter.

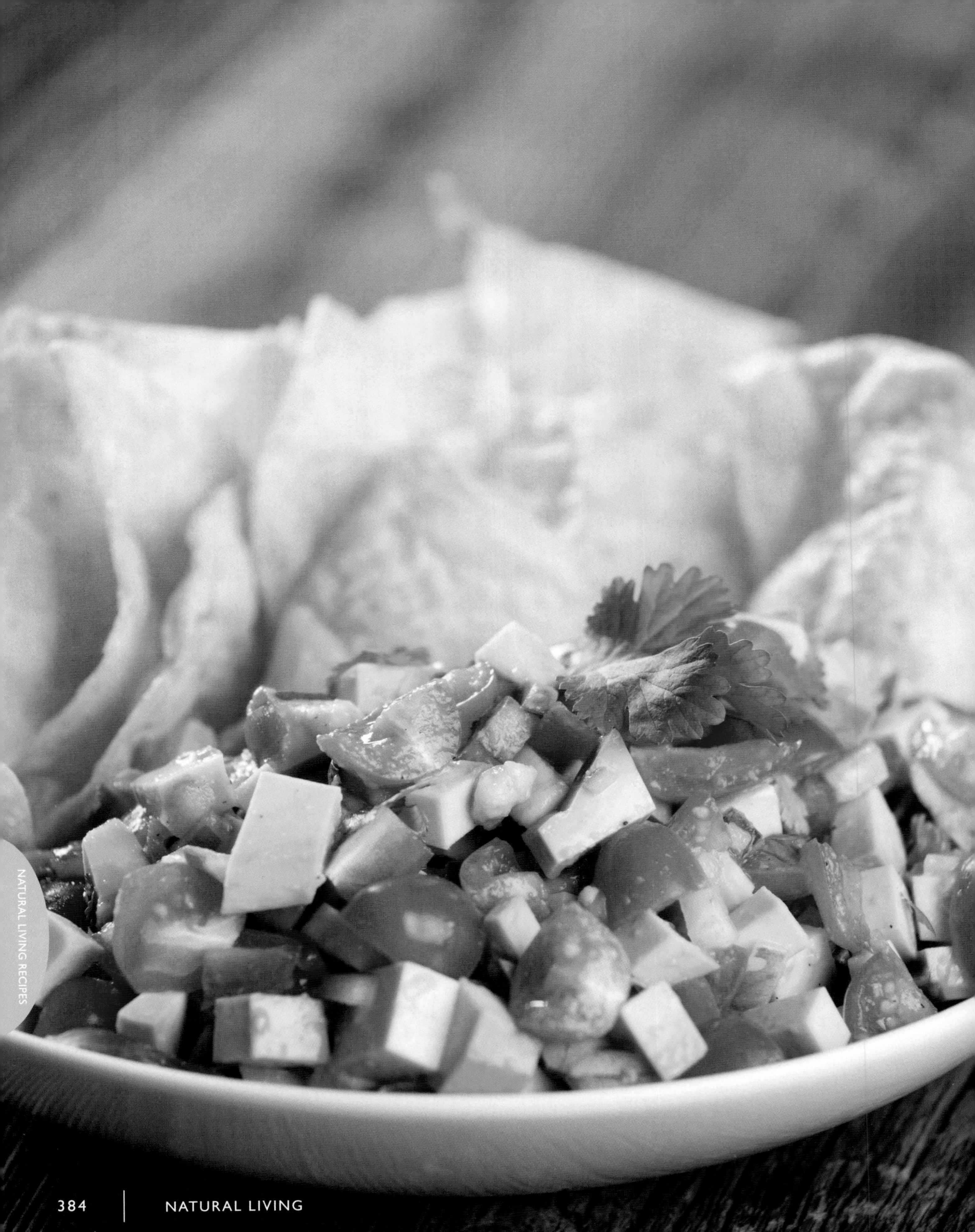

Avocado Salsa

6 medium roma tomatoes (20 ounces), seeded and diced
1 cup chopped red onion, chopped
1 large or 2 small jalapeños, seeded and chopped (1/4 cup. Leave seeds if you like heat)
3 medium avocados, semi-firm but ripe, peeled cored and diced
3 1/2 tablespoons olive oil
3 table spoons fresh lime juice
1 clove garlic, finely minced
1/2 teaspoons salt (more or less to taste as desired)
1/4 teaspoon freshly ground black pepper
1/2 cup loosely packed cilantro leaves, chopped

Place red onion in a strainer or sieve and rinse under cool water to remove harsh bite. Drain well. Add to a mixing bowl along with diced tomatoes, jalapeños and avocados.
In a separate small mixing bowl whisk together olive oil, lime juice, garlic, salt and pepper until mixture is well blended. Pour mixture over avocado mixture, add cilantro then gently toss mixture to evenly coat. Serve with tortilla chips or over Mexican entrees.

Italian Blend Salt

2 tablespoons sea salt
1 drop each: rosemary, basil, oregano, and thyme essential oils
Blend and reserve in airtight container.

5 Spice Sugar Blend

2 tablespoons cane sugar coarse
1 drop cinnamon essential oil
1 drop cardamom essential oil
1 drop black pepper essential oil
1 drop wild orange essential oil
1 drop clove essential oil
Blend and reserve in airtight container.

Asian Blend

2 tablespoons sea salt
2 drops ginger essential oil
2 drops lemongrass essential oil
1 drop basil essential oil
Blend and reserve in airtight container.

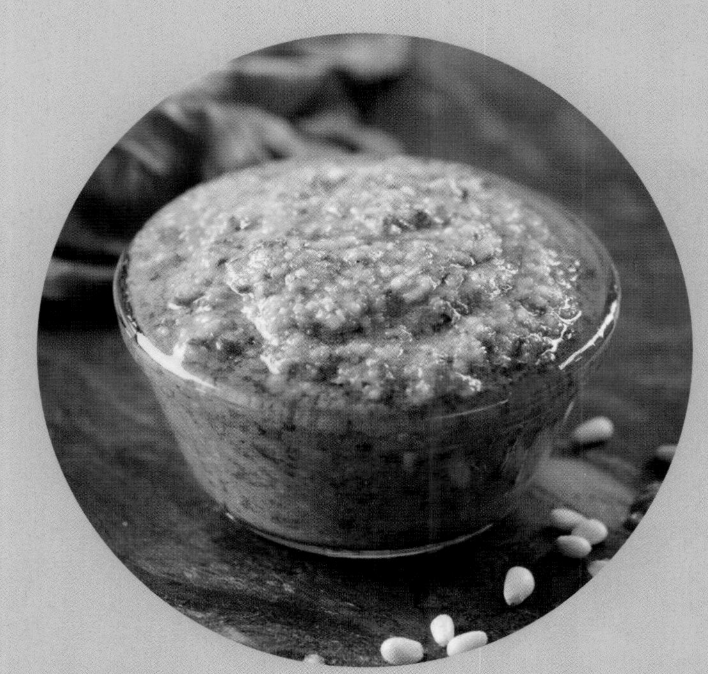

Pesto

3 cups basil leaves, loosely packed
3 small or 2 large cloves garlic
1/3 cup pine nuts
2/3 - 3/4 cup olive oil
1 toothpick dip black pepper essential oil
1 toothpick dip basil essential oil
1 toothpick dip lemon essential oil
1/2 cup freshly grated Parmesan cheese

Combine all ingredients in blender or food processor. If in blender, blend 1/2 the ingredients well, then add the rest and pulse-blend till pesto has reached desired consistency. Add more olive oil if too dry. If making in a food processor, add all ingredients and chop till well blended and has reached desired consistency. Store in refrigerator in airtight container. Excellent on pasta, fish, chicken, add to fresh salsa.

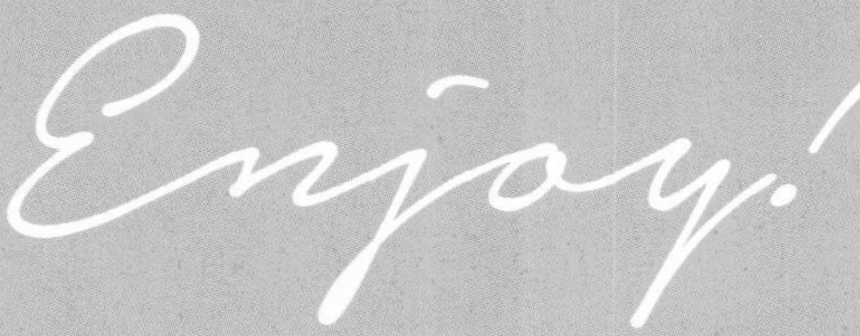

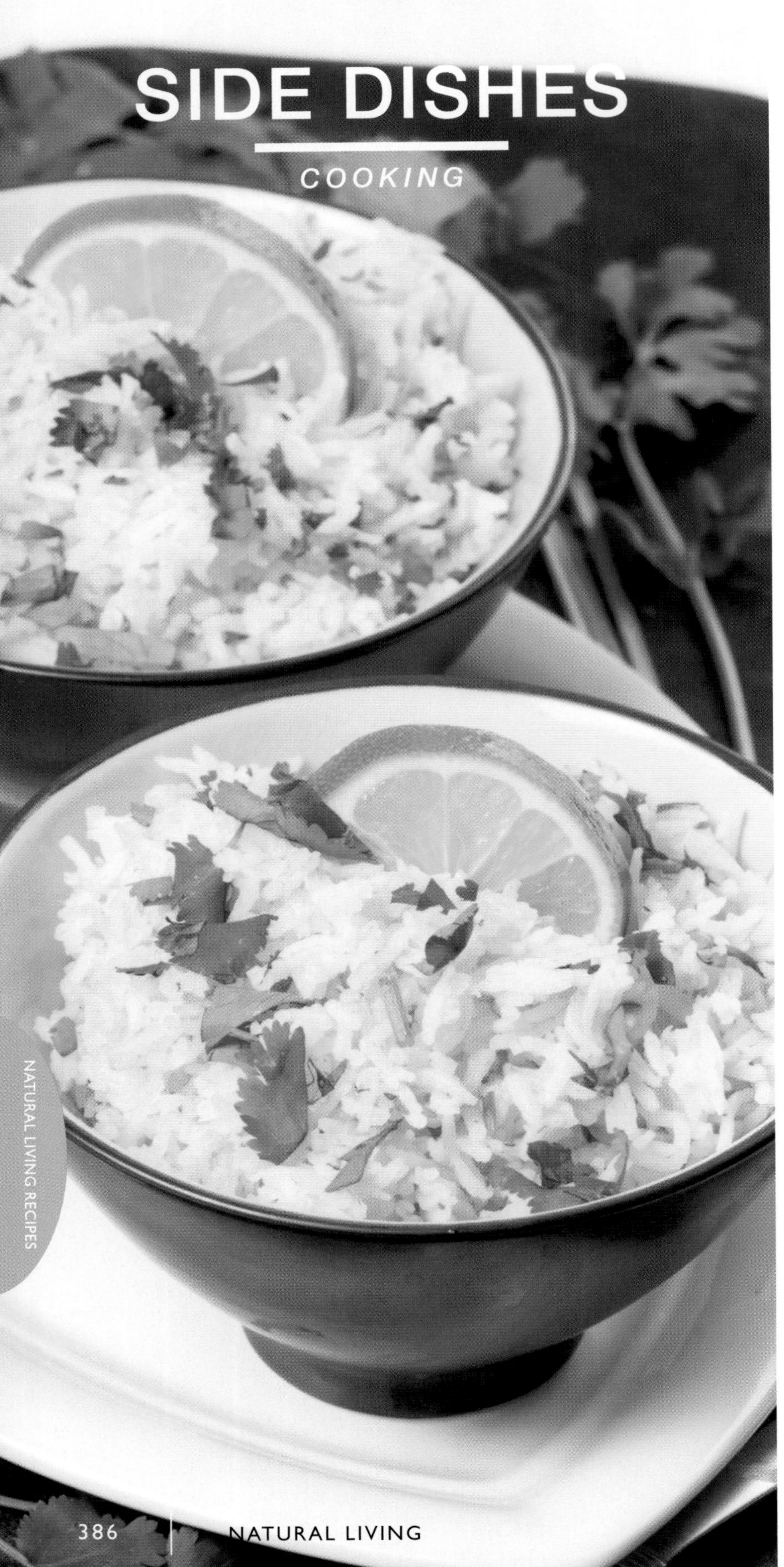

Lime Cilantro Rice

2 cups water
1 tablespoon coconut oil
2 drops lime essential oil
1 cup white rice
½ toothpick swirl cilantro essential oil
½ cup green chili salsa
Fresh cilantro

Dash of sea salt and ground pepper

Bring water to a boil, and add coconut oil, essential oils, and rice. Cover and reduce to low heat. Simmer until rice is tender, approximately 20 minutes. Stir in salsa and chopped cilantro, and add salt and pepper to taste.

Veggie & Pineapple Stir Fry

⅓ cup soy sauce
1 can pineapple chunks with juice (no sugar added)
2 teaspoons sesame oil
2 teaspoons peanut oil
2 red bell peppers, sliced
1 cup sliced squash
1 cup bok choy sliced in small pieces
½ cup snow peas
1 carrot, sliced thin
1 bunch green onions
1 drop ginger essential oil
1 toothpick dip lemongrass essential oil

You can also add 12 ounce pork, seitan or tofu strips.
Separate the pineapple chunks from the pineapple juice. In ½ cup of reserved pineapple juice, add soy sauce, sesame oil, ginger essential oil and grapefruit essential oil. In skillet, sauté carrots, squash, and peppers in peanut oil for about 5 minutes. Add in pineapple mix, and then add green onion, bok choy, snow peas and pineapple. Let cook for a few minutes.
**Protein version: If using pork, seitan or tofu, use all of the pineapple juice and add to sauce and let sit for 20-30 minutes. For cooking, if it's seitan or pork, sauté in oil before adding veggies then follow remaining steps as stated above. If using tofu, follow steps above and add with the sauce.

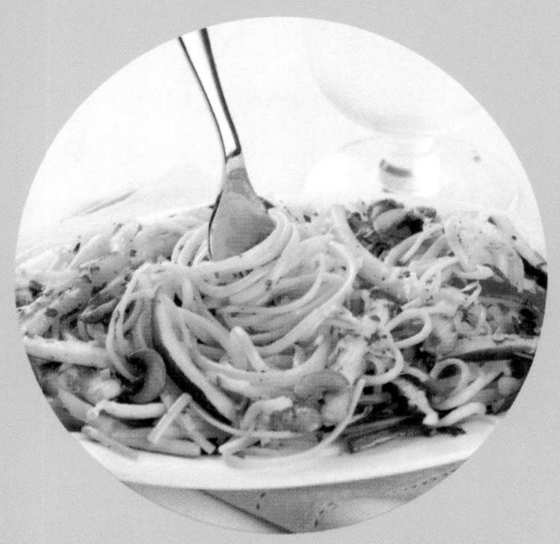

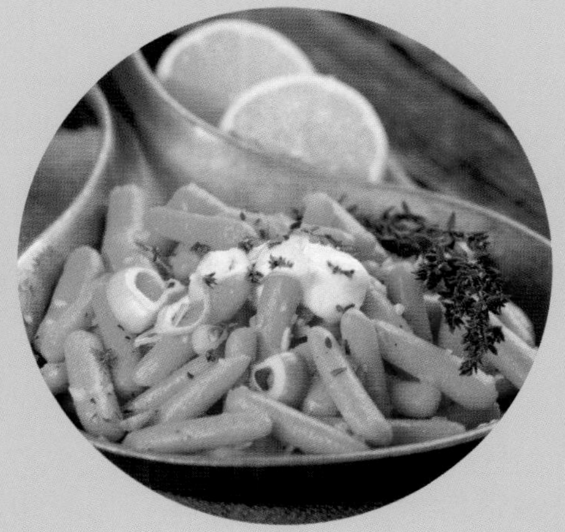

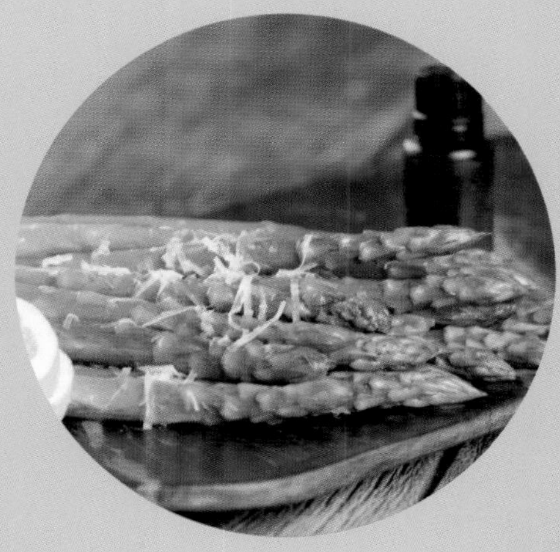

Zucchini Mushroom Pasta

- 1 pound medium zucchini, julienned
- 1 pound medium mushrooms, sliced thin
- 3 tablespoons olive oil
- 1 cup green onions, sliced thinly
- 2 cloves minced garlic
- 1-2 toothpick dips basil oil to taste
- 1 toothpick dip black pepper oil
- ½ teaspoon sea salt
- 3 tablespoon butter, softened
- ¼ teaspoon sea salt or to taste and pepper to taste
- 2 teaspoon parsley
- 1 ½ cups grated Parmesan cheese, divided
- 1 pound noodles of your choice

Start cooking pasta in a sauce pan. In a large skillet over medium heat, sauté onions until just tender. Add garlic and cook another minute. Add zucchini and cook until fork can be inserted, but still a little firm. Sprinkle salt and pepper, then add mushrooms, and sauté until tender. Remove from heat. When pasta is done, drain and put in serving bowl. Add essential oil to butter; toss butter in with warm pasta along with parsley, green onion, and ¾ cup grated Parmesan cheese. Once butter is melted, toss in veggies. Top with remaining freshly grated Parmesan cheese.

Carrots With Sweet & Spicy Yogurt

- 1 tablespoon + 2 teaspoons olive oil
- 2 ½ tablespoon finely chopped shallots
- ¼ teaspoon sea salt
- 1 toothpick dip thyme essential oil
- 1 toothpick dip black pepper essential oil
- Shake of ground pepper
- 2 pounds baby carrots
- Sweet and Spicy Yogurt Topping, recipe below

In bowl, mix all ingredients but carrots and yogurt topping. Add carrots and stir to coat. Transfer carrots onto baking pan and oven roast at 425 degrees for approximately 18-20 minutes or until tender. Remove from oven and transfer to serving dish. Top with the following dressing and serve.

Sweet & Spicy Yogurt Topping

- ⅔ cup plain yogurt
- 2-3 teaspoons olive oil
- 1 teaspoon honey
- Dash of ground red pepper
- Sea salt to taste

Mix together and serve over prepared carrots.

Lemon Parmesan Asparagus

- 12-16 asparagus spears
- 2 ½ tablespoons olive oil
- 1 toothpick dip or swirl (to taste) lemon essential oil
- Salt and pepper to taste
- 2 tablespoons shredded Parmigiano-Reggiano cheese

Wash asparagus spears, chop off ends, and place on baking sheet, preferably stone. Add lemon essential oil to olive oil and mix well. Drizzle over asparagus spears, place asparagus on pan, rub in oil until pan and spears are evenly coated. Salt and pepper to taste. Broil on high for 5-6 minutes on the middle oven rack. Sprinkle cheese evenly over spears and broil 1-2 minutes longer till cheese is melted. Serve.

tips

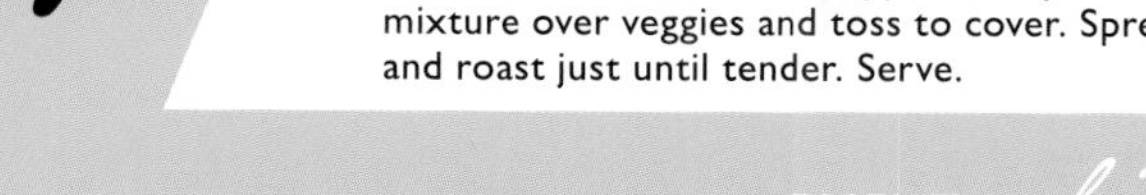

- Use a produce rinse for healthier and fresher tasting fruit, berries, and vegetables, including greens. Fill a clean glass or metal bowl with water. Add 1 tablespoon white vinegar and 2-3 drops lemon essential oil. Rinse produce, and place on clean paper towels or cotton cloth to dry.
- For oven-roasted veggies, add your favorite essential oils to taste to olive oil. Add salt and pepper until you like the flavor. Pour oil mixture over veggies and toss to cover. Spread out on cookie sheet and roast just until tender. Serve.

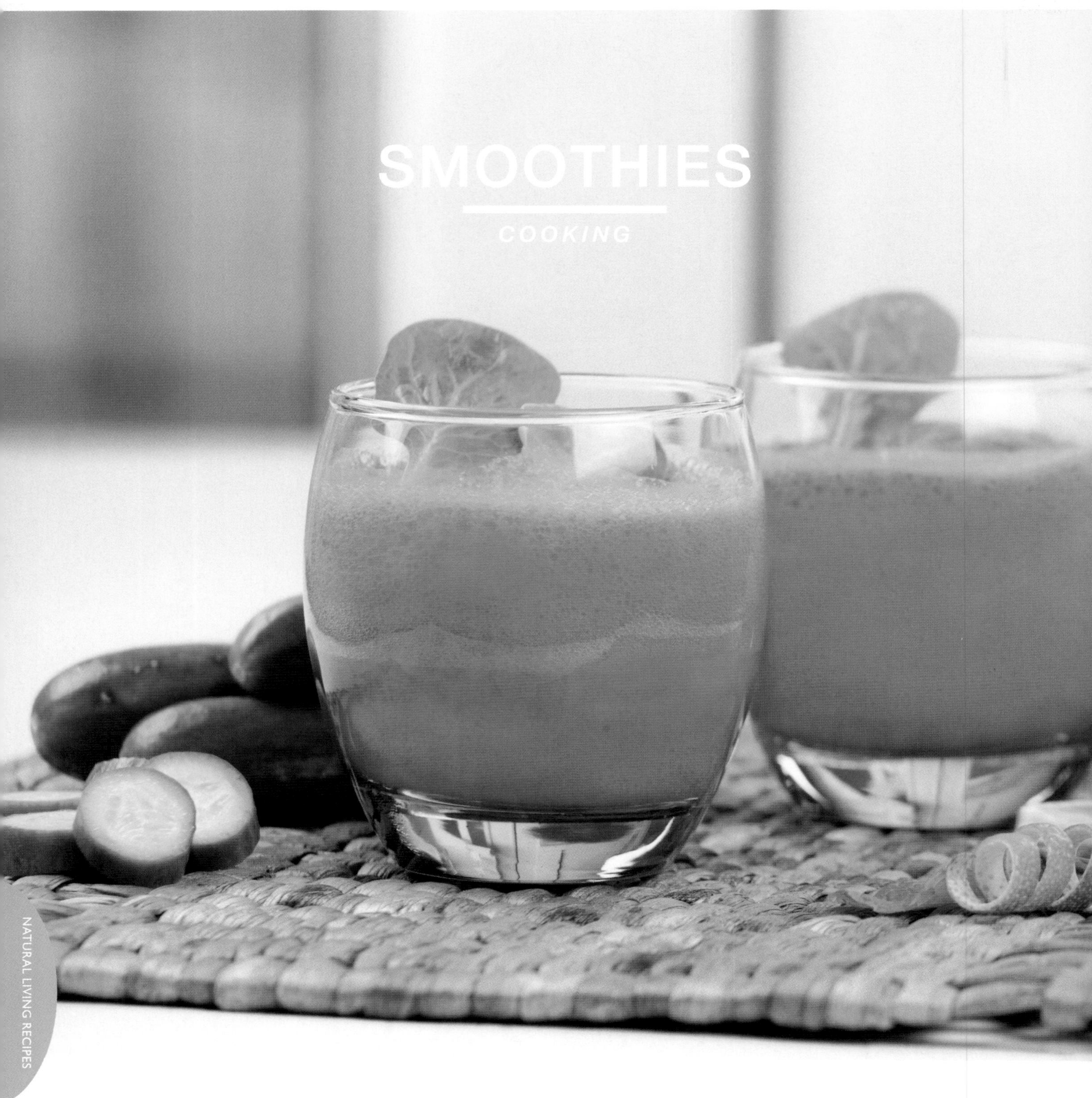

Basic formula:

2 cups liquid base
2 cups leafy greens
3 cups ripe or frozen fruit
Essential oils to taste

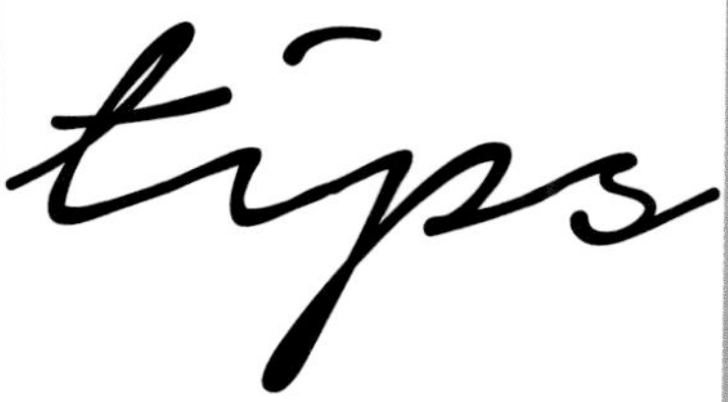

- You can use a glass regular-mouth jar (i.e. canning jar) in lieu of a regular blender container. Simply unscrew the base and blade from the blender container, put the blade over the mouth of the jar, then screw on the base. This is perfect for small portions, nuts, pestos, etc. It's a time saver too!
- Add extra nutrition to your smoothie by adding any of the following:
  - Ground flaxseed
  - Coconut oil
  - Chia seeds
  - Protein powder
- When blending, put liquid in first followed by greens and chunks of fruit and ice.

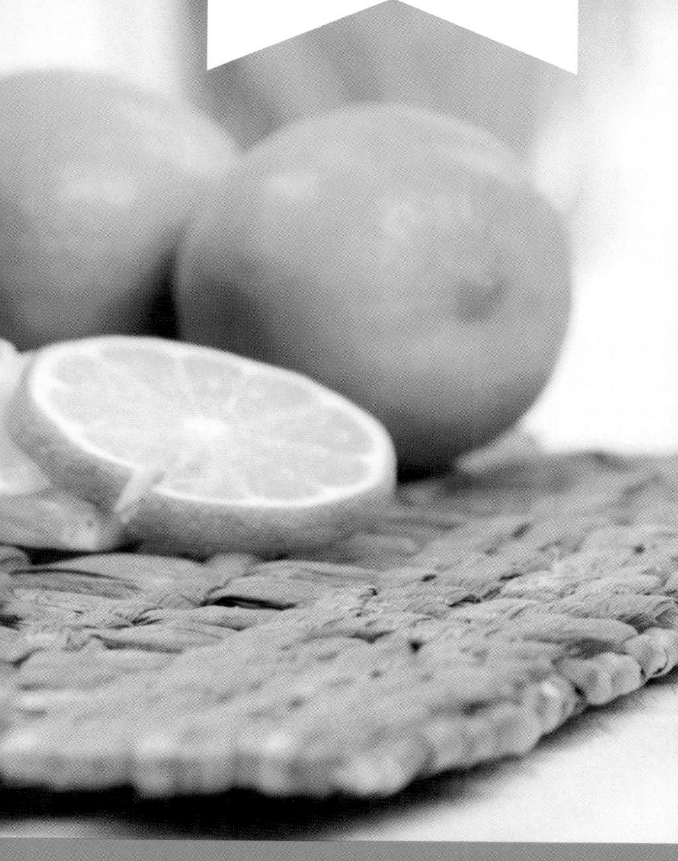

Tropical Green Smoothie

Blend together:
2 ½ cups spinach
1 mango, peeled and pit removed
⅔ cup vanilla almond milk
2-3 drops wild orange essential oil
1 toothpick swirled ginger essential oil (optional)
1 ¼ cups ice

Berry Banana Smoothie

Blend together:
2 cups spinach
1 cup frozen berries
1 banana
⅔ cup orange juice
⅔ cup vanilla almond milk
1-2 drops lemon essential oil
1 ½ cups ice

Apple & Green Smoothie

Blend together:
2 cups apple juice
1 cup spinach
1 cup kale
1 whole apple, cored
1 toothpick dip lime essential oil
½ avocado
1 cup ice

Paradise in a Glass Smoothie

Blend together:
½ cup coconut milk
1 toothpick dip lime essential oil
1 cup kale
1 cup spinach
1 cup chopped pineapple
½ cup frozen mango
4 frozen strawberries
1 banana
Water as needed for consistency

Simple Veggie Smoothie

Blend together:
2 cups kale
1 cup chopped tomato or grape tomatoes
¾ cup chopped cucumber
1 toothpick dip black pepper essential oil
1-2 cups water, as desired for consistency
1 cup ice
Dash salt

SNACKS

COOKING

Essential Popcorn

1 ½ quarts popped corn
3 tablespoons + 1 teaspoon butter
½ cup sugar
2 tablespoon water
½ teaspoon vanilla extract (only when using citrus oil)
1-2 dashes salt, to taste
Essential oil of your choice; the number of drops depends on which oil you use. Always start out with a few, taste, and add from there.
For cinnamon, add 4 drops (or to taste) and 1 teaspoon ground cinnamon for color. If desired, you can add spiced nuts to popcorn mixture (see recipe for honey spiced almonds).
For wild orange, add 4-5 drops to taste. If desired, you can drizzle white chocolate afterwards (see instructions)

Line a baking sheet with baking paper or foil. Place popcorn in a large bowl. In a saucepan, melt butter over low heat. Add the sugar, water, and salt; cook and stir over low heat until sugar is dissolved. Add essential oils and vanilla (if using citrus oil).
Pour mixture over the popcorn; toss and mix with a rubber spatula till popcorn is fully coated. Once coated, pour popcorn onto prepared baking sheet. Bake in the oven, uncovered, at 325° F for 10-15 minutes to crisp the popcorn and remove moisture. Stir mixture every 3-4 minutes. Take baking sheet out of the oven and keep stirring the mixture every few minutes. As the mixture cools, the popcorn will get nice and crispy. If using the citrus flavoring, you can add 1-2 drops wild orange to melted white chocolate. Drizzle over cooled popcorn. If using cinnamon flavoring, you can add spiced nuts to the mixture.

Spiced Roasted Almonds

Put roasted almonds in a zip-lock baggie or container with a lid. Add a couple drops of your essential oil preference – suggestions include protective blend, cassia, cinnamon, or black pepper together with lime. Seal the container; shake well, and let sit to allow flavor to permeate the almonds.

Citrus Cranberries

Add dried cranberries to a zip-lock baggie or container with a lid. Add a couple drops of wild orange essential oil. Seal the container, shake well, and let sit to allow flavor to permeate the cranberries. These flavored cranberries are excellent for use in salads, trail mixes, muffins/sweet breads, etc.

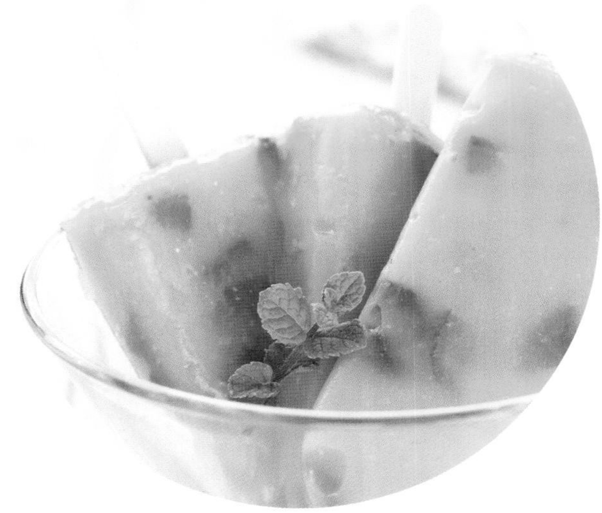

Popsicles

1 popsicle tray with sticks or ice cube tray and toothpicks
1 can frozen juice concentrate (orange or other juice of your choice)
½ can water
1 banana
2 ounces plain Greek yogurt
1 teaspoon vanilla
1 drop wild orange essential oil

Blend in blender and pour into tray. Add sticks or toothpicks and freeze.

Spiced Apple Slices

Add 4-6 drops protective blend essential oil to enough water to cover 2-5 apples, sliced. Swirl water. Add apple slices and let sit for 15+ minutes before serving.

Tropical Watermelon

In a 2-ounce glass spritzer bottle, combine 60 drops lime essential oil with water to fill. Shake and spritz on watermelon chunks just before serving.

Orange Chocolate Raisins

Add purchased chocolate-coated raisins to a zip-lock baggie or container with a lid. Add a couple drops of wild orange essential oil. Seal the container, shake well, and let sit to allow flavor to permeate the chocolate.

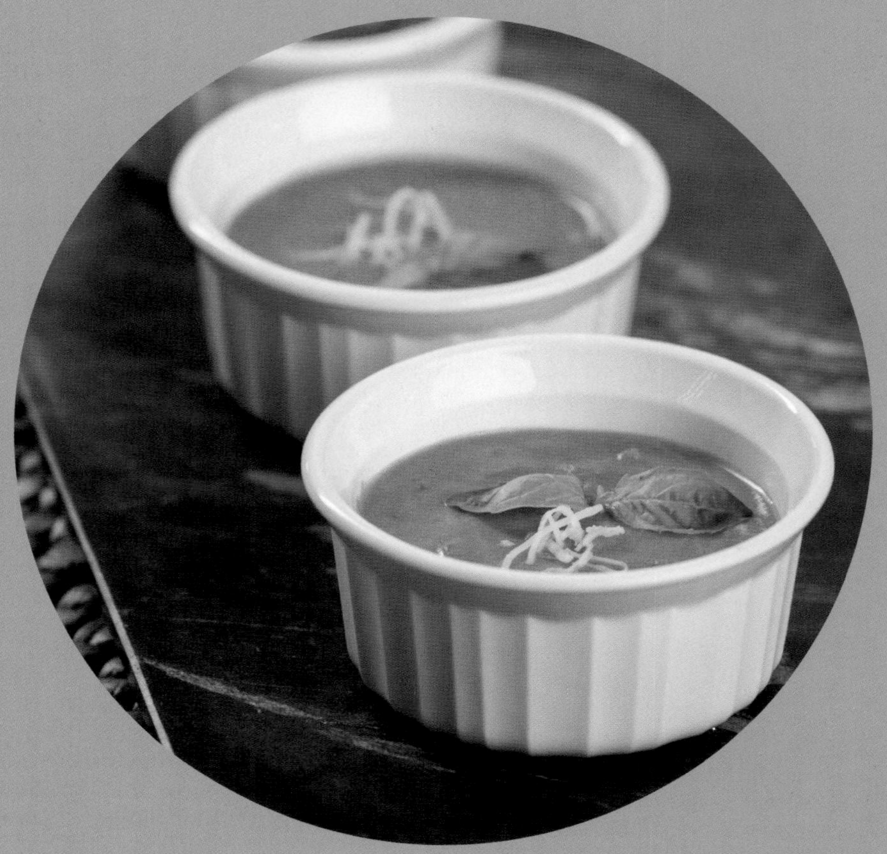

Quick & Easy Tomato Basil Soup

1 can diced stewed tomatoes roasted
¾ cup chicken broth
1 can tomato soup
8 ounces heavy cream or half and half
2 ounces butter
1 teaspoon sugar
1 shake of crushed dried basil
2 toothpick dips of basil essential oil
2 toothpick dips of black pepper essential oil
Ground pepper to taste
A few shakes of granulated garlic (optional)

Mix tomatoes and broth in a saucepan and heat to a boil. Reduce heat, cover, and simmer for about 10 minutes. Add soup, cream, butter, sugar, dried basil and essential oils. You can add more dried basil or ground pepper to taste, but do not add more essential oil, as it quickly becomes too powerful in flavor. Add garlic if desired. Cook on low heat until butter is melted and the soup is hot and bubbly.

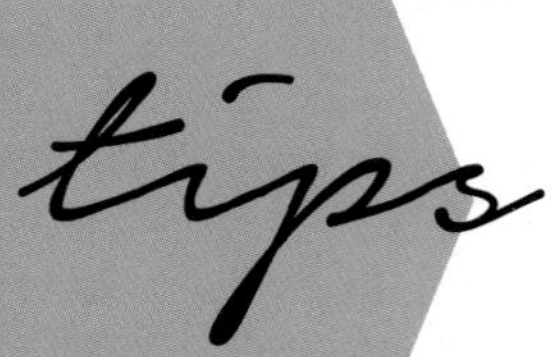

- It has been found that smelling essential oils helps curb the appetite. Every few hours, just take a sniff of a savory oil and trick the brain into feeling satiated.
- Asian soups are fantastic with a little lemongrass, lemon, and ginger essential oils.
- Remember, less is more. To retain the flavor of all of the ingredients in your dish, use the toothpick dip and add more to taste.

Chicken Tortilla Soup

Great way to use leftover chicken!

1 ½ pounds chicken, cooked and shredded
1 can (15 ounce) diced tomatoes
1 can (10 ounce) enchilada sauce
3 ½ tablespoons chicken base
1 medium onion, chopped
1 clove garlic, minced
3 ½ cups water
1 teaspoon chili powder
1 teaspoon salt
1 bay leaf (take out before serving)
1 package frozen corn
1 teaspoon cumin
1 toothpick dip cilantro oil
1 drop black pepper
Fresh cilantro (optional)
Grated cheese
Tortilla chips

In crockpot, combine all the ingredients and cover and cook on low for 6-8 hours or on high for 3-4 hours. Serve with avocado, shredded Monterey Jack cheese and tortilla chips. Top with fresh chopped cilantro also for extra flavor.

BBQ Chili

1 ½ pound ground turkey, browned and drained
1 cup 5 Star BBQ Sauce (see recipe on pg 383)
½ cup brown sugar
½ cup crispy bacon, crumbled
2 cans baked beans, drained
2 cans pork & beans, drained
1 can Northern beans, drained
1 can kidney beans, drained
2 cups water
1 tablespoon liquid smoke
1 tablespoon apple cider vinegar
1 toothpick swirl black pepper essential oil

Combine all ingredients and simmer in crockpot or warm on stove. Serve hot.

Enjoy!

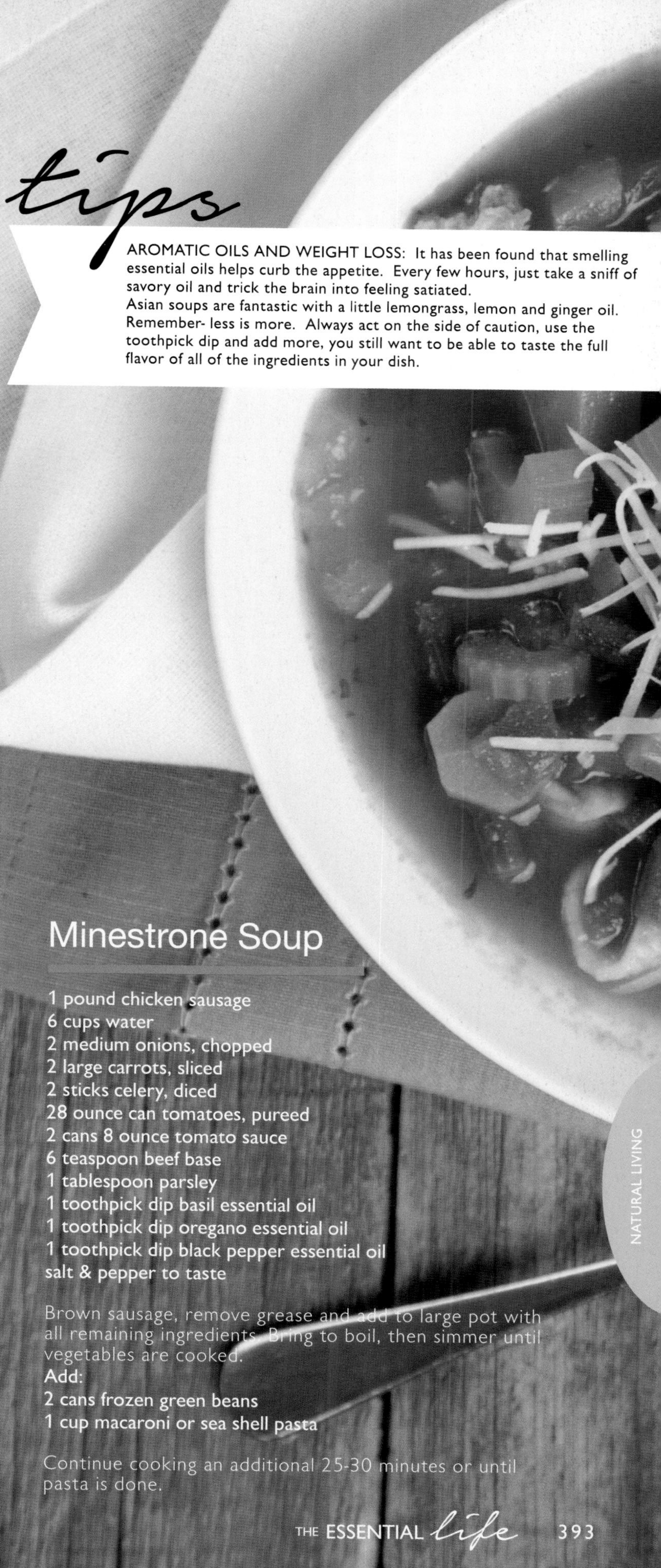

tips

AROMATIC OILS AND WEIGHT LOSS: It has been found that smelling essential oils helps curb the appetite. Every few hours, just take a sniff of savory oil and trick the brain into feeling satiated.
Asian soups are fantastic with a little lemongrass, lemon and ginger oil. Remember- less is more. Always act on the side of caution, use the toothpick dip and add more, you still want to be able to taste the full flavor of all of the ingredients in your dish.

Minestrone Soup

1 pound chicken sausage
6 cups water
2 medium onions, chopped
2 large carrots, sliced
2 sticks celery, diced
28 ounce can tomatoes, pureed
2 cans 8 ounce tomato sauce
6 teaspoon beef base
1 tablespoon parsley
1 toothpick dip basil essential oil
1 toothpick dip oregano essential oil
1 toothpick dip black pepper essential oil
salt & pepper to taste

Brown sausage, remove grease and add to large pot with all remaining ingredients. Bring to boil, then simmer until vegetables are cooked.
Add:
2 cans frozen green beans
1 cup macaroni or sea shell pasta

Continue cooking an additional 25-30 minutes or until pasta is done.

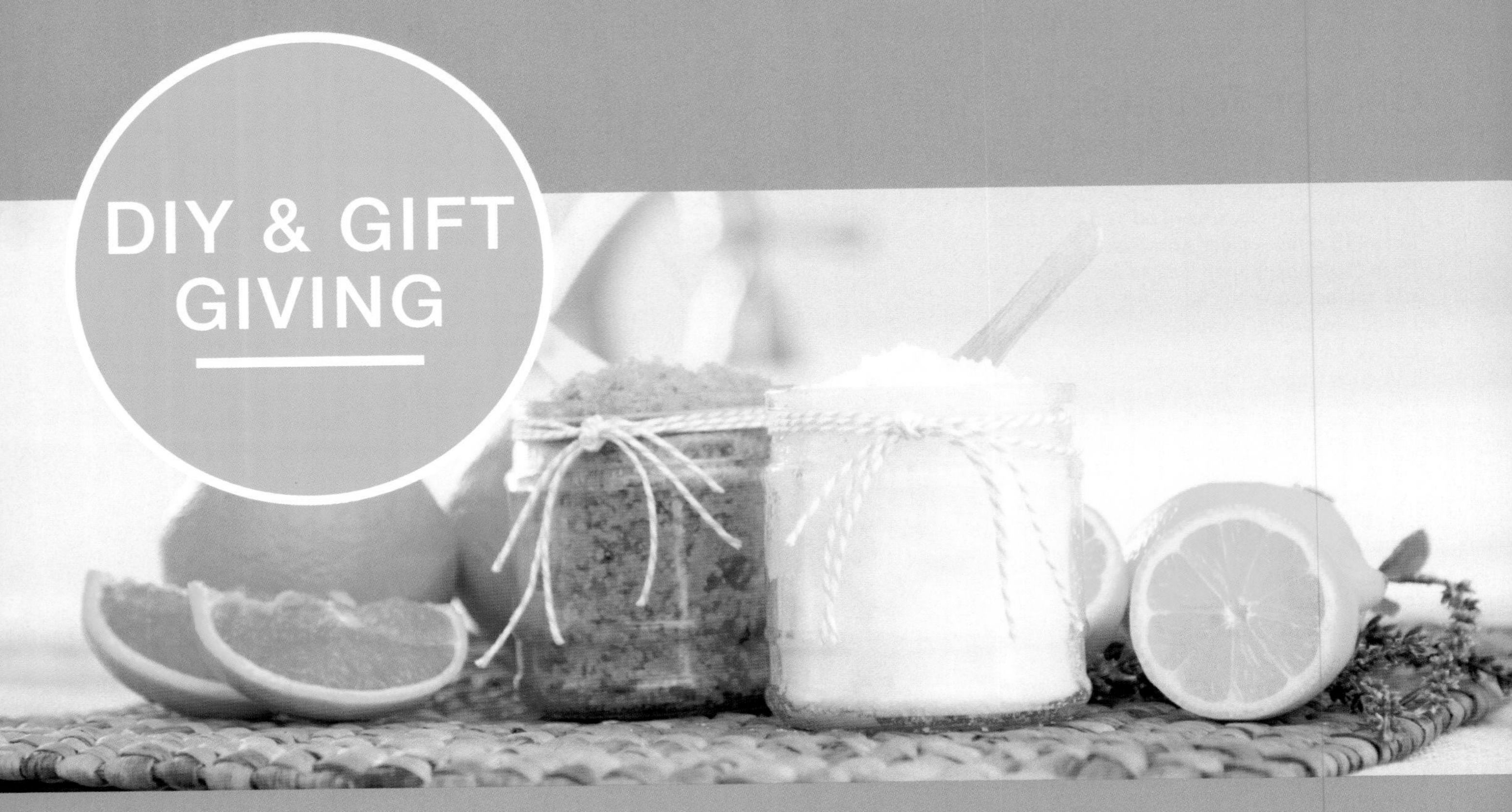

Sensory Play Dough

1 cup flour
¼ cup salt
1 tablespoon cream of tartar
½ cup warm water
5 drops lemon essential oil
Food coloring (optional)
Glitter (optional)

Mix flour, salt, and cream of tartar. Add water, essential oil, and food coloring. Mix well. Add glitter. Store in zip-lock bags. Reuse as desired.

Essential Oil Neck Wraps

Tube or dress socks or other fabric in the shape you desire
3 cups flaxseed or rice
2 drops desired essential oil(s)

Pour flaxseed or rice into sock and knot the end or sew fabric into the shape you desire. Fill and slip-stitch end closed. Warm in microwave for two to three minutes. Add 2 drops essential oil to the wrap. Place on neck and relax.

Festive Sugar Scrub

¾ cup white sugar, brown sugar, or sea salt
½ cup fractionated coconut or other oil
4 drops cassia essential oil
4 drops clove essential oil
4 drops ginger essential oil

Combine sugar and fractionated coconut oil in a bowl. Add essential oils. Stir until the mixture is the consistency of a slushy. Add more sugar or fractionated coconut oil to achieve desired consistency. Pour into an airtight container.

Mint Lime Foot Soak

2 ½ cup Epsom salts
Zest of 1 fresh lime
4 drops lime essential oil
3 drops peppermint essential oil
2 drops green food coloring (optional)

In medium bowl mix Epsom salts, lime zest, essential oils, and food coloring. Stir well. Place in jars and tie with a bow. Great for a summertime birthday, Mother's Day, or just because.

tip Simply mix your favorite essential oils together in a roller bottle to create your own unique aroma. Use for yourself or as a gift.

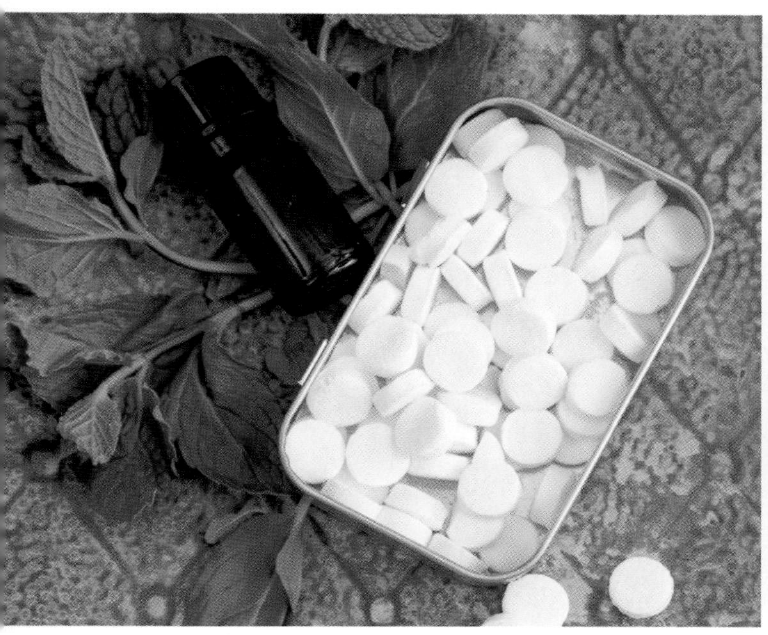

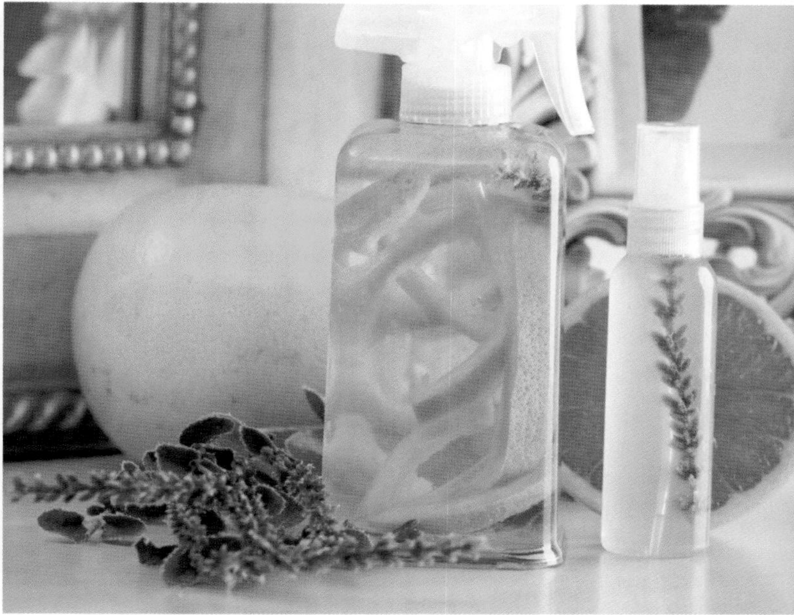

Homemade Mints

1 package gum paste (found with cake decorating supplies)
¼ cup powdered sugar
6 drops peppermint, cinnamon, or lemon essential oil (add more for stronger flavor)
Food coloring (optional)
Plastic straw

Pull off an egg-sized section of gum paste and knead it until soft. Add essential oil and a tiny bit of food coloring. Knead again, and roll out with rolling pin. Using the end of the straw, punch out shapes and roll in powdered sugar. This reduces sticking. Dry for 48 hours. Place mints in a decorative tin with lid.

Sweet Orange Scrub

1 cup brown sugar
¼ cup coconut oil
7-8 drops wild orange essential oil

Combine thoroughly in a glass jar, add a label and ribbon, and enjoy or share.

Embrace Fall Body Spray

8 ounces distilled water
1 tablespoon witch hazel
10 drops cinnamon essential oil
13 drops wild orange essential oil

Mix in a spray bottle.

Happy Grapefruit Body Spray

8 ounces distilled water
1 tablespoon witch hazel
13 drops grapefruit essential oil
4 drops lavender essential oil

Simply add ingredients to a spray bottle, shake, and enjoy or share.

Vanilla Lavender Sugar Scrub

1 cup white sugar
¼ cup coconut oil
1 teaspoon vanilla extract
5 drops lavender essential oil

Combine thoroughly in a glass jar, add a label and ribbon, and enjoy or share.

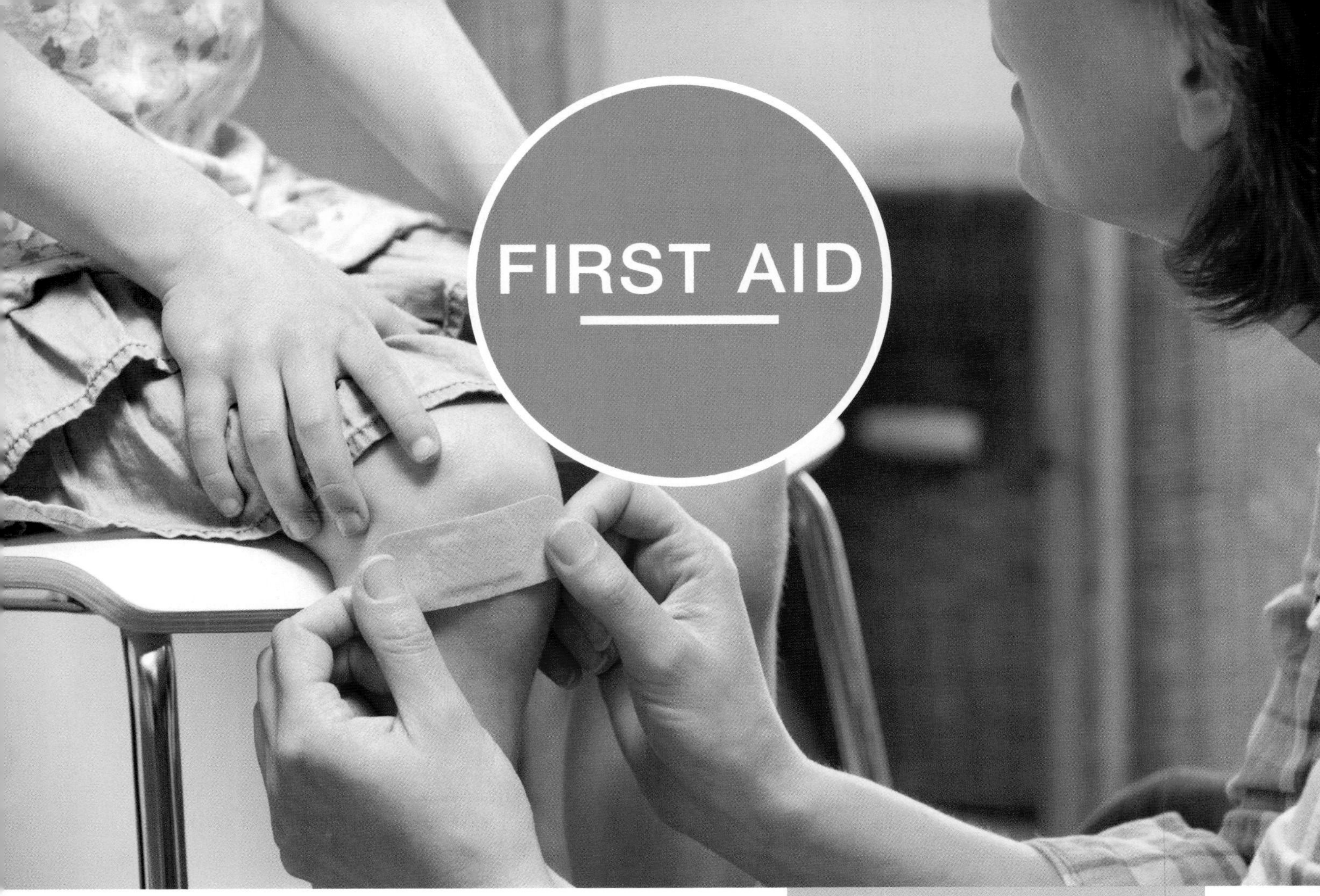

Flu Shot in a Bottle

40 drops lemon
30 drops protective blend
20 drops oregano
Fractionated coconut oil

Mix essential oils in roller bottle and fill with fractionated coconut oil. This is a great remedy for the onset of an illness. When you feel a scratchy throat or aches coming on, apply mixture to throat, bottoms of feet, and behind the ears. Because this mix contains oregano essential oil, it should be used for only five to seven days. Oregano essential oil can be hard on the liver when used for long periods of time. Protective blend essential oil should also be used along the spine (apply with coconut oil since it is a warm oil) and on bottoms of feet for prevention of illness.

Top reasons to include essential oils in your First Aid Kit

1. They're multi-faceted. You can disinfect a cut, stop bleeding, and soothe a child with a single application of a few drops of lavender essential oil.
2. They're affordable. They are pennies on the dollar for what you'd pay for most over-the-counter medications
3. They don't expire! They have an extended shelf-life that will keep you from wasting your oils.
4. They're all natural. So you'll avoid any negative side effects of synthetic medications by using nature's medicine cabinet.

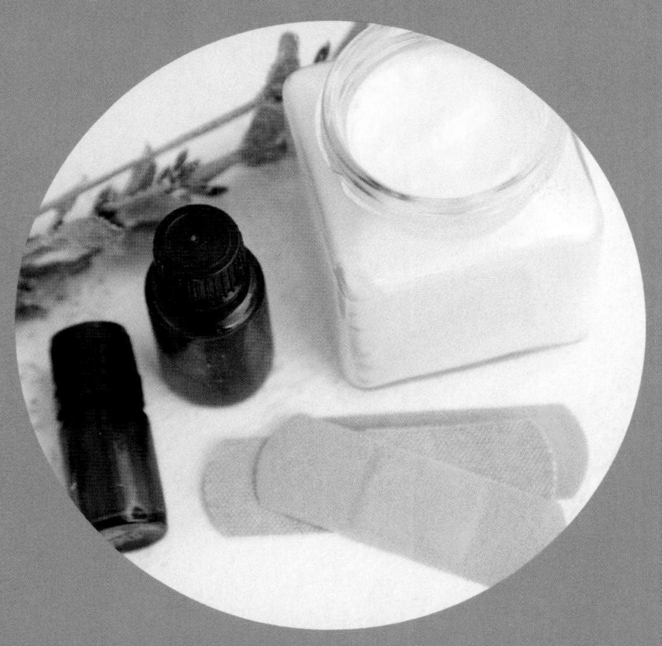

Bump & Bruise Spray

For bruise relief, roll on tension blend or soothing blend essential oils

30 drops geranium
15 drops lavender
10 drops cypress
5 drops frankincense
5 drops helichrysum
water

Mix ingredients together in a 2-ounce spray bottle and fill with water. Shake and spray to support normal circulation, soothe the skin, and support the body's natural healing process.

Sprain Tonic

½ cup apple cider vinegar
1 tablespoon sea salt
5 drops soothing blend
5 drops marjoram
5 drops lemongrass

In a small bowl mix all ingredients and apply to sprained area. Reapply as needed.

Ouchie Spray

2 drops roman chamomile
2 drops melaleuca
2 drops lavender
1 teaspoon fractionated coconut oil

Mix and apply directly to cuts or scrapes.

Allergy Relief

Try 1-3 seasonal blend softgels for quick allergy relief.

4 drops lemon
4 drops lavender
4 drops peppermint
Fractionated coconut oil

In a small roller bottle, mix essential oils and fill remainder with fractionated coconut oil. Shake and roll on as needed.

tips

- To clean a wound, apply lavender or corrective ointment to disinfect and promote healing.
- To stop bleeding quickly, apply lavender and then helichrysum essential oil.
- For splinters deep under the skin, apply clove to bring the splinter to the surface. For splinters near the surface, apply a piece of adhesive tape to the area of skin containing a splinter. Yank tape off quickly and the splinter should come out. Apply 1 drop of soothing blend essential oil to affected area.
- For stings, apply cleansing blend and then lavender to soothe.
- For blister relief, apply 2 drops lavender and 2 drops melaleuca. Repeat as necessary.

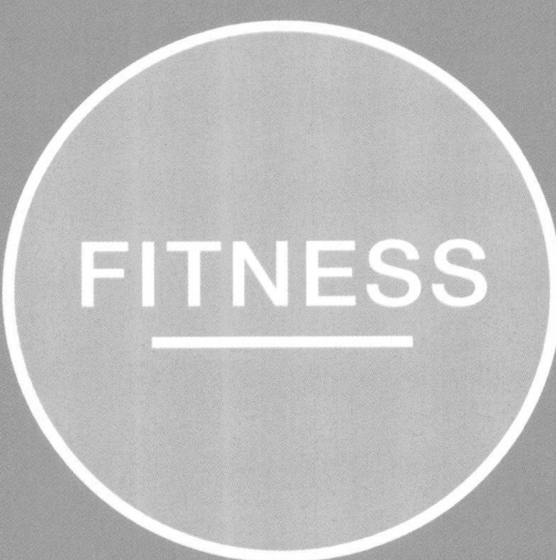

FITNESS

When it comes to health and fitness, isn't it nice to have cutting-edge natural products on your side?
Can you imagine the benefits of all-natural freshening and cleansing sprays for your body and workout equipment? Can you picture overcoming cravings and keeping your metabolism active with pure, zero-calorie essential oils?
Are you looking forward to more easily warming up and cooling down your muscles and effectively relieving muscle soreness? Get ready for essential oils to maximize your efforts and help you reach your fitness goals!

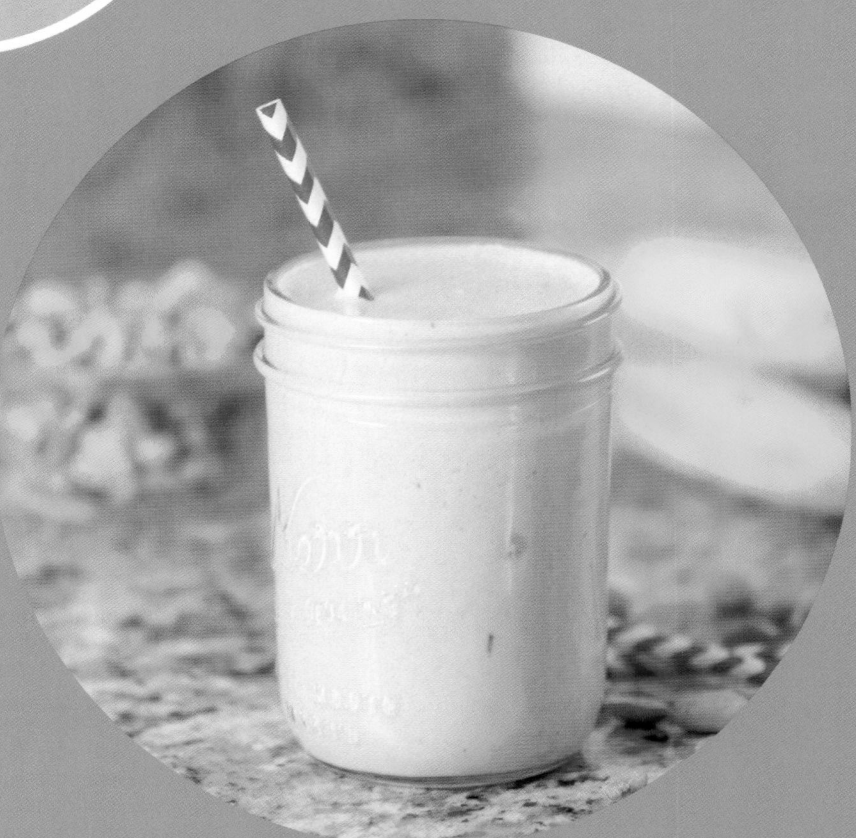

Peanut Butter Heaven Protein Shake

1 scoop vanilla meal replacement powder
¾ cup vanilla almond milk (or other non-fat milk)
1 tablespoon natural peanut butter
½ banana
1 cup ice

Mix in blender until smooth and creamy.

tips

- To help flush out toxins, add 1-2 drops of lemon essential oil in your water.
- To manage appetite between meals, use 3-5 drops of metabolic blend essential oil under tongue or in water.
- Open airways before, during, or after a workout by inhaling respiration blend essential oil.
- Increase your endurance by taking energy & stamina complex essential oil daily.
- For sore muscles, rub or massage soothing blend essential oil anywhere it aches.
- To improve clarity and focus, use grounding blend essential oil.
- To ease swimmers ear, rub clove essential oil behind, around, and on – but not in – the ear.
- To relieve pressure and tension, use massage blend essential oil on your back and shoulders.
- For quick relief of leg cramps, apply massage blend essential oil.

Leg Cramp Blend

3-4 drops soothing blend essential oil
3-4 drops lemongrass essential oil
1-2 drops helichrysum essential oil

Mix together and apply directly to affected area.

Post-Workout Bath

3 drops lavender essential oil
2 drops roman chamomile essential oil
2 drops marjoram essential oil
1 drop helichrysum essential oil

Add to bath and soak away your soreness.

Sanitizing Spray

½ cup water
2-6 drops protective blend essential oil

Add ingredients to a glass spray bottle. Shake well before each use to sanitize your yoga mat, hand weights, and other workout equipment.

Post-Workout Rub

1 ounce fractionated coconut oil
3 drops marjoram essential oil
2 drops thyme essential oil
4 drops roman chamomile essential oil
4 drops cypress essential oil
3 drops lemon essential oil
2 drops peppermint essential oil

Mix together and gently massage the mixture into your muscles and joints to prevent stiffness and pain.

Cellulite Reducing Spray

4 ounces fractionated coconut oil
15 ml grapefruit essential oil (one bottle)

Mixed together in a glass spray bottle. After bathing, spray on body to reduce the appearance of cellulite.

Refreshing Body Spray

6 drops lime essential oil
2 drops lavender essential oil
2 drops lemon essential oil
1 drop peppermint essential oil

Combine essential oils in a 2-ounce spray bottle and fill with water to refresh yourself in seconds.

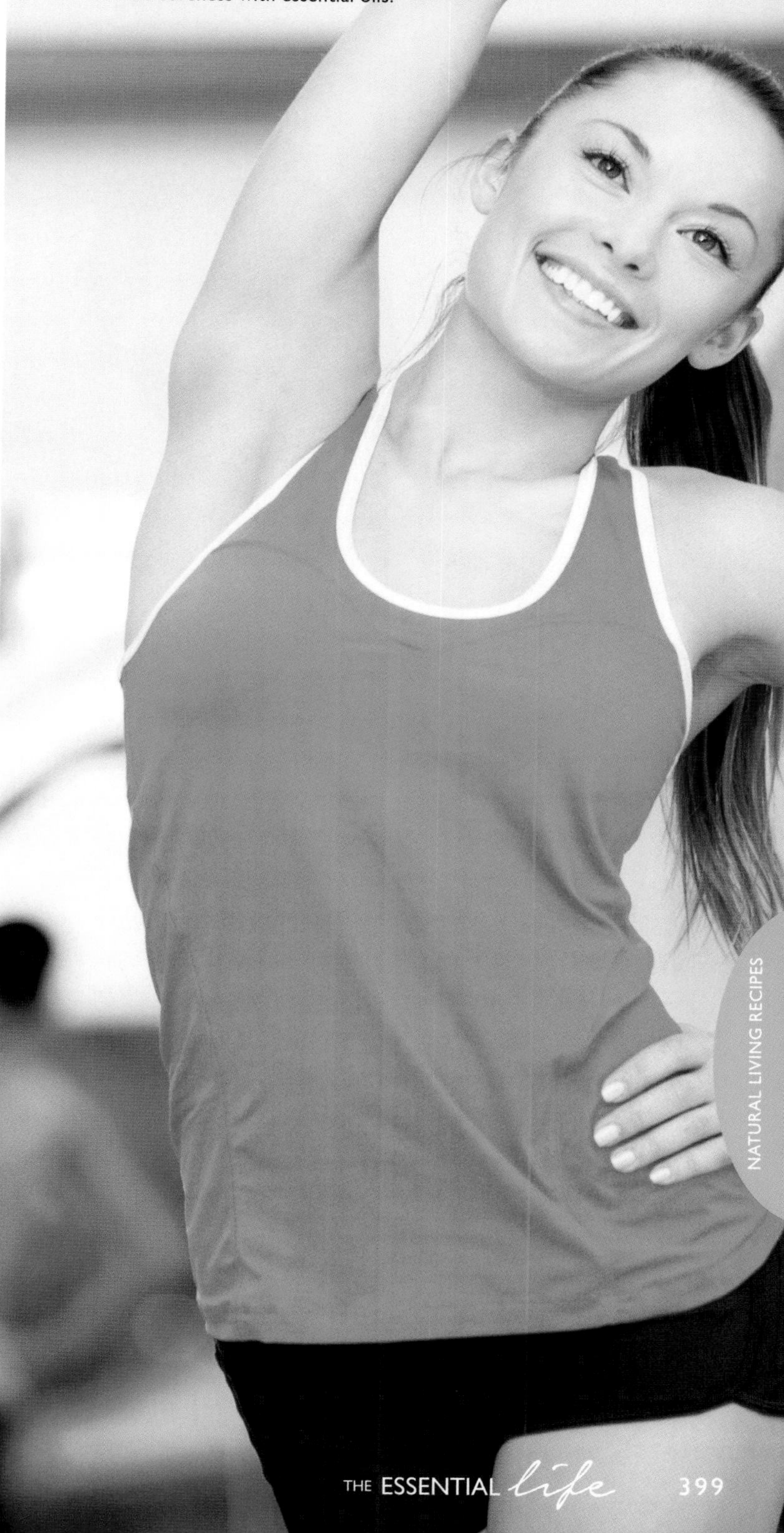

did you know?

- You can use cutting-edge natural products to help maximize your efforts and reach your fitness goals.
- Benefit from all-natural freshening and cleansing sprays for your body and workout equipment.
- Overcome cravings and keep your metabolism active with pure, zero-calorie essential oils.
- Easily warm up and cool down your muscles and effectively relieve muscle soreness with essential oils.

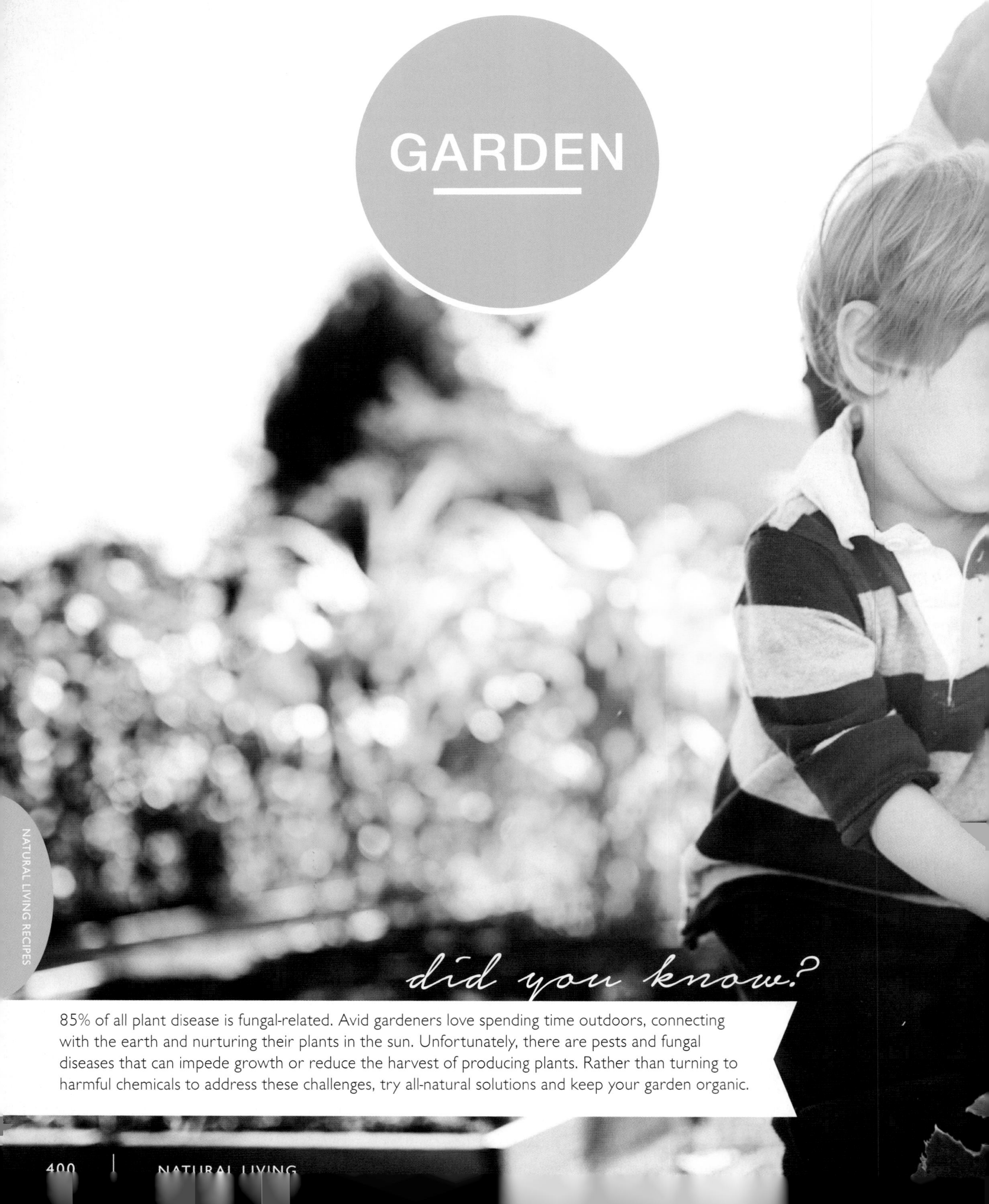

GARDEN

did you know?

85% of all plant disease is fungal-related. Avid gardeners love spending time outdoors, connecting with the earth and nurturing their plants in the sun. Unfortunately, there are pests and fungal diseases that can impede growth or reduce the harvest of producing plants. Rather than turning to harmful chemicals to address these challenges, try all-natural solutions and keep your garden organic.

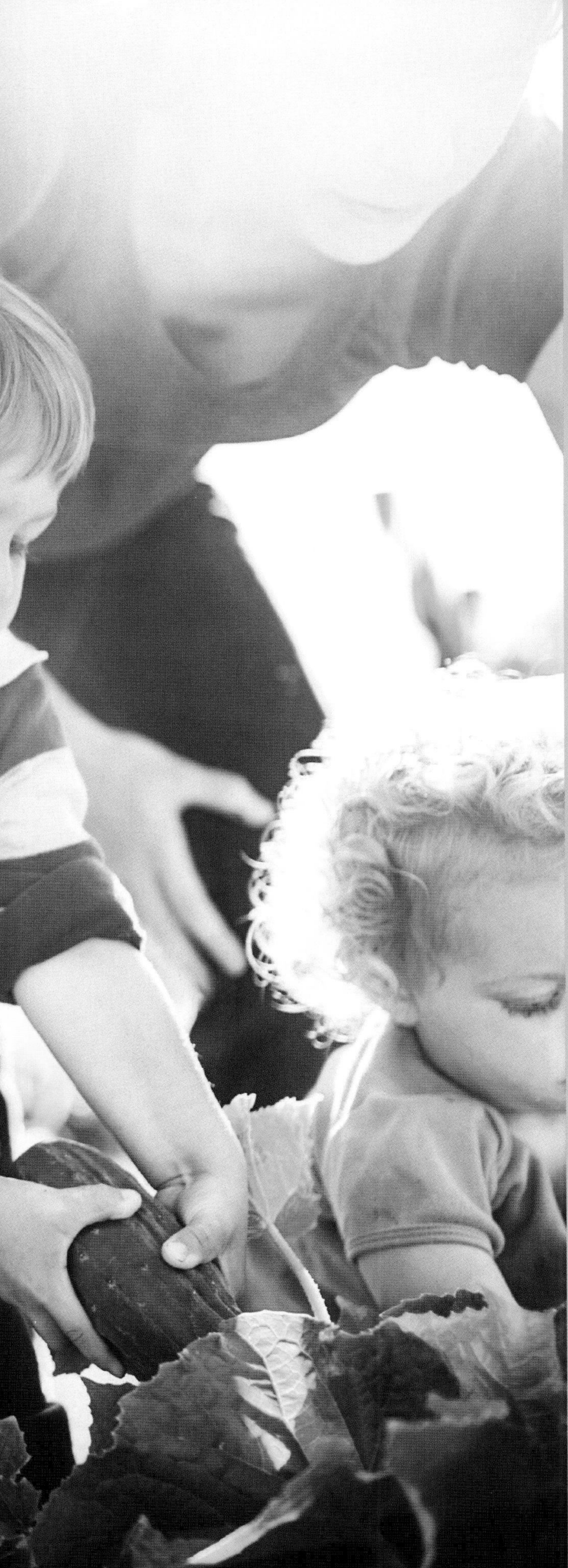

Garden Insect Deterrent

10 drops rosemary essential oil
10 drops peppermint essential oil
10 drops thyme essential oil
10 drops clove essential oil

Combine in a small spray bottle. Fill with water and shake well. Apply anywhere you want to get rid of insects.

Fungus Supressant

In a small spray bottle, combine 20 drops of melaleuca essential oil and water to fill. Spray directly onto infected plants once or twice weekly.

Veggie & Fruit Wash

Fill your kitchen sink up with cold water. Add 1/2 cup white vinegar and 6 drops of lemon essential oil. Soak fruits and vegetables, then rinse.

Pollinator Attractor

Add 5 to 6 drops of wild orange essential oil to a spray bottle filled with 1 cup water. Spray on flowers and buds to attract bees for pollination.

Pest Repellents

Scare rodents away with 2 drops of peppermint essential oil dropped on a cotton ball. Tuck balls into mouse holes, burrows and nests to encourage them to relocate.

Repel other pests with these essential oils:

Ants: peppermint, spearmint
Aphids: cedarwood, peppermint, spearmint
Beetles: peppermint, thyme
Caterpillars: spearmint, peppermint
Chiggers: lavender, lemongrass, sage, thyme
Fleas: peppermint, lemongrass, spearmint, lavender
Flies: lavender, peppermint, rosemary, sage
Gnats: patchouli, spearmint
Lice: cedarwood, peppermint, spearmint
Mosquitoes: lavender, lemongrass, arborvitae, repellent blend
Moths: cedarwood, lavender, peppermint, spearmint
Plant lice: peppermint, spearmint
Slugs: cedarwood
Snails: cedarwood, patchouli
Spiders: peppermint, spearmint
Ticks: lavender, lemongrass, sage, thyme
Weevils: cedarwood, patchouli, sandalwood

GUYS
Who said essential oils were only for women?
Most colognes and cleaners are both expensive and toxic.
Learn how real men can benefit from the power of pure essential oils.
Remove oil, grease stains, and sticky residue with lemon essential oil.
Clean the car battery and polish chrome wheels with melaleuca and lemon essential oils diluted with water in a spray bottle.
To support hair growth in thinning areas, apply rosemary essential oil directly to scalp or add to shampoo.

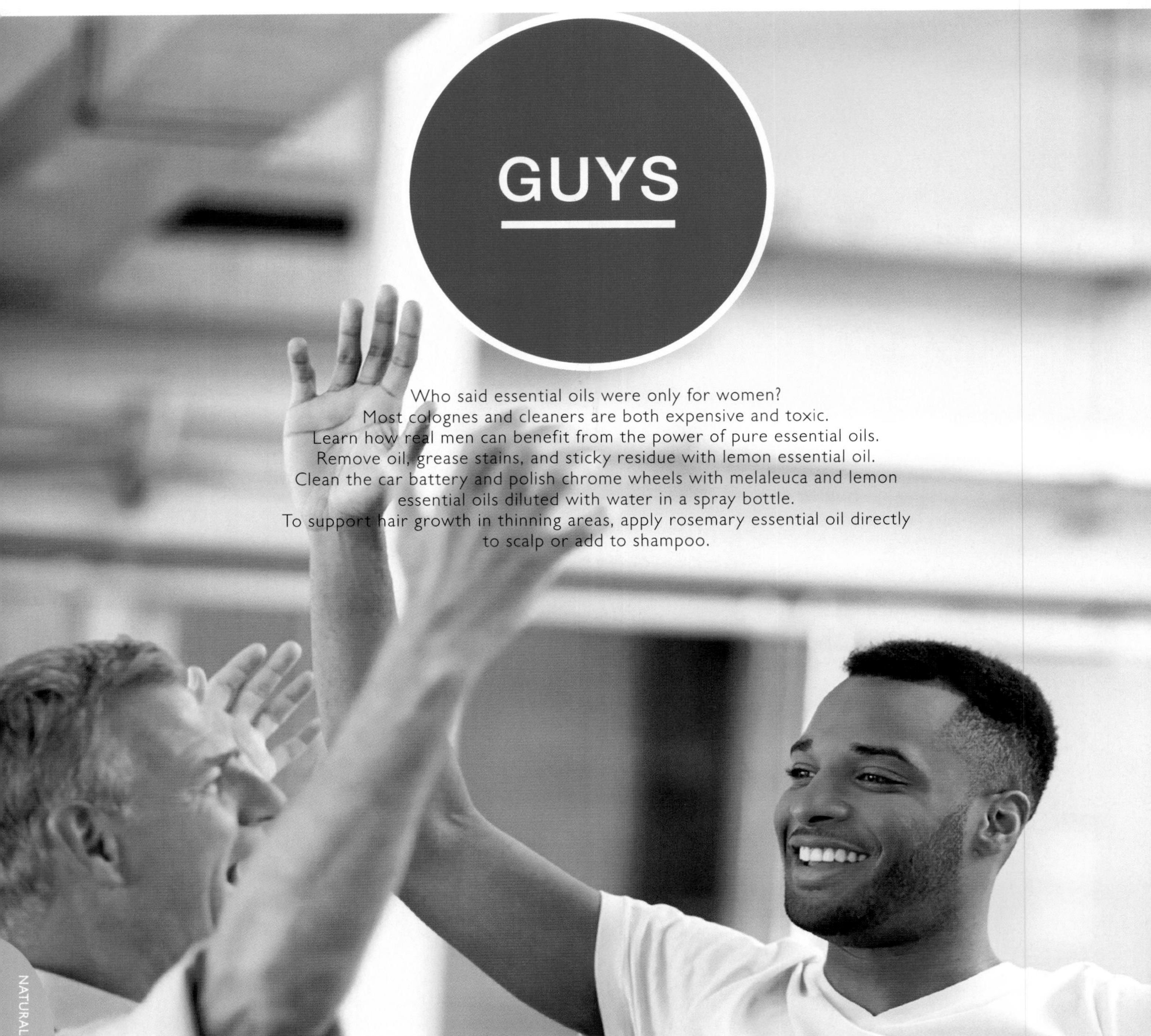

Shaving Cream

2/3 cup shea butter
2/3 cup cocoa butter
1/4 cup fractionated coconut oil
5 drops sandalwood essential oil
5 drops peppermint essential oil
5 drops melaleuca essential oil

Place butters and oil in double boiler to melt. Mix in essential oils. Let shaving cream cool. Whip with hand mixer.

Earthy Aftershave

3/4 cup witch hazel
1 tablespoon apple cider vinegar
10 drops sandalwood essential oil
5 drops peppermint essential oil
3 drops rosemary essential oil
2 drops melaleuca essential oil

Place all ingredients in a bottle. Shake well and pat onto skin after shaving for a natural, great-smelling antiseptic and anti-inflammatory aftershave.

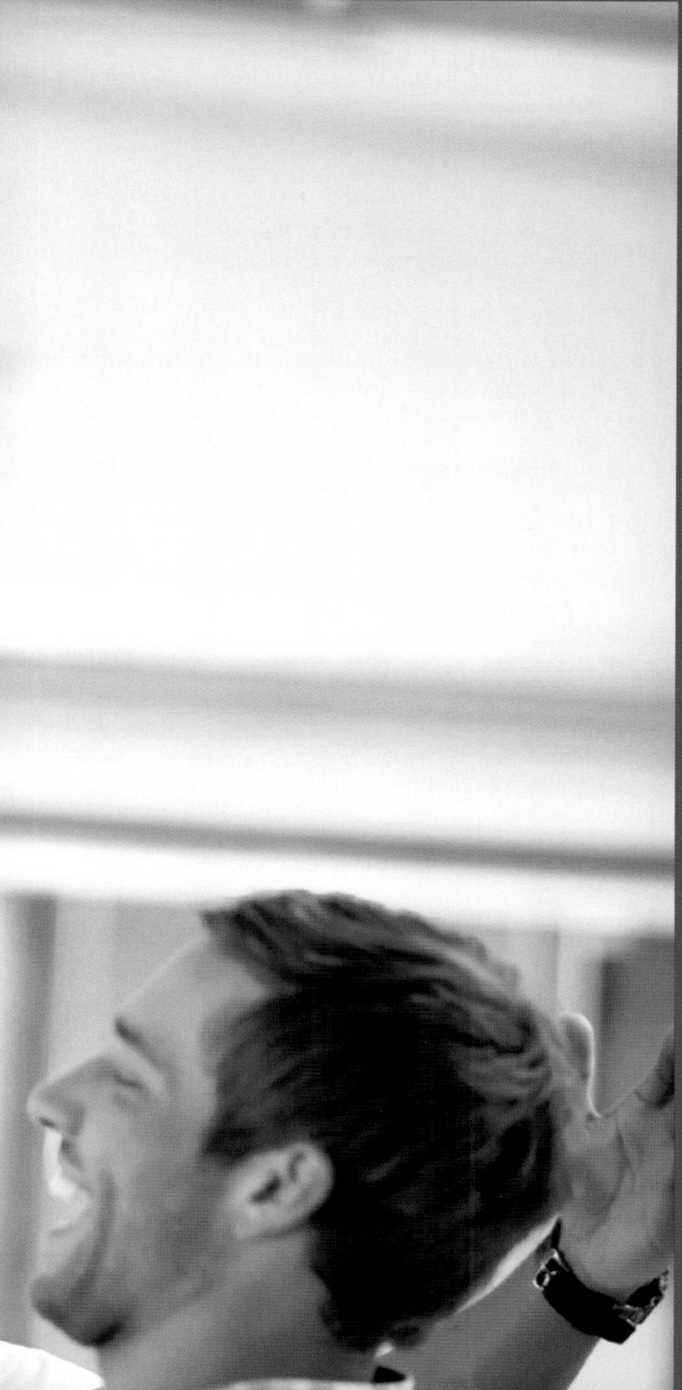

Spice Cologne

40 drops bergamot essential oil
10 drops clove essential oil
20 drops white fir essential oil
5 drops lemon essential oil
3 teaspoons fractionated coconut oil

Combine essential oils with fractionated coconut oil into a glass roller bottle. Attach the roll-on cap and shake the vial until the mixture is combined. Let mixture sit for at least 24 hours before use.

Musky Deodorant

15 drops cleansing blend essential oil
15 drops clary sage essential oil
10 drops frankincense essential oil
10 drops lime essential oil
5 drops lavender essential oil
5 drops patchouli essential oil
5 drops grounding blend essential oil
5 drops cedarwood essential oil
3 drops sandalwood essential oil
Fractionated coconut oil

Combine the essential oils in an empty 2-ounce glass spray bottle. Add fractionated coconut oil to fill the bottle. Shake well before each use.

Hair & Scalp Stimulator

½ cup fractionated coconut oil
40 drops rosemary essential oil
25 drops basil essential oil
20 drops lemon essential oil
15 drops lavender essential oil
15 drops lemongrass essential oil
10 drops peppermint essential oil

Drop essential oils and coconut oil into a storage bottle with lid. Shake vigorously for 2 minutes. Dip fingertips into mixture and gradually massage the entire amount into your dry scalp for three to five minutes. Wrap your hair completely with plastic wrap or a shower cap and cover with a very warm, damp towel. Replace towel with another warm towel once it has cooled. Leave on thirty to forty-five minutes. Follow with shampoo and light conditioner. Use up to two times per week if hair is thinning.

Antifungal Foot Roll-On

35 drops melaleuca essential oil
8 drops lavender essential oil

Combine essential oils in a glass bottle with a roller lid and apply topically to affected areas between toes and around toenails.

Shoe Deodorizer

2 drops peppermint essential oil
2 drops wild orange essential oil

Drop essential oils onto a paper towel or a used dryer sheet. Place in your shoes overnight.

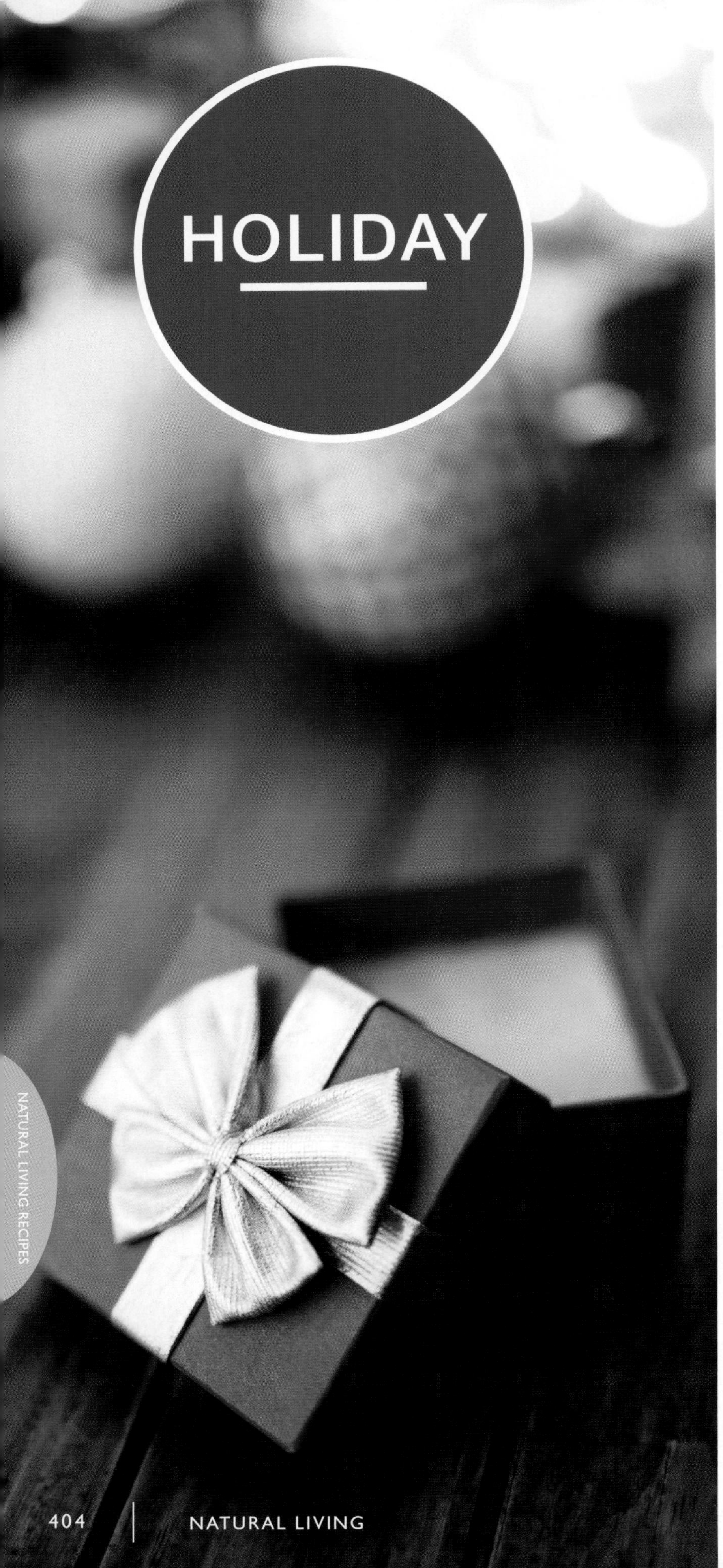

Scented Ornaments

1 cup baking soda
½ cup cornstarch
½ cup water
10-15 drops of cassia, white fir, holiday blend, wild orange, or peppermint essential oil

In a saucepan, heat together all ingredients but the oils over medium heat. Bring to a boil, stirring continuously. Once mixture has thickened into a dough-like consistency, remove from heat and mix in oils. Add glitter or food coloring, if desired. Roll cooled dough onto a cookie sheet and cut with cookie cutters. Use a large toothpick or skewer to make a hole in the top of each shape. String twine or ribbon through the hole to hang the ornament.

Mason Jar Candles

Lamp wicks (May be found at craft stores)
Small- to medium-sized mason jar with lid
Coconut oil
10 drops of orange, lemon, cassia, or white fir essential oil

Fill a mason jar almost to the top with coconut oil. Mix in desired essential oil. (If you want to add decorations such as pine cones, citrus fruit, cranberries, fir branches, food coloring, etc. add to jar before pouring in oil.)
Drill a small hole into the top of the mason jar lid, and slide the lamp wick through the hole, assuring that most of the wick is inside the jar. Tighten the lid and lighten the night.

Over-Indulgence Tea

You know we have all had the miserable feeling of overeating, also known as the food coma! Try this tea to help relieve the bloating, groggy, yucky feeling that is associated with it.

10 drops wild orange
2 drops peppermint
5 drops lemon
2 drops ginger
3 drops coriander

In a small bottle add all essential oils together. Keep the rest to get you through the holidays. In a tea cup add 1 cup hot water to 1 tablespoon honey, stir and then add 2 drops of essential oil mixture. mix well and sip until your tummy settles.

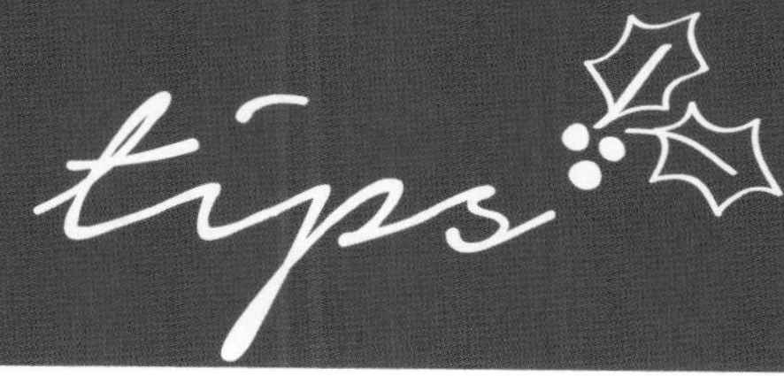

- Create the scent of Christmas by diffusing holiday blend essential oil.
- Create Christmas pine cones by adding 1-2 drops of cassia essential oil to a pine cone or spray a bowl of pine cones with holiday blend essential oil.
- Keep your Christmas tree smelling fresh all season long by filling a small glass spray bottle with 20 drops of white fir. Fill the remainder with water and spray on your Christmas tree.

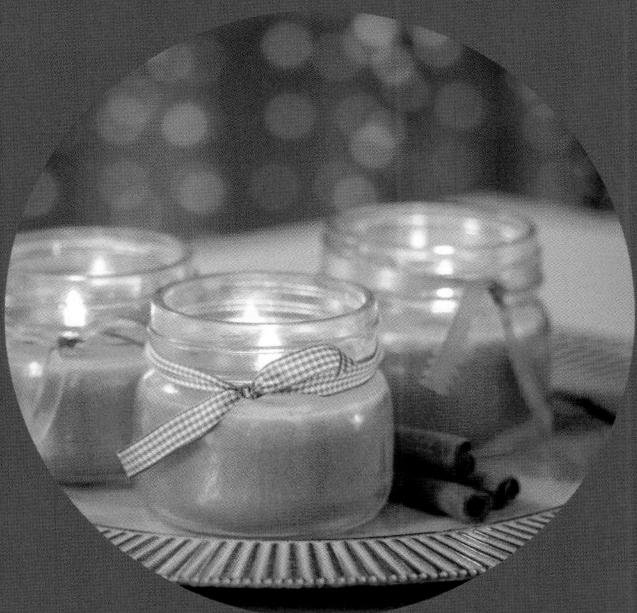

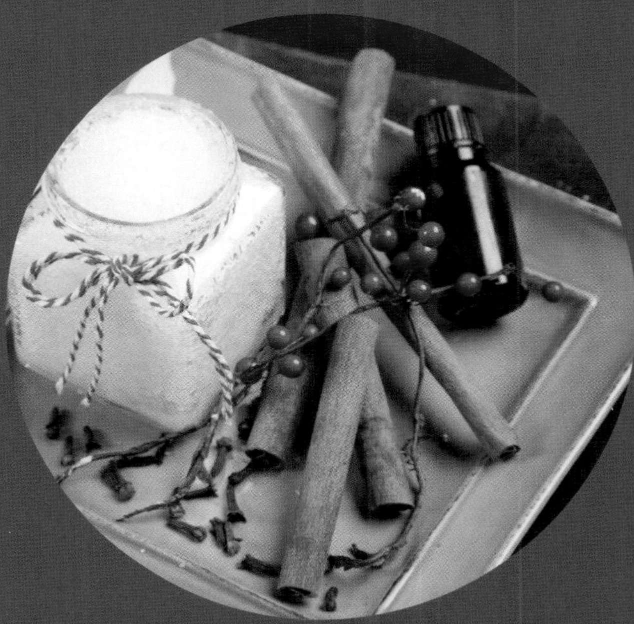

Festive Sugar Scrub

This sugar scrub is gentle on your skin and has a delicious, spicy aroma.

¾ cup white sugar (you can also use brown sugar or sea salt)
½ cup fractionated coconut oil (you could also use almond oil, grapeseed oil, or olive oil).
4 drops cassia essential oil
4 drops clove essential oil
4 drops ginger essential oil

Combine sugar and fractionated coconut oil into a bowl. Add essential oils. Stir until the mixture is the consistency of a slushy. You may need to add more sugar or oil for desired consistency. Pour into an air-tight container.

Fall Freshener

6 drops wild orange essential oil
1 drop patchouli essential oil
1 drop ginger essential oil

Combine oils in a 4-ounce spritzer bottle. Fill the bottle with water. Spray around the house.

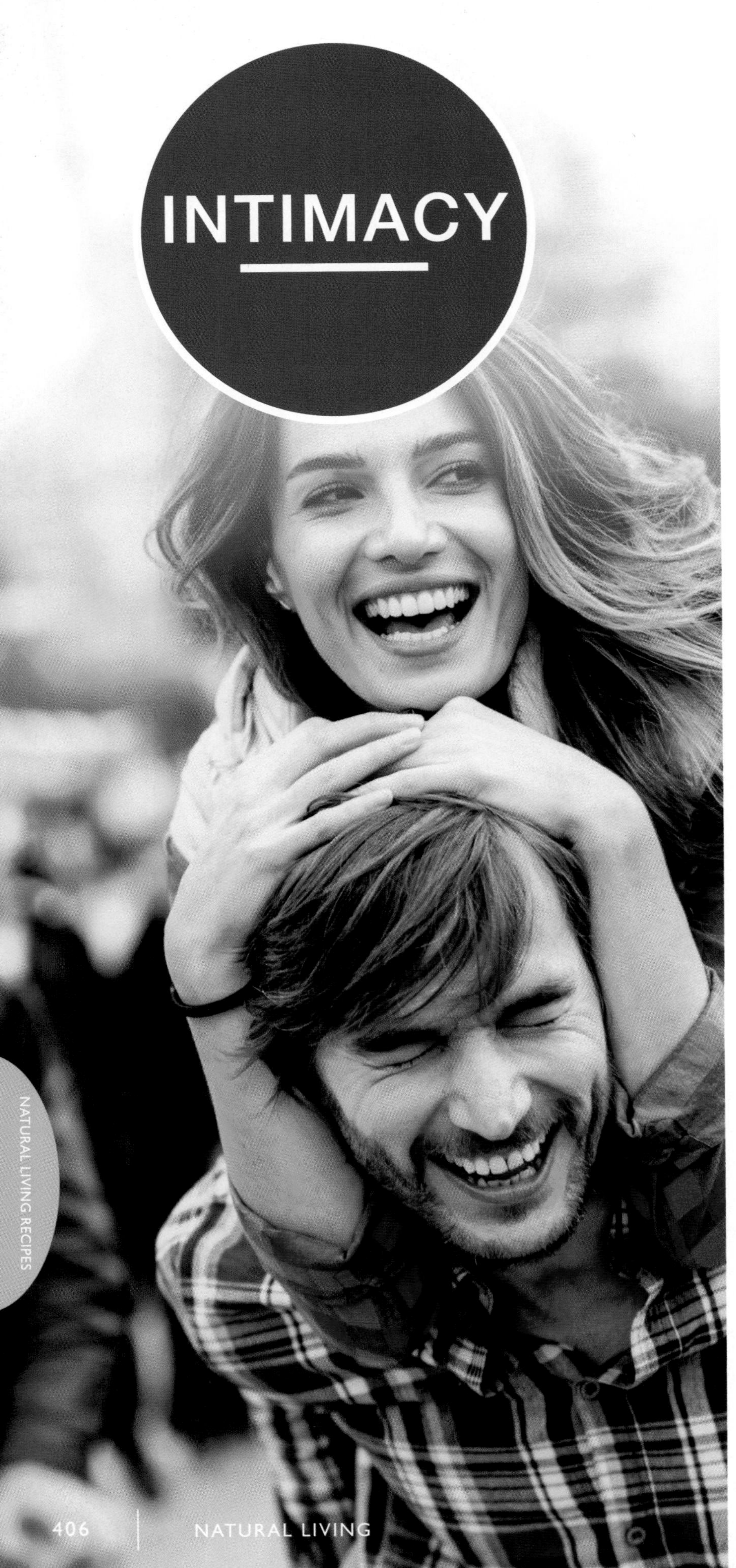

Sensual Sheets

10 drops sandalwood essential oil
10 drops bergamot essential oil
3 drops ginger essential oil
3 drops lime essential oil
2 drops ylang ylang essential oil

Add essential oils to a spray bottle and fill with water. Spray on bed sheets for a romantic evening.

Aphrodisiac Massage Blend

¼ cup fractionated coconut oil or unscented lotion
2 drops rose or geranium essential oil
3 drops sandalwood essential oil
2 drops ylang ylang essential oil
3 drops clary sage essential oil

Mix oils together and massage on skin to increase connection and arousal.

Aphrodisiac Blend For Diffusing

1 drop white fir essential oil
1 drop cinnamon essential oil
1 drop patchouli essential oil
1 drop rosemary essential oil
1 drop sandalwood essential oil
1 drop ylang ylang essential oil

Drop these essential oils into a diffuser and fill the air with excitement.

Erotic Massage Blend

¼ cup fractionated coconut oil
2 drops geranium essential oil
1 drop cinnamon essential oil
1 drop ginger essential oil
1 drop lemongrass essential oil
1 drop peppermint essential oil

Mix oils together and apply lightly on genitals. This blend helps to reach and prolong climax.

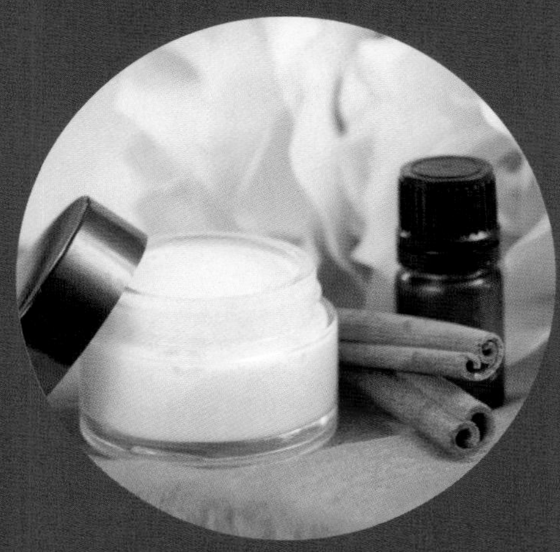

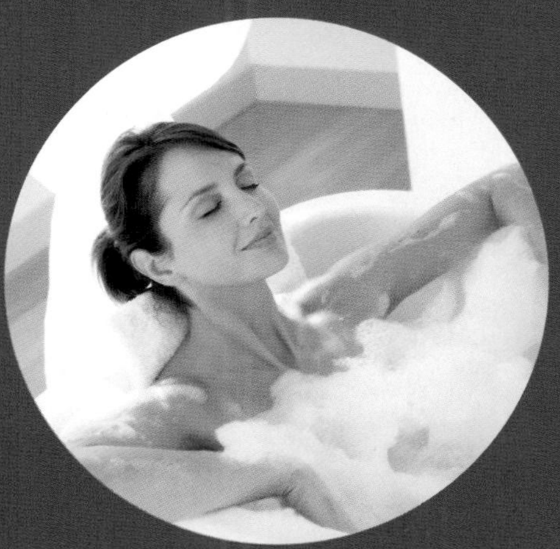

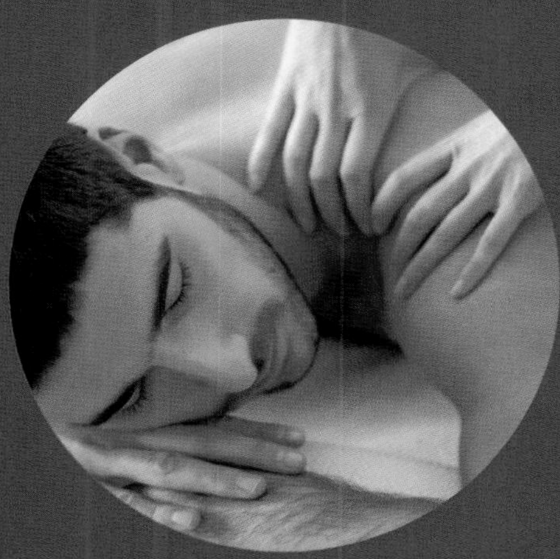

Exotic Cinnamon Love Balm

2 ½ tablespoons coconut oil
1 tablespoon cocoa butter
1 ½ teaspoons vegetable glycerin
1 teaspoons beeswax
6 drops cinnamon essential oil

Warm all ingredients, except essential oil, over low heat until the cocoa butter and beeswax are melted. Remove from heat and add the cinnamon essential oil. Beat the mixture for a few minutes until it begins to thicken and becomes opaque. Pour or spoon into a storage container. Cool for fifteen minutes before capping. Let mixture sit for four hours before use as a kissing or massage balm.

Ecstasy Bubble Bath

1 ½ cups liquid castile soap
2 tablespoons vegetable glycerin
½ tablespoon white sugar
30 drops cedarwood essential oil
20 drops clary sage essential oil
10 drops ylang ylang essential oil
6 drops patchouli essential oil

Stir together ingredients in a large glass or ceramic bowl until the sugar has dissolved. Pour into bottle, shake, and let sit for 24 hours before using. To use, pour about ¼ cup of bubble bath under hot running water.

Steamy After-Bath Rub

30 drops bergamot essential oil
10 drops sandalwood essential oil
5 drops juniper berry essential oil
4 drops ginger essential oil
4 drops ylang ylang essential oil
2 drops jasmine or lavender essential oil
4 ounces coconut oil

Combine ingredients and massage on skin. Combine the deep, intoxicating effects of essential oils with sensual touch and massage to arouse intense desire.

did you know?

- Essential oils have been used throughout history to increase sensuality and passion by helping provide a lovely ambience, relieve emotional exhaustion, and even increase libido.
- Essential oils, used for this purpose, are typically used topically and aromatically. Different oils appeal to different people; it's all about the journey of discovery to find out which oils work best for you and your partner.

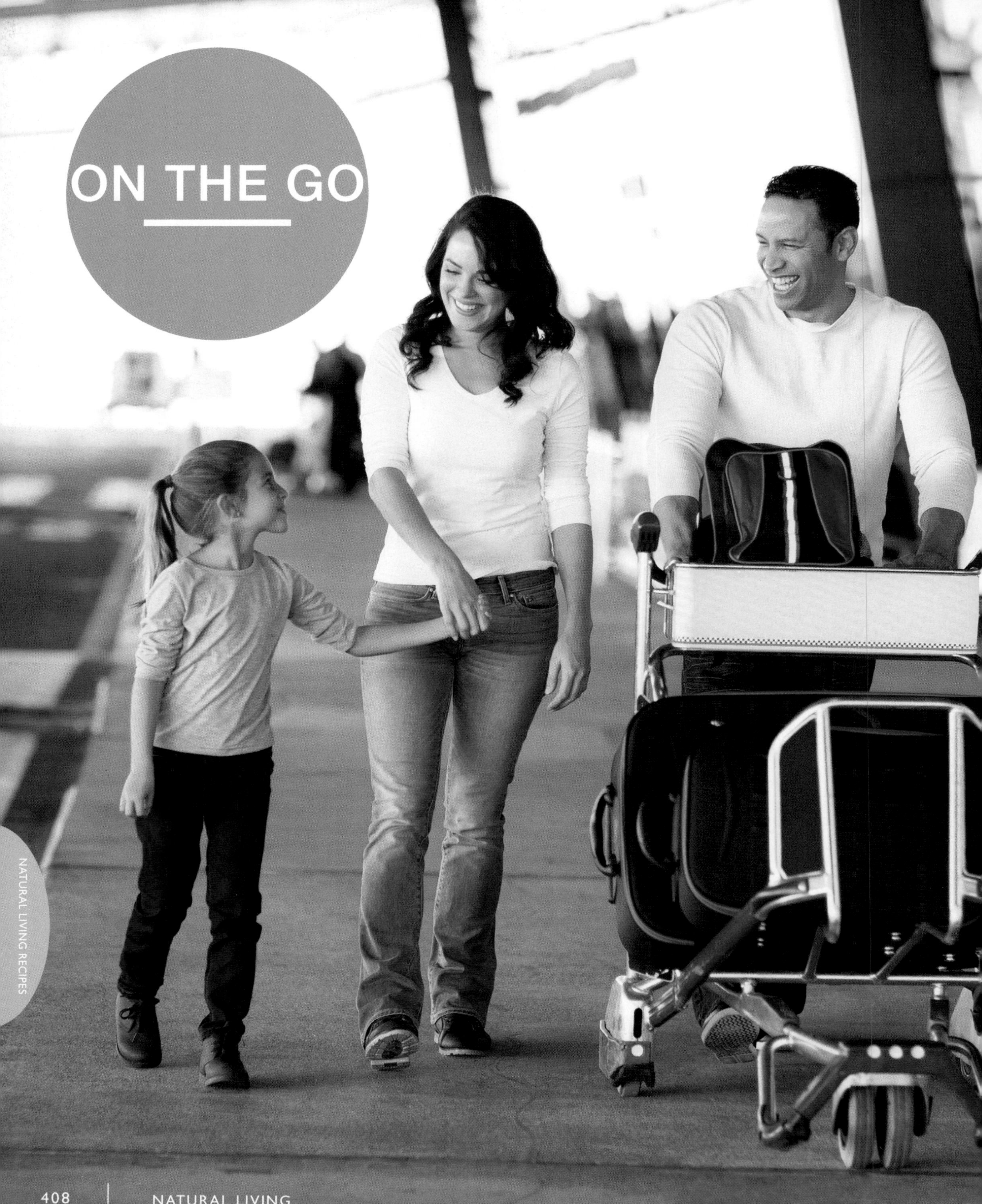

ON THE GO

Hand Sanitizer

5 tablespoons aloe vera gel
4 tablespoons water
½ teaspoon vitamin E oil
10 drops protective blend essential oil
5 drops wild orange essential oil

Combine all ingredients in a squeezable container. Shake well and you are ready to clean hands anywhere without stripping off your body's natural acid protection barrier.

Car Air Freshener

Wool Felt
Twine
10 drops of your favorite essential oils

Create non-toxic hanging car air fresheners in any shape, color, and scent you desire.
Cut a simple 4" shape from wool felt and drop the oil onto the felt.
Using a small hole punch, punch a hole into the top of your shape, thread twine through it, and knot. Hang on the rear view mirror.

Bedbugs Be Gone Spray

On your travels, bring a small spray bottle filled with 10 drops of melaleuca or peppermint essential oil mixed with water. Spray on bedding and seats before using to deter bedbugs. Spray suitcases too, so they can't stow away home with you.

Eye Glasses Cleaner

1 cup white vinegar
¼ cup water
5 drops lemon essential oil

Mix ingredients into a small spray bottle, shake, and spray directly onto glass. Wipe with a scratch-free cloth.

Jet Lag Help

Simply add 8 drops of lavender and 8 drops of rosemary essential oils to your tub water. Bathe and enjoy. Follow with a quick cold shower to help you feel refreshed and alive in no time.

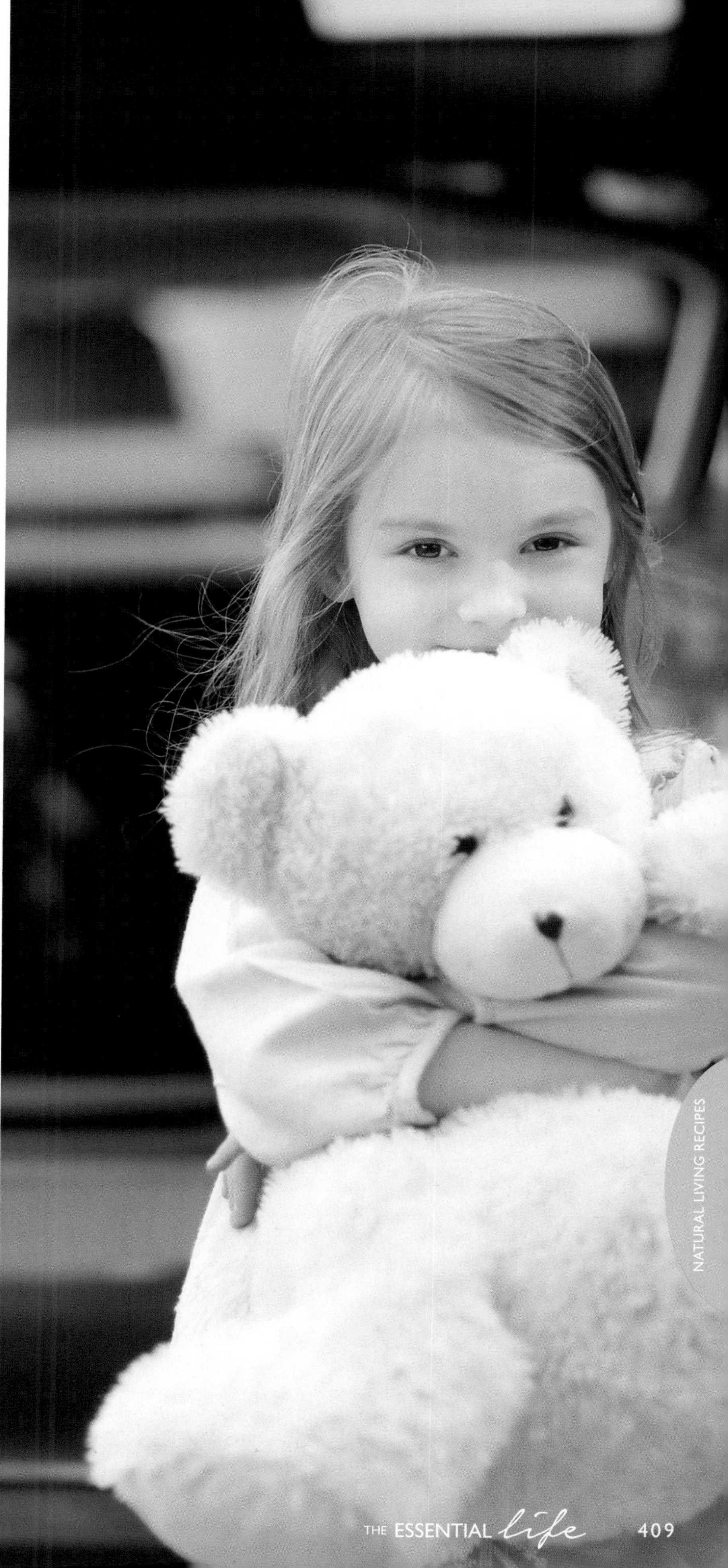

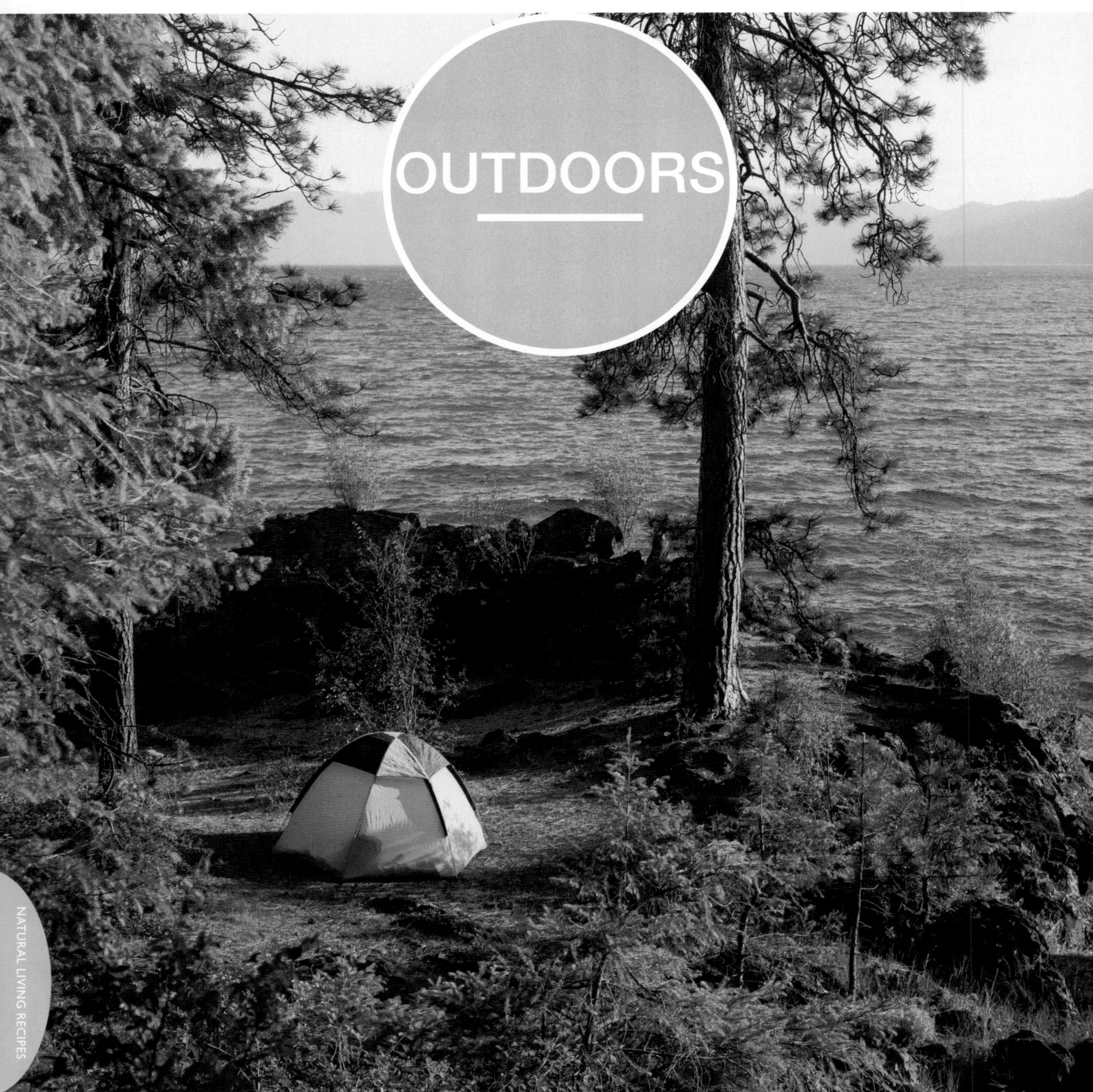

did you know?

- Out of 2,000 sunscreens reviewed, more than 75% were found to contain toxic chemicals.
- Common side effects for insect repellents include skin reactions, allergic rashes, and eye irritation.
- Many topical medicated creams for insect-bite itching and irritation have side effects causing redness, irritation, and swelling.

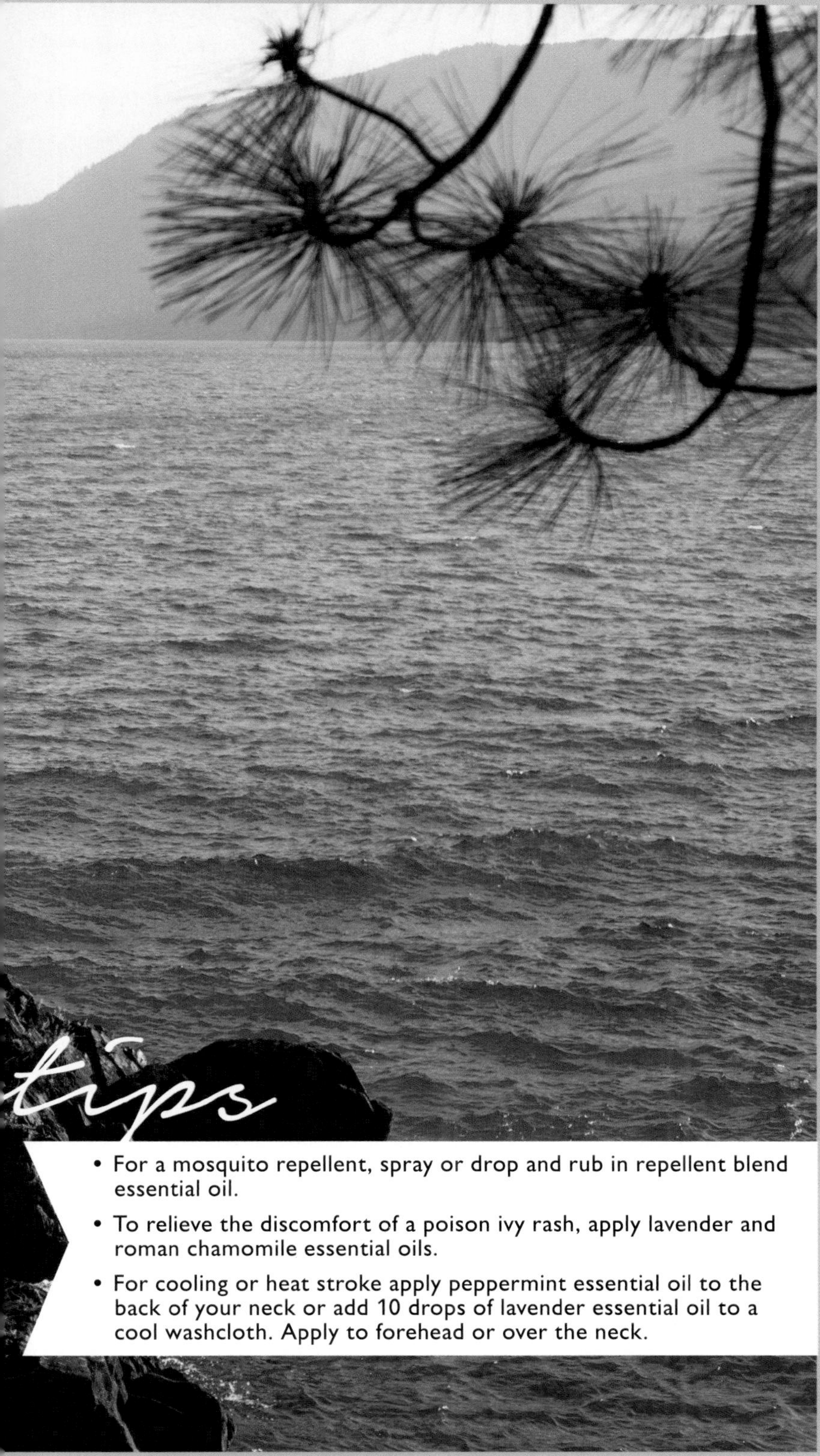

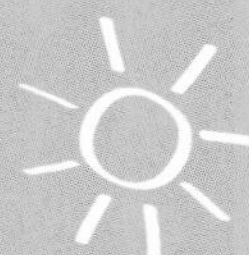

Sunburn Spray

1 cup aloe vera juice
¼ cup fractionated coconut oil
1 teaspoon vitamin E oil
8 drops lavender
8 drops melaleuca
8 drops roman chamomile

Combine ingredients in a 16-ounce glass spray bottle. Shake well and spray onto sunburned skin. Repeat as needed.

Bug Repellent

10 drops lemongrass
10 drops lavender
10 drops geranium
10 drops peppermint
Fractionated coconut oil

Mix essential oils in a small spray bottle, add coconut oil to fill. Shake well and spray on exposed areas of the skin.

Sunscreen

½ cup olive oil
¼ cup fractionated coconut oil
¼ cup beeswax
2 tablespoons shea butter
1 teaspoon vitamin E oil
2 tablespoons zinc oxide
12 drops helichrysum

Place all ingredients except zinc oxide and helichrysum essential oil into a glass mixing bowl. Fill saucepan with 2 to 3 inches of water and turn on medium heat. Place glass bowl in saucepan and stir as ingredients melt. Remove from heat and add the helichrysum essential oil and zinc oxide. Pour into a glass jar and store in a cool place. Apply lotion to skin before sun exposure. Reapply as needed.

Cooling Spray

8 ounces water
2 teaspoons witch hazel
10 drops peppermint

Combine in a small spray bottle for instant cooling and a reviving blast.

tips

- For a mosquito repellent, spray or drop and rub in repellent blend essential oil.
- To relieve the discomfort of a poison ivy rash, apply lavender and roman chamomile essential oils.
- For cooling or heat stroke apply peppermint essential oil to the back of your neck or add 10 drops of lavender essential oil to a cool washcloth. Apply to forehead or over the neck.

PERSONAL CARE

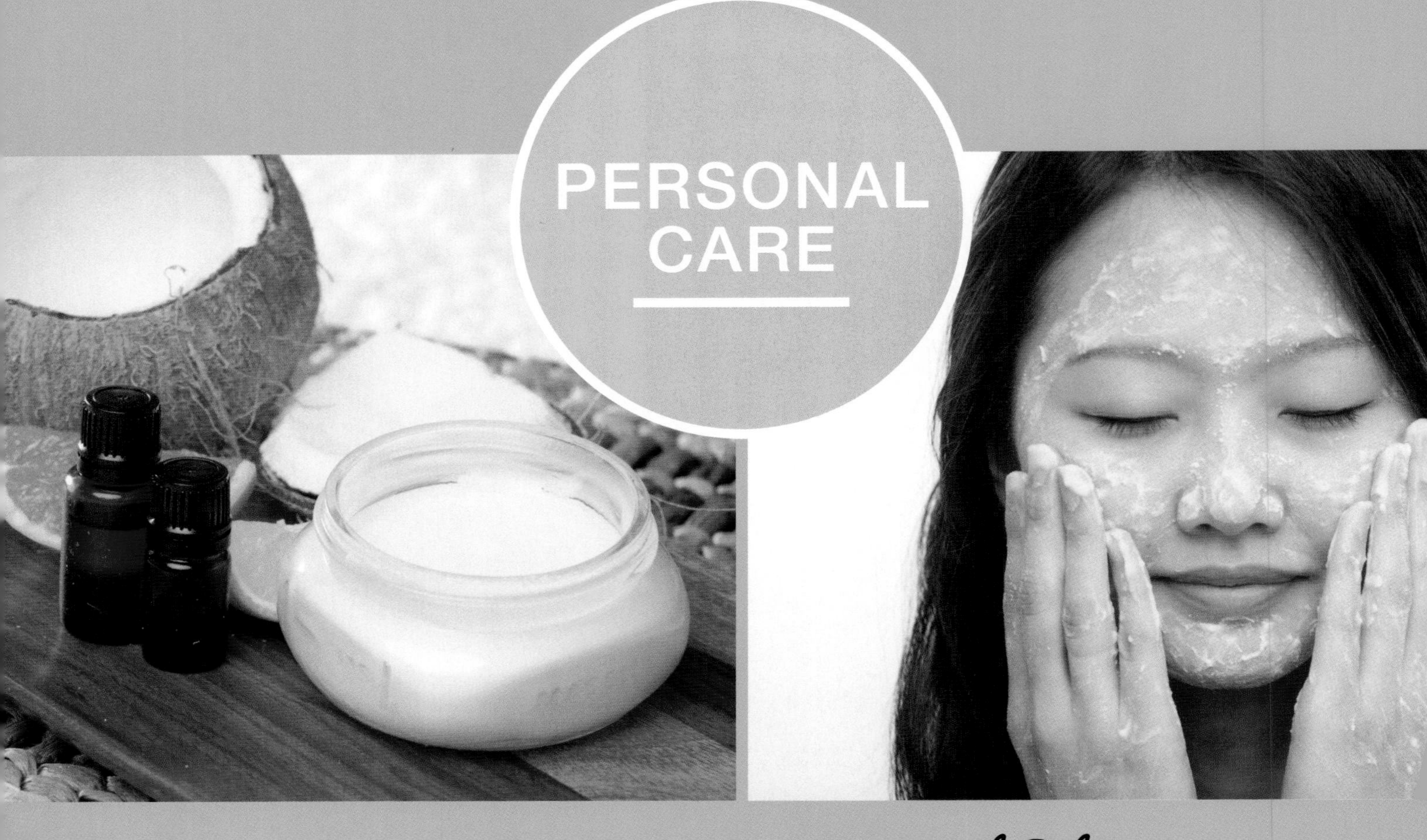

Natural Deodorant

6 tablespoons coconut oil
6 teaspoons baking soda
10 drops wild orange essential oil
3 drops helichrysum essential oil
2 drops rosemary essential oil

Mix coconut oil and baking soda together until a paste starts to form.
Add essential oils and mix well. Store in a glass jar with lid. Apply a thin layer of deodorant to underarms using finger, a cotton pad, or makeup sponge.

At Home Microdermabrasion

1 tablespoon baking soda
1 ½ teaspoons water
2 drops helichrysum essential oil

Mix ingredients in a small bowl until a watery paste forms. Dip clean fingers into paste and, using a circular motion, gently massage face and throat until covered with a thin coat. Rinse and moisturize. Safe for all skin types, but do not apply to sun/windburned skin. Microderm once or twice weekly to exfoliate and expel dead skin cells. The skin will feel refreshed and toned.

did you know?

- Most deodorants and antiperspirants contain ingredients linked to breast cancer and Alzheimer's disease.
- Teeth whitening products can cause sensitivity and lead to gum recession and irritation. Irritation of the oral mucous membranes, a burning feeling in the mouth, and potential to increase the risk of pharyngeal and oral cancers are common side effects from mouthwash use.
- Incorporate all-natural essential oils into your personal care regimen to bypass negative side effects and harmful chemicals.
- For easy eye and makeup remover use fractionated coconut oil.
- For a quick breath freshener, pop a peppermint essential oil beadlet.
- To pull toxins from the body and improve overall health, try oil pulling. Oil pulling has been said to help with overall oral health while pulling unwanted toxins out of the body. Apply 1-2 teaspoons fractionated coconut oil into mouth. Add desired essential oils and swish around for fifteen to twenty minutes, then spit out (in the trash, not down a drain). Rinse with warm water and brush teeth well.

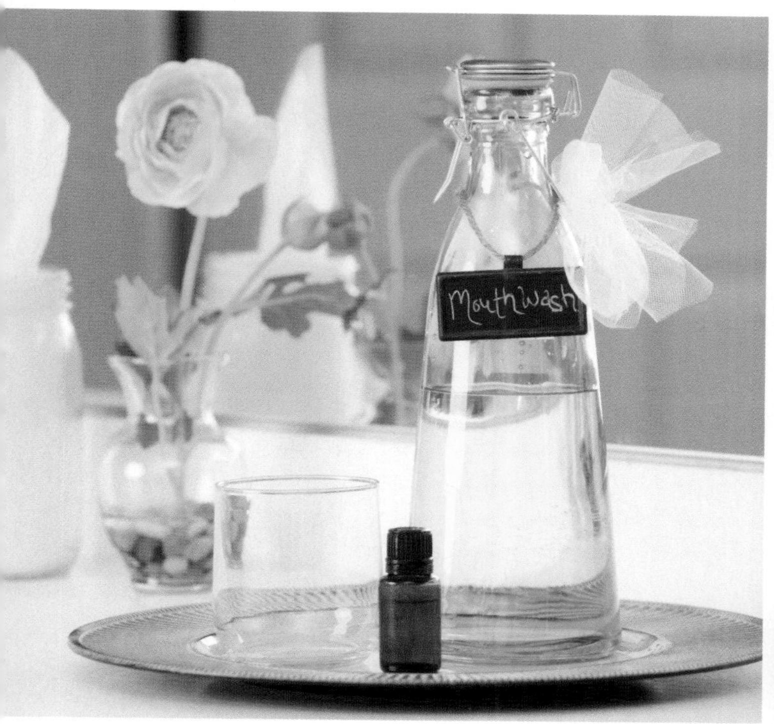

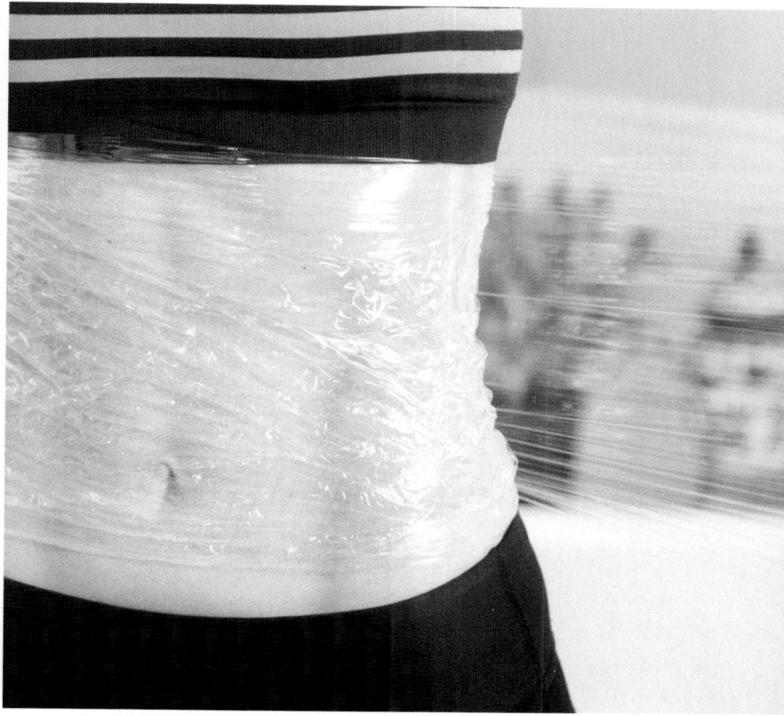

Minty Mouthwash

¾ cup water
3-4 drops peppermint essential oil

Put essential oil into a cup filled with water. Mix well and take small sips, swishing for twenty to thirty seconds. Spit or swallow and repeat.

Teeth Brightener

Strawberries have a slight bleaching effect and if used daily may help rid teeth of minor stains.

1 medium strawberry with stem
1 drop peppermint essential oil

Mash strawberry into a pulp. Add peppermint essential oil and mix well. Dip toothbrush into pulp mixture and brush normally. Rinse thoroughly

Skinny Wrap

40 drops massage blend essential oil
40 drops metabolic blend essential oil
40 drops cypress essential oil
40 drops geranium essential oil
40 drops lemongrass essential oil
40 drops grapefruit essential oil
15 drops eucalyptus essential oil
15 drops wintergreen essential oil
10 drops peppermint essential oil
Grapeseed oil

Place the oils into a 4-ounce spray bottle, top with grapeseed oil, and mix well. Spray over the area you are wrapping and cover with ace bandages or BPA-free plastic wrap. Allow wrap to sit for forty minutes. Remove wrapping and massage remaining oils into the skin. Wraps are most effective when you apply four or more, allowing two to three days between each wrap to decrease cellulite, improve circulation, and help tighten skin.

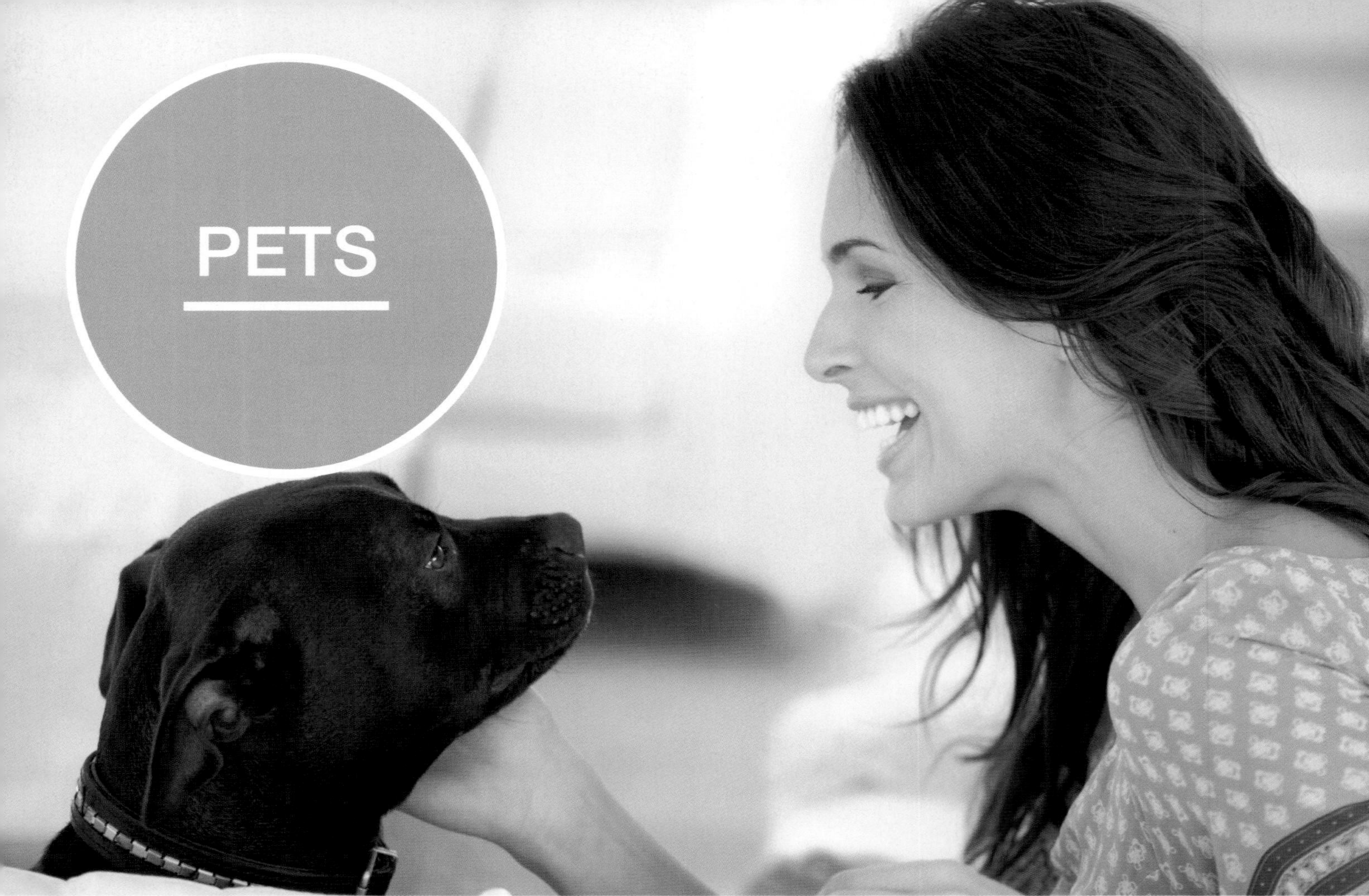

Bad Breath Biscuits

2 cups flour
½ cup oats
¼ teaspoon salt (optional)
2 bananas
3 eggs
2 tablespoons peanut butter
2 tablespoons coconut oil
3- 6 drops peppermint essential oil (depending on size of dog)
1 drop cinnamon essential oil

Mix dry ingredients together in a small mixing bowl. In another bowl mix bananas, eggs, peanut butter, and coconut oil. Mix thoroughly. Add essential oils and mix. Mix dry ingredients into banana mixture and stir until combined.

Using a spoon, scoop large balls onto a cookie sheet and bake at 350 degrees for 20 minutes to make about 1 dozen biscuits.

did you know?

- Common anti-flea solutions for dogs can cause adverse reactions such as skin irritation, hair loss, vomiting, diarrhea, tremors, and seizure.
- Medication commonly used to treat painful arthritis in cats and dogs often causes serious damage to the stomach, liver, and kidneys.
- Most people don't realize that pure essential oils can provide all-natural solutions for animals as well as humans.

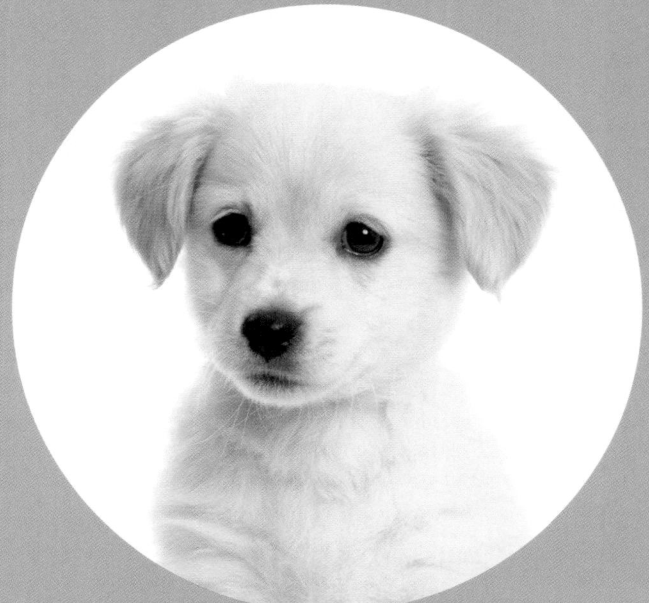

Flea Collar Repellent

½ teaspoon rubbing alcohol
4 garlic oil capsules
1 drop cedarwood essential oil
1 drop lavender essential oil
1 drop lemon essential oil
1 drop thyme essential oil

Mix ingredients in a medium bowl. Soak a pet collar in the mixture for 25 to 30 minutes. Lay out to dry; place on animal's neck. Repeat once or twice a month.

Pet Shampoo

1 cup water
1 tablespoon castile soap
¼ teaspoon vitamin E
3 drops peppermint essential oil
2 drops roman chamomile essential oil
2 drops cleansing blend essential oil
1 drop cedarwood essential oil

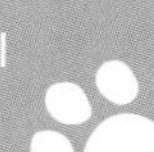

Place all ingredients in a glass jar and mix well. Apply a quarter-size amount to pet and scrub vigorously. Use more on a large pet, if needed. Shampoo will be a bit watery, but your pet will be clean and smell great for days.

Smell Good Pet Spray

10 drops cleansing blend
8 ounces water

Combine in a small glass spray bottle. Shake well and spray on pet for instant germ and smell relief.

No-Odor Kitty Litter

25 drops cleansing blend essential oil
4 cups baking soda.

Combine in a large bowl. Sprinkle 2 tablespoons onto kitty litter when cleaning box daily.

Cat Sratch Deterrent

10 drops eucalyptus essential oil
10 drops lemon essential oil
1 cup water

Fill an empty spray bottle with oils. Add, water shake well, and spray on areas you do not want your cat to scratch.

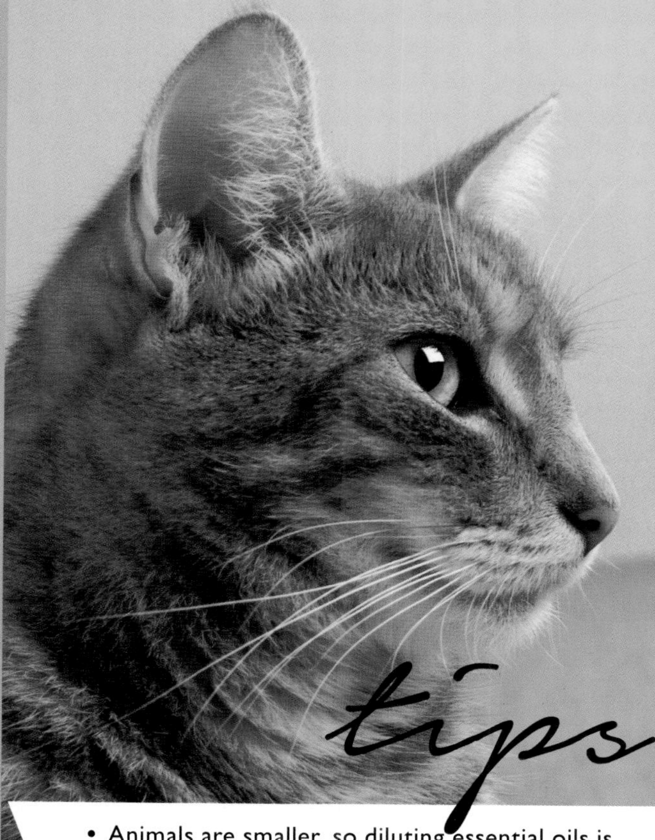

tips

- Animals are smaller, so diluting essential oils is important.
- Avoid using melaleuca for cats.
- Animals prefer certain aromas just as humans do—you can experiment with various oils to see how your pet responds to the aroma and the benefit of the oil.
- For joint pain relief, rub frankincense and soothing blend essential oils directly on joints.
- To help calm and relax a stressed pet, apply 2 to 3 drops of lavender essential oil to ears and paws.

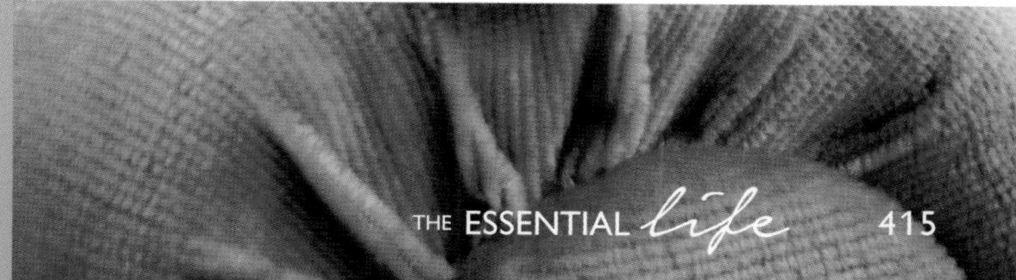

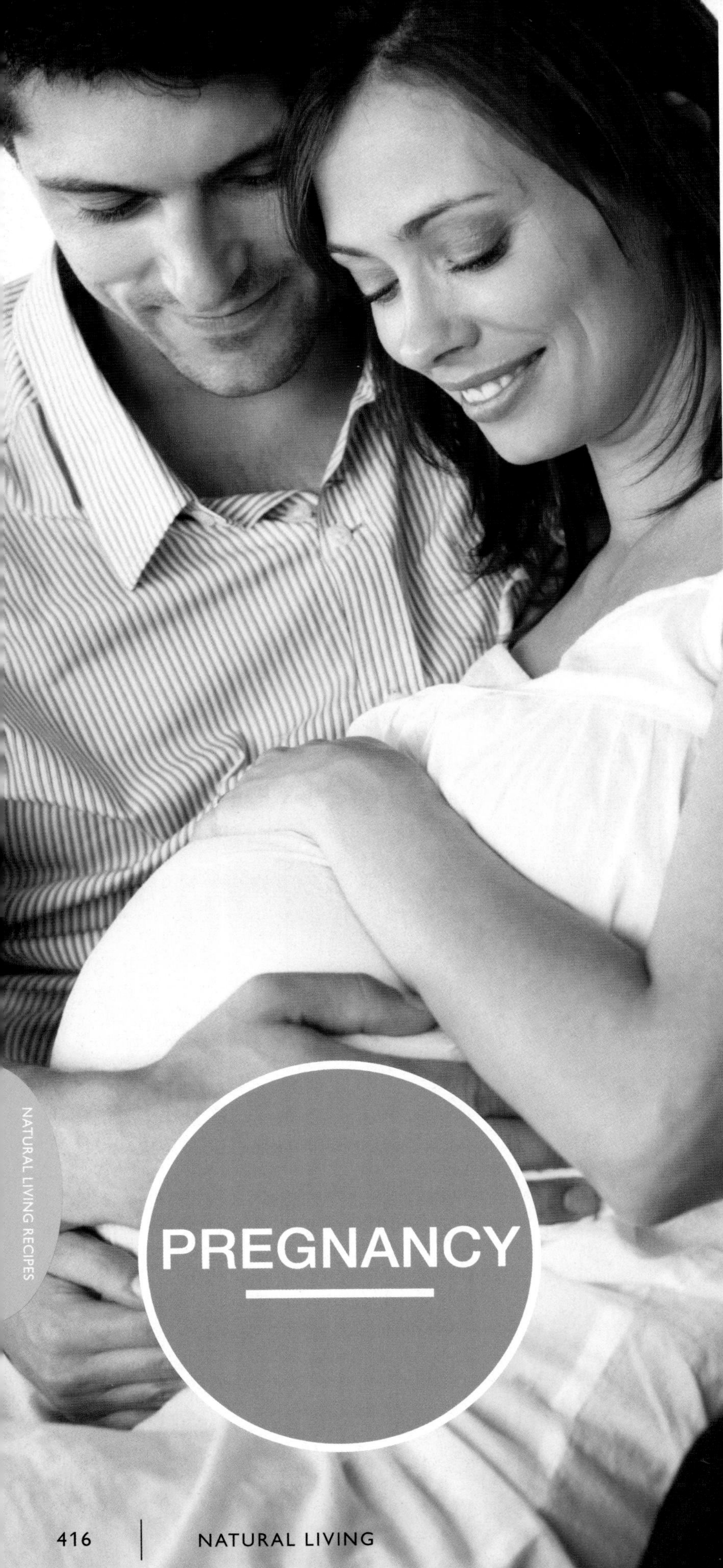

Pure essential oils are a powerful aid during pregnancy, especially since side effects from medication can be so detrimental. Essential oils support the general health of mom and baby, and go beyond to address other common discomforts.

Hemorrhoid Relief Spray

1 drop peppermint essential oil
2 drops helichrysum essential oil
2 drops geranium essential oil
2 drops cypress essential oil
fractionated coconut oil

Mix oils and fractionated coconut oil together in a spray bottle and apply.

After Birth Tear Relief

1 bottle of witch hazel
4 drops lavender essential oil
4 drops melaleuca essential oil

Add lavender and melaleuca to bottle of witch hazel and shake to mix. Then cut large menstrual pad into thirds. Spray the solution over the pads. Squirt aloe gel down the center and freeze them. Apply any remaining solution with peri bottle as needed.

Itchy Skin Belly Butter

½ cup shea butter
¼ cup coconut oil
¼ cup sweet almond oil
10 drops soothing blend

Add oil and shea butter and place in oven-safe glass bowl. Fill a pot with a couple inches of water and place glass bowl inside. Melt butter and oil over medium heat until translucent. Remove from heat and place in the refrigerator for about 2 hours until solid. Whip for about 2-3 minutes into buttery consistency. Spoon into jar, cover and refrigerate 1 more hour. Will store for 6 months at room temperature. Apply directly to belly or itchy spots to nourish and moisturize skin.
Another solution is to add coriander essential oil to your lotion.

Stretch Mark Blend

5 drops lavender essential oil
5 drops myrrh essential oil
5 drops helichrysum essential oil
10 drops fractionated coconut oil

Mix oils and apply on affected area. Repeat frequently as desired to lighten stretch marks.

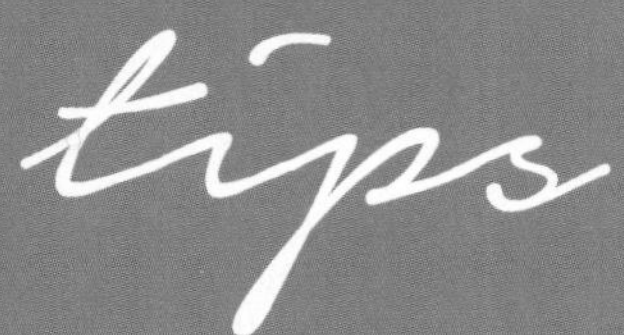

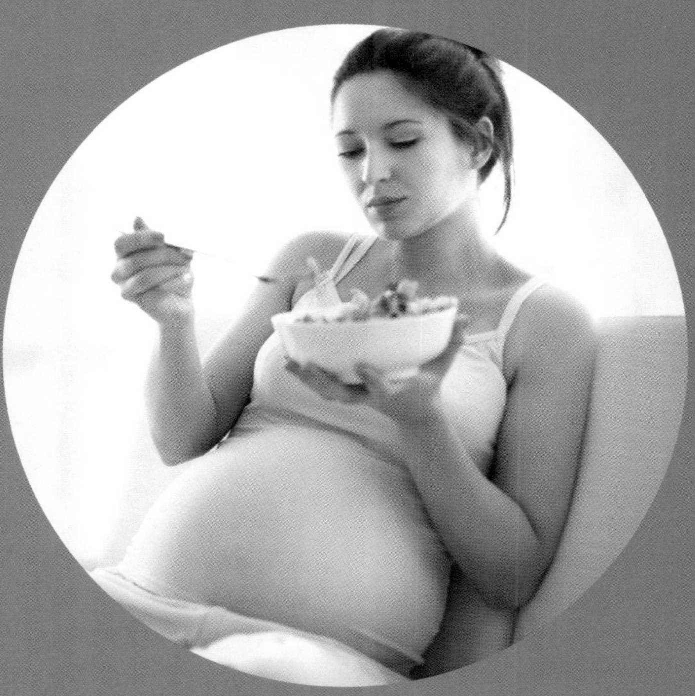

- When using superior grades of essential oils, use during pregnancy is expanded to most oils. For more information see the *Body Systems* section of this book under *Pregnancy, Labor & Nursing*
- Baby brain development: Take an additional 2-3 essential oil omega complex a day during pregnancy and nursing.
- Calming emotional support: apply grounding blend or frankincense to the bottoms of feet.
- Fatigue: add 2-3 drops of lemon, grapefruit, or wild orange in water, 2-3 times a day.
- Sleep support: apply lavender on feet at nap or bedtime, place a couple drops in bath water, or diffuse 30 minutes before bed. Add a few drops to a spray bottle with water and spray on sheets.
- Uplifting emotional support: apply joyful blend topically under nose, to ears, or bottoms of feet.

Pregnancy

- Allergy support: take 2 drops each of lemon and peppermint in a capsule or in water.
- Headache relief: apply tension blend or peppermint topically on forehead, temples, back of neck, and under nose.
- Heartburn: apply digestion blend, peppermint, or ginger directly on breastbone.
- Increase sex drive: diffuse or apply wild orange or ylang ylang topically.
- Morning sickness: apply detoxification blend and detoxification complex pre-pregnancy or during first trimester.
- Morning sickness: apply under nose or put in water or in a capsule. Use peppermint, digestion blend, fennel, or ginger.
- Relaxation and deep sleep: rub lavender or calming blend topically, under nose, forehead, heart, and/or feet.
- Sciatica and muscle pain: apply soothing blend topically to area of concern.
- Swelling: apply massage blend, soothing blend, or lemongrass to the bottoms of your feet or area of swelling. Add a few drops of lemon to your drinking water or take in a capsule.

Birth

- Back pain during labor: apply peppermint or massage blend on back to numb pain.
- Energy during labor: add peppermint topically or internally to drinking water or ice.
- Increase perineum elasticity: massage myrrh and or helichrysum on perineum prior to and during labor.
- Protect the birth canal from group B strep: add frankincense and oregano or basil to douche of water.
- Promote or induce labor: apply women's monthly blend to abdomen, ankles, and to pressure points when mother and baby are ready.
- To support labor: apply clary sage to ankles and other pressure points.

Post Partum

- After-birth pains: apply soothing blend to abdomen.
- Body aches and pains: apply soothing blend, massage blend, or clary sage to pain points.
- Bowels moving: take 2-3 drops of digestion blend in water or in a capsule.
- Engorgement: apply basil around breast.
- Depression: apply joyful blend, frankincense, melissa, or invigorating blend under nose and on ears
- Fatigue: take 6 drops of metabolic blend and 3 drops each of peppermint and wild orange in a capsule daily.
- Hemorrhoid relief: apply grounding blend directly to affected area.
- Increase milk production: apply fennel and/or rosemary to breasts.
- Prevent baby infection: combine frankincense with colloidal silver and spritz or apply over baby's whole body.
- Sore nipples: apply helichrysum directly to nipples to bring healing and elasticity.
- Tearing, inflammation and soreness: apply frankincense, helichrysum, and/or lavender topically. Put drops of lavender and frankincense on frozen feminine pads.

Newborn

- For swelling, baby blemishes, or skin discoloration: apply frankincense topically to any area of concern.
- To assist in baby's transition and release any trauma: diffuse or apply frankincense or grounding blend to baby's spine and bottom of feet.
- To help avoid infection and release umbilical cord remains: place several drops of myrrh on umbilical cord.

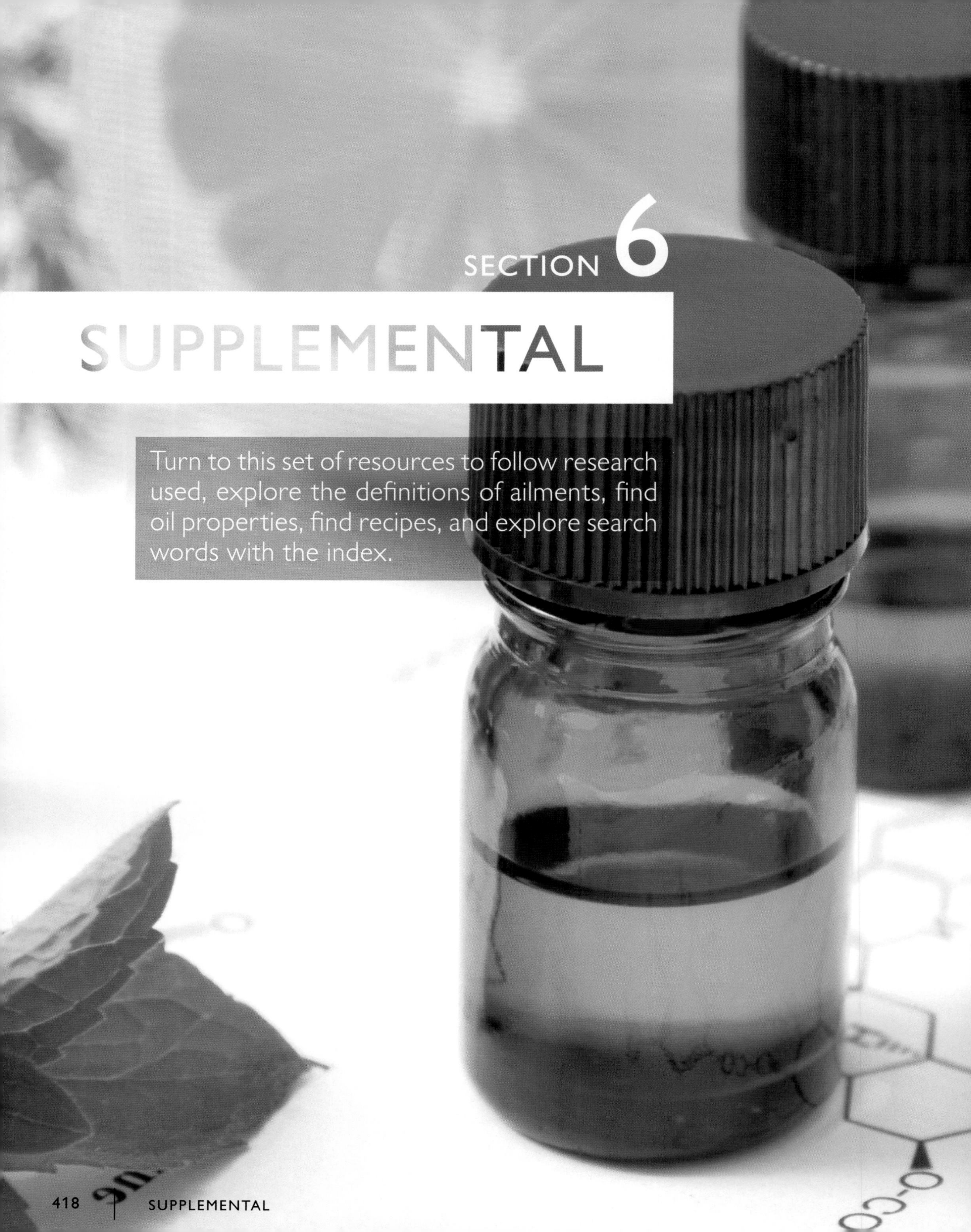

SECTION 6

SUPPLEMENTAL

Turn to this set of resources to follow research used, explore the definitions of ailments, find oil properties, find recipes, and explore search words with the index.

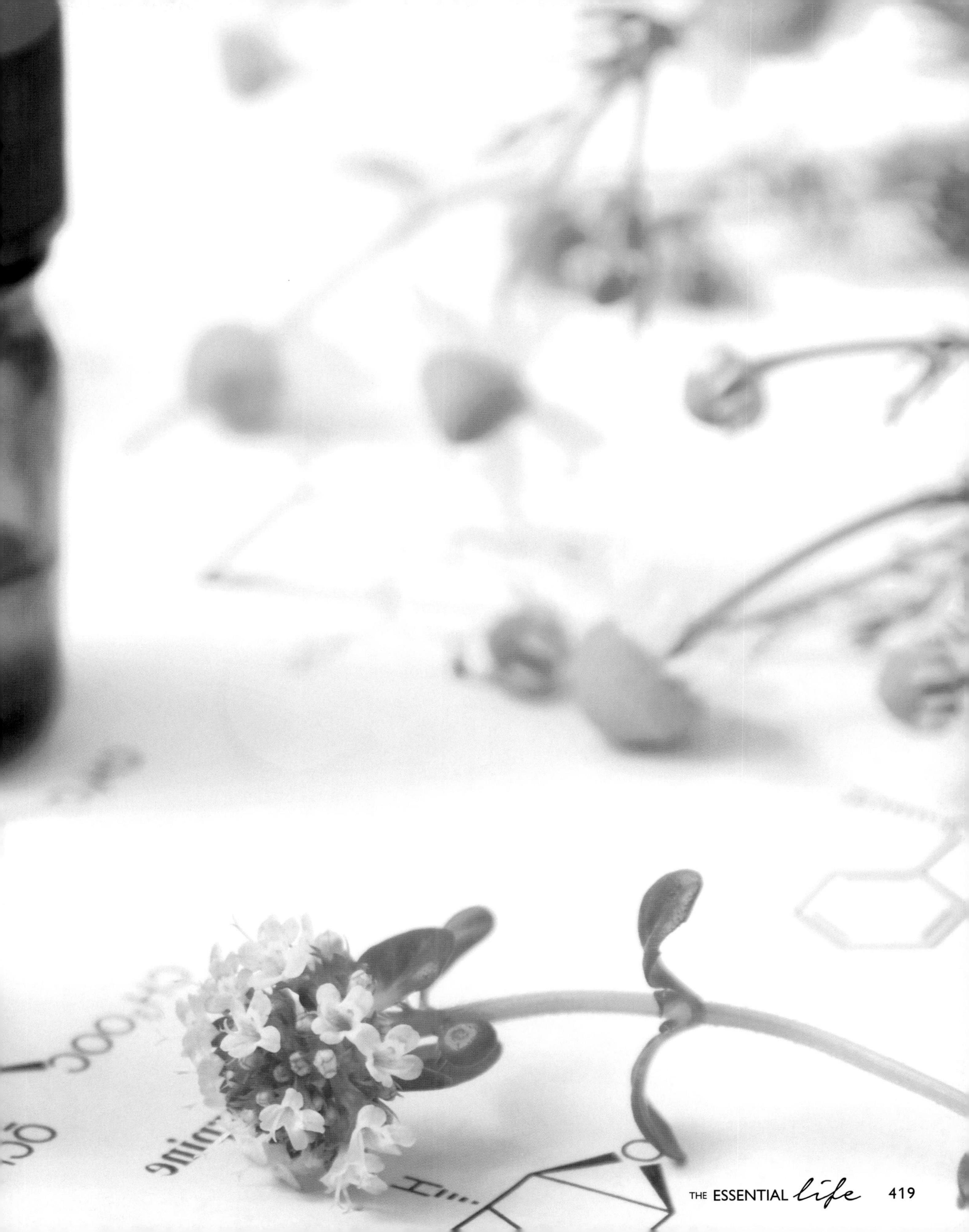

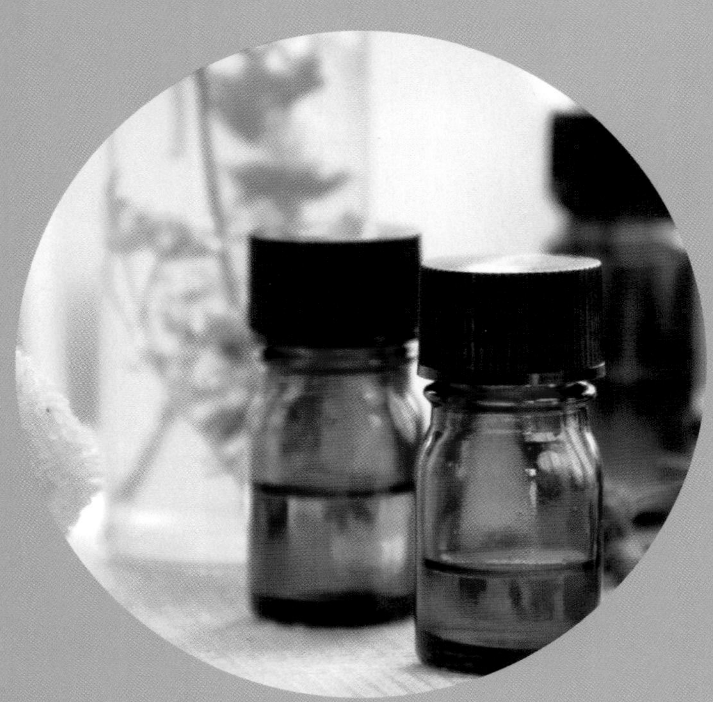

Be a Power User

The Essential Life is about focusing on the core elements of amazing wellness, and YOU hold the power to create this into your reality. This section will teach you how to become a confident power user of the healing tools that will elevate your essential life.

Live an Essential Lifestyle

To achieve elevated wellness, first understand the components that contribute to wellness, or if neglected, lack of wellness. The natural tools in this book can assist you in each of these key areas.

ESSENTIAL LIFESTYLE

BODY FUEL

What you put into your body becomes your body. If you want a high-energy, vibrant, high-functioning body, then put high-energy, vibrant, high-functioning food & fuel into your body! **Add vitality supplements and energizing oils to a great diet.**

ACTIVITY

Your body was built to move. As you enjoy some kind of active moment every day, your body systems will have good reason to stay active and healthy. **Enhance activity with oils for muscle, joint, and respiratory support**

REST

Meaningful rest is necessary for your systems to reset and regenerate. Commit to giving yourself adequate time to recover through meaningful sleep and personal care each day. **Learn the oils that your body responds to for great sleep.**

STRESS MANAGEMENT

Emotional and physical stressors are at the root of all illness and disease. Create space and use good tools to reduce stressors in your life. **Pause briefly throughout each day to enjoy emotional balancing with your oils.**

TOXIC REDUCTION

Toxicity can be found in our water, air, household cleaners and chemicals, and many things we put into our bodies. Minimize toxicity to create a clean environment inside your body. **Use oils to safely clean your home and detox your body.**

RESTORATIVE SELF-CARE

Knowing how to use safe, effective natural remedies is empowering. It allows you to restore health, prevent unwanted issues, and be prepared for the unexpected. **Learn the uses of the best oils for your health needs.**

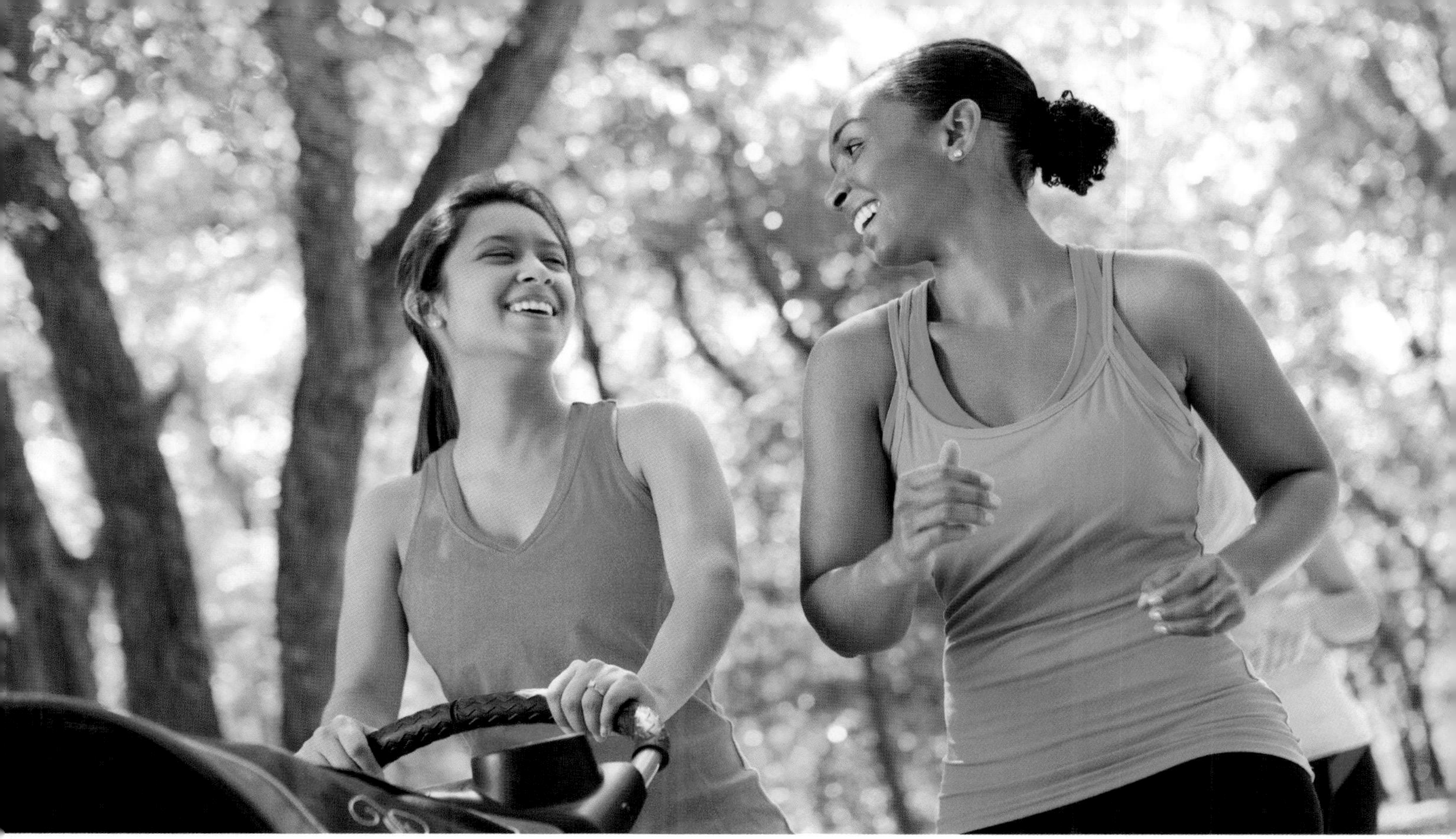

Good Health Loves Preparation

Be prepared for anything by having your essential oils and other remedies handy. Try a few of these:

- **Around the House** Keep frequently used oils handy by your bedside, in the bathroom, the kitchen, and main family living space. You'll use them more often and see better results, and your family will join in if they're easily accessible.
- **Purse or Keychain** Have a small bag of oils you need for mood support, digestive support, and immune protection when you're out and about. If you don't carry a purse or bag, get a keychain that holds small vials (5/8 dram) of your favorite oils.
- **Car** Keep oils for focus and stress management in your car to turn driving time into useful rejuvenation time.
- **Diaper Bag or Stroller** Kids love to do the unexpected, which is why you'll always be glad to have oils ready for bumps and bruises, skin irritations, and temper tantrums wherever you go.

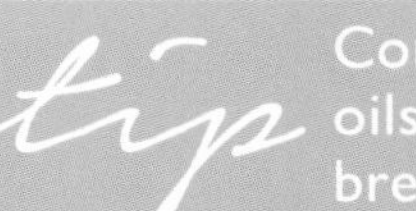

Consistency makes magic. While oils are fast-acting, consistency breeds the best long-term results.

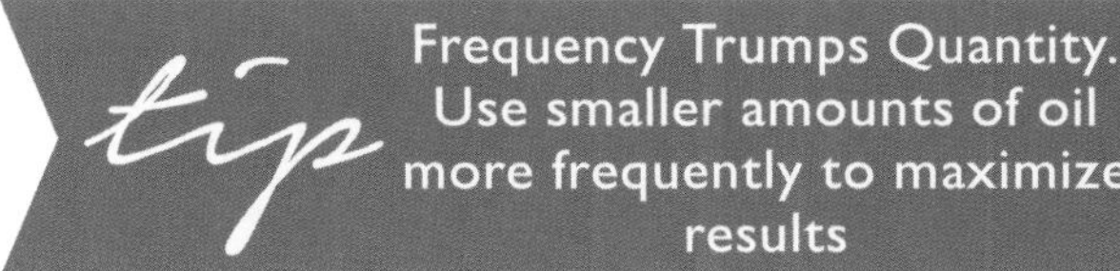

Frequency Trumps Quantity. Use smaller amounts of oil more frequently to maximize results

Find Brilliant Answers

Rather than stressing about becoming an expert on health and wellness, simply get familiar with where to find the answers you need for your health. If you develop the habit of turning to natural remedies first, and you know where to look for usage and other support, you'll have confidence in creating the wellness you desire. Try these resources:

- ***The Essential Life* Book**
- **Web Resources** There are good websites that allow you to look up ailments and essential oil usage. Bookmark your favorites for easy access.
- **Mobile Apps** Find an app you like, and enjoy having a good essential oil resource wherever you go.
- **Social Media Resources** There are many blogs and social media sites where you can find tips and tricks, recipes, and community support from other essential oil users. Follow bloggers you like, and join a Facebook group to connect with others.

Explore Different Usage Methods

- **Aromatic.** Keep a diffuser in high-traffic areas in the home and in sleeping areas. Diffusers are a great way to let everyone around enjoy the benefits of the oils.
- **Topical.** Have a carrier oil like fractionated coconut oil on hand for use on sensitive skin, and to use as a remedy if someone experiences sensitivity after an oil has been applied. Try recipes for skin creams and lotions with your oils.
- **Internal.** Keep veggie capsules near your oils for easy internal use. Try putting some in a small plastic baggie so you can have them ready on the go. Remember to only use oils internally if they are verified pure and therapeutic.

tip

Layering vs. Blending: While blending oils is a valuable art, you may have success with layering. Apply one oil topically, wait several seconds, and then apply the next one, etc.

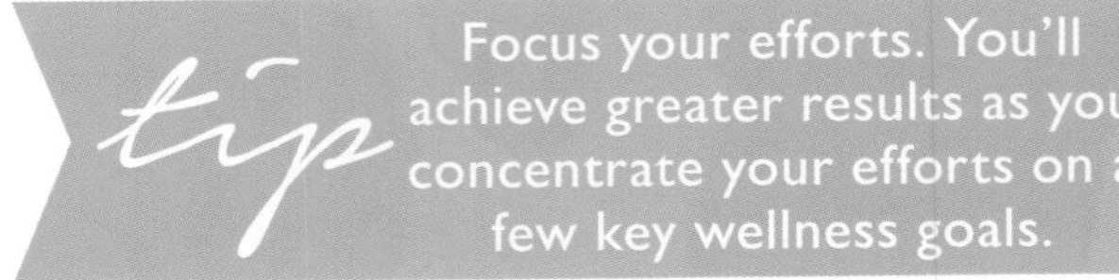

tip

Focus your efforts. You'll achieve greater results as you concentrate your efforts on a few key wellness goals.

Supercharge Your Oils

While you can use oils a seemingly infinite number of ways, you'll also find methods that work best for you and your family. Try some of these tips to enhance the effectiveness of your oils:

- **Add heat** Use a hot compress to drive the oils in deeper when using topically.
- **Add frankincense** Frankincense enhances the therapeutic effects of many protocols, and brings powerful healing properties.
- **Massage** Massaging oils into the needed area stimulates tissues and increases absorption. It also provides benefit for the person giving and the person receiving the massage.
- **Combine oils that complement each other** Don't be afraid to try different oil combinations. You can find an ocean of essential oil recipes and protocols because nature complements itself in so many ways. Try different combinations, and enjoy the process of discovering what resonates with your body.

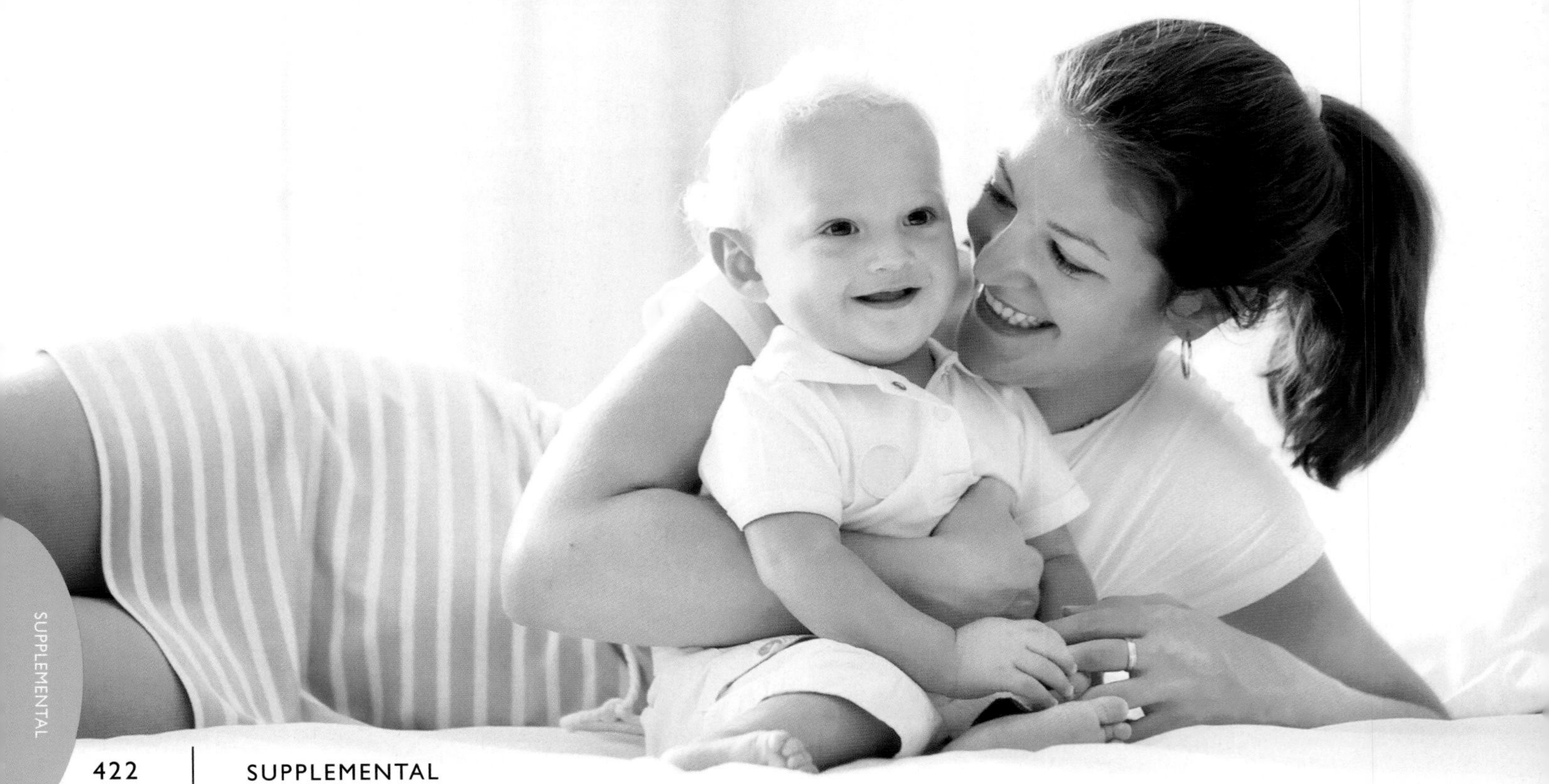

Oil Composition & Chemistry

Plants synthesize two types of oils: fixed oils and essential oils. Fixed oils consist of glycerol and fatty acids. Essential oils are a mix of volatile organic compounds that contribute to the fragrance and well being of the plant. Essential oils are made up of many compound constituents that serve several purposes for the plant:

- protection and responses to parasites such a bacteria, viruses, fungi, and other pests
- restoration from wounds and physical damage
- protection from sun and other elements
- communication through fragrance to insects or other plants of the same genus

Essential oils are volatile oils that have an intrinsic nature or essence of the plant. Essential oils are more soluble in lipophilic solvents than in water. They are complex mixtures of chemical compounds, and every biological effect displayed by an essential oil is due to the actions of one or more of its constituents.

Essential oils are secondary metabolites in plants. The oils are isolated from plants through a process called hydrodistillation: passing boiling water through the plant material and vaporizing the essential oil from the plant. As the steam rises and condenses, the water and essential oil separate and the oil product, the essential oil, is captured. The remaining water is aromatic and contains in much lower concentrations and in different ratios some of the constituents from the oil. This water is known as a hydrosol and is used and sold for its therapeutic benefits and its fragrance.

The chemical compounds in citrus essential oils come from the rind of the fruit. Most citrus essential oils are generally isolated by cold pressing rather than distillation. Citrus oils that are cold pressed also include relatively large, involatile molecules, including the phototoxic compounds. These compounds are not in distilled citrus oils.

Some fragrant oils such as rose or jasmine oil are at times extracted with organic solvents, which produces concretes, absolutes, or resinoids.

Essential oils typically contain dozens of constituents with related, but distinct, chemical structures. Each constituent has its own characteristic and has different effects when used. Even though an essential oil contains many different types of compounds, usually one or two compounds dominate their action. For example, alpha-Pinene is the main compound that is responsible for action of frankincense essential oil. Some constituents may comprise a small percentage of an oil but may play a significant role in its overall action. Because no two distillations are ever the same and because of many other variables such as elevation, harvest time, soil type, weather condition, etc., lists of compounds contained in an essential oil are usually stated as a range. For example, the compound alpha-Pinene may range from 41 percent to 80 percent of a frankincense essential oil (*Boswellia frereana*).

Because of their antimicrobial properties, essential oils are not generally subject to microbial contamination. Essential oils can be contaminated from unnatural constituents, distillation items, or adulterants. These include pesticides or herbicides, traces of solvent, and phthalates (plasticizing agents). Adulteration includes both intentional dilution and fabrication of an oil or parts of an essential oil. There are many ways and methods to test an essential oil for levels of purity. Testing by independent and properly equipped labs is critical to knowing of an oil's purity and complete profile. Adulteration could increase toxicity of an oil. Only essential oils that are tested and verified pure therapeutic grade should be used for therapeutic benefits.

It's a complex task to evaluate and unravel the chemistry of an essential oil. Many compounds in an essential oil are present in minute amounts. They may be hard to detect except through testing by laboratories with a large enough database to identify all of the constituents. Some of the modern methods and analyses that are used to determine the chemical profile of an essential oil include:

- Gas Chromatography (GC)
- Mass Spectrometry (MS)
- High Performance Liquid Chromatography (HPLC)
- Nuclear Magnetic Resonance Spectroscopy (NMR)
- Fourier Transform Infrared Spectroscopy (FTIS)
- Chiral GC Testing
- Isotope Carbon 14TPC/Microbial

The best testing involves a combination of several methods throughout the process from harvest to bottle.

Essential oils are made up of organic (carbon-based) compounds. The individual essential oil constituents contain atoms in addition to carbon(C), such as hydrogen(H) and oxygen(O). Learning the basics of essential oil chemical construction will help in understanding why different oils achieve different actions. For example, alpha-Pinene, a

[1] *Essential Oil Safety*, Robert Tisserand and Rodney Young, 2014, page 6.
[2] *Essential Oil Safety*, pg 7.
[3] *Essential Oil Safety*, pg 8.

compound in frankincense essential oil, is written chemically as $C_{10}H_{16}$ This means the alpha-Pinene consists of ten carbon atoms and sixteen hydrogen atoms. The compound can also be shown as a diagram. The double line indicates a double bond in that part of the compound. Essential oil molecules are three-dimensional but represented in this diagram as two-dimensional.

CH_3

CH_3

CH_3

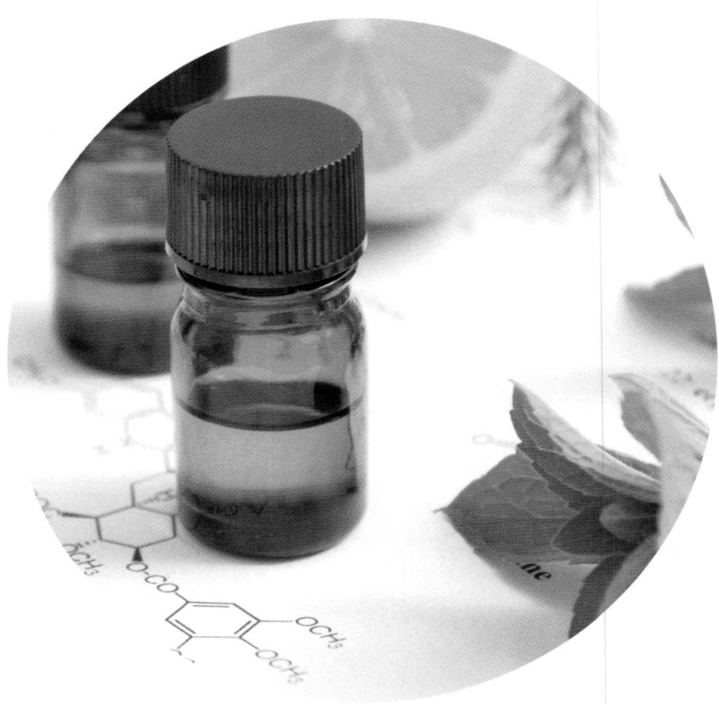

Essential oil constituents are built on a framework of isoprene units. Isoprene units consist of carbon and hydrogen atoms; their chemical makeup consists of five carbon atoms and eight hydrogen atoms. Their chemical signature is C_5H_8. Most of the compounds in essential oils consist of two to four isoprene units. These units are referred to as terpenes or terpenoids. Terpenoids are terpenes that have functional groups added to them. These functional groups are made up of mostly hydrogen and oxygen and include alcohols, phenols, aldehydes, esters, and ethers. Terpenes do not have a functional group added to them; they are often referred to as hydrocarbons. The simplest and most common class of terpenes found in essential oils is the monoterpene (a double isoprene unit with ten carbon atoms). The next group of terpenes is the sesquiterpenes, and the basic structure is composed of fifteen carbon atoms or three isoprene units. They have a larger molecular size than the monoterpenes and therefore are less volatile. See the following table for the classes of terpenes and the number of carbon atoms in each.

Monoterpene	10 carbon atoms	Most common
Sesquiterpenes	15 carbon atoms	Larger size molecule and less volatile
Diterpenes	20 carbon atoms	Only in some essential oils
Triterpenes	30 carbon atoms	Can be present in absolutes
Tetraterpenes	40 carbon atoms	Not part of essential oils but found in cold-pressed citrus oils (beta-carotene is an example)

All of the compounds or constituents in essential oils belong to a group. These groups are defined by the number of carbon atoms they have and the type of functional group assigned to them. For example alpha-Pinene is part of the monoterpene hydrocarbon group. It has ten carbon atoms and does not have a functional group as part of its molecular makeup, which makes it a hydrocarbon. It is unique from the other compounds in the group because of the number hydrogen atoms and how the carbon and hydrogen atoms are bonded together. Another example is alpha-Santalol, a major compound in sandalwood essential oil. Alpha-Santalol chemically is $C_{15}H_{24}O$ It has an oxygen functional group and fifteen carbon atoms, so it is part of the sesquiterpene alcohol group.

The compounds and the compound groups have been researched and found to exhibit certain common therapeutic benefits. Once a compound is identified as part of an essential oil and once the group to which it belongs is identified, the possible action of the essential oil can be determined. Essential oils are made up of many compounds. Some compounds make up a larger percentage of an oil, while others may only offer a trace of the total essential oil. Though compounds that comprise larger parts of an oil definitely help guide an oil's benefit, the smaller amounts play a part in the oil's actions.

The following table lists common groups of compounds in essential oils, examples of compounds in that group, the known therapeutic benefits of that group, and some of the essential oils that contain compounds in that group.

CHEMICAL COMPOUND GROUP AND EXAMPLES	THERAPEUTIC BENEFITS	OILS CONTAINING SOME OF THE GROUP	NOTES
Monoterpene Hydrocarbon (alpha & beta-pinene, limonene, sabinene, phellandrene)	Inhibit the accumulation of toxins and help discharge existing toxins, anti-inflammatory, antibacterial, soothing to irritated tissues, insect repellent, cancer-preventative properties	citrus oils, frankincense, ginger, thyme, cypress, white fir, black pepper, marjoram, melaleuca	10 carbon terpenes
Sesquiterpene Hydrocarbon (chamazulene, faresene, zingiberene)	Anti-inflammatory, sedative, soothing, antibacterial, soothing to irritated skin and tissue, liver and glandular stimulant	myrrh, ginger, vetiver, sandalwood, black pepper, patchouli, ylang ylang, helichrysum, cedarwood	15 carbon terpenes
Monoterpene Alcohols (borneol, geraniol, linalool)	Antimicrobial, supports the immune system, restorative to the skin, cleansing, antispasmodic, sedative, gentle, mild	geranium, lavender, melaleuca, frankincense	10 carbon terpenoids bound to a hydroxyl group, high resistance to oxidation
Sesquiterpene Alcohols	Anti-allergenic, antibacterial, anti-inflammatory, liver and glandular stimulant	sandalwood, patchouli, cedarwood, ginger	15 carbon terpenoids bound to a hydroxyl group bound to a carbon instead of a hydrogen
Esters (geranyl acetate, linalyl acetate, methyl salicylate)	Very calming, relaxing, and balancing, antifungal, antispasmodic, balancing to nervous system	cardamom, clary sage, helichrysum, lavender, roman chamomile, jasmine, ylang ylang, bergamot	Consists of a carboxyl group (carbon atom double-bonded to an oxygen atom)
Aldehydes (citral, geranial, neral)	Powerful aromas, calming to the emotions, anti-infectious, anti-inflammatory, calming to autonomic nervous system, fever-reducing, hypotensive, tonic	cassia, cinnamon, cilantro, lemongrass, melissa	Consists of a carboxyl group (carbon atom double-bonded to an oxygen atom). Slightly fruity odor, can cause skin irritation
Ketones (camphor, jasmone)	Mucolytic, stimulate cell regeneration, promote the formation of tissue, analgesic, sedative	helichrysum, peppermint, rosemary, fennel, vetiver, lavender, myrrh, roman chamomile, fennel, lemongrass	Consists of a carboxyl group (carbon atom double-bonded to an oxygen atom)
Phenols (carvacrol, eugenol, thymol)	Powerful antibacterial, anti-infectious, antiseptic, very stimulating to the autonomic nervous system, analgesic, antifungal, cancer preventative	oregano, thyme, clove	Consists of a benzene ring – 6 carbon atoms bound in a circle – and a hydroxyl group. May be irritating to the skin, some concerns at high dosages for liver toxicity. Use for short periods of time.
Oxides (1,8 cineole)	Expectorant, mildly stimulating, respiratory support, pain relief, anti-inflammatory	eucalyptus, rosemary, peppermint, cypress, clary sage, clove, cardamom, thyme, melaleuca, basil, peppermint, fennel	An oxygen atom has become bound between two carbon atoms.
Ethers (estragole, anethole)	Balancing to the autonomic nervous system, soothing, sedative	fennel, basil, ylang ylang, marjoram	Compounds in which an oxygen atom in the molecule is bonded to two carbon atoms.
Lactones (coumarin)	Expectorant properties	In very low amounts in some essential oils	Consists of an ester group integrated into a carbon ring system. Has a vanilla-like odor
Coumarins (bergamottin)		bergamot	phototoxic

Blending & Layering

When using essential oils, the desired outcome may best be accomplished by using more than one essential oil at a time. To do so, the oils may be layered topically, ingested separately, or placed together in a blend. Layering is defined as applying one essential oil to the skin, waiting for it to be absorbed, and then applying another oil over the first. This may be repeated several times until all the desired oils are applied. Massage expedites and improves this absorption process. Oils are absorbed rapidly into the skin, so the wait time can be short. A carrier oil, such as fractionated coconut oil, may be applied prior to or along with an oil application. In some cases, layering is a preferred method for topical use, as it requires less skill and knowledge than blending, and allows the oil selections to be varied at every application.

Layering is particularly useful when multiple concerns must be addressed simultaneously. For example, a sprained or twisted ankle may involve tendons or ligaments (connective tissue) as well as muscle or bone. Furthermore, bruising and swelling may be present. Increasing blood flow to the injury site would also be useful for healing. Each of these concerns may be addressed through the use of layering.

Here is an example of an injured tissue layering sequence:

1-2 drops of lemongrass – for connective tissue; apply, massage lightly if possible, wait for absorption

1-2 drops of marjoram – for muscle; apply, massage lightly if possible, wait for absorption

1-2 drops of cypress – for circulation; apply, massage lightly if possible, wait for absorption

1-2 drops of helichrysum – for pain; apply, massage lightly if possible, wait for absorption

1-2 drops of wintergreen – for bone; apply, massage lightly if possible, wait for absorption

This layering sequence would be repeatedly applied to expedite healing. For example, application every 30-60 minutes for the first four applications may be followed by application every 4-6 hours the following few days. Finally, twice-a-day application may be used once the pain has mostly subsided and until complete healing has occurred.

In addition to layering the oils, there are times when creating an essential oil blend is a good or better way to achieve an intended result such as calming a mood, relaxing muscles, or supporting a distressed respiratory system. Blending is the process of combining multiple selected essential oils together in one bottle. The chemical profile of a blend is very different from each of the individual oils it contains. Combining essential oils together creates a synergistic effect, forming a new, unique molecular structure.

There is an art to blending, which is enhanced and improved by practice and through applying proven techniques and principles. Artistry and skill combine to creating a blend that is aromatically pleasing and that accomplishes the desired therapeutic outcome or goal. Since essential oils are potent and often expensive, care should be taken to blend appropriately so as not to waste essential oils or to create a blend that may cause an adverse reaction, such as a headache or skin sensitivity. There are many resources and educational classes on the art of blending essential oils. One excellent resource is *Aromatherapy Workbook* by Marcel Lavabre. A study of the basic chemical makeup of essential oil aids in creating therapeutically effective blends. For a foundational understanding of the main chemical constituents in essential oils refer to the "Body Systems: Oil Composition & Chemistry" section in this book.

Blending Guidelines

Some basic guidelines help in blending regardless of the method used:

1. The "Blends Well With" listings under each oil description in the "Natural Solutions: Single Oils" assist in selecting oils that blend well together.
2. Blends that have been professionally created are best used as they are.
3. Essential oils from the same botanical family usually blend well together.
4. Essential oils with similar constituents usually mix well together.
5. A blend should be aromatically pleasing.
6. It is best to use the smallest amount of oil possible when experimenting with a blend.
7. It is helpful to label your blend.
8. Be specific in defining your desired outcome.
9. Keeping a blending journal serves as a reference for making adjustments or remembering what worked.
10. As a beginner, it is best to start with blending four to six essential oils for a total of fifteen to twenty drops in the blend.

There are differing opinions and experiences as to what order oils should be added to a blend. It is has been shown in a laboratory that in small amounts, such as blends for personal use, order doesn't matter. However, if blending in large amounts, i.e., companies that create their own blends en masse to sell, the order in which oils are added may be very important.

Blending Methods

There are three suggested techniques for creating essential oil blends:

1 Blending Classifications Method

2 Odor Types/Notes Method

3 Combination of Techniques (Chemical Compounds and Odor Types) Method

An in-depth description of each of these methods or techniques is beyond the scope of this book, though a summary is included here for each method. Practice and study improves the ability to create effective and aromatically pleasing blends.

Blending Classification Method

This method uses the four blending classifications: personifier, enhancer, equalizer, and modifier. Below is a description of each classification.

PLACE IN BLEND	NAME OF CLASSIFICATION	PERCENTAGE OF THE BLEND	CHARACTERISTICS	EXAMPLE OILS IN THIS CLASSIFICATION
First	Personifier	1-5%	Sharp, strong, and long-lasting aroma, dominant properties, strong therapeutic action	birch, black pepper, cassia, cardamom, cinnamon, clary sage, clove, coriander, ginger, helichrysum, orange, peppermint, roman chamomile, rose, spearmint, tangerine, vetiver, wintergreen, and ylang ylang
Second	Enhancer	50-80%	Enhances the properties of the other oils in the blend, not a sharp aroma; evaporates faster than the Personifier	arborvitae, basil, bergamot, birch, cassia, cedarwood, cinnamon, dill, eucalyptus, frankincense, geranium, grapefruit, jasmine, lavender, lemon, lemongrass, lime, marjoram, melaleuca, melissa, orange, oregano, patchouli, rose, rosemary, thyme, and wintergreen
Third	Equalizer	10-15%	Creates balance and synergy among the oils in the blend	arborvitae, basil,bergamot, cedarwood, cilantro, cypress, fennel, white fir, frankincense, geranium, ginger, jasmine, juniper berry, lavender, lemongrass, lime, marjoram, melaleuca, melissa, myrrh, oregano, rose, sandalwood, thyme, and white fir
Fourth	Modifier	5-8%	Mild; evaporates quickly, adds harmony to the blend	bergamot, black pepper, cardamom, coriander, eucalyptus, fennel, grapefruit, jasmine, lavender, lemon, melissa, myrrh, rose, sandalwood, tangerine, and ylang ylang

The table below provides an example of a blend for easing muscle strain using the Blending Classification Method. Using this recipe, mix the four oils in the order listed in a 10 ml roller bottle and fill with a carrier oil such as fractionated coconut oil for dilution.

CLASSIFICATION	AMOUNT*	ESSENTIAL OIL
Personifier	1 drop	cinnamon
Enhancer	8 drops	basil
Equalizer	2 drops	ginger
Modifier	4 drops	grapefruit

*based on a 15-drop blend

Odor Types/Notes

This second method focuses on the odor and odor intensity ascribed to each essential oil. The perfume industry has assigned perfume "notes" to essential oils. The three notes are base, middle, and top. These assignments can be used as a guide in creating a blend.

Top notes are light oils and often have fresh, sweet, citrusy, or fruity aromas. Middle notes are oils that have a floral, slight woody, or sweet aroma. Base notes are woody, heavy, earthy, rich, or deep. Some oils such as basil or fennel may be used in a blend as either a top or middle note. Clary sage and ylang ylang are examples of oils that may be used as either middle or base notes. When creating a blend, base notes are 5% to 20% of the blend, middle notes are 50% to 80%, and top notes are 5% to 20% of the blend. This blending method is more focused on aroma than therapeutic benefits.

Following is an example of a blend designed to ease muscle strain using the **Odor Types/Notes** method. Using this recipe, mix the four oils in the order listed in a 10 ml roller bottle and fill with a carrier oil such as fractionated coconut oil for dilution.

ODOR TYPE/NOTE	AMOUNT*	OIL
Base Note	3 drops	sandalwood
Middle Note	3 drops	ginger
Middle Note	4 drops	cypress
Top Note	5 drops	wild orange

*based on a 15-drop blend

Following is a table of single oils with their scent profile and assigned scent note. Knowing an oils scent note is critical in blending using the note type classification method.

OIL	SCENT PROFILE	SCENT NOTE
Arborvitae	Intense, medicinal, woody, earthy	Top to Middle
Basil	Herbaceous, spicy, anise-like, camphoraceous, lively	Top to Middle
Bergamot	Sweet, lively, citrusy, fruity	Top
Birch	Sweet, sharp, camphoraceous, fresh	Top
Black pepper	Spicy, peppery, musky, warm, with herbaceous undertones.	Middle
Cardamom	Sweet, spicy, balsamic, with floral undertones	Middle
Cassia	Spicy, warm, sweet	Middle
Cedarwood	Warm, soft, woody	Middle
Cilantro	Herbaceous, citrusy, fresh	Top
Cinnamon	Spicy, earthy, sweet	Middle
Clary sage	Herbaceous, spicy, hay-like, sharp, fixative	Middle to Base
Clove	Spicy, warming, slightly bitter, woody	Middle to Base
Coriander	Woody, spicy, sweet	Middle
Cypress	Fresh, herbaceous, slightly woody with evergreen undertones	Middle
Dill	Fresh, sweet, herbaceous, slightly earthly	Middle
Eucalyptus	Slightly camphorous, sweet, fruity	Middle
Fennel (sweet)	Sweet, somewhat spicy, licorice-like	Top to Middle
Frankincense	Rich, deep, warm, balsamic, sweet, with incense-like overtones	Base
Geranium	Sweet, green, citrus-rosy, fresh	Middle
Ginger	Sweet, spicy-woody, warm, tenacious, fresh, sharp	Middle
Grapefruit	Clean, fresh, bitter, citrusy	Top
Helichrysum	Rich, sweet, fruity, with tea and honey undertones	Middle
Jasmine	Powerful, sweet, tenacious, floral with fruity-herbaceous undertones	Base
Juniper berry	Sweet, balsamic, tenacious	Middle

OIL	SCENT PROFILE	SCENT NOTE
Lavender	Floral, sweet, herbaceous, balsamic, woody undertones	Middle
Lemon	Sweet, sharp, clear, citrusy	Top
Lemongrass	Grassy, lemony, pungent, earthy, slightly bitter	Top
Lime	Sweet, tart, intense, lively	Top
Marjoram	Herbaceous, green, spicy	Middle
Melaleuca	Medicinal, fresh, woody, earthy, herbaceous	Middle
Melissa	Delicate, lemony, spicy	Middle
Myrrh	Warm, earthy, woody, balsamic	Base
Orange	Fresh, citrusy, fruity, sweet	Top
Oregano	Spicy, warm, herbaceous, sharp	Middle
Patchouli	Earthy, herbaceous, sweet, balsamic, rich, with woody undertones	Base
Peppermint	Minty, sharp, intense	Middle
Roman chamomile	Fresh, sweet, fruity-herbaceous, apple-like, no tenacity	Middle
Rose	Floral, spicy, rich, deep, sensual, green, honey-like	Middle to Base
Rosemary	Herbaceous, strong, camphorous, with woody-balsamic and evergreen undertones	Middle
(Hawaiian) Sandalwood	Soft, woody, spicy, sweet, earthy, balsamic	Base
Spearmint	Minty, slightly fruity, less bright than peppermint	Top
Tangerine	Fresh, sweet, citrusy	Top
Thyme	Fresh, medicinal, herbaceous	Middle
Vetiver	Sweet undertones, heavy, earthy, woody, smoky, balsamic	Base
White fir	Fresh, woody, earthy, sweet	Middle
Wintergreen	Minty, camphorous, fresh	Top
Ylang ylang	Sweet, heavy, narcotic, cloying, tropical floral, with spicy-balsamic undertones	Middle to Base

Combination of Techniques (Chemistry Compounds and Odor Types)

The first two blending methods are primarily focused on creating a pleasing aroma with secondary consideration to the end therapeutic goal. The Combination of Techniques method allows for both aroma and therapeutic effectiveness to be considered. When a blend is created by first setting a specific end goal and then selecting essential oils based on the desired therapeutic benefits of the chemical compounds, a more effective blend is created. If odor types are also considered, then an effective and aromatically pleasing blend is created. Refer to Body Systems: Oil Composition & Chemistry.

The steps to create a blend by considering essential oil chemical compounds and odor types are listed below. Fine-tuning these steps necessarily includes intuitive action and experience.

1 Select the desired outcome. The more specific the outcome; the more effective the blend will be.

2 Select the essential oil chemical compound groups that will best meet the goal.

3 Select approximately eight to fifteen essential oils from these groups to draw from.

4 Note the odor type/notes for each of the selected oils.

5 Select one oil as the base note, two to three oils as the middle notes, and one oil to be the top note. (This is a guideline; use intuition and experience to alter.)

6 Decide how many drops will be used of each of the five oils selected. A fifteen-drop blend is a good ratio for a 5 ml or 10 ml bottle with a carrier oil.

7 Place the oils in the bottle and add the carrier oil. As the blend is used to meet the desired outcome, make notes in a blending journal.

The following is an example of using the steps to create a blend to ease muscle strain using Combination of Techniques Method. For **steps 1-2**, the following table is used to identify the most helpful chemical compound groups to meet the blend goal. In this example, aldehydes, esters, sesquiterpene hydrocarbons, and ethers would be helpful.

Steps 3-4: The following is an example of a list of oils chosen from the four selected chemical groups, which will help meet the desired outcome of easing muscle strain.

CHEMICAL COMPOUND GROUP	THERAPEUTIC BENEFITS	OILS
Monoterpene Hydrocarbon	Cellular protective, anti-inflammatory, antibacterial	citrus oils, frankincense, ginger, basil, thyme, cypress
Sesquiterpene Hydrocarbon	Anti-inflammatory, sedative, soothing, antibacterial	cedarwood, myrrh, white fir, black pepper, ginger, helichrysum, patchouli, ylang ylang
Monoterpene Alcohols	Antimicrobial, somewhat stimulating, tonifying and restorative to the skin, cleansing, antispasmodic, sedative, gentle, mild	geranium, lavender, melaleuca, frankincense
Sesquiterpene Alcohols	Anti-allergenic, antibacterial, anti-inflammatory, liver and glandular stimulant	cedarwood, geranium, patchouli, sandalwood
Esters	Very calming, relaxing, balancing, antifungal, antispasmodic	cardamom, bergamot, roman chamomile, helichrysum, clove, geranium, ylang ylang, peppermint, cassia
Aldehydes	Strong aroma; calming to the emotions, anti-infectious, anti-inflammatory, calming overall, fever-reducing, hypotensive, and tonic; some are vasodilators	cassia, lemongrass, lime, roman chamomile, melissa, marjoram
Ketones	Mucolytic, stimulate cell regeneration, promote the formation of tissue, analgesic, sedative	rosemary, fennel, vetiver, lavender, myrrh, roman chamomile, peppermint, helichyrsum
Phenols	Powerful antibacterial, anti-infective, and antiseptic, very stimulating to the autonomic nervous system	cinnamon, clove, oregano, thyme
Oxides	Expectorant, mildly stimulating	rosemary, peppermint, cypress, clary sage, clove, cardamom, thyme, melaleuca, basil, peppermint, fennel
Ethers	Balancing to the autonomic nervous system, soothing, sedative	fennel, basil, ylang ylang, marjoram

The letter next to each oil indicates the odor type assigned to that oil so as to assist with selection. (T) Top (M) Middle (B) Base

Aldehyde:	lemongrass (T), roman chamomile (M)
Esters:	roman chamomile (M), geranium (M), ylang ylang (M to B)
Sesquiterpene Hydrocarbons:	cedarwood (B), white fir (M), black pepper (M), ginger (M), ylang ylang (M to T)
Ethers:	basil (M to T), ylang ylang (M to T), marjoram (M)

Steps 5-7: Using the above list of selected oils, select five oils and the number of drops needed from each oil to create the blend that will equal a total of fifteen drops. The blend can be placed in a 5 ml or 10 ml roller bottle and topped off with a carrier oil to fill the bottle.

Base note:	cedarwood	(4 drops)
Middle note:	roman chamomile	(2 drops)
Middle note:	ginger	(2 drops)
Middle note:	black pepper	(3 drops)
Top note:	ylang ylang	(4 drops)

When using essential oils for a therapeutic goal, it is often helpful to use more than one oil. Layering these oils following the suggested steps in this section is beneficial to accomplish the desired outcome. When time permits, it may also be helpful to create a blend using oils selected based on their chemical compounds and their note type as outlined in this section. Intuition and experience improves blending skills.

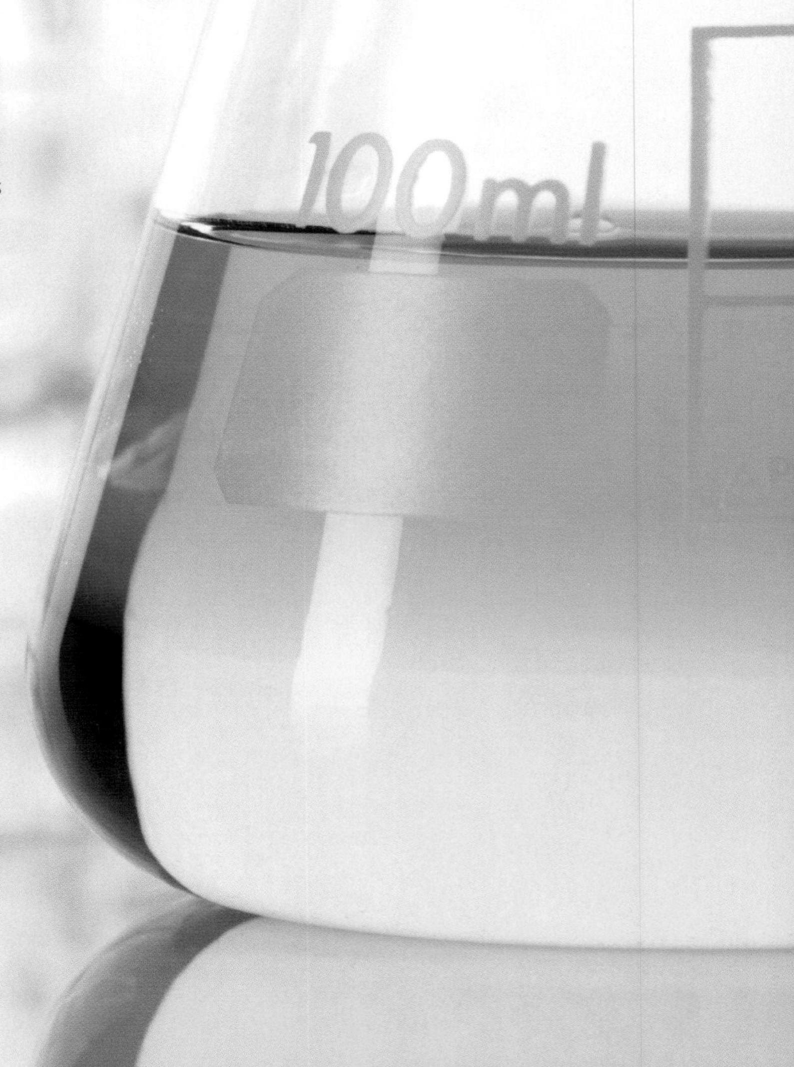

Massage with Oils

The application of essential oils topically, combined with massage, is simple to do but very powerful in the healing process. It increases the benefits of massage and the efficacy of essential oils on and within the body. Massage increases circulation and absorption, helps improve lymphatic flow, and aids in the release of toxins. It can also soothe nerve endings, relax muscles, and relieve stress and tension in the body.

Head

Apply essential oils to the fingertips and gently massage entire scalp. For headache, massage around the base of the neck and work upward to the base of the scalp.

Neck

Use circular movements, working from the base of the neck, up both sides of the vertebrae, to the base of the scalp. Work to the sides of the neck and repeat the movements, working down again.

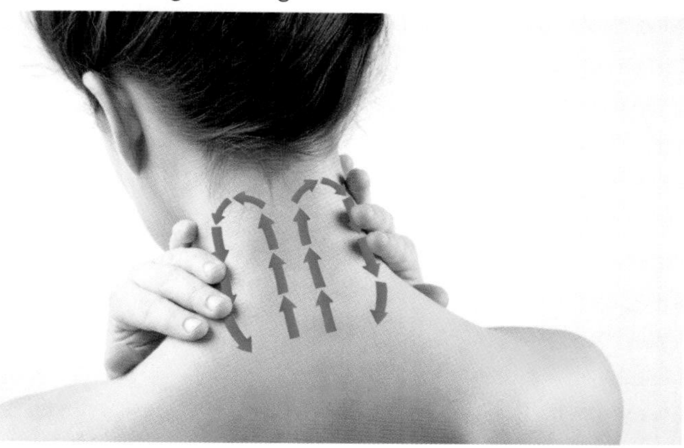

Shoulders

Using your thumbs and palms, make firm strokes from the shoulder to the neck and back again.

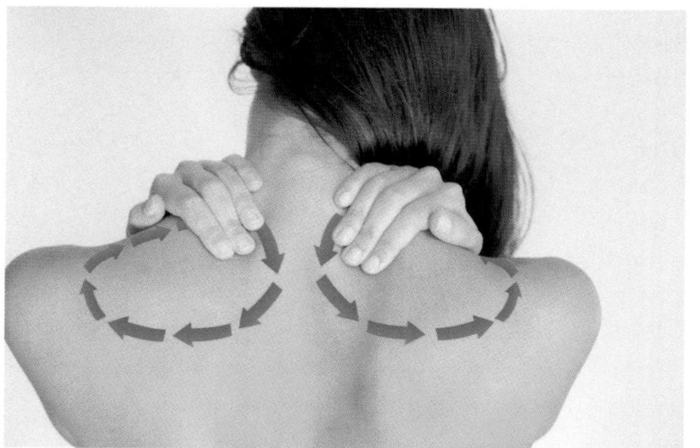

Arms

Massage up toward the armpit on the fatty or muscular areas only.

Back

Start from the lumbar region of the back, and with two hands stroke all the way up to the shoulders alongside the spine. Slide the hands over the shoulders and return down the sides of the back.

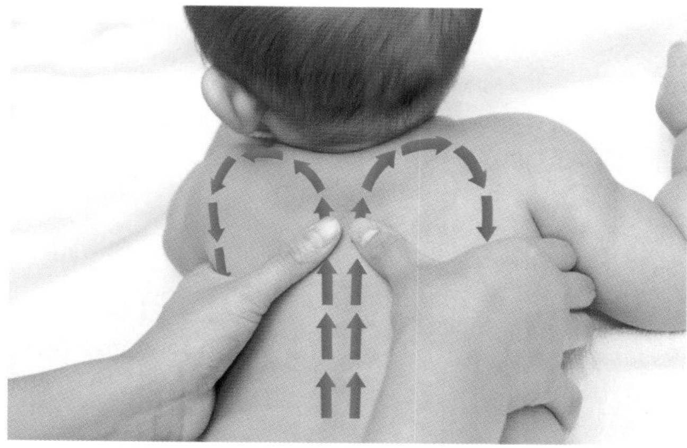

Abdomen

Use circular movements only, in a clockwise direction.

Legs

Always massage legs upward on the fatty or muscular areas only and avoid varicose veins.

Feet

Massage from the toes to the heel with thumbs under the foot and fingers on top.

- Massage is most effective when done with the flow of the body—and toward the heart, from hand to shoulder, foot to thigh, and so on.
- When massaging children and invalids, use gentle movements.

Reflexology

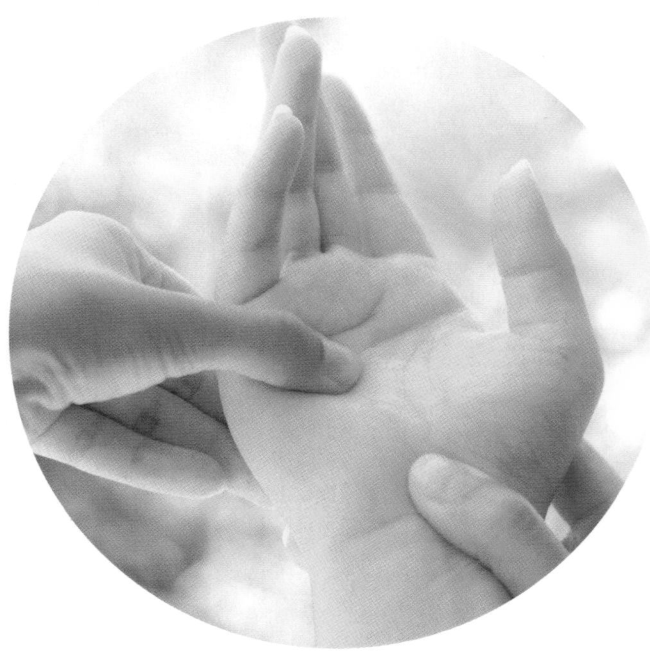

Reflexology is the application of pressure to the feet and hands with specific thumb, finger, and hand techniques without the use of oil or lotion. It is based on a system of zones and reflex areas that reflect an image of the body on the feet and hands, with the premise that such work effects a physical change to the body.

Ear Reflexology is a simple and efficient way to relieve stress and pain by applying minimal pressure to the reflex points on the ear. Each ear contains a complete map of the body, rich with nerve endings and multiple connectors to the central nervous system. For example, if the reflex point for the bladder is tender, the body may be in the beginning stages of a bladder infection. One can take preventative measures to head off the bladder infection by applying an essential oil to the reflex point on the ear followed by minimal pressure.

To begin treatment, start at the top of the right ear and slowly work your thumb and forefinger along the outer edges. Hold each point for five seconds before continuing to the end of the earlobe. For best results, repeat this procedure at least five times. Next, work the inner crevices of the ear using the pointer finger and applying minimal pressure. Repeat procedure on left ear. If any areas in and around the crevices of the ear are sensitive, consult the ear reflexology chart to pinpoint the area of the body that may be out of balance.

This a great technique to use personally, on family or friends, as well as with those whose hands and feet are not accessible for hand and foot reflexology. Young children are especially receptive to having their outer ears worked on, finding it calming and soothing.

Foot Reflexology is an effective method to bring the body systems into balance by applying pressure to specific places on the feet. Hand reflexology can be utilized in a similar manner. The nerves in the feet correspond with various parts of the body; thus, the entire body is mapped on the feet, telling a story of emotional and physical well being.

One way to find imbalances in the body is to massage all the areas noted on the foot reflexology chart and feel for triggers or small knots underneath the skin. When a trigger is found, apply an essential oil to the location on the foot and continue to massage the trigger until it releases. Another way to use reflexology is to address a specific ailment. For instance, if a person has a headache, locate the brain on the foot chart and the corresponding point on the foot. Apply an essential oil of choice and massage the pad of the big toe to reduce tension. If a person has a tight chest induced by stress, locate the lungs/chest on the foot chart and the corresponding point on the foot. Apply an essential oil of choice followed by medium to light circular massage on the ball of the foot.

The autonomic nervous system is then engaged, helping to alleviate symptoms and heal the body naturally.

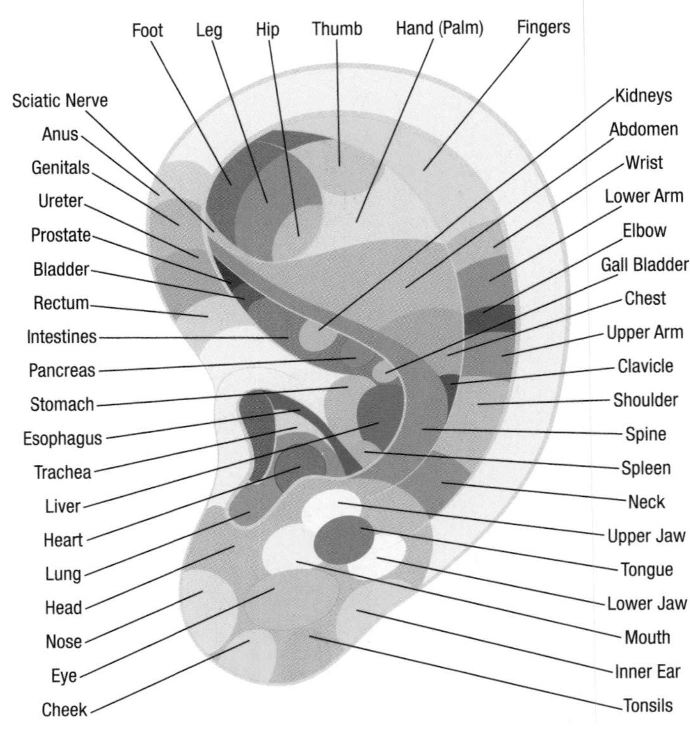

REFLEXOLOGY REFERENCE

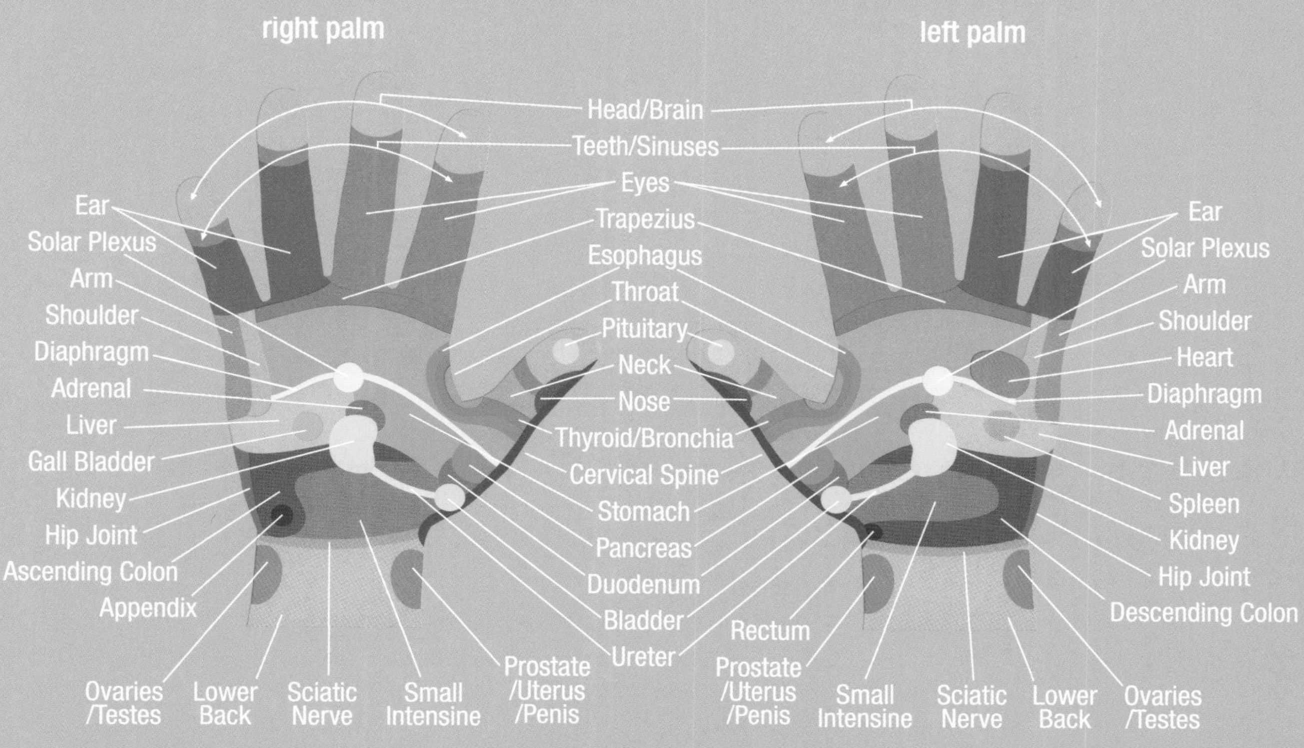

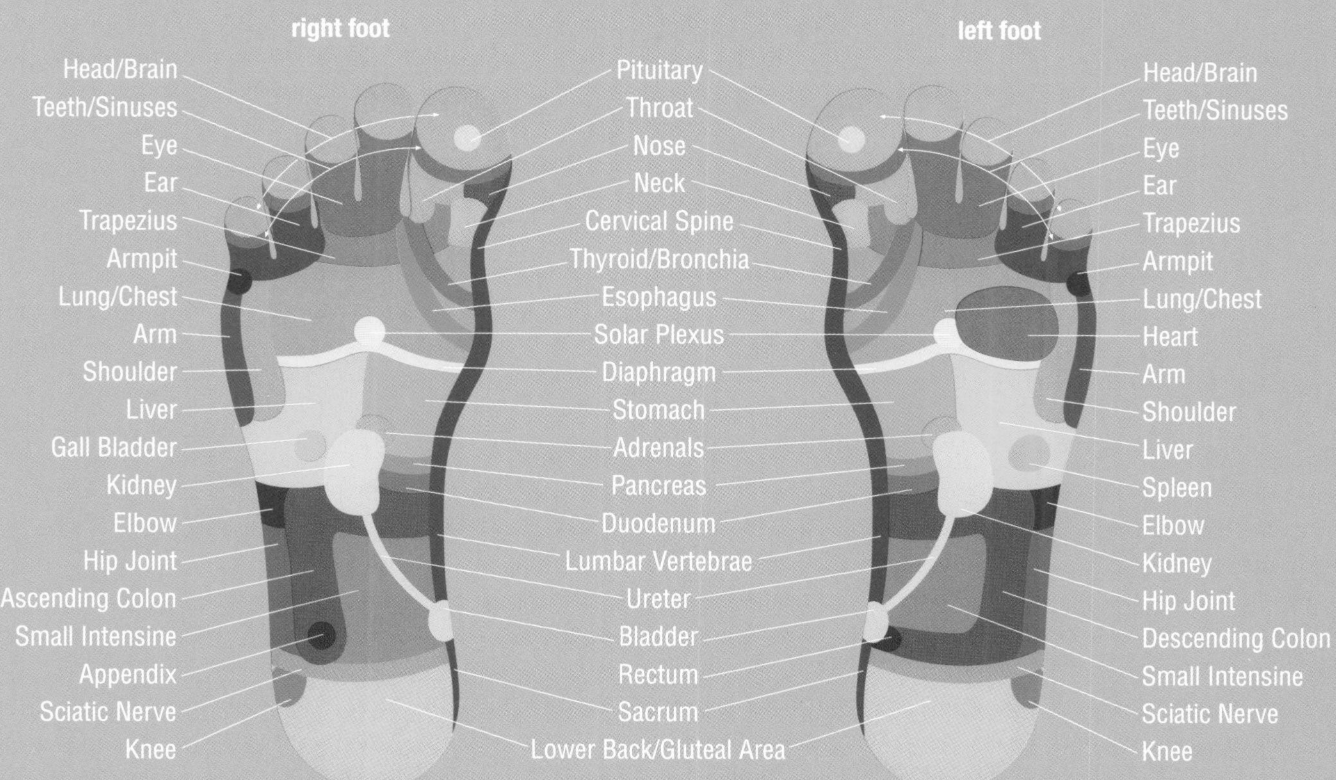

Cooking with Oils Chart

	Meat	Chicken	Fish	Eggs	Cheese	Vegetables	Rice	Pasta	Desserts	Pastries	Bread	Cakes	Sorbets	Ice Cream	Fruit	Dressings
Basil	•					•										•
Bergamot		•	•						•				•			
Black Pepper	•	•	•	•	•	•	•	•	•	•	•	•	•	•	•	
Cardamom	•	•	•	•		•	•		•	•	•	•	•	•	•	
Cassia			•		•	•	•	•	•		•				•	
Cilantro	•	•				•										
Cinnamon	•	•	•	•	•	•	•	•	•	•	•	•	•	•	•	
Clary Sage	•	•					•	•	•	•	•	•	•	•	•	
Clove	•	•														
Coriander	•															
Dill	•						•	•	•	•	•	•	•	•	•	•
Fennel			•			•	•	•			•				•	•
Geranium		•	•		•	•	•	•								
Ginger					•	•		•	•	•	•	•	•	•	•	
Grapefruit	•	•		•		•	•	•								
Jasmine		•	•			•	•	•	•	•	•	•	•	•	•	
Lavender		•		•	•		•	•	•	•	•	•	•	•	•	
Lemon	•	•	•		•	•	•	•			•	•	•	•	•	•
Lemongrass		•	•	•	•	•	•	•	•	•	•	•	•	•	•	•
Lime	•	•	•			•	•	•	•	•	•	•	•	•	•	•
Marjoram	•	•	•													•
Melissa		•	•	•	•	•	•						•	•	•	
Oregano	•	•	•	•	•	•	•	•	•	•	•	•	•	•	•	•
Peppermint						•			•	•		•	•	•	•	
Rose		•		•	•		•		•	•	•	•	•	•	•	
Rosemary	•	•														•
Spearmint						•			•	•		•	•	•	•	
Tangerine	•	•	•	•	•		•	•	•	•	•	•	•	•	•	•
Thyme	•	•														•
Wild Orange	•	•	•	•	•		•	•	•	•	•	•	•	•	•	•
Ylang Ylang		•					•	•	•	•	•	•	•	•	•	

Oil Properties Glossary

Analgesic - relieves or allays pain
Anaphrodisiac - reduces sexual desire
Anti-allergenic - reduces allergic response
Antiarthritic - effective in treatment of arthritis
Antibacterial - kills or inhibits growth of bacteria
Anticarcinogenic - inhibits development of cancer
Anti-carcinoma - destroys or inhibits cancer cells
Anticatarrhal - removes excess mucus
Anticoagulant - prevents clotting of blood
Anticonvulsant - reduces convulsions
Antidepressant - effective in treatment against depression
Antiemetic - effective against nausea and vomiting
Antifungal - inhibits growth of fungi
Antihemorrhagic - promotes hemostasis; stops bleeding
Antihistamine - blocks histamine receptors; reduces allergic response
Anti-infectious - reduces/prevents infection
Anti-inflammatory - reduces inflammation
Antimicrobial - kills or inhibits microorganisms
Antimutagenic - reduces rate of genetic variants/mutation
Antioxidant - mitigates damage by free radicals
Anti-parasitic - destroys or inhibits growth/reproduction of parasites
Anti-rheumatic - mitigates pain and stiffness
Antiseptic - destroys microorganisms to prevent or treat infection on living tissue/skin
Antispasmodic - relieves spasms of involuntary muscles
Antitoxic - neutralizes or counteracts toxins
Anti-tumoral - inhibits growth of tumors
Antiviral - destroys viruses or suppresses replication
Aphrodisiac - heightens sexual desire
Astringent - contracts tissues, generally of the skin; reduces minor bleeding
Calming - pacifying
Cardiotonic - tones and vitalizes the heart
Carminative - reduces gas or bloating
Cleanser - cleanses body and/or household surfaces
Cytophylactic - stimulates cell growth
Decongestant - reduces respiratory congestion; opens airways
Deodorant - stops formation of odors
Detoxifier - removes toxins from the body tissues and organs
Digestive stimulant - stimulates digestion
Disinfectant - mitigates growth of microorganisms on inorganic surfaces
Diuretic - increases production and excretion of urine
Emmenagogue - regulates and induces menstruation
Energizing - generates and enhances energy
Expectorant - promotes discharge of phlegm and other fluids from the respiratory tract
Galactagogue - promotes lactation and increases milk supply
Grounding - assists one's sense of feeling centered and secure
Hypertensive - raises blood pressure
Hypotensive - lowers blood pressure
Immunostimulant - induces activation of the body's protective ability
Insect repellent - deters insects and bugs
Insecticidal - kills insects and bugs
Invigorating - revitalizes and rejuvenates
Laxative - stimulates bowel excretion
Mucolytic - loosens, thins, and breaks down mucus
Nervine - beneficial effect on nerves
Neuroprotective - protects nerves
Neurotonic - improves tone or force of nervous system
Purifier - eliminates impurities
Refreshing - renews; promotes feeling of freshness
Regenerative - promotes regeneration of body tissue
Relaxant - promotes relaxation; reduces tension
Restorative - encourages repair, recovery, restoration
Revitalizer - uplifts and energizes
Rubefacient - increases circulation; increases skin redness
Sedative - promotes calm and sleep; reduces agitation; tranquilizing
Steroidal - stimulates cortisone-like action
Stimulant - increases activity
Stomachic - assists digestion, promotes appetite
Tonic - promotes a feeling of vigor or well being
Uplifting - elevating; promotes sense of happiness and hope
Vasoconstrictor - restricts blood vessels; decreases blood flow; can increase blood pressure
Vasodilator - relaxes/dilates blood vessels; increases blood flow; can decrease blood pressure
Vermicide - kills parasitic worms
Vermifuge - stuns parasites
Warming - raises body and/or specific body tissue temperature - referred to as "localized warming"

Oil Properties	anaphrodisiac	analgesic	anti-allergenic	antiarthritic	antibacterial	anticarcinogenic	anti-carcinoma	anticatarrhal	anticoagulant	anticonvulsant	antidepressant	antiemetic	antifungal	antihemorrhagic	antihistamine	anti-infectious	anti-inflammatory	antimicrobial	antimutagenic	antioxidant	anti-parasitic	anti-rheumatic	antiseptic	antispasmodic	antitoxic	anti-tumoral	antiviral	aphrodisiac	astringent	calming	cardiotonic	carminative	cleanser	cytophylactic	decongestant	deodorant	detoxifier
Arborvitae	•	•		•	•	•	•						•		•	•	•	•		•			•			•	•		•				•	•			•
Basil		•			•			•			•	•				•	•	•		•			•	•			•			•		•			•		
Bergamot		•			•						•		•			•	•				•		•	•	•					•		•				•	
Birch		•			•												•					•	•	•					•								
Black pepper		•			•			•									•			•	•		•	•	•			•		•							
Cardamom					•							•				•	•	•					•	•				•				•			•		
Cassia		•		•	•							•	•				•	•		•		•		•			•		•	•	•	•			•		•
Cedarwood					•								•			•	•						•						•								
Cilantro					•								•					•		•												•	•				•
Cinnamon		•			•						•		•			•	•	•	•	•	•		•	•	•		•	•	•			•					
Clary sage		•			•				•	•	•		•				•	•					•	•				•	•	•		•				•	
Clove		•			•							•	•		•	•	•			•	•	•	•	•		•	•	•				•					
Coriander		•			•						•	•	•				•	•		•		•		•	•			•		•		•				•	
Cypress		•			•								•			•	•	•				•	•	•					•		•	•			•	•	•
Dill					•						•		•				•	•						•			•					•					
Douglas Fir		•			•															•			•						•								
Eucalyptus		•			•			•					•			•	•	•		•		•		•			•						•		•	•	
Fennel		•								•		•	•				•	•			•		•	•	•					•		•					
Frankincense		•				•	•	•			•					•	•	•		•	•		•			•			•	•				•			
Geranium			•		•					•	•		•	•		•	•						•	•	•				•	•				•		•	•
Ginger		•		•	•							•	•				•		•	•		•	•				•				•	•			•		
Grapefruit					•		•				•									•			•		•				•				•		•		
Helichrysum		•	•		•			•	•				•	•			•	•		•			•	•			•		•								
Jasmine		•									•						•						•	•				•		•		•					
Juniper berry		•																		•	•	•	•	•	•			•	•	•		•	•				•
Lavender		•							•	•	•	•	•		•	•	•	•	•		•	•	•	•	•	•			•	•	•	•		•		•	
Lemon							•				•		•					•		•		•	•	•	•		•					•	•		•		•
Lemongrass		•			•		•				•		•				•	•	•	•		•	•		•							•			•	•	
Lime					•												•			•		•	•	•			•										•
Marjoram	•	•			•											•							•	•							•						
Melaleuca		•			•								•			•	•			•	•		•				•								•		
Melissa					•						•				•		•	•					•	•			•			•		•					
Myrrh					•	•	•	•					•			•	•	•					•			•	•		•			•					
Oregano		•			•						•		•				•	•		•	•	•	•				•			•		•					
Patchouli					•						•	•	•			•	•	•					•	•	•			•	•	•		•			•	•	•
Peppermint		•			•	•						•					•						•	•			•	•				•					
Ravensara		•			•						•		•					•					•	•			•	•									
Roman chamomile																•	•				•			•						•		•					
Rose											•					•							•	•			•	•				•					
Rosemary		•			•		•	•					•			•	•	•		•	•	•	•	•				•	•			•		•			•
Sandalwood					•		•	•			•		•				•						•	•		•		•	•	•		•					
Spearmint					•			•					•				•						•	•				•				•					
Spikenard					•								•				•																			•	
Tangerine					•					•			•					•					•	•						•				•			
Thyme					•								•					•		•	•	•	•	•	•		•	•				•	•				
Vetiver																				•			•	•				•		•		•					
White fir		•		•				•														•	•				•		•						•	•	
Wild orange		•			•		•				•		•				•			•			•	•				•				•	•				•
Wintergreen		•															•					•	•	•					•			•					
Yarrow																	•					•	•	•					•	•		•					
Ylang ylang					•						•												•	•				•									

	digestive stimulant	disinfectant	diuretic	emmenagogue	energizing	expectorant	galactagogue	grounding	hypertensive	hypotensive	immunostimulant	insect repellant	insecticidal	invigorating	laxative	mucolytic	nervine	neuroprotective	neurotonic	purifier	refreshing	regenerative	relaxing	restorative	revitalizer	rubefacient	sedative	steroidal	stimulant	stomachic	tonic	uplifting	vasoconstrictor	vasodilator	vermicide	vermifuge	warming
Arborvitae		•	•	•		•					•	•							•	•									•		•					•	
Basil	•	•	•	•	•	•	•	•							•	•	•		•			•	•	•			•	•	•	•	•					•	
Bergamot	•		•		•										•				•							•	•		•		•	•				•	
Birch		•	•									•														•			•		•						•
Black pepper	•					•				•					•				•							•			•								•
Cardamom	•		•			•																							•	•	•	•					
Cassia				•							•												•														•
Cedarwood			•	•		•		•				•	•			•						•	•				•		•		•	•				•	
Cilantro																																					
Cinnamon	•			•							•	•								•									•	•						•	•
Clary sage	•			•			•	•		•						•	•		•				•				•			•	•	•			•		•
Clove		•			•	•					•						•					•							•							•	•
Coriander	•												•									•			•		•		•	•	•						
Cypress			•		•			•								•			•		•		•						•		•	•	•				
Dill	•			•		•	•			•																			•								
Douglas Fir			•			•									•												•		•	•							
Eucalyptus		•	•			•				•	•	•	•							•						•			•							•	•
Fennel	•		•	•		•	•				•				•	•							•						•	•	•					•	
Frankincense	•	•	•			•					•							•				•		•			•				•						
Geranium			•									•									•	•	•				•				•					•	
Ginger				•		•					•				•				•							•			•	•	•						•
Grapefruit	•	•	•		•									•						•	•								•		•	•					
Helichrysum	•		•			•										•	•					•				•							•				
Jasmine				•		•	•															•	•				•										
Juniper berry	•		•	•													•								•	•	•		•	•	•						
Lavender			•	•						•			•				•	•				•	•			•	•				•				•	•	
Lemon		•	•		•					•	•		•	•		•					•				•	•					•	•				•	
Lemongrass	•				•		•					•	•				•			•		•			•		•				•			•			•
Lime		•	•		•						•									•	•			•	•				•		•	•					
Marjoram	•			•		•				•										•			•				•			•	•			•			•
Melaleuca	•					•		•			•		•						•	•	•	•							•							•	
Melissa									•		•						•										•			•	•	•					
Myrrh	•			•		•										•						•	•						•		•						
Oregano	•	•		•		•					•									•															•		•
Patchouli	•		•						•			•	•				•					•		•			•		•		•						
Peppermint				•		•								•			•				•									•			•			•	•
Ravensara		•	•			•					•												•								•						
Roman chamomile				•														•					•				•				•					•	
Rose				•											•		•										•			•	•						
Rosemary			•	•	•	•			•		•						•							•		•		•	•	•	•			•		•	
Sandalwood			•			•			•				•									•		•			•				•	•					
Spearmint	•			•							•		•	•										•					•								
Spikenard															•												•										
Tangerine					•																									•	•	•					
Thyme			•	•		•			•		•	•	•				•	•								•			•		•			•		•	•
Vetiver								•			•	•	•					•								•	•		•		•					•	
White fir			•		•	•				•	•												•			•			•		•		•				
Wild orange	•		•		•						•			•						•	•	•								•	•	•				•	
Wintergreen		•	•	•			•							•							•								•						•	•	•
Yarrow	•									•																				•	•						
Ylang ylang								•		•		•											•				•		•		•	•	•				

SUPPLEMENTAL

Recipe Index

Research Index

ADDICTION

The effects of aromatherapy on nicotine craving on a U.S. campus: a small comparison study, Cordell B, Buckle J, *The Journal of Alternative and Complementary Medicine*, 2013

ALERTNESS

Effects of Peppermint and Cinnamon Odor Administration on Simulated Driving Alertness, Mood and Workload, Raudenbush B, Grayhem R, Sears T, Wilson I., *North American Journal of Psychology*, 2009

The influence of essential oils on human attention. I: alertness, Ilmberger J, Heuberger E, Mahrhofer C, Dessovic H, Kowarik D, Buchbauer G, *Chemical Senses*, 2001

The influence of essential oils on human vigilance, Heuberger E, Ilmberger J, *Natural Product Communications*, 2010

Volatiles emitted from the roots of Vetiveria zizanioides suppress the decline in attention during a visual display terminal taskvi, Matsubara E, Shimizu K, Fukagawa M, Ishizi Y, Kakoi C, Hatayama T, Nagano J, Okamoto T, Ohnuki K, Kondo R, *Biomedical Research*, 2012

ALLERGIES

Cytological aspects on the effects of a nasal spray consisting of standardized extract of citrus lemon and essential oils in allergic rhinopathy, Ferrara L, Naviglio D, Armone Caruso A, *ISRN Pharm*, 2012

ALZHEIMER'S DISEASE

Effect of arborvitae seed on cognitive function and α7nAChR protein expression of hippocampus in model rats with Alzheimer's disease, Cheng XL, Xiong XB, Xiang MQ, *Cell Biochem Biophys*, 2013

Effect of aromatherapy on patients with Alzheimer's disease, Jimbo D, Kimura Y, Taniguchi M, Inoue M, Urakami K, *Psychogeriatrics*, 2009

Inhalation of coriander volatile oil increased anxiolytic-antidepressant-like behaviors and decreased oxidative status in beta-amyloid (1-42) rat model of Alzheimer's disease, Cioanca O, Hritcu L, Mihasan M, Trifan A, Hancianu M, *Physiology & Behavior*, 2014

ANTIBACTERIAL

Activity of Essential Oils Against Bacillus subtilis Spores, Lawrence HA, Palombo EA, *Journal of Microbiology and Biotechnology*, 2009

Antibacterial activity of essential oils and their major constituents against respiratory tract pathogens by gaseous contact, Inouye S, Takizawa T, Yamaguchi H, *The Journal of Antimicrobial Chemotherapy*, 2001

Antibacterial activity of the essential oil from Rosmarinus officinalis and its major components against oral pathogens, Bernardes WA, Lucarini R, Tozatti MG, Flauzino LG, Soutza MG, Turatti IC, Andrade e Silva ML, Martins CH, da Silva Filho AA, Cunha WR, *Zeitschrift Fur Naturforschung C-A Journal of Biosciences*, 2010

Antibacterial and antioxidant properties of Mediterranean aromatic plants, Piccaglia R, Marotti M, Giovanelli E, Deans SG, Eaglesham E, *Industrial Crops and Products*, 1993

Antibacterial Effects of the Essential Oils of Commonly Consumed Medicinal Herbs Using an In Vitro Model, SokoviĐ M, GlamoĐlija J, Marin PD, BrkiĐ D, van Griensven LJ, *Molecules*, 2010

Atomic force microscopy analysis shows surface structure changes in carvacrol-treated bacterial cells, La Storia A, Ercolini D, Marinello F, Di Pasqua R, Villani F, Mauriello G, *Research in Microbiology*, 2011

Bactericidal activities of plant essential oils and some of their isolated constituents against Campylobacter jejuni, Escherichia coli, Listeria monocytogenes, and Salmonella enterica, Friedman M, Henika PR, Mandrell RE, *Journal of Food Protection*, 2002

Chemical composition and antibacterial activity of selected essential oils and some of their main compounds, Wanner J, Schmidt E, Bail S, Jirovetz L, Buchbauer G, Gochev V, Girova T, Atanasova T, Stoyanova A, *Natural Product Communications*, 2010

Coriander (Coriandrum sativum L.) essential oil: its antibacterial activity and mode of action evaluated by flow cytometry, Silva F, Ferreira S, Queiroz JA, Domingues FC, *Journal of Medical Microbiology*, 2011

Effects of Helichrysum italicum extract on growth and enzymatic activity of Staphylococcus aureus, Nostro A, Bisignano G, Angela Cannatelli M, Crisafi G, Paola Germanò M, Alonzo V, *International Journal of Antimicrobial Agents*, 2001

Eugenol (an essential oil of clove) acts as an antibacterial agent against Salmonella typhi by disrupting the cellular membrane, Devi KP, Nisha SA, Sakthivel R, Pandian SK, *Journal of Ethnopharmacology*, 2010

Evaluation of bacterial resistance to essential oils and antibiotics after exposure to oregano and cinnamon essential oils, Becerril R, Nerín C, Gómez-Lus R, *Foodborne Pathogens and Disease*, 2012

Growth inhibition of pathogenic bacteria and some yeasts by selected essential oils and survival of L. monocytogenes and C. albicans in apple-carrot juice., Irkin R, Korukluoglu M, *Foodborne Pathogens and Disease*, 2009

Helichrysum italicum extract interferes with the production of enterotoxins by Staphylococcus aureus., Nostro A, Cannatelli MA, Musolino AD, Procopio F, Alonzo V, *Letters in Applied Microbiology*, 2002

In vitro antibacterial activity of some plant essential oils, Prabuseenivasan S, Jayakumar M, Ignacimuthu S, *BMC Complementary and Alternative Medicine*, 2006

Inhibition by the essential oils of peppermint and spearmint of the growth of pathogenic bacteria, Imai H, Osawa K, Yasuda H, Hamashima H, Arai T, Sasatsu M, *Microbios*, 2001

Investigation of antibacterial activity of rosemary essential oil against Propionibacterium acnes with atomic force microscopy, Fu Y, Zu Y, Chen L, Efferth T, Liang H, Liu Z, Liu W, *Planta Medica*, 2007

Origanum vulgare subsp. hirtum Essential Oil Prevented Biofilm Formation and Showed Antibacterial Activity against Planktonic and Sessile Bacterial Cells, Schillaci D, Napoli EM, Cusimano MG, Vitale M, Ruberto A, *Journal of Food Protection*, 2013

Potential of rosemary oil to be used in drug-resistant infections, Luqman S, Dwivedi GR, Darokar MP, Kalra A, Khanuja SP, *Alternative Therapies in Health and Medicine*, 2007

Screening of the antibacterial effects of a variety of essential oils on microorganisms responsible for respiratory infections, Fabio A, Cermelli C, Fabio G, Nicoletti P, Quaglio P, *Phytotherapy Research*, 2007

Screening of the antibacterial effects of a variety of essential oils on respiratory tract pathogens, using a modified dilution assay method, Inouye S, Yamaguchi H, Takizawa T, *Journal of Infection and Chemotherapy: Official Journal of the Japan Society of Chemotherapy*, 2001

Some evidences on the mode of action of Cinnamomum verum bark essential oil, alone and in combination with piperacillin against a multi-drug resistant Escherichia coli strain, Yap PS, Krishnan T, Chan KG, Lim SH, *Journal of Microbiology and Biotechnology*, 2014

Tea tree oil-induced transcriptional alterations in Staphylococcus aureus, Cuaron JA, Dulal S, Song Y, Singh AK, Montelongo CE, Yu W, Nagarajan V, Jayaswal RK, Wilkinson BJ, Gustafson JE, *Phytotherapy Research*, 2013

The anti-biofilm activity of lemongrass (Cymbopogon flexuosus) and grapefruit (Citrus paradisi) essential oils against five strains of Staphylococcus aureus, Adukwu EC, Allen SC, Phillips CA, *Journal of Applied Microbiology*, 2012

The antibacterial activity of geranium oil against Gram-negative bacteria isolated from difficult-to-heal wounds, Sienkiewicz M, PoznaĐska-Kurowska K, Kaszuba A, Kowalczyk E, *Burns*, 2014

The effect of lemongrass EO highlights its potential against antibiotic resistant Staph. aureus in the health-care environment, Adukwu EC, Allen SC, Phillips CA, *Journal of Applied Microbiology*, 2012

The potential of use basil and rosemary essential oils as effective antibacterial agents, Sienkiewicz M, Łysakowska M, Pastuszka M, Bienias W, Kowalczyk E, *Molecules*, 2013

ANTIFUNGAL

Antibacterial, antifungal, and anticancer activities of volatile oils and extracts from stems, leaves, and flowers of Eucalyptus sideroxylon and Eucalyptus torquata, Ashour HM, *Cancer Biology and Therapy*, 2008

Antifungal activity of clove essential oil and its volatile vapour against dermatophytic fungi, Chee HY, Lee MH, *Mycobiology*, 2007

Antifungal mechanism of essential oil from Anethum graveolens seeds against Candida albicans, Chen Y, Zeng H, Tian J, Ban X, Ma B, Wang Y, *Journal of Medical Microbiology*, 2013

Antifungal, anti-biofilm and adhesion activity of the essential oil of Myrtus communis L. against Candida species, Cannas S, Molicotti P, Usai D, Maxia A, Zanetti S, *Natural Product Research*, 2014

Chemical composition, bio-herbicidal and antifungal activities of essential oils isolated from Tunisian common cypress (Cupressus sempervirens L.), Ismail A, Lamia H, Mohsen H, Samia G, Bassem J, *Journal of Medicinal Plants Research*, 2013

Coriandrum sativum L. (Coriander) Essential Oil: Antifungal Activity and Mode of Action on Candida spp., and Molecular Targets Affected in Human Whole-Genome Expression, Freires Ide A, Murata RM, Furletti VF, Sartoratto A, Alencar SM, Figueira GM, de Oliveira Rodrigues JA, Duarte MC, Rosalen PL, *PLoS One*, 2014

Dill (Anethum graveolens L.) seed essential oil induces Candida albicans apoptosis in a metacaspase-dependent manner, Chen Y, Zeng H, Tian J, Ban X, Ma B, Wang Y, *Fungal Biology*, 2014

In vitro antagonistic activity of monoterpenes and their mixtures against 'toe nail fungus' pathogens, Ramsewak RS, Nair MG, Stommel M, Selanders L, *Phytotherapy Research*, 2003

In-vitro and in-vivo anti-Trichophyton activity of essential oils by vapour contact, Inouye S, Uchida K, Yamaguchi H, *Mycoses*, 2001

Oil of bitter orange: new topical antifungal agent, Ramadan W, Mourad B, Ibrahim S, Sonbol F, *International Journal of Dermatology*, 1996

ANTIMICROBIAL

A novel aromatic oil compound inhibits microbial overgrowth on feet: a case study, Misner BD, *Journal of the International Society of Sports Nutrition*, 2007

Antimicrobial activities of cinnamon oil and cinnamaldehyde from the Chinese medicinal herb Cinnamomum cassia Blume, Ooi LS, Li Y, Kam SL, Wang H, Wong EY, Ooi VE, *The American Journal of Chinese Medicine*, 2006

Antimicrobial Activities of Clove and Thyme Extracts, Nzeako BC, Al-Kharousi ZS, Al-Mahrooqui Z, *Sultan Qaboos University Medical Journal*, 2006

Antimicrobial activity against bacteria with dermatological relevance and skin tolerance of the essential oil from Coriandrum sativum L. fruits, Casetti F, Bartelke S, Biehler K, Augustin M, Schempp CM, Frank U, *Phytotherapy Research*, 2012

Antimicrobial activity of clove oil and its potential in the treatment of vaginal candidiasis, Ahmad N, Alam MK, Shehbaz A, Khan A, Mannan A, Hakim SR, Bisht D, Owais M, *Journal of Drug Targeting*, 2005

Antimicrobial activity of essential oils and five terpenoid compounds against Campylobacter jejuni in pure and mixed culture experiments, Kurekci C, Padmanabha J, Bishop-Hurley SL, Hassan E, Al Jassim RA, McSweeney CS, *International Journal of Food Microbiology*, 2013

Antimicrobial activity of individual and mixed fractions of dill, cilantro, coriander and eucalyptus essential oils, Delaquis PJ, Stanich K, Girard B, Mazza G, *International Journal of Food Microbiology*, 2002

Antimicrobial activity of juniper berry essential oil (Juniperus communis L., Cupressaceae), Pepeljnjak S, Kosalec I, Kalodera Z, BlazeviĐ N, *Acta Pharmaceutica*, 2005

Antimicrobial activity of the bioactive components of essential oils from Pakistani spices against Salmonella and other multi-drug resistant bacteria, Naveed R, Hussain I, Tawab A, Tariq M, Rahman M, Hameed S, Mahmood MS, Siddique AB, Iqbal M, *BMC Complementary and Alternative Medicine*, 2013

Antimicrobial Effect and Mode of Action of Terpeneless Cold Pressed Valencia Orange Essential Oil on Methicillin-Resistant Staphylococcus aureus, Muthaiyan A, Martin EM, Natesan S, Crandall PG, Wilkinson BJ, Ricke SC, *Journal of Applied Microbiology*, 2012

Antimicrobial effects of essential oils in combination with chlorhexidine digluconate, Filoche SK, Soma K, Sissons CH, *Oral Microbiology and Immunology*, 2005

Chemical composition and in vitro antimicrobial activity of essential oil of Melissa officinalis L. from Romania, HĐncianu M, Aprotosoaie AC, Gille E, PoiatĐ A, TuchiluĐ C, Spac A, StĐnescu U, *Revista Medico-Chirurgicala a Societatii de Medici si Naturalisti din Iasi*, 2008

Comparison of essential oils from three plants for enhancement of antimicrobial activity of nitrofurantoin against enterobacteria, Rafii F, Shahverdi AR, *Chemotherapy*, 2007

Evaluation of the antimicrobial properties of different parts of Citrus aurantifolia (lime fruit) as used locally, Aibinu I, Adenipekun T, Adelowotan T, Ogunsanya T, Odugbemi T, *African Journal of Traditional, Complementary, and Alternative Medicines*, 2006

Immune-Modifying and Antimicrobial Effects of Eucalyptus Oil and Simple Inhalation Devices, Sadlon AE, Lamson DW, *Alternative Medicine Review: A Journal of Clinical Therapeutic*, 2010

Microbicide activity of clove essential oil (Eugenia caryophyllata), Nuñez L, Aquino MD, *Brazilian Journal of Microbiology*, 2012

Oregano essential oil as an antimicrobial additive to detergent for hand washing and food contact surface cleaning, Rhoades J, Gialagkolidou K, Gogou M, Mavridou O, Blatsiotis N, Ritzoulis C, Likotrafiti E, Journal of Applied Microbiology, 2013

Study of the antimicrobial action of various essential oils extracted from Malagasy plants. II: Lauraceae, Raharivelomanana PJ, Terrom GP, Bianchini JP, Coulanges P, *Arch Inst Pasteur Madagascar*, 1989

The additive and synergistic antimicrobial effects of select frankincense and myrrh oils–a combination from the pharaonic pharmacopoeia, de Rapper S, Van Vuuren SF, Kamatou GP, Viljoen AM, Dagne E, *Letters in Applied Microbiology*, 2012

The battle against multi-resistant strains: Renaissance of antimicrobial essential oils as a promising force to fight hospital-acquired infections, Warnke PH, Becker ST, Podschun R, Sivananthan S, Springer IN, Russo PA, Wiltfang J, Fickenscher H, Sherry E, *Journal of Cranio-Maxillo-Facial Surgery*, 200

Volatile composition and antimicrobial activity of twenty commercial frankincense essential oil samples, Van Vuurena SF, Kamatoub GPP, Viljoenb, AM, *South African Journal of Botany*, 2010

ANTIOXIDANT

Antioxidant activities and volatile constituents of various essential oils, Wei A, Shibamoto T, Journal of Agriculture and Food Chemistry, 2007

Antioxidant activity of rosemary (Rosmarinus officinalis L.) essential oil and its hepatoprotective potential, Ra Kovi A, Milanovi I, Pavlovi NA, Ebovi T, Vukmirovi SA, Mikov M, *BMC Complementary and Alternative Medicine*, 2014

Antioxidant and antimicrobial activities of essential oils obtained from oregano, Karakaya S, El SN, Karagözlü N, Sahin S, *Journal of Medicinal Food*, 2011

Antioxidant and Hepatoprotective Potential of Essential Oils of Coriander (Coriandrum sativum L.) and Caraway (Carum carvi L.) (Apiaceae), Samojlik I, LakiĐ N, Mimica-DukiĐ N, DakoviĐ-Svajcer K, Bozin B, *Journal of Agricultural and Food Chemistry*, 2010

Antioxidant potential of the root of Vetiveria zizanioides (L.) Nash, Luqman S, Kumar R, Kaushik S, Srivastava S, Darokar MP, Khanuja SP, *Indian Journal of Biochemistry and Biophysics*, 2009

Antioxidative effects of lemon oil and its components on copper induced oxidation of low density lipoprotein, Grassmann J, Schneider D, Weiser D, Elstner EF, *Arzneimittel-Forschung*, 2001
Biological effects, antioxidant and anticancer activities of marigold and basil essential oils, Mahmoud GI, *Journal of Medicinal Plants Research*, 2013
Evaluation of in vivo anti-hyperglycemic and antioxidant potentials of α-santalol and sandalwood oil, Misra BB, Dey S, *Phytomedicine*, 2013
In Vitro Antioxidant Activities of Essential Oils, Veerapan P, Khunkitti W, *Isan Journal of Pharmaceutical Sciences*, 2011
Minor Furanocoumarins and Coumarins in Grapefruit Peel Oil as Inhibitors of Human Cytochrome P450 3A4, César TB, Manthey JA, Myung K, *Journal of Natural Products*, 2009

ANTIVIRAL
Antiviral activities in plants endemic to madagascar, Hudson JB, Lee MK, Rasoanaivo P, *Pharm Biol.* 2000
Antiviral activity of the volatile oils of Melissa officinalis L. against Herpes simplex virus type-2, Allahverdiyev A, Duran N, Ozguven M, Koltas S, *Phytomedicine*, 2004
Antiviral efficacy and mechanisms of action of oregano essential oil and its primary component carvacrol against murine norovirus, Gilling DH, Kitajima M, Torrey JR, Bright KR, *Journal of Applied Microbiology*, 2014
Immunologic mechanism of Patchouli alcohol anti-H1N1 influenza virus may through regulation of the RLH signal pathway in vitro, Wu XL, Ju DH, Chen J, Yu B, Liu KL, He JX, Dai CQ, Wu S, Chang Z, Wang YP, Chen XY, *Current Microbiology*, 2013
Oral administration of patchouli alcohol isolated from Pogostemonis Herba augments protection against influenza viral infection in mice, Li YC, Peng SZ, Chen HM, Zhang FX, Xu PP, Xie JH, He JJ, Chen JN, Lai XP, Su ZR, International Immunopharmacology, 2012

ANXIETY
Ambient odor of orange in a dental office reduces anxiety and improves mood in female patients, Lehrner J, Eckersberger C, Walla P, Pötsch G, Deecke L, *Physiology and Behavior*, 2000
Anxiolytic-like effects of rose oil inhalation on the elevated plus-maze test in rats, de Almeida RN, Motta SC, de Brito Faturi C, Catallani B, Leite JR, *Pharmacology Biochemistry and Behavior*, 2004
Effect of sweet orange aroma on experimental anxiety in humans, Goes TC, Antunes FD, Alves PB, Teixeira-Silva F, *The Journal of Alternative and Complementary Medicine*
Essential oils and anxiolytic aromatherapy, Setzer WN, *Natural Product Communications*, 2009
The effects of prolonged rose odor inhalation in two animal models of anxiety, Bradley BF, Starkey NJ, Brown SL, Lea RW, *Physiology & Behavior*, 2007
The GABAergic system contributes to the anxiolytic-like effect of essential oil from Cymbopogon citratus (lemongrass), Costa CA, Kohn DO, de Lima VM, Gargano AC, Flório JC, Costa M, *Journal of Ethnopharmacology*, 2011

ARTHRITIS
Anti-arthritic effect of eugenol on collagen-induced arthritis experimental model, Grespan R, Paludo M, Lemos Hde P, Barbosa CP, Bersani-Amado CA, Dalalio MM, Cuman RK, *Biological and Pharmaceutical Bulletin*, 2012
The effects of aromatherapy on pain, depression, and life satisfaction of arthritis patients, Kim MJ, Nam ES, Paik SI, *Taehan Kanho Hakhoe Chi*, 2005

BEHAVIOR
Immunological and Psychological Benefits of Aromatherapy Massage, Kuriyama H, Watanabe S, Nakaya T, Shigemori I, Kita M, Yoshida N, Masaki D, Tadai T, Ozasa K, Fukui K, Imanishi J, *Evidence-based Complementary and Alternative Medicine*, 2005
The effect of gender and ethnicity on children's attitudes and preferences for essential oils: a pilot study, Fitzgerald M, Culbert T, Finkelstein M, Green M, Johnson A, Chen S, *Explore (New York, N.Y.)*, 2007

BLOOD
Antioxidative Properties and Inhibition of Key Enzymes Relevant to Type-2 Diabetes and Hypertension by Essential Oils from Black Pepper, Oboh G, Ademosun AO, Odubanjo OV, Akinbola IA, *Advances in Pharmacological Sciences*, 2013
Black pepper essential oil to enhance intravenous catheter insertion in patients with poor vein visibility: a controlled study, Kristiniak S, Harpel J, Breckenridge DM, Buckle J, *Journal of Alternative and Complementary Medicine*, 2012
Comparative screening of plant essential oils: Phenylpropanoid moiety as basic core for antiplatelet activity, Tognolini M, Barocelli E, Ballabeni V, Bruni R, Bianchi A, Chiavarini M, Impicciatore M, *Life Sciences*, 2006
Comparison of oral aspirin versus topical applied methyl salicylate for platelet inhibition, Tanen DA, Danish DC, Reardon JM, Chisholm CB, Matteucci MJ, Riffenburgh RH, *Annals of Pharmacotherapy*, 2008
Effects of a novel formulation of essential oils on glucose-insulin metabolism in diabetic and hypertensive rats: a pilot study, Talpur N, Echard B, Ingram C, Bagchi D, Preuss H, Diabetes, *Obesity and Metabolism*, 2005
Essential oil inhalation on blood pressure and salivary cortisol levels in prehypertensive and hypertensive subjects, Kim IH, Kim C, Seong K, Hur MH, Lim HM, Lee MS, *Evidence-Based Complementary and Alternative Medicine*, 2012
Inhibitory potential of omega-3 fatty and fenugreek essential oil on key enzymes of carbohydrate-digestion and hypertension in diabetes rats, Hamden K, Keskes H, Belhaj S, Mnafgui K, Feki A, Allouche N, *Lipids in Health and Disease*, 2011
Mechanism of changes induced in plasma glycerol by scent stimulation with grapefruit and lavender essential oils, Shen J, Niijima A, Tanida M, Horii Y, Nakamura T, Nagai K, *Neuroscience Letters*, 2007
Suppression of neutrophil accumulation in mice by cutaneous application of geranium essential oil, Maruyama N, Sekimoto Y, Ishibashi H, Inouye S, Oshima H, Yamaguchi H, Abe S, *Journal of Inflammation (London, England)*, 2005
The effects of the inhalation method using essential oils on blood pressure and stress responses of clients with essential hypertension, Hwang JH, *Korean Society of Nursing Science*, 2006

BLOOD PRESSURE
Antioxidative Properties and Inhibition of Key Enzymes Relevant to Type-2 Diabetes and Hypertension by Essential Oils from Black Pepper, Oboh G, Ademosun AO, Odubanjo OV, Akinbola IA, *Advances in Pharmacological Sciences*, 2013
Effects of Aromatherapy Massage on Blood Pressure and Lipid Profile in Korean Climacteric Women, Myung-HH , Heeyoung OH, Myeong SL, Chan K, Ae-na C, Gil-ran S, *International Journal of Neuroscience*, 2007
Effects of Ylang-Ylang aroma on blood pressure and heart rate in healthy men, Jung DJ, Cha JY, Kim SE, Ko IG, Jee YS, *Journal of Exercise Rehabilitation*, 2013
Essential oil inhalation on blood pressure and salivary cortisol levels in prehypertensive and hypertensive subjects, Kim IH, Kim C, Seong K, Hur MH, Lim HM, Lee MS, *Evidence-Based Complementary and Alternative Medicine*, 2012
Olfactory stimulation with scent of essential oil of grapefruit affects autonomic neurotransmission and blood pressure, Tanida M, Niijima A, Shen J, Nakamura T, Nagai K, *Brian Research*, 2005
Randomized controlled trial for Salvia sclarea or Lavandula angustifolia: differential effects on blood pressure in female patients with urinary incontinence undergoing urodynamic examination, Seol GH, Lee YH, Kang P, You JH, Park M, Min SS, *The Journal of Alternative and Complementary Medicine*, 2013
The effects of the inhalation method using essential oils on blood pressure and stress responses of clients with essential hypertension, Hwang JH, *Korean Society of Nursing Science*, 2006

BRAIN
Effects of fragrance inhalation on sympathetic activity in normal adults, Haze S, Sakai K, Gozu Y, *The Japanese Journal of Pharmacology*, 2002
Essential oil from lemon peels inhibit key enzymes linked to neurodegenerative conditions and pro-oxidant induced lipid peroxidation, Oboh G, Olasehinde TA, Ademosun AO, *Journal of Oleo Science*, 2014
Inhibition of acetylcholinesterase activity by essential oil from Citrus paradisi, Miyazawa M, Tougo H, Ishihara M, *Natural Product Letters*, 2001
Neuropharmacology of the essential oil of bergamot, Bagetta G, Morrone LA, Rombolà L, Amantea D, Russo R, Berliocchi L, Sakurada S, Sakurada T, Rotiroti D, Corasaniti MT, *Fitoterapia*, 2010
Olfactory receptor neuron profiling using sandalwood odorants., Bieri S, Monastyrskaia K, Schilling B, *Chemical Senses*, 2004
Plasma 1,8-cineole correlates with cognitive performance following exposure to rosemary essential oil aroma, Moss M, Oliver L, *Therapeutic Advances in Psychopharmacology*, 2012
The essential oil of bergamot enhances the levels of amino acid neurotransmitters in the hippocampus of rat: implication of monoterpene hydrocarbons, Morrone LA, Rombolà L, Pelle C, Corasaniti MT, Zappettini S, Paudice P, Bonanno G, Bagetta G, *Pharmacological Research*, 2007

CANCER
Alpha-santalol, a chemopreventive agent against skin cancer, causes G2/M cell cycle arrest in both p53-mutated human epidermoid carcinoma A431 cells and p53 wild-type human melanoma UACC-62 cells, Zhang X, Chen W, Guillermo R, Chandrasekher G, Kaushik RS, Young A, Fahmy H, Dwivedi C, *BMC Research Notes*, 2010
Anticancer activity of an essential oil from Cymbopogon flexuosus (lemongrass), Sharma PR, Mondhe DM, Muthiah S, Pal HC, Shahi AK, Saxena AK, Qazi GN, *Chemico-Biological Interactions*, 2009
Anticancer activity of liposomal bergamot essential oil (BEO) on human neuroblastoma cells, Celia C, Trapasso E, Locatelli M, Navarra M, Ventura CA, Wolfram J, Carafa M, Morittu VM, Britti D, Di Marzio L, Paolino D, *Colloids and Surfaces*, 2013
Antioxidant and Anticancer Activities of Citrus reticulate (Petitgrain Mandarin) and Pelargonium graveolens (Geranium) Essential Oils, Fayed SA, *Research Journal of Agriculture and Biological Sciences*, 2009
Apoptosis-mediated proliferation inhibition of human colon cancer cells by volatile principles of Citrus aurantifolia, Patil JR, Jayaprakasha GK, Chidambara Murthy KN, Tichy SE, Chetti MB, Patil BS, Food Chemistry, 2009
Biological effects, antioxidant and anticancer activities of marigold and basil essential oils, Mahmoud GI, *Journal of Medicinal Plants Research*, 2013
Composition and potential anticancer activities of essential oils obtained from myrrh and frankincense, Chen Y, Zhou C, Ge Z, Liu Y, Liu Y, Feng W, Li S, Chen G, Wei T, *Oncology Letters*, 2013
Conservative surgical management of stage IA endometrial carcinoma for fertility preservation, Mazzon I, Corrado G, Masciullo V, Morricone D, Ferrandina G, Scambia G, *Fertil Steril*, 2010
Differential effects of selective frankincense (Ru Xiang) essential oil versus non-selective sandalwood (Tan Xiang) essential oil on cultured bladder cancer cells: a microarray and bioinformatics study, Dozmorov MG, Yang Q, Wu W, Wren J, Suhail MM, Woolley CL, Young DG, Fung KM, Lin HK, *Chinese Medicine*, 2014
Effect of Vetiveria zizanioides Essential Oil on Melanogenesis in Melanoma Cells: Downregulation of Tyrosinase Expression and Suppression of Oxidative Stress, Peng HY, Lai CC, Lin CC, Chou ST, *The Scientific World Journal*, 2014
Medicinal plants as antiemetics in the treatment of cancer: a review, Haniadka R, Popouri S, Palatty PL, Arora R, Baliga MS, *Integrative Cancer Therapies*, 2012
Protective effects of lemongrass (Cymbopogon citratus STAPF) essential oil on DNA damage and carcinogenesis in female Balb/C mice, Bidinotto LT, Costa CA, Salvadori DM, Costa M, Rodrigues MA, Barbisan LF, *Journal of Applied Toxicology*, 2011
Sesquiterpenoids from myrrh inhibit androgen receptor expression and function in human prostate cancer cells, Wang XL, Kong F, Shen T, Young CY, Lou HX, Yuan HQ, *Acta Pharmacologica Sinica*, 2011
Skin cancer chemopreventive agent, {alpha}-santalol, induces apoptotic death of human epidermoid carcinoma A431 cells via caspase activation together with dissipation of mitochondrial membrane potential and cytochrome c release, Kaur M, Agarwal C, Singh RP, Guan X, Dwivedi C, Agarwal R, *Carcinogenesis*, 2005
Terpinen-4-ol, the main component of Melaleuca alternifolia (tea tree) oil inhibits the in vitro growth of human melanoma cells, Calcabrini A, Stringaro A, Toccacieli L, Meschini S, Marra M, Colone M, Salvatore G, Mondello F, Arancia G, Molinari A, *Journal of Investigative Dermatology*, 2004
Topically applied Melaleuca alternifolia (tea tree) oil causes direct anti-cancer cytotoxicity in subcutaneous tumour bearing mice, Ireland DJ, Greay SJ, Hooper CM, Kissick HT, Filion P, Riley TV, Beilharz MW, *Journal of Dermatological Science*, 2012
α-Santalol, a derivative of sandalwood oil, induces apoptosis in human prostate cancer cells by causing caspase-3 activation, Bommareddy A, Rule B, VanWert AL, Santha S, Dwivedi C, *Phytomedicine*, 2012

CELLULAR REPAIR AND CELLULAR HEALTH
Carvacrol and rosemary essential oil manifest cytotoxic, DNA-protective and pro-apoptotic effect having no effect on DNA repair, Melusova M, Slamenova D, Kozics K, Jantova S, Horvathova E, *Neoplasma*, 2014
Effectiveness of aromatherapy with light thai massage for cellular immunity improvement in colorectal cancer patients receiving chemotherapy, Khiewkhern S, Promthet S, Sukprasert A, Eunhpinitpong W, Bradshaw P, *Asian Pacific Journal of Cancer Prevention*, 2013
Protective effect of basil (Ocimum basilicum L.) against oxidative DNA damage and mutagenesis, BeriĐ T, NikoliĐ B, StanojeviĐ J, VukoviĐ-GaciĐ B, KnezeviĐ-VukceviĐ J, *Food and Chemical Toxicology*, 2008

CHEMICAL COMPOSITION AND PROPERTIES
Anethum graveolens: An Indian traditional medicinal herb and spice, Jana S, Shekhawat GS, Pharmacognosy Review, 2010
Antioxidant activities and volatile constituents of various essential oils, Wei A, Shibamoto T, *Journal of Agriculture and Food Chemistry*, 2007
Application of near-infrared spectroscopy in quality control and determination of adulteration of African essential oils, Juliani HR, Kapteyn J, Jones D, Koroch AR, Wang M, Charles D, Simon JE., Phytochem Anal. 2006 Mar-Apr
Botanical perspectives on health peppermint: more than just an after-dinner mint, Spirling LI, Daniels IR, *Journal for the Royal Society for the Promotion of Health*, 2001
Chamomile: A herbal medicine of the past with bright future, Srivastava JK, Shankar E, Gupta S, *Molecular Medicine Reports*, 2010
Chemical composition and antibacterial activity of selected essential oils and some of their main compounds, Wanner J, Schmidt E, Bail S, Jirovetz L, Buchbauer G, Gochev V, Girova T, Atanasova T, Stoyanova A, *Natural Product Communications*, 2010
Chemical composition and biological activity of the essential oil from Helichrysum microphyllum Cambess.

ssp. tyrrhenicum Bacch., Brullo e Giusso growing in La Maddalena Archipelago, Sardinia., Ornano L, Venditti A, Sanna C, Ballero M, Maggi F, Lupidi G, Bramucci M, Quassinti L, Bianco A, *Journal of Oleo Science*, 2014

Chemical composition of the essential oils of variegated pink-fleshed lemon (Citrus x limon L. Burm. f.) and their anti-inflammatory and antimicrobial activities, Hamdan D, Ashour ML, Mulyaningsih S, El-Shazly A, Wink M, *Zeitschrift Fur Naturforschung C- A Journal of Biosciences*, 2013

Constituents of south Indian vetiver oils, Mallavarapu GR, Syamasundar KV, Ramesh S, Rao BR, *Natural Product Communications*, 2012

Determination of the absolute configuration of 6-alkylated alpha-pyrones from Ravensara crassifolia by LC-NMR., Queiroz EF, Wolfender JL, Raoelison G, Hostettmann K, *Phytochem Anal.* 2003

Evaluation of the chemical constituents and the antimicrobial activity of the volatile oil of Citrus reticulata fruit (Tangerine fruit peel) from South West Nigeria, Ayoola GA, Johnson OO, Adelowotan T, Aibinu IE, Adenipekun E, Adepoju AA, Coker HAB, Odugbemi TO, *African Journal of Biotechnology*, 2008

The Essential Oil of Bergamot Stimulates Reactive Oxygen Species Production in Human Polymorphonuclear Leukocytes, Cosentino M, Luini A, Bombelli R, Corasaniti MT, Bagetta G, Marino F, *Phytotherapy Research*, 2014

The essential oil of ginger, Zingiber officinale, and anaesthesia, Geiger JL, *International Journal of Aromatherapy*, 2005

Two 6-substituted 5,6-dihydro-alpha-pyrones from Ravensara anisata., Andrianaivoravelona JO, Sahpaz S, Terreaux C, Hostettmann K, Stoeckli-Evans H, Rasolondramanitra J, *Phytochemistry*. 1999

Volatile composition and biological activity of key lime Citrus aurantifolia essential oil, Spadaro F, Costa R, Circosta C, Occhiuto F, *Natural Product Communications*, 2012

Volatiles from steam-distilled leaves of some plant species from Madagascar and New Zealand and evaluation of their biological activity, Costa R, Pizzimenti F, Marotta F, Dugo P, Santi L, Mondello L, *Nat Prod Commun*, 2010

CHOLESTEROL

Hypolipidemic activity of Anethum graveolens in rats, Hajhashemi V, Abbasi N, *Phytotherapy Research*, 2008

Protective effect of lemongrass oil against dexamethasone induced hyperlipidemia in rats: possible role of decreased lecithin cholesterol acetyl transferase activity, Kumar VR, Inamdar MN, Nayeemunnisa, Viswanatha GL, *Asian Pacific Journal of Tropical Medicine*, 2011

Protective role of arzanol against lipid peroxidation in biological systems, Rosa A, Pollastro F, Atzeri A, Appendino G, Melis MP, Deiana M, Incani A, Loru D, Dessì MA, Chemical and Physics of Lipids, 2011

DECONGESTANT

Effect of inhaled menthol on citric acid induced cough in normal subjects, Morice AH, Marshall AE, Higgins KS, Grattan TJ, *Thorax*, 1994

Remedies for common family ailments: 10. Nasal decongestants, Sinclair A, *Professional Care of Mother and Child*, 1996

DEMENTIA

Aromatherapy as a safe and effective treatment for the management of agitation in severe dementia: the results of a double-blind, placebo-controlled trial with Melissa, Ballard CG, O'Brien JT, Reichelt K, Perry EK, *The Journal of Clinical Psychiatry*, 2002

DEPRESSION (INCLUDING POSTPARTUM)

Antidepressant-like effect of carvacrol (5-Isopropyl-2-methylphenol) in mice: involvement of dopaminergic system, Melo FH, Moura BA, de Sousa DP, de Vasconcelos SM, Macedo DS, Fonteles MM, Viana GS, de Sousa FC, *Fundamental and Clinical Pharmacology*, 2011

Antidepressant-like effect of Salvia sclarea is explained by modulation of dopamine activities in rats, Seol GH, Shim HS, Kim PJ, Moon HK, Lee KH, Shim I, Suh SH, Min SS, *Journal of Ethnopharmacology*, 2010

Effects of Aroma Hand Massage on Pain, State Anxiety and Depression in Hospice Patients with Terminal Cancer, Chang SY, *Journal of Korean Academy of Nursing*, 2008

Effects of lavender aromatherapy on insomnia and depression in women college students, Lee IS, Lee GJ, *Taehan Kanho Hakhoe Chi*, 2006

The effects of clinical aromatherapy for anxiety and depression in the high risk postpartum woman – a pilot study, Conrad P, Adams C, *Complimentary Therapy in Clinical Practice*, 2012

DIABETES

Ameliorative effect of the cinnamon oil from Cinnamomum zeylanicum upon early stage diabetic nephropathy, Mishra A, Bhatti R, Singh A, Singh Ishar MP, *Planta Medica*, 2010

Cinnamon bark extract improves glucose metabolism and lipid profile in the fructose-fed rat, Kannappan S, Jayaraman T, Rajasekar P, Ravichandran MK, Anuradha CV, *Singapore Medical Journal*, 2006

Comparative effects of Artemisia dracunculus, Satureja hortensis and Origanum majorana on inhibition of blood platelet adhesion, aggregation and secretion, Yazdanparast R, Shahriyary L, *Vascular Pharmacology*, 2008

Effects of a novel formulation of essential oils on glucose-insulin metabolism in diabetic and hypertensive rats: a pilot study, Talpur N, Echard B, Ingram C, Bagchi D, Preuss H, Diabetes, *Obesity and Metabolism*, 2005

From type 2 diabetes to antioxidant activity: a systematic review of the safety and efficacy of common and cassia cinnamon bark., Dugoua JJ, Seely D, Perri D, Cooley K, Forelli T, Mills E, Koren G, *Canadian Journal of Physiology and Pharmacology*, 2007

Hypoglycaemic effects of myrtle oil in normal and alloxan-diabetic rabbits, Sepici A, Gürbüz I, Cevik C, Yesilada E, *Journal of Ethnopharmacology*, 2004

Hypoglycemic and antioxidant effects of leaf essential oil of Pelargonium graveolens L'Hér. in alloxan induced diabetic rats, Boukhris M, Bouaziz M, Feki I, Jemai H, El Feki A, Sayadi S, *Lipids in Health and Disease*, 2012

Inhibitory potential of ginger extracts against enzymes linked to type 2 diabetes, inflammation and induced oxidative stress, Rani MP, Padmakumari KP, Sankarikutty B, Cherian OL, Nisha VM, Raghu KG, *International Journal of Food Sciences and Nutrition*, 2011

DIGESTION

Antigiardial activity of Ocimum basilicum essential oil, de Almeida I, Alviano DS, Vieira DP, Alves PB, Blank AF, Lopes AH, Alviano CS, Rosa Mdo S, *Parasitology Research*, 2007

Enteric-coated, pH-dependent peppermint oil capsules for the treatment of irritable bowel syndrome in children, Kline RM, Kline JJ, Di Palma J, Barbero GJ, *The Journal of Pediatrics*, 2001

Gastroprotective activity of essential oils from turmeric and ginger, Liju VB, Jeena K, Kuttan R, *Journal of Basic and Clinical Physiology and Pharmacology*, 2014

Gastroprotective effect of cardamom, Elettaria cardamomum Maton. fruits in rats., Jamal A, Javed K, Aslam M, Jafri MA, *Journal of Ethnopharmacology*, 2006

Olfactory stimulation using black pepper oil facilitates oral feeding in pediatric patients receiving long-term enteral nutrition, Munakata M, Kobayashi K, Niisato-Nezu J, Tanaka S, Kakisaka Y, Ebihara T, Ebihara S, Haginoya K, Tsuchiya S, Onuma A, *The Tohoku Journal of Experimental Medicine*, 2008

Peppermint oil for the treatment of irritable bowel syndrome: a systematic review and meta-analysis, Khanna R, MacDonald JK, Levesque BG, *Journal of Clinical Gastroenterology*, 2014

Randomized clinical trial of a phytotherapic compound containing Pimpinella anisum, Foeniculum vulgare, Sambucus nigra, and Cassia augustifolia for chronic constipation, Picon PD, Picon RV, Costa AF, Sander GB, Amaral KM, Aboy AL, Henriques AT, *BMC Complementary and Alternative Medicine*, 2010

Reversal of pyrogallol-induced delay in gastric emptying in rats by ginger (Zingiber officinale), Gupta YK, Sharma M, *Methods and Findings in Experimental and Clinical Pharmacology*, 2001

Systematic Review of Complementary and Alternative Medicine Treatments in Inflammatory Bowel Diseases, Langhorst J, Wulfert H, Lauche R, Klose P, Cramer H, Dobos GJ,Korzenik,J, *Journal of Crohn's & Colitis*, 2015

The cinnamon-derived dietary factor cinnamic aldehyde activates the Nrf2-dependent antioxidant response in human epithelial colon cells, Wondrak GT, Villeneuve NF, Lamore SD, Bause AS, Jiang T, Zhang DD, *Molecules*, 2010

Treatment of irritable bowel syndrome with herbal preparations: results of a double-blind, randomized, placebo-controlled, multi-centre trial, Madisch A, Holtmann G, Plein K, Hotz J, *Alimentary pharmacology and & therapeutics*, 2004

FIBROMYALGIA

Cutaneous application of menthol 10% solution as an abortive treatment of migraine without aura: a randomised, double-blind, placebo-controlled, crossed-over study, Borhani Haghighi A, Motazedian S, Rezaii R, Mohammadi F, Salarian L, Pourmokhtari M, Khodaei S, Vossoughi M, Miri R, *The International Journal of Clinical Practice*, 2010

Lavender essential oil in the treatment of migraine headache: a placebo-controlled clinical trial, Sasannejad P, Saeedi M, Shoeibi A, Gorji A, Abbasi M, Foroughipour M, *European Neurology*, 2012

HERPES

Inhibitory effect of essential oils against herpes simplex virus type 2, Koch C, Reichling J, Schneele J, Schnitzler P, *Phytomedicine*, 2008

Susceptibility of drug-resistant clinical herpes simplex virus type 1 strains to essential oils of ginger, thyme, hyssop, and sandalwood, Schnitzler P, Koch C, Reichling J, *Antimicrobial Agents and Chemotherapy*, 2007

IMMUNE SYSTEM

Chemistry and immunomodulatory activity of frankincense oil, Mikhaeil BR, Maatooq GT, Badria FA, Amer MM, *Zeitschrift fur Naturforschung C*, 2003

INFLAMMATION AND PAIN

A review on anti-inflammatory activity of monoterpenes, de Cássia da Silveira e Sá R, Andrade LN, de Sousa DP, *Molecules*, 2013

An experimental study on the effectiveness of massage with aromatic ginger and orange essential oil for moderate-to-severe knee pain among the elderly in Hong Kong, Yip YB, Tam AC, *Complementary Therapies in Medicine*, 2008

Anti-inflammatory activity of patchouli alcohol in RAW264.7 and HT-29 cells, Jeong JB, Shin YK, Lee SH, *Food and Chemical Toxicology*, 2013

Anti-inflammatory and analgesic activity of different extracts of Commiphora myrrha, Su S, Wang T, Duan JA, Zhou W, Hua YQ, Tang YP, Yu L, Qian DW, *Journal of Ethnopharmacology*, 2011

Anti-inflammatory and anti-ulcer activities of carvacrol, a monoterpene present in the essential oil of oregano, Silva FV, Guimarães AG, Silva ER, Sousa-Neto BP, Machado FD, Quintans-Júnior LJ, Arcanjo DD, Oliveira FA, Oliveira RC, *Journal of Medicinal Food*, 2012

Anti-inflammatory and antioxidant properties of Helichrysum italicum, Sala A, Recio M, Giner RM, Máñez S, Tournier H, Schinella G, Ríos JL, *The Journal of Pharmacy and Pharmacology*, 200

Anti-inflammatory effects of Melaleuca alternifolia essential oil on human polymorphonuclear neutrophils and monocytes, Caldefie-Chézet F, Guerry M, Chalchat JC, Fusillier C, Vasson MP, Guillot J, *Free Radical Research*, 2004

Antihypernociceptive activity of anethole in experimental inflammatory pain, Ritter AM, Domiciano TP, Verri WA Jr, Zarpelon AC, da Silva LG, Barbosa CP, Natali MR, Cuman RK, Bersani-Amado CA, *Inflammopharmacology*, 2013

Antiinflammatory effects of essential oil from the leaves of Cinnamomum cassia and cinnamaldehyde on lipopolysaccharide-stimulated J774A.1 cells., Pannee C, Chandhanee I, Wacharee L, *Journal of Advanced Pharmaceutical Technology & Research*, 2014

Antiinflammatory effects of ginger and some of its components in human bronchial epithelial (BEAS-2B) cells, Podlogar JA, Verspohl EJ, *Phytotherapy Research*, 2012

Antioxidant components of naturally-occurring oils exhibit marked anti-inflammatory activity in epithelial cells of the human upper respiratory system, Gao M, Singh A, Macri K, Reynolds C, Singhal V, Biswal S, Spannhake EW, *Respiratory Research*, 2011

Antioxidant, anti-inflammatory and antinociceptive activities of essential oil from ginger, Jeena K, Liju VB, Kuttan R, *Indian Journal of Physiology and Pharmacology*, 2013

Arzanol, a prenylated heterodimeric phloroglucinyl pyrone, inhibits eicosanoid biosynthesis and exhibits anti-inflammatory efficacy in vivo, Bauer J, Koeberle A, Dehm F, Pollastro F, Appendino G, Northoff H, Rossi A, Sautebin L, Werz O, *Biochemical Pharmacology*, 2011

Arzanol, an anti-inflammatory and anti-HIV-1 phloroglucinol alpha-Pyrone from Helichrysum italicum ssp. microphyllum, Appendino G, Ottino M, Marquez N, Bianchi F, Giana A, Ballero M, Sterner O, Fiebich BL, Munoz E, *Journal of Natural Products*, 2007

Assessment of the anti-inflammatory activity and free radical scavenger activity of tiliroside., Sala A, Recio MC, Schinella GR, Máñez S, Giner RM, Cerdá-Nicolás M, Rosí JL, *European Journal of Pharmacology*, 2003

Boswellia frereana (frankincense) suppresses cytokine-induced matrix metalloproteinase expression and production of pro-inflammatory molecules in articular cartilage., Blain EJ, Ali AY, Duance VC, *Phytotherapy Research*, 2012

Ginger: An herbal medicinal product with broad anti-inflammatory actions, Grzanna R, Lindmark L, Frondoza CG, *Journal of Medicinal Food*, 2005

Identification of proapoptopic, anti-inflammatory, anti-proliferative, anti-invasive and anti-angiogenic targets of essential oils in cardamom by dual reverse virtual screening and binding pose analysis, Bhattacharjee B, Chatterjee J, *Asian Pacific Journal of Cancer Prevention*, 2013

In vitro cytotoxic and anti-inflammatory effects of myrrh oil on human gingival fibroblasts and epithelial cells, Tipton DA, Lyle B, Babich H, Dabbous MKh, *Toxicology in Vitro*, 2003

In Vivo Potential Anti-Inflammatory Activity of Melissa officinalis L. Essential Oil, Bounihi A, Hajjaj G, Alnamer R, Cherrah Y, Zellou A, *Advances in Pharmacological Sciences*, 2013

Inhibitory effect of anethole in nonimmune acute inflammation, Domiciano TP, Dalalio MM, Silva EL, Ritter AM, Estevão-Silva CF, Ramos FS, Caparroz-Assef SM, Cuman RK, Bersani-Amado CA, *Naunyn-Schmiedeberg's Archives of Pharmacology*, 2013

Lavender essential oil inhalation suppresses allergic airway inflammation and mucous cell hyperplasia in a murine model of asthma, Ueno-Iio T, Shibakura M, Yokota K, Aoe M, Hyoda T, Shinohata R, Kanehiro A, Tanimoto M, Kataoka M, *Life Sciences*, 2014

Rose geranium essential oil as a source of new and safe anti-inflammatory drugs, Boukhatem MN, Kameli A, Ferhat MA, Saidi F, Mekarnia M, *The Libyan Journal of Medicine*, 2013

Supercritical fluid extraction of oregano (Origanum vulgare) essentials oils: anti-inflammatory properties based on cytokine response on THP-1 macrophages, Ocaña-Fuentes A, Arranz-Gutiérrez E, Señorans FJ, Reglero G, *Food and Chemical Toxicology*, 2010

INSECT REPELLENT
Bioactivity-guided investigation of geranium essential oils as natural tick repellents, Tabanca N, Wang M, Avonto C, Chittiboyina AG, Parcher JF, Carroll JF, Kramer M, Khan IA, *Journal of Agricultural and Food Chemistry*, 2013
Essential oils and their compositions as spatial repellents for pestiferous social wasps., Zhang QH, Schnidmiller RG, *Hoover DR, Pest Management Science*, 2013
Field evaluation of essential oils for reducing attraction by the Japanese beetle (Coleoptera: Scarabaeidae), Youssef NN, Oliver JB, Ranger CM, Reding ME, Moyseenko JJ, Klein MG, Pappas RS, *Journal of Economic Entomology*, 2009
Fumigant toxicity of plant essential oils against Camptomyia corticalis (Diptera: Cecidomyiidae), Kim JR, Haribalan P, Son BK, Ahn YJ, *Journal of Economic Entomology*, 2012
Insecticidal properties of volatile extracts of orange peels, Ezeonu FC, Chidume GI, Udedi SC, *Bioresource Technology*, 2001
Repellency of Essential Oils to Mosquitoes (Diptera: Culicidae), Barnard DR, Journal of Medical Entomology, 1999
Repellency to Stomoxys calcitrans (Diptera: Muscidae) of Plant Essential Oils Alone or in Combination with Calophyllum inophyllum Nut Oil, Hieu TT, Kim SI, Lee SG, Ahn YJ, *Journal of Medical Etomology*, 2010
Repelling properties of some plant materials on the tick Ixodes ricinus L, Thorsell W, Mikiver A, Tunón H, *Phytomedicine*, 2006

MENOPAUSE
Aromatherapy Massage Affects Menopausal Symptoms in Korean Climacteric Women: A Pilot-Controlled Clinical Trial, Myung-HH, Yun Seok Y, Myeong SL, *Evidence-based Complementary and Alternative Medicine*, 2008
Changes in 5-hydroxytryptamine and Cortisol Plasma Levels in Menopausal Women After Inhalation of Clary Sage Oil, Lee KB, Cho E, Kang YS, *Phytotherapy Research*, 2014
Effect of aromatherapy massage on abdominal fat and body image in post-menopausal women, Kim HJ, *Taehan Kanho Hakhoe Chi*, 2007

MENSTRUAL
Effect of aromatherapy on symptoms of dysmenorrhea in college students: A randomized placebo-controlled clinical trial, Han SH, Hur MH, Buckle J, Choi J, Lee MS, *The Journal of Alternative and Complementary Medicine*, 2006
Pain relief assessment by aromatic essential oil massage on outpatients with primary dysmenorrhea: a randomized, double-blind clinical trial, Ou MC, Hsu TF, Lai AC, Lin YT, Lin CC, *The Journal of Obstetrics and Gynecology Research*, 2012

MIGRAINE
Cutaneous application of menthol 10% solution as an abortive treatment of migraine without aura: a randomised, double-blind, placebo-controlled, crossed-over study, Borhani Haghighi A, Motazedian S, Rezaii R, Mohammadi F, Salarian L, Pourmokhtari M, Khodaei S, Vossoughi M, Miri R, *The International Journal of Clinical Practice*, 2010
Lavender essential oil in the treatment of migraine headache: a placebo-controlled clinical trial, Sasannejad P, Saeedi M, Shoeibi A, Gorji A, Abbasi M, Foroughipour M, *European Neurology*, 2012

MOOD
Effects of fragrance inhalation on sympathetic activity in normal adults, Haze S, Sakai K, Gozu Y, *The Japanese Journal of Pharmacology*, 2002
Evaluation of the harmonizing effect of ylang-ylang oil on humans after inhalation, Hongratanaworakit T, Buchbauer G, *Planta Medica*, 2004
Relaxing effect of rose oil on humans, Hongratanaworakit T, *Natural Product Communications*, 2009
Relaxing Effect of Ylang ylang Oil on Humans after Transdermal Absorption, Hongratanaworakit T, Buchbauer G, *Phytotherapy research*, 2006

NAUSEA
A brief review of current scientific evidence involving aromatherapy use for nausea and vomiting, Lua PL, Zakaria NS, *The Journal of Alternative and Complementary Medicine*, 2012
Aromatherapy as a Treatment for Postoperative Nausea: A randomized Trial, Hunt R, Dienemann J, Norton HJ, Hartley W, Hudgens A, Stern T, *Divine G, Anesthesia and Analgesia*, 2013
Controlled breathing with or without peppermint aromatherapy for postoperative nausea and/or vomiting symptom relief: a randomized controlled trial, Sites DS, Johnson NT, Miller JA, Torbush PH, Hardin JS, Knowles SS, Nance J, Fox TH, Tart RC, *Journal of PeriAnesthesia Nursing*, 2014
The effect of lemon inhalation aromatherapy on nausea and vomiting of pregnancy: a double-blinded, randomized, controlled clinical trial, Yavari Kia P, Safajou F, Shahnazi M, Nazemiyeh H, *Iranian Red Crescent Medical Journal*, 2014
The palliation of nausea in hospice and palliative care patients with essential oils of Pimpinella anisum (aniseed), Foeniculum vulgare var. dulce (sweet fennel), Anthemis nobilis (Roman chamomile) and Mentha x piperita (peppermint), Gilligan NP, *International Journal of Aromatherapy*, 2005

ORAL HEALTH
Efficacy of grapefruit, tangerine, lime, and lemon oils as solvents for softening gutta-percha in root canal retreatment procedures, Jantarat J, Malhotra W, Sutimuntanakul S, *Journal of Investigative and Clinical Dentistry*, 2013
Essential oil of Melaleuca alternifolia for the treatment of oral candidiasis induced in an immunosuppressed mouse model, de Campos Rasteiro VM, da Costa AC, Araújo CF, de Barros PP, Rossoni RD, Anbinder AL, Jorge AO, Junqueira JC, *BMC Complementary and Alternative Medicine*, 2014
Susceptibility to Melaleuca alternifolia (tea tree) oil of yeasts isolated from the mouths of patients with advanced cancer, Bagg J, Jackson MS, Petrina Sweeney M, Ramage G, Davies AN, *Oral Oncology*, 2006
Synergistic effect between clove oil and its major compounds and antibiotics against oral bacteria, Moon SE, Kim HY, Cha JD, *Archives of Oral Biology*, 2011
Topical lavender oil for the treatment of recurrent aphthous ulceration, Altaei DT, *American Journal of Dentistry*, 2012

PHYSICAL AGILITY
Effects of lavender (lavandula angustifolia Mill.) and peppermint (Mentha cordifolia Opiz.) aromas on subjective vitality, speed, and agility, Cruz AB, Lee SE, Pagaduan JC, Kim TH, *The Asian International Journal of Life Sciences*, 2012
The effects of peppermint on exercise performance, Meamarbashi A, Rajabi A, *Journal of International Society of Sports Nutrition*, 2013

PREGNANCY
Clinical trial of aromatherapy on postpartum mother's perineal healing, Hur MH, Han SH, *Journal of Korean Academy of Nursing*, 2004

REPRODUCTIVE SYSTEM
Effect of different terpene-containing essential oils on permeation of estradiol through hairless mouse skin, Monti D, Chetoni P, Burgalassi S, Najarro M, Saettone MF, Boldrini E, *International Journal of Pharmaceutics*, 2002
Effect of olfactory stimulation with flavor of grapefruit oil and lemon oil on the activity of sympathetic branch in the white adipose tissue of the epididymis, Niijima A, Nagai K, *Experimental Biology and Medicine*, 2003
The Effects of Herbal Essential Oils on the Oviposition-deterrent and Ovicidal Activities of Aedes aegypti (Linn.), Anopheles dirus (Peyton and Harrison) and Culex quinquefasciatus (Say), Siriporn P, Mayura S, *Tropical Biomedicine*, 2012

SEIZURES
Anticonvulsant and neuroprotective effects of Pimpinella anisum in rat brain, Fariba K, Mahmoud H, Diana M, Hassan A, Gholam RH, Mohamad B, Maryam J, Hadi K, Ali G, *BMC Complementary and Alternative Medicine*, 2012
Increased seizure latency and decreased severity of pentylenetetrazol-induced seizures in mice after essential oil administration, Koutroumanidou E, Kimbaris A, Kortsaris A, Bezirtzoglou E, Polissiou M, Charalabopoulos K, Pagonopoulou O, *Epilepsy Research and Treatment*, 2013

SKIN
A comparative study of tea-tree oil versus benzoylperoxide in the treatment of acne, Bassett IB, Pannowitz DL, Barnetson RS, *Medical Journal of Australia*, 1990
Activities of Ten Essential Oils towards Propionibacterium acnes and PC-3, A-549 and MCF-7 Cancer Cells, Zu Y, Yu H, Liang L, Fu Y, Efferth T, Liu X, Wu N, *Molecules*, 2010
Cinnamomum cassia essential oil inhibits α-MSH-induced melanin production and oxidative stress in murine B16 melanoma cells, Chou ST, Chang WL, Chang CT, Hsu SL, Lin YC, Shih Y, *International Journal of Molecular Sciences*, 2013
Cooling the burn wound: evaluation of different modalites., Jandera V, Hudson DA, de Wet PM, Innes PM, Rode H, Burns: *Journal of the International Society for Burn Injuries*, 2000
Coriandrum sativum L. protects human keratinocytes from oxidative stress by regulating oxidative defense systems, Park G, Kim HG, Kim YO, Park SH, Kim SY, Oh MS, *Skin Pharmacology and Physiology*, 2012
Essential oil of Australian lemon myrtle (Backhousia citriodora) in the treatment of molluscum contagiosum in children, Burke BE, Baillie JE, Olson RD, *Biomedicine & Pharmacotherapy*, 2004
Randomized trial of aromatherapy: successful treatment for alopecia areata, Hay IC, Jamieson M, Ormerod AD,, *Archives of Dermatology*, 1998
Tea tree oil as a novel anti-psoriasis weapon, Pazyar N, Yaghoobi R, *Skin Pharmacology and Physiology*, 2012
Tea tree oil reduces histamine-induced skin inflammation, Koh KJ, Pearce AL, Marshman G, Finlay-Jones JJ, Hart PH, *British Journal of Dermatology*, 2002
The effect of clove and benzocaine versus placebo as topical anesthetics, Alqareer A, Alyahya A, Andersson L, *Journal of Dentistry*, 2006
Two US practitioners' experience of using essential oils for wound care, Hartman D, Coetzee JC, *Journal of Wound Care*, 2002

SLEEP
An olfactory stimulus modifies nighttime sleep in young men and women, Goel N, Kim H, Lao RP, *Chronobiology International*, 2005
Preliminary investigation of the effect of peppermint oil on an objective measure of daytime sleepiness, Norrish MI, Dwyer KL, *International Journal of Psychophysiology: Official Journal of the International Organization of Psychophysiology*, 2005
Sedative effects of the jasmine tea odor and (R)-(-)-linalool, one of its major odor components, on autonomic nerve activity and mood states, Kuroda K, Inoue N, Ito Y, Kubota K, Sugimoto A, Kakuda T, Fushiki T, *European Journal of Applied Physiology*, 2005
Stimulating effect of aromatherapy massage with jasmine oil, Hongratanaworakit T, *Natural Product Communications*, 2010
Stimulative and sedative effects of essential oils upon inhalation in mice, Lim WC, Seo JM, Lee CI, Pyo HB, Lee BC, *Archives of Pharmacal Research*, 2005

STRESS
Effect of "rose essential oil" inhalation on stress-induced skin-barrier disruption in rats and humans, Fukada M, Kano E, Miyoshi M, Komaki R, Watanabe T, *Chemical Senses*, 2012
Effect of flavour components in lemon essential oil on physical or psychological stress, Fukumoto S, Morishita A, Furutachi K, Terashima T, Nakayama T, Yokogoshi H, *Stress and Health*, 2008
The physical effects of aromatherapy in alleviating work-related stress on elementary school teachers in taiwan, Liu SH, Lin TH, Chang KM, *Evidence-Based Complementary and Alternative Medicine*, 2013

STROKE
Effect of lavender oil (Lavandula angustifolia) on cerebral edema and its possible mechanisms in an experimental model of stroke,Vakili A, Sharifat S, Akhavan MM, Bandegi AR, *Brain Research*, 2014

TUMORS
Chemopreventive effects of alpha-santalol on skin tumor development in CD-1 and SENCAR mice, Dwivedi C, Guan X, Harmsen WL, Voss AL, Goetz-Parten DE, Koopman EM, Johnson KM, Valluri HB, Matthees DP, Cancer Epidemiology, *Biomarkers and Prevention*, 2003
Frankincense oil derived from Boswellia carteri induces tumor cell specific cytotoxicity, Frank MB, Yang Q, Osban J, Azzarello JT, Saban MR, Saban R, Ashley RA, Welter JC, Fung KM, Lin HK, *BMC Complementary and Alternative Medicine*, 2009
Sandalwood oil prevent skin tumour development in CD1 mice, Dwivedi C, Zhang Y, *European Journal of Cancer Prevention*, 1999

WEIGHT LOSS AND WEIGHT MANAGEMENT
Effect of aromatherapy massage on abdominal fat and body image in post-menopausal women, Kim HJ, *Taehan Kanho Hakhoe Chi*, 2007
Effects of herbal essential oil mixture as a dietary supplement on egg production in quail, Çabuk M, Eratak S, Alçicek A, Bozkurt M, *The Scientific World Journal*, 2014
Essential oil from Citrus aurantifolia prevents ketotifen-induced weight-gain in mice, Asnaashari S, Delazar A, Habibi B, Vasfi R, Nahar L, Hamedeyazdan S, Sarker SD, *Phytotherapy Research*, 2010
Low level of Lemon Balm (Melissa officinalis) essential oils showed hypoglycemic effects by altering the expression of glucose metabolism genes in db/db mice, Mi Ja Chung, Sung-Yun Cho and Sung-Joon Lee, *The Journal of the Federation of American Societies for Experimental Biology*, 2008
Olfactory stimulation with scent of grapefruit oil affects autonomic nerves, lipolysis and appetite in rats, Shen J, Niijima A, Tanida M, Horii Y, Maeda K, Nagai K, *Neuroscience Letters*, 2005
Safety assessment of Ylang-Ylang (Cananga spp.) as a food ingredient., Burdock GA, Carabin IG, *Food and chemical toxicology*, 2008
The effects of inhalation of essential oils on the body weight, food efficiency rate and serum leptin of growing SD rats, Hur MH, Kim C, Kim CH, Ahn HC, Ahn HY, *Korean Society of Nursing Science*, 2006
The metabolic responses to aerial diffusion of essential oils, Wu Y, Zhang Y, Xie G, Zhao A, Pan X, Chen T, Hu Y, Liu Y, Cheng Y, Chi Y, Yao L, Jia W, *PLOS One*, 2012

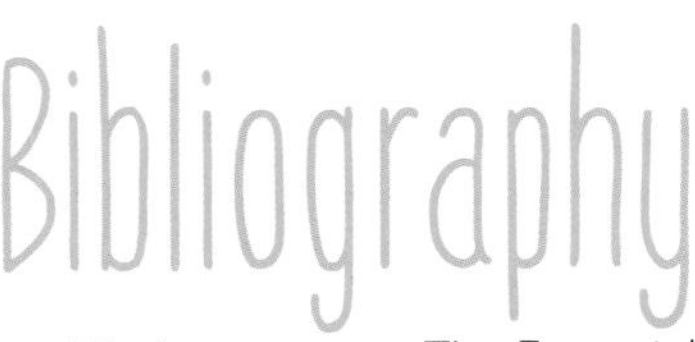

About Brain Tumors. Barrow Neurological Institute. Thebarrow.org, 2014.

The American Heritage Medical Dictionary. Boston: Houghton Mifflin Co., 2007.

The Aromatic Practitioners Reference. Australia: Maria Mitchell, 2011.

The Aromatherapy Encyclopedia: A Concise Guide to Over 385 Plant Oils. Basic Health Publications, Inc.: Schiller, C. and Schiller, D., 2008.

Aromatherapy Workbook. London: Price, Shirley, Thorsons, 2000 .

The Art of Aromatherapy. Essex: The C W Daniel Company Ltd, Tisserand, Robert, 2009.

The Aromatherapy Encyclopedia. Laguna Beach, CA: Basic Health Publications Inc, Schiller, Carol & Schiller, David, 2008.

Aromatherapy for Health Professionals, 3rd ed. London: Churchhill Livingstone Elsevier, Price, Shirley & Price, Len, 2007

Aromatherapy A-Z. London, England: Random House, Davis Patricia, 2005.

BabyMed.com, 2014.

Churchill Livingstone Dictionary of Sport and Exercise Science and Medicine. Philadelphia: Churchill Livingstone, 2008.

Clinical Aromatherapy Essential Oils in Healthcare, 3rd ed. St Louis, MO: Elsevier, Buckle, Jane 2015.

Collins English Dictionary. London: Collins, 2000.

The Columbia Electronic Encyclopedia. New York, NY: Columbia University Press, 2012.

The Complete Aromatherapy & Essential Oils Handbook for Everyday Wellness. Toronto: Robert Rose Inc, Purchon, Nerys & Cantele, Lora, 2014.

The Complete Guide to Aromatherapy, 2nd ed. Brisbane, QLD: The International Centre of Holistic Aromatherapy, Battaglia, Salvatore, 2003.

The Directory of Essential Oils. London: Vermillion, Sellar, Wanda, 2005.

Dorland's Medical Dictionary for Health Consumers. 2014

Emotions & Essential Oils 3rd Edition. American Fork, Utah: Enlighten Alternative Healing, 2014.

The Encyclopedia of Essential Oils. London: Thorsons, Lawless, Julia, 2002.

Essential Oil Safety, 2nd ed. London: Churchill Livingstone Elsevier, Tisserand, Robert & Young, Rodney, 2013.

Essential Oils Desk Reference, 5th ed. USA: Life Science Publishing, 2011.

The Essential Oils Handbook. London: Duncan Baird Publishers Ltd, Harding, Jennie, 2008

Essential Oils Integrative Medical Guide. USA: Essential Science Publishing, Young, D Gary, 2006.

Essentials of the Earth, 2nd ed. Idaho USA: Essential Oils Books LLC, James, R L, 2013.

Farlex Partner Medical Dictionary. Huntingdon Valley, PA: Farlex Inc. 2014.

The Fragrant Pharmacy. Moorebank, NSW: Transworld Publishers Ltd, Wormwood, Valerie A, 1993.

Gale Encyclopedia of Medicine. Farmington Hills, MI: Gale, 1999

The Healing Intelligence of Essential Oils. Rockester, Vermont: Healing Arts Press, Schnacbelt Kurt, 2011.

The Huffington Post; HuffingtonPost.com, 2014.

The Human Body. New York, New York: Dorling Kindersley Publishing, Inc., 2001.

Illustrated Dictionary of Podiatry and Foot Science. New York: Churchill Livingstone, 2009.

MayoClinic.org, 2014 & 2015.

McGraw-Hill Concise Dictionary of Modern Medicine. New York: McGraw-Hill, 2006.

McGraw-Hill Dictionary of Scientific & Technical Terms 6th ed., New York: McGraw-Hill, 2003.

Mind Over Medicine. Hay House, Inc.: Rankin Lissa, 2014.

Molecules of Emotion. Simon & Schuster, Pert Candance B. Ph.D., 1999.

The Mood Cure. London, England: Penguin Books, Ross Julia MA, 2003.

Mosby's Dental Dictionary, 2nd ed. C.V. Mosby Co, 2008

Mosby's Dictionary of Complementary and Alternative Medicine. St. Louis, MO: Elsevier Mosby, 2005.

Mosby's Medical Dictionary 9th ed., Philadelphia: Elsevier, 2013

Miller-Keane Encyclopedia and Dictionary of Medicine, Nursing, and Allied Health, 7th ed. Philadelphia: Saunders, 2003.

Patient.co.uk, 2014.

Random House Kernerman Webster's College Dictionary. New York: Random House, 1997.

Saunders Comprehensive Veterinary Dictionary. Edinburgh [Scotland]: Saunders Elsevier, 2012.

Segen's Medical Dictionary. New York: McGraw-Hill, 2006.

Stedman's Medical Dictionary for the Health Professions and Nursing. Philadelphia: Lippincott Williams & Wilkins, 2005

WebMD.com, 2014.

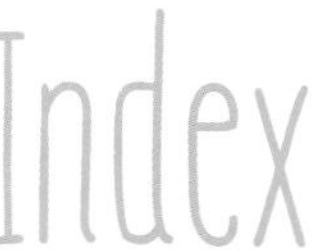

SUPPLEMENTAL

SUPPLEMENTAL